MATERNAL AND CHILD HEALTH PRACTICES

THIRD EDITION

MATERNAL AND CHILD HEALTH PRACTICES

THIRD EDITION

EDITORS

HELEN M. WALLACE, M.D., M.P.H.
PROFESSOR OF MATERNAL AND CHILD HEALTH
GRADUATE SCHOOL OF PUBLIC HEALTH
SAN DIEGO STATE UNIVERSITY
SAN DIEGO, CALIFORNIA

GEORGE M. RYAN, JR., M.D., M.P.H.
PROFESSOR, DEPARTMENT OF OBSTETRICS
AND GYNECOLOGY
UNIVERSITY OF TENNESSEE COLLEGE OF MEDICINE
MEMPHIS, TENNESSEE

ALLAN C. OGLESBY, M.D., M.P.H.
PROFESSOR AND HEAD, DIVISION OF MATERNAL
AND CHILD HEALTH
GRADUATE SCHOOL OF PUBLIC HEALTH
SAN DIEGO STATE UNIVERSITY
SAN DIEGO, CALIFORNIA

 THIRD PARTY PUBLISHING COMPANY
OAKLAND, CALIFORNIA

ACKNOWLEDGMENT

The editors wish to express their deep appreciation of the contributions of the authors who have given generously of their expertise, time, and effort.

In addition, a very special acknowledgment is made of the contributions by Mary Hafner, whose commitment to the project and whose determination and unfailing good spirits made this book possible.

MATERNAL AND CHILD HEALTH PRACTICES, THIRD EDITION
International Standard Book Number **0-89914-028-9**
Library of Congress Number **88-050643**

Printed in the United States of America
First Impression 1988
Third Party Publishing Company
A Division of Third Party Associates, Inc.
P.O. Box 13306, Montclair Station E
Oakland, California 94661+0306, U.S.A.

Managing Editor and Designer, Paul R. Mico
Electronic Page Composition and Graphics, Marilynn Collin, Argent Enterprises

TABLE OF CONTENTS

SECTION I   POLICIES AND ISSUES IN MATERNAL AND CHILD HEALTH

SECTION III   REPRODUCTIVE HEALTH CARE

SECTION IV   CHILD HEALTH CARE

❙ PREFACE

Many changes have taken place since the previous edition of this textbook was published in 1982. These changes have been social, technical, programmatic, and political. Examples in the *social* arena include the emergence of large numbers of female-headed families in poverty, with young children; the large numbers of teenagers who are pregnant; the large numbers of working mothers with young children; and the need for more day care services for young children.

Examples of *technology* changes include the significant advances in the field of genetics and its application as a preventive tool; improved survival of low birthweight and very-low birthweight infants; and the current survival of high-technology infants and children, with the need for organized home care assistance for them and their families.

In the *programmatic* arena, one example is the development and implementation of the concept of high risk, with efforts to identify early high-risk mothers and children and provide special services for them. Another example is the emergence of Medicaid as the major source of funding-of-care of some poor pregnant women and children. An additional trend is the current interest in cost-containment and development of the DRG (diagnostic related group) approach to it. Public-funding costs and expenditures continue to focus on the problem of quality of care, in addition to paying bills.

In the *political* arena, one example is the continuing struggle over funding for support of MCH and family planning education and services, including information, referral, and services for abortion.

Health professionals need continuous help in keeping abreast of current trends in the health care of mothers and children. The field of MCH/CC is a dynamic, moving series of activities, programs, and services. It requires a deep sense of commitment, dedication, and effort to improve and expand the concept of comprehensive health care of women, children, and families. The editors hope that this book will continue to play a role in the education of MCH/CC health professionals, and aid them in meeting that commitment.

Helen M. Wallace, M.D., M.P.H.
George M. Ryan, Jr., M.D., M.P.H.
Allan C. Oglesby, M.D., M.P.H.

‖ CONTRIBUTORS

Joel J. Alpert, M.D.   Professor and Chair, Department of Pediatrics, Boston University School of Medicine, Boston, Massachusetts

Kathryn E. Barnard, Ph.D.   Professor, University of Washington School of Nursing, Seattle, Washington

Mark A. Belsey, M.D., M.P.H.,T.M.   Chief, Maternal and Child Health, World Health Organization, Geneva, Switzerland

Robert William Blum, M.D., Ph.D.   Associate Professor of Pediatrics and Maternal and Child Health, University of Minnesota, Minneapolis, Minnesota

Sarah S. Brown, M.S.P.H.   Institute of Medicine, National Academy of Sciences, Washington, D.C.

Sylvia Cerel Bowen   Teaching Fellow, Program in Human Biology, Stanford University, Palo Alto, California

Willard Cates, Jr., M.D., M.P.H.   Director, Sexually Transmitted Diseases, Center for Infectious Diseases, Centers for Disease Control, Atlanta, Georgia

James O. Cleveland, Ed.D.   Regional Center for the Developmentally Disabled, San Diego, California

Anne H. Cohn, Dr. P.H.   Executive Director, National Committee for Prevention of Child Abuse, Chicago, Illinois

Donald A. Cornely, M.D., M.P.H.   Professor and Chairman, Department of Maternal and Child Health, The Johns Hopkins University School of Hygiene and Public Health, Baltimore, Maryland

James W. Curran, M.D., M.P.H.   Director, AIDS Program, Center for Infectious Diseases, Centers for Disease Control, Atlanta, Georgia

Deborah Dawson, Ph.D.   National Center for Health Statistics, Hyattsville, Maryland

Joy G. Dryfoos, M.A.   Hastings On Hudson, New York City, New York

Johanna T. Dwyer, D.Sc., R.D.   Director, Frances Stern Nutrition Center, Tufts University Medical School, Boston, Massachusetts

Thomas E. Elkins, M.D.   Associate Professor of Obstetrics and Gynecology, University of Michigan Medical School, Ann Arbor, Michigan

Judith Freedland, B.S.   Frances Stern Nutrition Center, Boston, Massachusetts

Susan S. Gallagher, M.P.H.   Director, Childhood Injury Prevention Resource Center, Harvard University School of Public Health, Boston, Massachusetts

A. Joanne Gates, M.D.   Medical Director, Ventilator Assisted Care Program, Children's Hospital, New Orleans, Louisana

Josephine Gittler, J.D.   Director, National Maternal and Child Health Resources Center, University of Iowa College of Law, Iowa City, Iowa

David A. Grimes, M.D.   Professor, Departments of Obstetrics & Gynecology and Preventive Medicine, University of Southern California School of Medicine, Los Angeles, California

Felicia Jane Guest, B.A.   Regional Training Center for Family Planning, Department of Gynecology and Obstetrics, Emory University School of Medicine, Atlanta, Georgia

Bernard Guyer, M.D., M.P.H.   Associate Professor, Department of Maternal and Child Health, Harvard University School of Public Health, Harvard, Massachusetts

Janet B. Hardy, M.D., C.M.   Professor Emeritus of Pediatrics, The Johns Hopkins University Hospital, Baltimore, Maryland

Robert A. Hatcher, M.D., M.P.H.   Professor of Gynecology and Obstetrics, Director of the Family Planning Program, Emory University School of Medicine, Atlanta, Georgia

Alan R. Hinman, M.D., M.P.H.   Director, Center for Prevention Services, Centers for Disease Control, Atlanta, Georgia

Charlotte T. Houde, C.N.M.   Assistant Professor of Clinical Maternal and Child Health, Department of Maternal and Child Health, Dartmouth University Medical School, Hanover, New Hampshire

Dana Hughes   Children's Defense Fund, Washington, D.C.

Henry T. Ireys, Ph.D.   Associate Professor of Pediatrics and Psychiatry, Albert Einstein College of Medicine, Bronx, New York

Kay Johnson   Children's Defense Fund, Washington, D.C.

Jean F. Kelly, Ph.D.   Child Development and Mental Retardation Center, Department of Parent and Child Nursing, University of Washington, Seattle, Washington

Elhamy F. Khalil, M.D., M.P.H.   Program Director, Lanterman Developmental Center, Pomona, California; Assistant Clinical Professor, Psychiatry and Behavorial Sciences, Neuropsychiatric Institute, University of California, Los Angeles, California

Douglas Kirby, Ph.D.   Director of Research, Center for Population Options, Washington, D.C.

Kathryn A. Kirkhart, Ph.D.   Coordinator, Ventilator Program, Children's Hospital, New Orleans, Louisana

Mary Grace Kovar, Dr.P.H.   Special Assistant for Data Policy and Analysis, National Center for Health Statistics, Hyattsville, Maryland

Ruth A. Lee   Assistant to the Director, National Committee for Prevention of Child Abuse, Chicago, Illinois

George A. Little, M.D.   Professor and Chair, Department of Maternal and Child Health, Dartmouth University Medical School, Hanover, New Hampshire

Donald Ian Macdonald, M.D.   Special Assistant to the President, and Director, Drug Abuse Policy Office; and Administrator, Alcohol, Drug Abuse, and Mental Health Administration, U.S. Department of Health and Human Services, The White House, Washington, D.C.

Charles S. Mahan, M.D.   Professor, Department of Obstetrics and Gynecology, University of Florida College of Medicine, and Director of Maternal Health, State of Florida Department of Health, Gainesville, Florida

Donald McNellis, M.D., M.S.P.H.   Special Assistant for Obstetrics, Pregnancy and Perinatology Branch, National Institute of Child Health and Human Development, Bethesda, Maryland

C. Arden Miller, M.D.   Professor and Chairman, Department of Maternal and Child Health, University of North Carolina School of Public Health, Chapel Hill, North Carolina

David Muram, M.D.   Chief, Section of Pediatric and Adolescent Gynecology, Department of Obstetrics and Gynecology, University of Tennessee College of Medicine, Memphis, Tennessee

Philip R. Nader, M.D.   Professor of Pediatrics, University of California Medical School, San Diego, California

Patrick W. O'Carroll, M.D., M.P.H.   Medical Epidemiologist, Intentional Injuries Section, Epidemiology Branch, Division of Injury Epidemiology and Control, Center for Environmental Health and Injury Control, Centers for Disease Control, Atlanta, Georgia

Allan C. Oglesby, M.D., M.P.H.   Professor and Head, Division of Maternal and Child Health, School of Public Health, San Diego State University, San Diego, California

Margaret J. Oxtoby, M.D.   Medical Epidemiologist, AIDS Program, Center for Infectious Diseases, Centers for Disease Control, , Atlanta, Georgia

Mary D. Peoples-Sheps, R.N., Dr.P.H.   Associate Professor, Department of Maternal and Child Health, University of North Carolina School of Public Health, Chapel Hill, North Carolina

Raymond M. Peterson, M.D.   Director, Regional Center for the Developmentally Disabled, San Diego, California

Margaret W. Pratt   President, Information Sciences Research Institute, Vienna, Virginia

Elvoy Raines, J.D.   President, Square One Consulting Group, Inc., Durham, North Carolina

Julius B. Richmond, M.D.   John D. MacArthur Professor of Health Policy, Harvard University Medical School, Boston, Massachusetts

Daniel K. Roberts, M.D., Ph.D.   Professor and Chairman, Department of Obstetrics and Gynecology, Wesley Medical Center, Wichita Kansas

Sara Rosenbaum   Children's Defense Fund, Washington, D.C.

Erica Royston   Statistician, Division of Family Health, World Health Organization, Geneva, Switzerland

George M. Ryan, Jr., M.D., M.P.H.   Professor, Department of Obstetrics and Gynecology, University of Tennessee College of Medicine, Memphis, Tennessee

Stephen E. Saunders, M.D., M.P.H.   Assistant Director, State of Arizona Department of Health Services, Phoenix, Arizona

Patricia T. Schloesser, M.D.   Director, Division of Health, State of Kansas Department of Health and Environment, Topeka, Kansas

William M. Schmidt, M.D.   Professor Emeritus of Maternal and Child Health, Harvard University School of Public Health, Boston, Massachusetts

Lowell E. Sever, Ph.D.   Assistant Director for Science, Division of Birth Defects and Developmental Disabilities, Center for Environmental Health and Injury Control, Centers for Disease Control, Atlanta, Georgia

Ruth Sidel, Ph.D.   Professor of Sociology, Department of Sociology, Hunter College/City University of New York, New York, New York

Joe Leigh Simpson, M.D.   Professor and Chairman, Department of Obstetrics and Gynecology, University of Tennessee College of Medicine, Memphis, Tennessee

Jack C. Smith, M.S.   Chief, Research and Statistics Branch, Division of Reproductive Health, Center for Health Promotion and Education, Centers for Disease Control, Atlanta, Georgia

Felicia Hance Stewart M.D.   Associate Medical Director, Planned Parenthood Association of Sacramento, and Clinical Instructor in Obstetrics and Gynecology, University of California at Davis, School of Medicine, Sacramento, California

Gary K. Stewart, M.D., M.P.H.   Medical Director, Planned Parenthood Association of Sacramento, and Clinical Assistant Professor in Obstetrics and Gynecology, University of California at Davis, School of Medicine, Sacramento, California

Phyllis E. Stubbs, M.D., M.P.H.   Medical Director, U.S. Head Start Program, Bureau of Maternal and Child Health, U.S. Department of Health and Human Services, Rockville, Maryland

Patrick J. Sweeney, M.D., M.P.H., Ph.D.   Associate Professor of Obstetrics and Gynecology, Brown University Program in Medicine, Providence, Rhode Island

James Trussell, Ph.D.   Professor, Office of Population Research, Princeton University, Princeton, New Jersey

Carl W. Tyler, Jr., M.D.   Director, Epidemiology Program Office, Centers for Disease Control, Atlanta, Georgia

Kenneth C. Troutman, D.D.S., M.P.H.   Professor, Pediatric Dentistry, Louisiana State University School of Dentistry, New Orleans, Louisana

Helen M. Wallace, M.D., M.P.H.   Professor of Maternal and Child Health, Graduate School of Public Health, San Diego State University, San Diego, California

Paul H. Wise, M.D., M.P.H.   Director of Perinatal Epidemiology, Division of Health Policy Research and Education, Harvard University Medical School, Boston, Massachusetts

❙❙ FOREWORD

This is the third edition of the **Maternal and Child Health** textbook. This edition differs considerably from the previous one published in 1982, reflecting the changes that are occurring in the health care of women, infants, children, and youth.

One of the differences in this new edition includes the increased emphasis on the health needs and care of adolescents, with their special problems related to risk-taking behavior. Another is the expanded section on the health care of women, bolstering the argument for comprehensive health care and strengthening the *M* in *MCH*. Recognition of the importance of injury prevention in childhood and adolescence is presented. The continued disadvantaged position of the United States in infant mortality is stressed by the authors as one of the major public health problems demanding solution. Case management, as a concept, has been rediscovered, developed, and strengthened. To assure quality of services and control their costs, it is becoming a service for families with children who have complex medical needs.

In another vein, this edition contains other evidence of society's ways of dealing with some MCH problems. Detailed discussions of ethical issues in the provision of services, and the resurgence of care at home for the new populations of technology-dependent children are included. Advocacy for improved health care for women, children, and families is one way society expresses its concerns toward the goals of making it possible for all women, children, and families to have health care which is available, accessible, and of high quality.

Old standbys from previous editions, such as legislation, demographics, health status, nutrition, day care, and evaluation can be found updated in the text.

This third edition of **Maternal and Child Health Practices** is a documentation of where we are and what some of the future directions are for MCH in the United States.

Vince L. Hutchins, M.D., M.P.H.
Deputy Director
Bureau of Maternal and Child Health
and Resources Development
U.S. Department of Health and
Human Services
Rockville, Maryland, U.S.A.

MATERNAL AND CHILD HEALTH PRACTICES

THIRD EDITION

SECTION I

POLICIES AND ISSUES IN MATERNAL AND CHILD HEALTH

THE DEVELOPMENT OF HEALTH SERVICES FOR MOTHERS AND CHILDREN IN THE UNITED STATES

1

William M. Schmidt and Helen M. Wallace

In this chapter, events occurring from about 1890 into the 1960s are the main focus of interest. The earlier sources for development of programs of health care for mothers and children are outlined briefly and then only those occurring in the U.S. The child health movement in the U.S., however, owes much to the ideas and practices in France, England, and other European countries around the turn of the century. We have continued to borrow from these countries and we should be taking greater advantage of their efforts, often apparently more successful than ours, to serve the interests of maternal and child health. [1,2]

Advances in the application of knowledge to the protection of health of mothers and children have not occurred in a pattern of smooth incremental development. On the contrary, there have been advances and setbacks. Different views as to public responsibility for children and to methods of discharging this responsibility have prevailed at different periods of time. The constituencies sponsoring more generous support for extension and improvement of health care, broadly defined for mothers and children, are not constant, and in recent years new groupings have been emerging. The poor, the minority groups, and the dependent are making their voices heard.

New impetus for social action may be expected to support a more effective application of the notable advances that are occurring in the medical sciences and in practice. This will require the strengthening of state and local health organizations since public responsibility for children—requiring the substantial support of

3

public funds from tax revenues—can be made available to the whole population only through governmental organizations.

It was not until the end of the nineteenth and the early years of the twentieth centuries that the idea of attempting to assure health services for mothers and children as a public responsibility finally took hold. In the seventeenth and eighteenth centuries, the concepts and practices of child health in America varied in accordance with the great variety of inhabitants and colonizers. Indian children were protected against sickness and treated for diseases by combinations of medicine, magic, and religion that characterized the particular tribes to which they belonged. Children who were brought as slaves from Africa or were born into slavery had only the care that their owners were able and willing to provide for them. Children of European origin were tended to according to the knowledge and limitations of their parents and their community.

> What did slave children, immigrant children in city slums, children of a proud aristocrat on a plantation or those of a wealthy New England merchant really have in common? Little more, one suspects, than the land itself—a mere geographical location—and even in that simple respect there was greater diversity in the American environment than in any of the many nations and provinces from which the ancestors of the American young had come. [3]

There were some advances in knowledge of measures necessary for the protection of child health. Zabdiel Boylston introduced smallpox inoculation in 1721 (trying it on his own son) and started to stir up physicians to explain its value to the people. An effort to overcome the risks arising from unskilled and ignorant midwives led Shippen to establish a course in midwifery in Philadelphia, in 1765. Lying-in and foundling hospitals were created. Waterhouse introduced smallpox vaccination in the beginning of the nineteenth century.

For the most part, there was little basis for community child health programs, and no great effort was made to apply the knowledge that was available. "It is hard to recall Americans who crusaded for child health" in the eighteenth century. "No doubt the chief beneficiaries of better child care were the upper class families."[4]

In the latter half of the nineteenth century, social action for the welfare of children was one source of a gradually emerging concept of maternal and child health. A second stimulus came from the more rapid pace of advances in medicine, especially in pediatrics and obstetrics, and in medical education. A third element was the development of state and local health departments, which provided the governmental framework within which pediatric and obstetric knowledge and the broad concern with social action for children could join to form programs that were new to public health.

SOCIAL ACTION FOR THE WELFARE OF CHILDREN

In the expanding industrial development, children formed a large proportion of the labor force. They were employed in mines, mills, and factories, often as young as seven or eight years, for long hours and under poor or hazardous working conditions. While factory and mill owners and their political allies opposed restrictions on child labor, social reformers led the movement for effective child labor legislation. Trade unions joined the reform movement, recognizing the limitation of child labor as essential to improving the condition of the working class generally. The adverse effect of premature child labor on the health and development of children as well as the child's need for schooling were the central issues for many voluntary groups, which lead to the organization of the National Child Labor Committee in 1904. Efforts on state and federal levels to protect children from the harm of oppressive and exploitative labor were met with opposition at every step, and it was not until the Fair Labor Standards Act of 1937 that national regulation of a substantial proportion of occupations was achieved.

Among the leaders of the National Child Labor Committee were Jane Addams of Hull House, Florence Kelley of the National Consumers League, and Lillian Wald, head of the Henry Street Settlement and its visiting nurse service.

Slum housing, undernourishment, and depressing social conditions of family life among the poor led to anxious speculation as to the consequences for the future generation. Within the struggles against poverty carried on by social reformers, children had high priority. They could hardly be held responsible for their condition, whatever the stereotypes of their parents that may have arisen from the social biases of the times.

Philanthropic organizations were formed to improve the condition of children who were at special risk of neglect or abuse and those who, because of poverty, experienced excessive sickness and high mortality.

ADVANCES IN MEDICINE

The founding of the Children's Hospital of Philadelphia (1855) and the organized teaching on diseases of children that came with the establishment of the first department of pediatrics headed by Abraham Jacobi (1860) heralded advances that would become incorporated into child health programs later. Pediatrics, as a special branch of medicine, was recognized by the formation of a section on Diseases of Children of the American Medical Association in 1879 and by the establishment of the American Pediatric Society in 1888.

Leaders of the pediatric thought deplored the relative neglect of problems of child health and illness. Early meetings of the American Pediatric Society served to expose the "dead platitudes concerning children" and the "off-hand opinions and advice... to the credulous mother of the suffering child." [5]

At the turn of the century, diarrheal disease was still one of the leading causes of death of infants and young children, although it was well known that it was caused by contaminated milk.

Observations on rickets and scurvy had already shown that cod liver oil prevented rickets, that epidemics of scurvy among children occurred when the potato crop failed, and that orange and tomato juices were effective in prevention.

The series of fundamental discoveries in bacteriology during the last quarter of the nineteenth century gave way to new approaches to the prevention and control of infectious diseases.

STATE AND LOCAL HEALTH ORGANIZATIONS

The development of state and local health departments provided the third element—the governmental framework within which pediatric knowledge and the broad concern with social action for children could join to form public programs of maternal and child health. As early as 1869, a state board of health had been established (Massachusetts). By 1890, many states had set up state health agencies, and a few counties and larger cities had established their own public health authorities. For the most part, their activities focused upon environmental sanitation, communicable disease control, and vital statistics. The possibility of extending the work of health agencies to include services for mothers and children was beginning to be appreciated.

BEGINNING OF MCH PROGRAMS

Milk stations (first in New York in 1893), medical services in schools (first undertaken in Boston in 1894), and the reported experiences of visiting nurses were evidence of the readiness of laymen and professionals for advances in the public sector.

What was needed to launch programs of health services for mothers and children was initiative to prove the feasibility of community-wide application of preventive measures. The problem of eliminating heavily contaminated milk as an infant food and supplying bacteriologically clean milk was an outstanding example.

What Rosenau called the milk question..."illustrates, better than any single subject, many of the fundamental factors in preventive medicine." [6]

Infants and young children were supplied with milk of a satisfactory quality in so-called infant milk depots beginning in New York in 1893; similar efforts were soon made in other parts of the country. Mothers were shown and taught how to prepare and safeguard feedings and other aspects of child care.

These initial efforts under voluntary auspices came to be incorporated into the public agencies' programs. "I have done as much as one man and one purse can do to save the lives of the children of this city," Nathan Straus said, in addressing the aldermen in 1909. "Now I must put the work up to the city."

Before the Boston program of school medical inspectors, there had been isolated activities. Soon after Boston, other cities followed: Chicago, 1895; Philadelphia, 1895; New York, 1897. All of these efforts were of limited significance and were focused mainly on suspects of communicable disease.

The idea for educational work along with school medical inspection led to a request from the health commissioner of New York City to Lillian Wald of the Henry Street Settlement for the loan of a nurse, Lina L. Rogers—the first full-time school nurse. Soon others were employed to try to teach parents and children about the prevention of or need for treatment of minor skin conditions, malnutrition, and other impairments or illnesses that might be identified or suspected.

In Massachusetts, in 1906, responsibility for school health services was assigned to local school committees (boards of education). Absence of local health departments in most towns was one of the main reasons for this step, which separated services for school-age children from those for infants and preschool children. This pattern is still widely followed except where comprehensive child health services are beginning to create more fully integrated and more nearly adequate plans of child health care.

The promotion of the health of children and other family members by nursing care in their own homes developed initially as a service of voluntary agencies in several large cities. After the Henry Street Visiting Nurse Association, in 1902, assigned a nurse to the New York City Health Department for work in schools, other nurses were employed; health departments elsewhere also adopted the practice of appointing public health nurses. Some were assigned to specific disease-category programs, some to infant and child health work. The idea of a generalized type of service took time to develop. Many parts of the country, especially rural areas, lacked such services.

The first Bureau of Child Hygiene was established in New York City in 1908. Dr. S. Josephine Baker was the first chief of the bureau. With enormous vigor she organized a group of nurses to visit the tenement homes of newborn babies to teach and help care for school children, conducted child health clinics, supervised midwives, and was responsible for regulating children's institutions and boarding homes.[7] In the view of Jane Addams, the move from private charity to public responsibility was a step forward. The next step would be the acceptance of broad national responsibility by the federal government.

THE ESTABLISHMENT OF
THE U.S. CHILDREN' S BUREAU

The first nationwide meeting to examine the causes and prevention of infant mortality was followed by the founding of an association for this purpose (1909). In the same year, and with many of the same people taking the lead, a conference of some 100 professional and lay leaders interested in the care of dependent children was held in Washington, D.C. The conference, which was called by President Theodore Roosevelt, came to be known as the first White House Conference on Children. One of its major recommendations was the call for a Federal Children's Bureau.

The first bill to establish a Children's Bureau had been introduced in 1906, and six years of sometimes heated debate followed. Opponents challenged the constitutionality of the bill, holding that the responsibility for children's health and welfare was solely that of the states. Senator Borah, who introduced the bill that was finally enacted in 1912, granted that 50 years earlier the problems of children could well be left to the states, but "economic conditions have changed and the responsibilities and duties of government must necessarily change with those changes." [8] As the debates drew to a close, one of the opposing senators declared that if a children's bureau were established,

> a $900 clerk, 'drest in a little brief authority,' inflated with self-importance and puffed with impertinence, can knock at the door of an American and demand admission and, if denied, can force his way in. I presume he would almost have the warrant to kick open the door and assemble the family around the hearthstone to propound such questions as he might think important and within the range of his authority.[9]

The bill passed in the Senate by a vote of 54 to 20, with 17 not voting, and in the House by a vote of 177 to 17, with 190 not voting. It was approved by President Taft and became effective April 9, 1912. This marked the beginning of a period of studies of economic and social factors related to infant mortality, of maternal deaths, of maternal and infant care in rural counties, as well as other investigations that created the basis for stimulating better standards of care for mothers and children. In discharging its statutory obligation to investigate and report on all matters affecting children in child life, the staff of the Children's Bureau and its consultants reported these studies both to professional audiences and to the general public. Such reports informed and encouraged a logical step, the first Maternity and Infancy Act (Sheppard-Towner) in 1921, providing grants to states to develop health services for mothers and children. By 1920, all cities with a population of more than 100,000, and many others, carried on some aspects of maternal and child health. In many, this function was established as a unit of the health department. With rare exceptions, every state had established, or would soon do so, a Division of Maternal and Child Health. The principle of public responsibility for child health had been established, but not without doubts and opposition.

Some leaders of pediatrics thought it ill-advised to engage in activities of sociologic interest. Some considered higher infant mortality in certain population groups beneficial. One health officer wrote:

> Infants born into subnormal families fortunately suffer a greater handicap in their struggle to survive infanthood, else the more fecund subnormal class would soon outnumber the high normal citizenry and the population would soon become one of mental degenerates.[10]

"Conservative opinion held that cooperation at private expense rather than expansion of public agencies ..." [11] was the real need in bringing about a complete program of child health services.

The Sheppard-Towner Bill was assailed and opposed in Congress as "socialistic" and denounced as "drawn chiefly from the radical, socialistic, bolshevistic philosophy of Germany and Russia." It was condemned because it included a requirement that services provided under the Act "be available for all residents of the state," which was interpreted, rightly, as a move toward eliminating racial discrimination. The American Medical Association, in a formal resolution, declared firm opposition to it as an "imported socialistic scheme." The Commonwealth of Massachusetts unsuccessfully challenged the Act, on constitutional grounds, in the Supreme Court.

By the end of the 1920s, those who opposed grants-in-aid for maternity and infant care prevailed for the time being, and in 1929 the Sheppard-Towner Act lapsed.

During this remarkable period, roughly from 1890 to 1930, of sustained effort and recurrent counterattack, other developments affecting the health and welfare of children were taking place. The American Association for the Study and Prevention of Infant Mortality* in the annual meetings drew upon local and state experience to encourage improvement of MCH services. The birth registration area was established in 1915, with the promotion and interest of many groups, not the least being the General Federation of Women's Clubs. State after state qualified for inclusion in the area by reaching an acceptable level of completeness of birth registration. The first appropriation by states for care of handicapped children was in Minnesota, in 1897.

Progress in medical education received historic impetus with the publication of the Flexner Report (1919). The limited role of health departments began to be enlarged, and more broadly trained personnel became available as schools of public health began to be organized (1918-1923). The broadened infant welfare movement emerged in the form of the Child Welfare League of America, a national

---

*Successor organizations of the Association were the American Child Hygiene Association (1919) and, by merger with the Child Hygiene Organization of America in 1923, the American Child Health Association.

nongovernmental educational organization with expert staff helping to advance the standards of agencies serving children. Other organizations, particularly the Consumer's League and the National Child Labor Committee, continued their leadership and support of legislation and public action protecting child development.

The year 1919 followed two years of U.S. involvement in World War I. The Children's Bureau was determined to show the need and to take the opportunity for bettering both public and private child welfare activities, using the term child welfare in its inclusive sense, embracing health and social well-being. This was done in a series of eight regional conferences, of which Grace Abbott was secretary, beginning with one in Washington. These conferences on Standards of Child Welfare came to be known as the Second White House Conference on Children. The report includes perhaps the first substantial series of proposals for standards of programs for the health of mothers and children. The recommendations were put forward in plain language.*

In contrast to the steady and marked decrease in infant mortality during these years, the maternal death rate remained at a high level. In 1927 and 1928, there-fore, the Children's Bureau conducted the first extensive studies of the problem in the U.S. [13] A series of concrete recommendations to the medical profession and to the general public was adopted by the Obstetric Advisory Committee. These were major guidelines preparing the way for the great improvements in maternity care that were to follow in a few years. One of the recommendations of particular in-terest was, "Medical societies and departments of health in cooperation should in-vestigate each maternal death within a few weeks of the death". [13] This recommen-dation was adopted in one state after another.

The New York Academy of Medicine began its study of maternal deaths in 1930, patterned after the Fifteen States Study and using the same questionnaires.[14] In 1937 the maternal death rate began a fall that continued steadily into the 1950s. The series of maternal death studies had played an important part in this, and they continue to contribute to better practice of maternity care.

THE AMERICAN ACADEMY OF PEDIATRICS AND
THE AMERICAN COLLEGE OF OBSTETRICIANS AND GYNECOLOGISTS

The American Academy of Pediatrics (AAP) was founded in 1930. As with so many other developments in the child health movement, controversy concerning public responsibility for children was one factor leading to its formation. The Pediatric Section of the American Medical Association favored continuation of the

---

* For example, J. Whittridge Williams, Professor of Obstetrics at the Johns Hopkins University, wrote: To make progress trying to meet minimum standards would require "(a) a campaign of education in which women and their husbands are taught that it is their right and duty to demand reasonable care during pregnancy and at the time of labor; (b) the institution of State aid and National subventions, partly for educational purposes, but particularly for carrying out of such minimal standards as seem essential." [12]

Sheppard-Towner Act, while the House of Delegates opposed it and ruled that the section could not publish its views independently. Members of the section thereupon prepared to organize the AAP and adopted as its motto, "For the Welfare of Children". [15] The Academy had been a most important influence on the standards of child health care by continuing education in pediatrics, providing educational materials for parents, and sponsoring special studies among which the study of child health services and pediatric education in 1949 is especially noteworthy.

A recent contribution, the AAP's studies of pediatric practice and the use of non-physician personnel, is basic to planning for some extensive child health services. Parallel studies in maternity care have been sponsored by the American College of Obstetricians and Gynecologists, which, since its founding in 1951, has had a role in its field somewhat comparable to that of the AAP in child health.

Local societies of obstetrics and gynecology had been in existence since the 1860s, and a section on Obstetrics and Diseases of Women of the AMA first met in 1903. The American College of Obstetricians and Gynecologists was organized in 1951 to advance the standards of practice, the educational interests of the profession, and the obstetric and gynecologic care of women.*

NUTRITION AND MCH

Since the earliest child health activities of modern times, largely built around the idea of milk stations, nutrition has had a central place in MCH services. Concern at first centered on maintenance of breast feeding, cleanliness and adequacy of artificial cow's milk feeding, and weaning foods. As discoveries of the vitamins were added to the growing body of knowledge about the chemical and physiological characteristics of foods, nutrition studies and dietary advice in services for mothers and children became standard practice. The first edition of Infant Care[16]—the popular Children's Bureau booklet addressed to the average mother of this country—included a detailed section on infant feeding and the food for older children. By the second edition (1926), Vitamin D had been demonstrated to be effective in the prevention and treatment of rickets.

> The conquest of rickets, once the most common affliction of childhood, ranks with the prevention of diarrheal diseases of infancy and of diphtheria as triumphs of combined medical research and public health administration. [17] In studies of the methods of achieving prevention on a community scale and in evaluating the methods, Martha Eliot contributed to the disappearance of rickets as a public health problem. [18]

Dietary surveys and studies of the nutritional status of children established the prevalence of insufficient food and impaired nutritional status. [19] Poverty was the main problem, although not the only one.

---

*Originally named the American Academy of Obstetrics and Gynecology; the name was changed in 1956.

Recognizing the need to have special health workers for nutrition in public health programs, funds available from federal grants under the Sheppard-Towner Act enabled Connecticut, Illinois, Michigan, and Mississippi to appoint nutritionists, a practice that became general in health agencies.

MCH IN THE SOCIAL SECURITY ACT

With the end of the Sheppard-Towner Act and the beginning of the Great Depression, the states had reduced budgets for programs for mothers and children, while the needs were greater than ever. The Children's Bureau collected data during the first years of the Depression and prepared a suggested plan for children's health and welfare programs.

The plan, which was to become the basis for the child health and welfare sections of the Social Security Act, comprised three major program proposals: (1) aid to dependent children, (2) MCH services, including services for crippled children, and (3) child welfare services for children needing special care. The first part of the plan contained a requirement that state plans for aid to dependent children must furnish "assistance at least great enough to provide, when added to the income of the family, a reasonable subsistence compatible with decency and health."* [20]

The second part of the Children's Bureau plan was for a maternal and child health program broader than the Sheppard-Towner Act and with a doubling of the appropriation. A provision allowing for direct appropriation to the Children's Bureau was to be used in collaboration with the states for demonstrations. This was later converted by the Congress into the so-called B Fund, which was the foundation of experience for innovative project grant amendments a generation later.

An entirely new development was the proposed program of federal grants to states for Crippled Children's Services. Grace Abbott, chief of the Children's Bureau, suggested this as a start of a medical care program for children. The Children's Bureau had done studies that showed that certain aspects of care were being provided for crippled children but the program was inadequate in most parts of the country. What might be gained, for example, by providing orthopedic surgery for a child could be in large measure nullified if there was a failure to meet other related needs, such as physical therapy and appliances, social services, and special education. There was enough evidence to conclude that thousands of children would go through life with severe handicaps if more public funds were not made available.

The grants were not intended simply to pay medical bills. They were to enable states to organize new and better programs of care and, as the Act stated, "to

---

*This provision was struck out before passage of the bill. Miss Abbott's explanation was: "There was much objection to federal determination of adequacy on the part of Southern members who feared that Northern standards would be forced on the South in providing for Negro and white tenant families."

extend and improve ... services for crippled children." This is why programs proposed by the states would be approved only if they fulfilled the requirement for provision of an entire array of services, beginning with finding the crippled children and including the medical, surgical, and other needed services and aftercare.

Another important innovation was the inclusion in the statement of purpose of the phrase, "children who are suffering from conditions which lead to crippling." Thus, the idea was established that this new medical care program would include preventive services as well as needed medical and surgical treatment.

The third proposal was for grants to enable states to establish, extend, and strengthen child welfare services for children needing special care. Close relation to family welfare and relief programs were needed, but these programs in themselves did not provide many services needed by children. The need for services, over and above financial assistance, was repeatedly emphasized.

It is interesting to speculate that if the administration of aid-to-dependent children programs had been placed in the Children's Bureau, as originally intended, instead of the Social Security Board, an earlier start would have been made to develop skilled social services for the families of all needy children, as well as specialized social services for children with special needs. It is also possible that with the advantage of a close link with the MCH programs and the medical care in the Crippled Children's programs, comprehensive health care for children and youth in low-income families might have been made available two or even three decades sooner than was actually the case.

The Ways and Means Committee of the House of Representatives in hearings on the Social Security Bill, considered whether assignment of the child health grant-in-aid programs should be to the Public Health Service (as the AMA preferred) or to the Children's Bureau. The committee recommended that the program should go to the Children's Bureau, having heard testimony on the relation of child health and child welfare services, on the fact that the Crippled Children's Program was a medical care program, and the Public Health Service showed no enthusiasm for entering into the provision of medical care. The past record of the Children's Bureau, both in investigating and reporting and in administering the Sheppard-Towner Act, was also taken into account.

THE BEGINNING OF THE GRANT-IN-AID
PROGRAM UNDER THE SOCIAL SECURITY ACT

At first, the MCH programs were largely devoted to such services as pre- and postnatal clinics and child health clinics, and to the training of professional personnel. By 1937, however, the Bureau's advisory committee on maternal welfare recommended that the program be enlarged to provide medical and hospital care of mothers during labor and delivery. A quarter of a million women delivered in 1936 without the advantage of a physician's care; more than 15,000 of them had no care except that of family or neighbors. [21]

The American Birth Control League had been founded in 1921. A bill to remove a prohibition against contraceptives and information about contraception failed to pass in Congress, in 1924. A Conference on Better Care for Mothers and Babies, organized by the Children's Bureau, was the first national conference of the federal government at which a participant was given the floor to speak on family planning.

In a review, in 1939, of the accomplishments under the Social Security Act, Martha Eliot, then assistant chief of the Children's Bureau, Jessie Bierman, and A. L. Van Horn, who were responsible for the MCH and Crippled Children's programs, urged the extension of these programs to provide more nearly complete medical care of mothers and children. [22] They wrote:

> The utter futility of providing means of assessing the health and welfare of children and of mothers, and of not providing the means to maintain them in health or to restore them to health if sick, or in the case of maternity to make available complete medical and nursing care of mother and infant, has forced itself upon health and welfare workers and upon the people.

"A courageous attack on the problem of maternity care and care of newborn infants that would meet the need with no half-way measure" was urged.

As for crippled children's services, they declared that funds were "wholly inadequate" to meet the need, to include such conditions as rheumatic fever, rheumatic heart disease, and impairments of vision and hearing, or to improve the notably inadequate care of the hopelessly crippled child.

This effort to move ahead toward more comprehensive medical care programs for mothers and children came at a time when organized medicine was in an active campaign against the first Wagner National Health Bill—a national medical care program that was based upon the proposals of an interdepartmental committee—with Martha M. Eliot as chairman of its technical committee. Despite this intense campaign against public medical care, Congress approved in the next year an amendment [23] authorizing an additional appropriation of one million dollars for handicapped children with the understanding that it would be used, in part, in developing programs for care of children with rheumatic heart disease. In adding provision for care of children with chronic illness to a program that previously concentrated on children with physical handicaps, a step was taken toward a broadly inclusive medical care program for children. The next step was a nationwide program of care for childbearing mothers and their infants. It was a temporary, emergency measure, but it had a profound impact.

THE EMERGENCY MATERNITY AND INFANT CARE PROGRAM

World War II brought about a rapid, large-scale increase in the numbers of enlisted men. Many wives came to live near posts where their husbands were temporarily stationed. The capacity of station hospitals to provide maternity care was soon found to be insufficient.

An emergency program developed with great rapidity, extending to servicemen's wives wherever they lived, and providing care for one and one-fourth million mothers and 230,000 infants by the time it was terminated after the end of the war. This was the largest public medical care program known by the country, and dealt with the state health departments. It was entirely supported by general tax funds. There was no state matching, and there was no means test required or permitted for designated beneficiaries. It enabled states to make great progress in licensing and upgrading hospital maternity care, and further aided hospitals in improving standards by establishing a basis of payment related to the cost of care—a principle later adopted by other federal agencies and by the Blue Cross Insurance Plans.

The rapidity of expansion of this program, its widespread acceptance, and the general participation of physicians and hospitals overshadowed the scattered opposition initially encountered and a short-lived attempt of one state medical association to encourage a boycott of the program.

RESEARCH RELATING TO CHILDREN

Responsibility for research relating to children was placed upon the Children's Bureau under the basic act of 1912, in which it was stated that the Bureau "shall investigate and report...all matters pertaining to the welfare of children and child life among all classes of our people." In the early years, there were studies of infant and maternal mortality and birth registration, childhood accidents, employment of children, and social problems, such as child neglect.

The investigative work of the Children's Bureau was carried out entirely from the modest appropriations available to the Bureau itself. Small amounts of the grants to state health and crippled children's agencies were occasionally utilized for studies. The staff of the Children's Bureau attempted to encourage and stimulate research relating to children, not only in state agencies but also in institutions of higher learning and in teaching hospitals. Despite administrative innovations, however, and despite the Bureau's effort to stretch its funds to the very limit, it was obvious that research relating to children was badly undernourished financially.

In the 1930s, research was far from being as popular in the public mind and in the minds of legislators, as it was to become. Even as late as 1949, the proposal for a National Child Research Act was defeated. [24] The 1930 White House Conference on Children focused upon child development, including child development research. But it was not until the National Institute of Child Health and Human Development was established in 1961 that a national center for basic research in child development came into being.

There was an ebb and flow of relative emphasis over the years on program-related research and service programs. [25] Although the Children's Bureau never ceased to recognize and to encourage research relating to children side-by-side with service programs, there were periods during which its heavy responsibilities in extending and improving services for mothers and children had to take precedence over its promotion of child health and welfare research. Happily, the establishment of specific authorization for program-related research in child health and child welfare, in Title V of amendments enacted in 1963 and 1965, restored the balance and emphasized the relationship.

THE WHITE HOUSE CONFERENCES OF 1940 AND 1950

The fourth White House Conference for children was again held in the midst of world war. This time, the conference focused attention on problems of nutrition, urged a national program of maternity care by 1950, and pressed for the elimination of discrimination on the basis of race or creed.

The 1950 conference brought a demand to ban racial public school segregation. Kenneth Clark's excellent document, *Prejudice and Your Child*, commissioned for the White House Conference, became a part of the U.S. Supreme Court's opinion in Brown v Board of Education, in 1954. At this Conference, too, more attention began to be given to the needs of retarded children, and following the Conference the National Association for Retarded Children was formed, helping to educate the public, foster research, and stimulate support for better services.

It is, of course, impossible to assess the effect of conferences such as these amidst all of the forces acting with or against each other on efforts to contribute to the welfare of children. At the least, they seem to have widened moral support for progressive programs.

SPECIAL PROJECTS FOR MATERNITY AND INFANT CARE
AND FOR CHILDREN AND YOUTH

In 1934, when the Social Security Act was under consideration, questions were raised about the possibility of including services for children with mental retardation. In the light of existing knowledge on which programs for the mentally retarded could be based, however, the problems involved seemed too vast at that time.

The services were not included until, in the early 1950s, the Children's Bureau began to pioneer efforts in making grants from maternal and child health funds for community services for mentally retarded children. In 1954, one million dollars of the appropriation for MCH was earmarked for this purpose. These grants helped to educate the public and the professions; later, the concern of President Kennedy stimulated nationwide interest. In 1962, a task force on mental retardation brought together experts in medical, social, educational, and other related aspects of mental retardation. One of the proposals of the task force drew upon the advancing knowledge of the relationship of complications of childbirth to mental retardation. To reduce the risk of complications, grants for comprehensive maternity and infant care projects were authorized in 1963, an important step to meeting the need with no halfway measures, as proposed some 25 years earlier.

The 1965 amendments providing for comprehensive health care for children and youth were incorporated into PL 89-87. In the same Act, Medicare and Medicaid (Titles XVIII and XIX) commanded the greatest attention and provoked the most discussion. These programs, of course, are far greater in magnitude than were the maternity care and children's projects.

However, programs under Title XIX did not include organization of services to assure comprehensive care. The great significance of the maternity and infant care and children and youth projects is that they are founded on the idea of comprehensive provision of care.

THE WHITE HOUSE CONFERENCES ON
CHILDREN AND YOUTH OF 1960 AND 1970

The White House Conference on Children and Youth of 1960 (with youth participation for the first time) seemed to some observers to have produced only a confusing mass of varied recommendations. This superficial view overlooks the fact that this conference directed attention to the great change in the relative importance of major problems affecting child health and development. The old problems, by no means overcome, were now seen in the context of poverty, deprivation, denial of civil rights, and racial discrimination. Profound concern also arose about drug abuse, increases in the incidence of venereal diseases, illegitimate births, inadequate opportunities for youth employment, and concern for the environment. The response of state and federal governments and of the public generally to these issues, at that time, was inadequate. Only when the problems grew in magnitude were they to receive wider, if still insufficient, attention. The urgent concern for extension of health services for mothers and children was followed by the design, enactment, and launching of maternal and infant care, and children and youth projects referred to in an earlier section.

The 1970 White House Conferences were held separately for children and for youth. Some of the reports originating in the 25 forums embodied concrete proposals for a national program of health care for mothers and children and for handicapped children. Others pointed out the way in which gross deficits could be corrected in services such as early childhood education and day care for children. Assurance of a decent standard of living for families was widely supported.

Perhaps most significant for the future was the impression left by the unofficial caucuses of black participants, Indians, persons of Spanish language and cultural heritage, and others. These caucuses gave strong reminders that children of minority groups are still at significant disadvantage in health and development. Improvement in their status has occurred, but their relative position in measurements of health and development is still unchanged. It is the relative position that counts. The coexistence of slum and suburb, deficit and surfeit—so the caucuses seemed to say—forms the seedbed of the ills that beset children and youth of the 1970s.

NEIGHBORHOOD HEALTH CENTERS AND HEAD START PROGRAMS

Comprehensive neighborhood health centers were created under the Office of Economic Opportunity (OEO) and as part of the Partnership for Health Act. Some of the Maternity and Infant Care programs and Children and Youth Centers were able to tap this source of funding to add medical care for adults to the other family health services provided under their initial plans. Altogether, by the end of the 1960s, there were 150 such centers publicly supported or largely so. Many are described as offering family-focused health care, evidently with somewhat varied definitions of this term.

Taken together, however, these centers still fall far short of meeting the needs of mothers and children who are not cared for in private practices or in other suitable public centers.

In 1965, Head Start programs were launched by the Office of Economic Opportunity. Set up primarily in areas where children have had little to build upon, Head Start centers are planned for learning, social development, and health care. They have been based upon planning, guided by expert knowledge of child health development and welfare. New extensions to provide needed care for younger infants and children are under way.

DISMEMBERMENT OF THE CHILDREN'S BUREAU

In August 1967, a reorganization of the Department of Health, Education and Welfare was announced by administrative order, under which the health and welfare components of the Children's Bureau were split apart, and some of the functions were distributed among other agencies. The Children's Bureau itself, of course, could be abolished only by an act of Congress. What remained of the statutory responsibilities under the Act of 1912 came to form a subdivision of a new agency, the Office of Child Development, establishment of which, by executive order, was announced April 9, 1969. The Head Start program was delegated by OEO to the new office.

The splitting apart of child health, child welfare, youth services, and the basic mandate to "investigate and report...upon all matters pertaining to the welfare of children and child life" is the most recent turn of events in the clash of conflicting concepts of public responsibility for children. One view—which has been called the vertical approach—assumes that a general health program will fully meet the needs of children; a general welfare program will admit no errors of commission or omission as to child welfare; and the various correctional, judicial, and public safety structures and programs of government will suitably protect the public from delinquent acts of children and foster the care of the delinquent equally well. All this may be proved true in time, although we must wait to see what in fact a general health care program and a general welfare plan will look like in actual practice.

Meanwhile, the words of Grace Abbott, written over 30 years ago, are still relevant:

> Children, it should be repeated, are not pocket editions of adults. Because childhood is a period of physical growth and development, a period of preparation for adult responsibility in public and private life, a program for children cannot be merely an adaptation of the program for adults, nor should it be curtailed during periods of depression or emergency expansion of other programs. [26]

This viewpoint assumes the importance of attending to see to the needs of children and their families across the rigid lines of professional disciplines and the constraints imposed by administrative boundaries.

FAMILY PLANNING AND FAMILY HEALTH

In 1970, the Family Planning Services and Population Research Act of 1970 was passed. Although family planning services had long been an accepted part of maternity care in MCH programs and maternity care projects and in projects funded by the Office of Economic Opportunity, this Act is the first U.S. statute specifically to provide authority and funds for family planning.

The Act provides support for comprehensive programs of voluntary family planning services. The grants may be made to private nonprofit as well as to public agencies. While some see in this legislation primarily a design to "deal with this country's own population problem," [27] others regard voluntary family planning as one element in family health care. The director of the National Center for Family Planning Services considers that it has become:

> almost too easy to look toward reducing population growth as the panacea to our country's problems...The family planner's work is to provide a basic health service far more closely tied to infant and maternal morbidity and mortality, and family health and stability, than to the implications of population patterns. [28]

Barriers of state legislation limiting access to family planning services have largely (but not entirely) fallen away. Voluntary family planning counseling and services are increasingly a standard part of maternity care, including postpartum and interpregnancy care, but are as yet insufficiently available because such health care is itself insufficiently available.

THE RIGHTS OF CHILDREN

It is not common today, as it was in the early period of the child health movement, for overt opposition to be expressed to the extension and improvement of child health services or even to federal support for these purposes. The declarations of children's rights, as they appeared in the Children's Charter of 1930, are now asserted with little disagreement. The Joint Commission on Mental Health of Young Children [29] asserts in its final report that every infant must be granted:

The right to be wanted
The right to be healthy
The right to live in a healthy environment
The right to satisfaction of basic needs
The right to continuous loving care
The right to acquire the intellectual and emotional skills necessary to achieve individual aspirations and to cope effectively in our society

The 1970 White House Conference on Children adopted positions similar to these and produced proposals for programs intended to make these asserted rights genuine entitlements. To confer rights that are available is to give a generous check with no funds in the bank.

Whether the next period is one of slow or rapid progress remains to be seen.

REFERENCES

1. Miller HC. Health services for children in some Western European Countries: Their significance for the United States. Pediatrics 42:845, 1968.

2. Eliot MM. An American looks at European child health. Pediatrics 42:727, 1968.

3. Bremner RH. Children and Youth in America, Vol 1. Cambridge, Mass. Harvard University Press, 1970, p. 343.

4. Shyrock RH. Medicine and Society in America 1660-1860. New York. New York University Press, 1960.

5. Rotch TM. Iconoclasm and original thought in the study of pediatrics. Transactions of the American Pediatric Society, III. 1891, pp.6-9. A document in Bremner, R.: Children and Youth in America, Vol. 2, pt. 2. Cambridge, Mass. Harvard University Press, 1970, p. 819.

6. Rosenau MJ. The Milk Question. Boston and New York. Houghton Mifflin Co., 1912.

7. Baker SJ. Fighting for Life. New York. Macmillan. 1939.

8. The Senate Congressional Record: 702-705 (Jan 8) 1912.

9. The Senate Congressional Record: 1564-1579 (Jan 31) 1912.

10. Wood HB. Sanitation Practically Applied. New York. John Wiley and Sons, Inc. 1917.

11. Emerson H. The part of the general public in bringing about a complete program of child health services. Transactions, American Child Health Association, 1923, pp. 63-70.

12. Williams JW. Standards of Child Welfare. Bureau Publication 60, Children's Bureau, U.S. Department of Labor. 1919. p. 146.

13. Maternal Mortality in Fifteen States: Bureau Publication 223, Children's Bureau, U.S. Department of Labor. 1934. (A summary report of this study appeared as: Maternal Deaths, a Brief Report of a Study Made in Fifteen States. Bureau Publication No. 221, 1933.)

14. Maternal Mortality in New York City: New York. The Commonwealth Fund. New York Academy of Medicine, Committee on Public Health Relations, 1933. (A popular account is Gladston, I.: Maternal Deaths - The Pathways to Prevention. New York. The Commonwealth Fund. 1937.)

15. Beaven PW. For the Welfare of Children. Springfield. Thomas. 1955. pp. xiv and xv.

16. Infant Care - Care of Children: Series No. 2. Bureau Publication No. 8. Children's Bureau, U. S. Department of Labor. 1914.

17. Harrison HE. The disappearance of rickets. Am. J. Public Health 56:734-737, 1966.

18. Eliot MM. The Control of rickets-Preliminary discussion of the demonstration in New Haven. JAMA 85:656, 1925.

19. For an example of one early study: Roberts, L. The Nutrition and Care of Children in a Mountain County of Kentucky. U.S. Children's Bureau Publication 110. 1922.

20. Abbott G. The Child and the State. Chicago. University of Chicago Press. 1938. p. 240.

21. Proceedings of Conference on Better Care for Mothers and Babies, January 17-18, 1938.

22. Eliot MM. Bierman, J.M., and Van Horn, A.L.: Accomplishments in maternal and child health and crippled children's services under the Social Security Act, J Pediatr 13:678-691. 1938.

23. Social Security Act Amendment of 1939, approved August 10, 1939.

24. National Child Research Act, Hearings before the Subcommittee on Health Legislation of the Committee on Labor and Public Welfare. 81st Congress, First Session, 1949, pp. 1, 19, S-904.

25. Advocacy and inquiry: Their roles in the development of health services for mothers and children. Am. J. Public Health 56, 1966.

26. Abbott G. The Child and the State. Vol. II. Chicago. University of Chicago Press. 1938. p. 619.

27. New York Times, Editorial, January 11, 1971.

28. Beckles FN. Federal policies and services in family planning. Memo-prepared for presentation April 28, 1971, to the Association of Teachers of Maternal and Child Health, New Orleans, La.

29. Crisis in child mental health: Challenge for the 1970s. Report of the Joint Commission on Mental Health of Children. Washington, D.C. 1969.

ADDENDUM FOR
THE 1970s AND 1980s

Helen M. Wallace

For the field of MCH/handicapped children in the U.S., the 1970s and 1980s represent several types of efforts:

1. The extensive collection of facts on the status of infants, children, youth, parents, and families;

2. The production of authoritative statements about some special problems in regard to the MCH population, such as low birth weight, teenage pregnancy;

3. Marked extension of services for handicapped children, first of school age and more recently of infancy and preschool age;

4. Increased efforts to improve the immunization level of infants and children;

5. Some steps to incorporate the concept of high risk in maternal health services, leading to regionalization of perinatal infant care and, to a lesser extent, of perinatal maternal care;

6. Extension of family planning services to about two-thirds of the women in need, but more recently a reduction of federal funds to support family planning services;

7. Evidence of increased concern about the special problems of the adolescent population, but insufficient support to assist states and local com-

communities to provide adequate preventive services, and services to properly care for adolescents with special problems;

8. Concern about the problem of child abuse and neglect, and of sexual abuse in children;

9. Concern about the many-faceted problems of children and families in poverty, and especially the plight of female-headed families;

10. Recognition of the fact that Title 19 of the Social Security Act (Medi caid) has emerged as the largest source of public sector funds for the health care of mothers and children;

11. Increased recognition of the need for maternity leave for both the pre- and post-delivery phases of mother and child care for the large number of women who work.

While there has been evidence of these special efforts and concerns listed above, this has occurred in a climate of reduced federal funding for the MCH/ Crippled Children's field and for the federal support of family planning services; a consistent effort to eliminate the availability of legal abortion services; the polarized public controversies about teaching family life education in the schools, and about school-based clinics to prevent pregnancy in teenagers. Some of the more negative stances taken by the present Presidential administration have included efforts to withdraw federal support from those family planning clinics which also provide abortion counseling and referral; and they have included the Adolescent Family Life Act, which epitomizes the prevention of teenage pregnancy, by just saying "no."

Some of these trends and concerns will be discussed in greater detail in the remainder of this chapter.

RESTRUCTURING MCH AT THE FEDERAL LEVEL

As Dr. Schmidt pointed out in the previous section of this Chapter, the dismemberment of the U.S. Children's Bureau represented a significant step in muting the voice and leadership for children in our federal government. Nevertheless, steps are slowly being taken to integrate some of the federal fragments in the MCH field to begin to reconstitute MCH at the federal level. For example, the Bureau of Maternal and Child Health and Resource Development has been created, thus giving MCH a higher voice in the federal government. The health program of Head Start has been moved into the new federal MCH Bureau. The new federal MCH Bureau has been given the responsibility for publication of *Infant Care*, the national best seller, as well as for *Prenatal Care*, and *Child Care Ages One to Six*, and *Six to Twelve*. These are all signs of specific steps to strengthen MCH at the federal level, and give the field of MCH the opportunity to be heard more effectively.

THE SELECT PANEL FOR THE PROMOTION OF CHILD HEALTH

The Select Panel for the Promotion of Child Health was established in the late 1970s by Congress, during the Carter Administration, to redesign the foundations of a national effort to improve the health of children in the U.S. It completed its report in December 1980, "Better Health for Our Children: A National Strategy."[1] This four-volume report consists of (1) Major Findings and Recommendations; (2) Analysis and Recommendations for Selected Federal Programs; (3) A Statistical Profile; (4) A Series of Background Papers.

The report of the Select Panel is a valuable set of four documents, summarizing the concensus of the facts and "state of the art" in the health care of women, children and families at that time. It served as a basis for discussion and for the blueprint for health, social, nutritional care of women and children for the early 1980s. While it contains a large number of specific recommendations, the fundamental needed services are that "it should not longer be considered acceptable that an individual be denied access to prenatal, delivery, and postnatal care; comprehensive health care for children from birth through age five; family planning services." A second category of services which merits special attention includes mental health and related psychosocial services, dental services, genetic services, and services that promote access to care.

WORKING WOMEN

The World Wide Picture

Employment of women is a world-wide necessity and requires special attention. Most women who work do so for financial reasons. Employment of women needs to consider the special needs of the woman, her fetus, her children, and her family. The principal objective of measures of maternity protection is to protect the health of the future mother and child; it is also to guarantee a continuing source of income and security of employment. An analysis of the national legislation of 127[2] countries for which information is available shows that the average length of maternity leave in the world is between 12 and 14 weeks. Over half the countries (69) stipulate maternity leave of this duration. Thirty one countries provide less than the average, while the rest exceed this average. The shorter period of leave is prevalent mostly in developing countries, while longer maternity leave has been the national policy of socialist countries for a long time.

United Nations Decade for Women (1975-1985)

The UN Decade for Women was a worldwide effort to improve the status of women. It culminated in the 1985 Conference in Nairobi on The UN Decade for Women. There were concerns and statements about the status of women, including their socioeconomic status; support systems in society; women in the labor force; unemployment; maternity benefits; health status of working women; child care; training; education; legal rights; family planning.

WOMEN IN THE LABOR FORCE AND THEIR CHILDREN
IN THE UNITED STATES [3]

The proportion of women who are working full time in the United States has increased from 29 percent in 1975 to 41 percent in 1986. For those with children aged three-five years, it increased from 27 percent to 39 percent, and for those with children three years of age, it increased from 19 percent to 30 percent. The proportions of mothers who work part time have also been increasing, but more modestly.

In 1986, half of all married mothers with infants one year old or under were working or looking for work, compared with 31 percent in 1975. Nearly 60 percent of married women are in the work force by the time their youngest child is four years of age. Divorced and separated mothers are more likely to be in the labor force than are married mothers. Never married mothers are less likely than married mothers to be in the labor force.

Children under five years of age with employed mothers are more likely to be cared for outside their own home, particularly if their mothers work fulltime. Much of the increase in out-of-home care has been due to increasing the use of group care centers or of care provided in the home of non-relatives. In 1982, 27 percent of children under five years of mothers employed fulltime were cared for in the child's own home; 46 percent were cared for in another home; 20 percent were in a group care center; and seven percent were in other arrangements. For children under five years of age, where the mother was employed part-time, the percentages were 41 percent, 36 percent, eight percent, and 15 percent respectively.

Concerns About the Health Status, Working Conditions of Women and About the Care of Their Children

For several decades in the U.S., there have been concerns about various aspects of employment of women before, during, and after pregnancy, and about the care of their children. These concerns have been expressed by efforts to introduce federal legislation about child care in the early 1970s, and more recently about parental leave.

Concerns include the need for preventive and protective measures against health hazards at work, including heavy labor during pregnancy; work in industries that manufacture and use potentially toxic substances; with the recommendations that women be re-assigned to be more protected working conditions. Maternity leave benefits adopted by some countries include paid time off (usually two months) prior to the expected date of confinement; encouragement of time off for prenatal care when scheduled; concern about the woman's general health and nutrition status; preparation for the care of the baby. Maternity benefits also include the allowance of time off up to one year after delivery with full salary; additional time without salary may be available; protection of the job and seniority rights of the women. It also includes concerns about the care of the child, and provision of child care, either by government or by industry at the work site. Breast feeding is encouraged. There have been recent efforts to broaden maternity leave to parental leave. Family planning education and services are a part of the maternity leave package.

It is clear that the U.S. has fallen behind modern trends in protection and concerns about the working woman, maternity leave, and the care of children in society. At this writing (1987), only seven states guarantee some form of maternity leave through disability law, and five more do so through anti-discrimination statute.

ADOLESCENT HEALTH

The 1970s and 1980s, in the U.S., have been a period of development in the field of adolescent medicine and of adolescent health as a specific field. The reasons for this are several: the recognition that the adolescent population is large in size; that their health and social needs are serious for themselves, their families, and for society; and that society efforts must be organized to deal with them. Examples of the special health and social problems of adolescents include: drug abuse; alcohol abuse; smoking; suicide; homicide; accidents, especially motor vehicle; crime; earlier sexual activity; pregnancy; sexually transmitted diseases; delinquency; runaways; school drop out. One of the main themes underlying much of these problems is their disenchantment and alienation from family and society; another one is their risk-taking behavior.

While research has added considerable to our understanding and knowledge about their development and risk-taking behavior, we seem not yet to have found an effective way of preventing the problems from occurring or of effectively working with many adolescents in difficulty to assist them in resolving them. Furthermore, the polarization of society about teenage sexuality, contraception, and pregnancy has prevented the U.S. from taking steps to prevent and curb the present epidemic of teenage pregnancy.

There is evidence reported by Klerman [5] of the health needs of adolescents not being adequately met. At present there are 43 adolescent medicine training programs in the U.S., representing some growth in the last two decades. [6] Nevertheless, a recent survey of health professionals—physicians (family practice, internal medicine, and pediatrics), nurses, nutritionists, psychologists, social workers, and special educators—revealed that only a modest percentage of them feel competent to manage adolescent health issues; a considerable percentage feel insufficiently trained and would like more training.

The field of adolescent health represents one of the priority areas requiring more attention and support by society and by the field of MCH.

TEENAGE PREGNANCY

Pregnancy in teenagers is one of the most serious problems in the field of MCH today (1987). It is serious for the young woman who is pregnant, and equally serious for her child. In spite of this, teenage pregnancy has been one of the fields of MCH without any agreed-upon blueprint for a comprehensive program to prevent it and to provide services for those who become pregnant. The absence of such an agreed-upon comprehensive program is a reflection of the polarization of society in the U.S. about what needs to be done.

Comparison of Teenage Pregnancy In The U.S. With Other Developed Countries [8]

A recent report comparing the U.S. and other "developed countries" revealed that teenage fertility is considerably higher in the U.S. While there is a large differential within the U.S. between the rates of white and black teenagers, even if one considers whites only, the rates in the U.S. are much higher than in most of the other countries. The gap between the U.S. and the other countries is greater among younger adolescents. Abortion rates are also higher among U.S. teenagers. Policies regarding maternity leave and benefits are broader and more protective in most of these other countries. There is more openness in discussing sex in most of these other countries.

The Consequences of Teenage Pregnancy [9-13]

The consequences of teenage pregnancy upon the teenager are well known and have been well summarized. These include a higher maternal mortality rate; a higher incidence of anemia; a higher incidence of toxemia. They receive late and less prenatal care.

In addition, pregnant teenagers have a higher rate of dropout from school and interruption of education; higher unemployment; higher subsequent poverty; a high utilization of AFDC (Aid to Families with Dependent Children); a pattern of repeat pregnancies; if married, a higher rate of marital disruption.

The babies born of teenage mothers have a higher perinatal and infant mortality, and a higher incidence of low birth weight. Some studies indicate possible lower scores in intelligence testing and cognitive tests among children of teenage mothers. Babies born to teenage mothers are more likely to be hospitalized subsequently and have an increased risk of accidents.

Economic Costs [14]

In addition to the issues of emotional, social, psychological, health, educational, and vocational consequences and costs for the individuals involved, there is also the cost of teenage pregnancy to society. In the U.S., over half the budget for AFDC (Aid to Families with Dependent Children) is expended on families in which the mother was a teenager when she had her first child, and nearly three-quarters of AFDC recipients younger than 30 were teenagers at first birth. Since fewer than one-quarter of all U.S. women born between 1945 and 1959 bore a child by age 20, it is clear that teenagers are disproportionately high among welfare recipients. In addition to costs incurred under AFDC, there are also costs for health care under Medicaid, and for nutrition assistance under the food stamp program.

Prevention of Teenage Pregnancy

Prevention of pregnancy in teenagers includes a series of steps, services, and programs required of U.S. society.

BROAD SOCIETAL STEPS AT PREVENTION

This type of preventive approach includes pinpointed efforts to strengthen family life in the U.S., and to strengthen parent-child relationships and ability to communicate. It also includes the need to promote closer teacher-pupil relationships within the schools.

The preventive approach includes the need to devise more employment opportunities for youth, the need for meaningful work-study programs, and for strengthening career and vocational counseling.

Family Life Education As a Preventive Step [15-22]

There has been no consensus developed in the U.S. on the role of family life education in the schools, as one measure to prevent teenage pregnancy. And yet sex education has existed for several decades in Sweden. In Sweden, it is a required program and has been compulsory since 1964. It is taught openly in the schools from the time of entrance to graduation. Efforts are made to educate teachers in the teacher training schools and through refresher courses. There is a manual on sex education.

Family life education/sex education is required in three states (New Jersey, Maryland, and the District of Columbia) in the U.S. In most states, the option of performance of family life education is left up to the states, and in turn in most states is left up to local school districts.

A recent study [16,17] of the programs in six districts in New Jersey revealed some variation among the districts. All six districts include family life education and sexuality. Most include human reproduction. All include sex education in the lower grades. Relatively few parents exercised the option to remove their children from the family life education classes.

A review of the literature on the effects of school sex education by Kirby [18] indicates that instruction does increase knowledge, and does modify attitudes toward sexual practices of others. However, there is no conclusive evidence that instruction changes sexual behavior.

School-Based Clinics [23-31]

School-based clinics to serve adolescents in the schools represent one approach to prevent and reduce the incidence of pregnancy in teenagers. The first school-based clinic to serve teenagers in the field of pregnancy and its prevention was begun in St. Paul, Minnesota, in 1973. At this writing, there are at least 71 such clinics in large cities in the U.S. They offer comprehensive health care, as well as information, counseling and contraception. They are staffed by a team of health and education personnel. Confidentiality is maintained. Funding has been secured from a variety of sources, including foundations, Medicaid, Title 10 of the Public Health Service Act, Title 5 of the Social Security Act, education funds, etc. They have been endorsed by such organizations as the American Academy of Pediatrics.

Availability of Family Planning Information and Services

In addition to programs of family life education in the schools and in the community for students and parents, another essential service is the provision of family planning information and services to teenagers, so that these services will be freely and easily available. This includes the timing and location of such services to make them easily available to the teenagers; the provision of a friendly climate, including telephone service as the first contact for some; inclusion of the male partner; maintenance of confidentiality; provision of free contraceptive supplies; counseling and referral for abortion services when appropriate; and not requiring written consent of the teenagers' parents.

Working With the Male Partner [32]

One of the major problems in preventing teenage pregnancy is having effective access and impact on the male partner. It is clear that not enough attention has been paid to this, nor has sufficient effort been made with the male. In U.S. society, males need to play a much more active role in preventing teenage pregnancy, in staff roles in agencies serving teenagers, and in working with young teenage males.

ABORTION

In 1973, the Supreme Court legalized abortion by a 7-2 vote, in Roe V. Wade, ruling that women have a constitutional right of privacy in deciding whether to bear a child. Since then, the number of reported legal abortions in the U.S. has risen almost steadily through 1985.

Year	# Legal Abortions	Abortion Rate*	Year	# Legal Abortions	Abortion Rate
1973	744,600	16.3	1980	1,553,900	29.3
1974	898,600	19.3	1981	1,557,300	29.3
1975	1,034,200	21.7	1982	1,573,900	28.8

Year	# Legal Abortions	Abortion Rate*	Year	# Legal Abortions	Abortion Rate
1976	1,179,300	24.2	1983	1,575,000	28.5
1977	1,316,700	26.4	1984	1,577,300	28.1
1978	1,409,600	27.7	1985	1,588,600	28.0
1979	1,497,700	28.8			

* per 1,000 women aged 15-44 years

Early safe abortion has contributed to the marked reduction in maternal mortality rates. Since 1976, the Hyde Amendment to an appropriation bill has barred the use of federal Medicaid funds for abortion, unless the mother's life is endangered by the pregnancy. This decision was relaxed in 1977 to allow funding of abortions to protect the mother's long-term health, then tightened again in 1979, and upheld 5-4 by the Supreme Court in 1980. Fifteen states (California, Washington, Massachusetts, New Jersey, Oregon, Michigan, Alaska, North Carolina, West Virginia, District of Columbia, New York, Connecticut, Vermont, Delaware, Maryland) provide full Medicaid funding for abortions. An additional four states (Iowa, Wisconsin, Pennsylvania, Virginia) have Medicaid coverage of abortions in some circumstances, usually including pregnancies that result from rape or incest, life endangerment of the mother, or severe fetal deformity. Most states pay for abortions only if the mother's life is endangered.

Since the early 1980s, several attempts to ban abortion have failed. For example, in 1981-1982, several Congressional efforts to permit states to ban abortion were voted down. A bill seeking to rescind Roe v Wade through statute rather than constitutional amendment failed to reach the floor of the U.S. Senate. In 1983, the Supreme Court reaffirmed the Roe v Wade decision in a ruling denying abortion restrictions in three states.

The Reagan administration attempted, by executive order, to block access to abortion services by proposing to withhold federal family planning funds from any clinic which provides information about abortion. In 1988, the Federal courts ruled this proposal unconstitutional.

Abortion Services In The U.S., 1984 and 1985 [33]

In 1984 and 1985, the number of abortions, the abortion rate, and the abortion ratio stayed at approximately the same levels as in the previous three years. Just under 1.6 million abortions were performed annually. About three percent of women of reproductive age obtained an abortion, and about 30 percent of pregnancies were terminated by an abortion.

The geographic distribution of services continued to be very uneven. 82 percent of all U.S. counties lacked an abortion provider in 1985. The long-term trend away from hospital abortions continued. Eighty-seven percent of the abortions in 1985 were done in non-hospital facilities. Although abortion clinics constituted only 15 percent of all providers, they were responsible for 60 percent of the procedures performed in 1985. In 1985, 14 states and the District of Columbia covered the cost of some 187,500 abortions obtained by indigent women.

Women Having Abortions in 1982-1983 [34]

In 1982 and 1983, the majority of abortions in the U.S. were obtained by young women (62 percent), white women (70 percent) and unmarried women (81 percent). Ninety-one percent of all abortions were performed at 12 weeks or earlier after the last menstrual period. The rate of abortion, 29 per 1,000, has remained essentially the same since 1981. Women aged 18-19 continue to have the highest abortion rate of any age group (60 per 1,000). While most abortions are obtained by white women, the nonwhite abortion rate is more than twice that of whites.

Thirty percent of all pregnancies were terminated by abortion in 1983, the same as in 1982 and 1981. The highest abortion ratios are found in unmarried women (63 percent), women 40 and over (51 percent), teenagers (42 percent) and non-whites (40 percent). Teenage nonwhites and whites have about the same abortion ratios.

AIDS IN WOMEN AND CHILDREN [35-37]

AIDS (acquired immunodeficiency syndrome) is increasing in the U.S. in women, from several sources: from exposure to infected bisexual men, from intravenous drug use, from blood transfusion, and as prostitutes. In the U.S., approximately seven percent of adult cases of AIDS are women.

The methods of transmission of AIDS to children include (1) from the infected mother (transplacental, from vaginal secretions, and possibly from breast milk); (2) infected blood products; (3) sexual contact/abuse of the child; (4) intravenous drug use.

The question of admission of children with AIDS to school or to day care has been an emotionally debated issue. Generally, recommendations have included the establishment of criteria for consideration of children for admission; the appraisal of each child by a panel, with individualization of the decision; and educational programs for parents, staff, teachers, and the public. Also an intensive educational program in sex education/family life education in the schools for pupils.

Prevention [38,39]

Prevention of AIDS is the objective of any program directed towards AIDS. The basic ingredients of a prevention program include an active educational program for the public, for parents, teachers and other providers of human services for adults and children. An active family life education/sex education program in the schools is essential. Among approaches to be emphasized include efforts to decrease sexual transmission, transmission among IV drug users, and perinatal transmission from infected mothers. The use of the condom is recommended. Efforts to decrease drug use are essential, as are efforts to modify and decrease the pattern of multiple sexual partners. Avoidance of use of sharing of unsterilized needles is essential. Women known to be infected with AIDS virus should postpone pregnancy. Voluntary screening should be encouraged. Counseling resources should be made available.

Comments on Current Status of AIDS

At this writing (April, 1988), AIDS represents a serious general public health problem in the health care of mothers, children, and families.In the beginning, AIDS represented a serious problem in adolescents and male homosexual adults, as well as in drug abusers and in individuals receiving blood transfusion. It is currently extending to women, including pregnant women, to fetuses, and infants and children. There is already discussion in Scandinavia of possible effects on perinatal and infant mortality.

In a broad sense, AIDS is beginning to have additional impact on current thinking regarding sexual behavior, practices and discussion. For example, it is being recommended that U.S. society conduct itself with fewer and preferably one sexual partner, rather than multiple ones. There is already a much more open discussion of sex, sexual practices, and sex education/family life education in the media, and the Surgeon General has recommended a more active sex education/ family life education program in the schools. The condom is recommended as one measure to prevent the spread of AIDS, in addition to its general contraceptive role.

CHILD ABUSE AND NEGLECT

The federal Child Abuse Prevention and Treatment Act Amendments and Reform Act was enacted in 1978. This legislation provides funds for the National Center on Child Abuse, which has the mandate to receive reports of child abuse and to disseminate information on activities and research on child abuse and neglect. Funds are available for grants to states and to support and monitor research and demonstration projects. A new program on the sexual abuse of children was established; at least three treatment centers for sexually abused children, their parents, and sexual abusers have been established. This legislation also contains funds regarding adoptions to locate children who are potential adoptees and to assist in their placement; to gather and analyze data at national and statewide levels; to conduct educational and training programs; to provide technical assistance; and to conduct a study of unlicensed adoptions.The appropriation for fiscal year 1987 is $26 million.

In 1986, there were 1.9 million reports of child abuse, and at least 1,200 deaths in children from maltreatment.

RECENT EFFORTS TO MONITOR THE HEALTH AND
HEALTH CARE OF MOTHERS, CHILDREN AND FAMILIES

During the last decade, there has been increasing interest in quantifying the field of MCH to a greater degree. Reasons for this are several: (1) planning services and programs must be based upon facts about the needs; (2) with the current shortage of funds for MCH/CC services, it is essential that not only must MCH/CC programs and services be well planned, but also there must be information about their outcome, end results, costs, and benefits; (3) there must be answers to such questions as "Did the program or service accomplish what was intended?" "Did the curtailment of funds or of a program have a deleterious effect on the health status of mothers and children?" An assessment of need must precede planning. Evaluation of both process and outcome must be an integral part of planning, management, and administration of programs and services.

Examples to monitor and evaluate specific services, programs, and events include the following over time: (1) efforts to evaluate the effects of the Children and Youth Projects in the 1960s and 1970s;[40] (2) effort to evaluate an Improved Pregnancy Outcome Project;[41] (3) effort to evaluate the effects of the budgetary reductions of the present national Administration;[42] (4) assessment of need on a statewide basis under the MCH Services Block Grant;[43] (5) development of indicators within the field of maternal and child health;[44] survey of data capability in the eight southeastern states;[45] (6) setting objectives for 1990 is another step.

At the same time, there has also been evidence of beginning steps to prepare MCH personnel to become more capable in these activities, such as incorporating the teaching of methods to assess need and to evaluate outcome in MCH training programs in Schools of Public Health; incorporating content on needs assessment and evaluation in MCH Continuing Education Programs, and providing consultation to State MCH/CC Programs in the establishment of state data systems. Each of these represents a small step in the development of methods to determine needs and to evaluate outcome of program efforts.

HEALTH INSURANCE

The vast majority of the U.S. population have some type of health insurance which covers all or part of the cost of health care. But a large number of people have no such coverage. Between 1979 and 1984, the number of people in the U.S. without health insurance increased to 35.1 million. Of the uncovered, the majority are poor or near-poor, and have limited funds to purchase care. Of these, a large proportion are women of child bearing age and children. In 1984, 17 percent of all women aged 15-44 and 16 percent of all poor women in this age group had no health insurance. One third of all poor and near-poor children have no insurance for all or part of the year.

The reasons for the increase in lack of health insurance coverage is due to an increase in poverty; the recession of the early 1980s, with an increase in unemployment; re-employment in lower paying jobs without health insurance as a benefit; curtailment of health insurance benefits by employers; loss of Medicaid coverage by about one million children, due to reductions in AFDC and Medicaid in 1981; reduction of eligibility for Medicaid by a number of states in 1981 and 1982. Also during the early 1980s, funding was reduced in the MCH Block Grant, and in community health centers.

Beginning Steps To Improve Medicaid Coverage [46]

Beginning in July 1986, steps were taken to improve coverage of poor pregnant women and children under the age of five years.

The Consolidated Omnibus Budget Reconciliation Act of 1986 (COBRA), PL 99-272 included the following:

- Mandates Medicaid coverage of all pregnant women with family incomes and resources below state AFDC financial eligibility levels.

- Mandates an additional 60 days' postpartum coverage for all women whose Medicaid eligibility is based solely on pregnancy, even if they would not otherwise be eligible for Medicaid once their pregnancies end.

- Permits states to provide pregnant women with enriched Medicaid benefits without having to provide these additional benefits to other Medicaid recipients.

- Builds key protections for mothers and children into Medicaid's so called "third party liability" recovery program.

- Clarified states' option to immediately provide Medicaid coverage to all financially needy children under age five without having to phase-in coverage on a year-by-year basis.

- Permits states to provide "case management" services to Medicaid recipients.

- Prohibits any Medicare-funded hospital from refusing to treat or appropriately transfer emergency patients including those in active labor.

In the fall of 1986, Congress approved the Sixth Omnibus Budget ReconciliationAct (SOBRA), PL 99-507. Reforms in this Act include options to states to:

- Provide Medicaid coverage to pregnant women and children under age five years with incomes above the states' AFDC payment levels, but below the federal poverty level. States may also eliminate the use of any resource test in determining eligibility of pregnant women and children under five.

- Establish programs of "presumptive eligibility" whereby women believed to be Medicaid-eligible may be enrolled immediately upon seeking care from certain types of prenatal care providers while their applications are processed.

- Provide continuous coverage of pregnant women under Medicaid through the 60th day following the end of their pregnancies, even if they become ineligible due to increased family income.

PROVISION AND COVERAGE OF MOTHERS, CHILDREN, AND FAMILIES OF HEALTH CARE AND SERVICES

At this writing (1987), the U.S. has not yet set or achieved the goal of providing comprehensive health and social care for women of childbearing age, children, and families. These objectives have been established and are well on the way in Scandinavia. Furthermore, in the U.S., we are much further along in the fields of education (universal free education for all from school entrance through secondary education), special education of handicapped children and youth (from birth to 21 years of age) and the provision of services and coverage to handicapped infants, children, and youth than is the field of MCH, the basic preventive arm of health and social services.

In the field of MCH, we have made progress made by incremental steps, adding a "category" or segment of the population of women, children, and families here and there—a part of a group here this year, and another part of another group there the next year. And so it is in 1988, when the Medicaid Program has just been extended to cover more pregnant women and young children—picking up a little more of the poverty group of pregnant women, and a year by year age level group of young children of poor disadvantaged families. Medicaid is a payment program, and not a program primarily concerned about quality of care, about early case management, and the need for stengthening and support of basic preventive health services. Until we have a "national health service" and "national health insurance" program for women, children, and families, we will continue the present pattern of paying bills and not being able to deliver comprehensive health and social care to women and children, the most vulnerable part of of our population.

REFERENCES

1. The Report of The Select Panel For the Promotion of Child Health. Better Health For Our Children: A National Strategy Volume I. Major Findings & Recommendations. Volume II. Analysis and Recommendations for Selected Federal Programs. Volume III. A Statistical Profile. Volume IV. Background Papers. U.S. Government Printing Office, Washington, D.C. 1981.
2. International Labor Office. Maternity Benefits In The Eighties. 1985. Geneva, Switzerland.

3. Select Committee on Children, Youth, and Families. U.S. Children & Their Families: Current Conditions and Recent Trends, 1987. U.S. House of Representatives, Washington, D.C. March 1982.

4. Blum RW. Health Futures of Adolescents. Report of the National Invitational Conference held in Daytona Beach, Florida. April 2-5, 1986. Available from the University of Minnesota School of Public Health, Minneapolis. 1986.

5. Klerman LV and Stack MR. Problems In The Organization of Health Services for Adolescents. Report of the National Invitational Conference held in Daytona Beach, Florida. April 2-5, 1986.

6. Jellinek P. The Integration of Adolescent Health Services: What Works, What Doesn't, What Next. Report of the National Invitational Conference held in Daytona Beach, Florida. April 2-5, 1986.

7. Blum RW. Continuing Education In Adolescent Health Care: Reaching Professionals in Practice. Report of the National Invitational Conference held in Daytona Beach, Florida. April 2-5, 1986.

8. Jones EF; Forrest JD; Goldman N; Henshaw S; Lincoln R; Rosoff JI; Westoff CF; and Wulff D.

   A. Teenage Pregnancy In Industrialized Countries. Yale University Press. New Haven, Conn. 1986.

   B. Teenage Pregnancy In Developed Countries. Determinants and Policy Implications. Family Planning Perspectives 17:53-63, March/April, 1985.

9. Polit DF and Kahn JR. Early Subsequent Pregnancy Among Economically Disadvantaged Teenage Mothers. American Journal of Public Health 76:171-176, 1986.

10. O'Connell M and Rogers CC. Out-of-Wedlock Births, Premarital Pregnancies and Their Effect on Family Formation & Dissolution. Family Planning Perspectives 16:157-162, 1984.

11. Mott FL and Marsiglio W. Early Childbearing and Completion of High School. Family Planning Perspectives 17:234-237, 1985.

12. Mott FL. The Pace of Repeated Childbearing Among Young American Mothers. Family Planning Perspectives 18:5-12, 1986.

13. Makinson C. The Health Consequences of Teenage Fertility. Family Planning Perspectives 17:132-139, 1985.

14. Moore KA and Wertheimer RI. Teenage Childbearing and Welfare: Preventive and Ameliorative Strategies. Family Planning Perspectives 16:285-289, 1984.

15. The National Swedish Board of Education. Instructions Concerning Interpersonal Relations. 1977. English Translation 1981. Ulbildnings forlaget, / 68 69. Stockholm, Sweden.

16. Muraskin LD. Sex Education Mandates: Are They The Answer? Family Planning Perspectives 18:171-174, 1986.

17. Muraskin LD and Jargowsky PA. Creating and Implementing Family Life Education in New Jersey. National Association of State Boards of Education, Washington, DC, 1985.

18. Kirby D. The Effects of School Sex Education Programs: A Review of The Literature. Family Planning Perspectives 18:162-170, 1986.

19. Dawson DA. The Effects of Sex Education on Adolescent Behavior. Family Planning Perspectives 18:162-170, 1986.

20. Marsiglio W and Mott FL. The Impact of Sex Education on Sexual Activity, Contraceptive Use and Premarital Pregnancy Among American Teenagers. Family Planning Perspectives 18:151-162, 1986.

21. Sonenstein FL and Pittman KJ. The Availability of Sex Education in Large City School Districts. Family Planning Perspectives 16:19-25, 1984.

22. Macdonald DI. An Approach To The Problem of Teenage Pregnancy. Public Health Reports 102:377-385, 1987.

23. Steinman ME. Reaching and Helping the Adolescent Who Becomes Pregnant. The American Journal of Maternal & Child Health Nursing 4:35-37, 1979.

24. Edwards LE; Steinman ME; Arnold KA; and Hakanson EY. Adolescent Pregnancy Prevention Services in High School Clinics. Family Planning Perspectives 12:6-14, 1980.

25. Berg M; Taylor B; Edwards LE; and Hakanson EY. Prenatal Care for Pregnant Adolescents In A Public High School. Journal of School Health 32-39, 1979.

26. Edwards LE; Steinman ME and Hakanson EY. An Experimental Comprehensive High School Clinic. American Journal of Public Health. 67:765-766, 1977.

27. Zabin LS; Hirsch MB; Smith EA; Streett R; and Hardy JB. Evaluation of a Pregnancy Prevention Program for Urban Teenagers. Family Planning Perspectives 18:119-126, 1986.

28. Dryfoos J. School-Based Health Clinics: A New Approach To Preventing Adolescent Pregnancy? Family Planning Perspectives 17:70-75, 1985.

29. Successful Programs to Prevent Pregnancy In Adolescents. Morbidity and Mortality Weekly Report Vol. 29, No. 2, January 18, 1980.

30. Kirby D. School-Based Health Clinics. Center For Population Options, Washington, DC. April 1985.

31. American Academy of Pediatrics. School-Based Health Clinics. AAP Guidelines. Printed in AAP News. April 1987. Page 7.

32. Sander JH and Rosen JL. Teenage Fathers: Working With The Neglected Partner in Adolescent Childbearing. Family Planning Perspectives 19:107-110, 1987.

33. Henshaw SK; Forrest JD: and Van Vort J. Abortion Services In The United States, 1984 and 1983. Family Planning Perspectives 19:63-70, 1987.

34. Henshaw SK. Characteristics of U.S. Women Having Abortions, 1982-1983. Family Planning Perspectives 19:5, 1987.

35. Committee on Infectious Diseases, American Academy of Pediatrics. Health Guidelines for the Attendance in Day Care and Foster Care Settings of Children Infected with Human Immunodeficiency Virus. Pediatrics 79:466-471, 1987.

36. Surgeon General Workshop on Children with HIV Infection and Their Families. April 6-8, 1987. Work Group Recommendations. Pages 51-70.

37. Rutherford GW, et al. Guidelines For The Control of Perinatally Transmitted Human Immunodeficiency Virus Infection and Care of Infected Mothers, Infants and Children. Western Journal of Medicine 147:104-108, 1987.

38. Francis DP and Chin J. The Prevention of Acquired Immunodeficiency Syndrome in the United States. JAMA 257:1357-1366, 1987.

39. Macdonald DI. Coolfont Report: a PHS Plan for Prevention and Control of AIDS and the AIDS Virus. Public Health Reports 101:341-348, 1986.

40. De Geynt W and Sprague LM. Differential Patterns In Comprehensive Health Care Delivery For Children and Youth. American Journal of Public Health 60:1402-1420, 1970.

41. Peoples MD; Grimson RC; and Daughtry GL. Evaluation of the Effects of the North Carolina Improved Pregnancy Outcome Project. American Journal of Public Health 74:549-554, 1984.

42. Wallace HM and Smith JC. Monitoring The Effects of Budgetary Reductions On The Health Status and Health Care of Mothers and Children. Clinical Pediatrics 21:421-423, 1982.

43. Guyer B; Schor L; Messenger KP; Prenney B; and Evans F. Needs Assessment Under The Maternal and Child Health Services Block Grant: Massachusetts. American Journal of Public Health 74:1014-1019, 1984.

44. Miller CA; Fine A; Adams-Taylor S; and Schorr LB. Monitoring Children's Health: Key Indicators. American Public Health Association, Washington, DC 20005. 1986.

45. Peoples-Sheps MD; Siegel E; Guild PA; and Cohen SR. The Management and Use of Data on Maternal and Child Health and Crippled Children: A Survey. Public Health Reports 101:320-329, 1986.

46. Hughes D. Advocacy For Maternal and Child Health. Dated June 14, 1987. Children's Defense Fund, Washington, D.C.

DEVELOPMENT OF MCH SERVICES AND POLICY IN THE UNITED STATES

2

C. Arden Miller

Development of MCH services and policy in the United States is characterized by an uneasy dynamic of competing influences. The first weighs societal responsibility for the wellbeing of infants and children against the presumed rights of parents to provide for, or neglect, their own children. Another dynamic seeks to locate societal responsibility, whatever its extent, in either federal or state government. Changes in prevailing political ideologies have caused each of these dynamics to shift policy uncertainly in one direction or the other to the detriment of strong and stable maternal and child health programs. Local variations in the quality and scope of services are exceedingly great. In aggregate they are less adequate than in other nations of the western world. [1]

Considerations of public policy require attention to one further circumstance. What we as a nation say we do (nominal policy) may differ greatly from our performance (operative policy). No clear synoptic expression of public policy for MCH, (such as pronouncements in statutes, court actions, or in the rhetoric of the nation's leaders), bears up as faithful representation of services that are actually available in support of MCH. An understanding of public policy, therefore, must derive from inferences drawn from careful analysis of how our society actually distributes its goods, services, and influence as they impact on the health of infants, children, youth, women of childbearing years, and families. Insofar as patterns for those distributions can be identified, operational policy can be said to be defined. Those definitions may vary over time, but many of them are exceed-

ingly durable (operational policy) and contradictory of popular public pronouncements (nominal policy).

SCOPE OF SOCIETAL RESPONSIBILITY

Arguments in favor of a societal role for the protection of children are
largely a product of twentieth century social reforms. They are best exemplified
by debate over establishment of the U.S. Children's Bureau. Wald argued as follows in support of establishing the bureau: "...whereas the Federal Government
concerned itself with the conservation of material wealth, mines and forests, hogs
and lobsters, and had long since established bureaus to supply information concerning them, citizens who desired instruction and guidance for the conservation
and protection of the children of the nation had no responsible governmental body
to which to appeal.[2] Wald's emphasis on conservation of children as a national
resource represented a departure from prior policies that regarded children only
as a resource for their own parent's concern. Social reformists of the early twentieth century, like Wald, identified the health and vigor of children as important
for the progress of society. [3]

The reformists' view was bitterly contested out of fear by some leaders that
the Children's Bureau would usurp the role of the family. Senator Heyburn declared, "The jurisdiction established over the children of mankind in the beginning
of the human race has worked out very well. It is in accord with the rules of
nature... The mother needs no admonition to care for the child, nor does the
father." [4]

Senator Heyburn's views did not prevail, but when the Children's Bureau
was established important constraints defined its activities. The Bureau was
charged to "...investigate and report... upon all matters pertaining to the welfare
of children and child life..." [5] No authorization was given for direct sponsorship
of services. That bold governmental role would not be sanctioned until passage
of the Social Security Act in 1935. Debate on the Children's Bureau had clearly
established that no direct responsibility for implementing new services would fall
under authority of the Bureau. The enabling Act further cautioned that ...no official, or agent, or representative of said bureau shall, over the objection of the
head of the family, enter into any house used exclusively as a family residence."[5]

A perspective on child health within recent decades has moved away from
defining its importance as a social good, and toward a formulation which holds
that children have rights independent from either the interests of their parents or
the prospects for improving society at large. [6] Opposition to government action for
protecting rights that are presumed for children is no less intensive in recent years
than in the early part of the century. Restraints on child labor provide a useful
example. A restrictive law was passed by Congress in 1916 and later declared
unconstitutional. Child labor was not successfully constrained until the years of

the Great Depression, when adults needed the jobs that might be held by children. The issue of child labor continues to be re-argued every summer when arguments in favor of de-regulation are raised with relation to migrant workers. Some voices argue the character building benefits of hard work against the hazards of shiftless children having too much unscheduled time on their hands.

Another interesting example of recent tension between the roles of government and family was provided by consideration of the Comprehensive Child Development Act of 1971. Senator Walter Mondale had introduced the legislation in an effort to strengthen and support families by providing them with expanded community services including funding for day care centers. President Nixon vetoed the Act, claiming "... for the federal government to plunge headlong financially into supporting child development would commit the vast moral authority of the National Government to the side of communal approaches to child rearing over against the family-centered approach." [7]

Tension between parental and societal roles for the protection of children is striking when considering issues of child abuse. For many decades the condition of abused children was overlooked, inadequately documented, and not addressed by statute or organized community action. Control of parents over their children was generally regarded as absolute, even at the expense of occasional neglect and abuse. The matter became a legitimate cause for societal action only when Helfer and Kempe[8] defined abuse as a plea of the parent for help. When the victim was defined as the parent rather than the child, societal intervention became acceptable without threat of interfering with parental rights.

Governmental programs for the maternal and child health population were reduced more than any others in the budget reductions after 1981. [9] Getting government off our backs became a prevailing theme of President Reagan's New Federalism. The cause was pursued more vigorously against programs for the MCH population than, for example, against farm subsidies, retirement pensions, or health care for the elderly. President Reagan declared, "There is no question that many well-intentioned great society-type programs (referring to the domestic initiatives of the Johnson administration in the 1960s) contributed to family break-ups, welfare dependency, and a large increase in births out of wedlock."[10] That statement derives from ideologic conviction bearing a controversial relationship to the available data. The statement articulates a policy orientation that has waxed and waned throughout most of the twentieth century.

Federal-State Interactions

Progress toward establishing a societal role for protecting and promoting MCH has not been steady but it has grown substantially. Uneven growth has come from the vacillations over time and among programs concerning the kinds of responsibilities that attach to different levels of government. The scope and quality of MCH services come close to being regarded as matters of state option. Within some states that option is further delegated to local agencies with great unevenness of performance within those states.

Grad's Public Health Law Manual analyzes the constitutional and legal bases for the regulation of public health in ways that contribute to an understanding of the confused dynamic between federal and state authority. He emphasizes that the 50 states are repositories of police power, while the national government, being a government of delegated power, does not possess such power. Grad further identifies police power with a role"...to enact and enforce laws to protect and promote the health, safety, morals, order, peace, comfort, and general welfare of the people.[11] State and local public health agencies derive their power by delegation from state legislatures. That formulation leaves to the national government a narrow domain for action relying heavily on roles that are limited to investigating and reporting *(vide supra)*, demonstrating, financing, and importantly, regulating interstate commerce.

As a device for national action to protect children's health, federal power to regulate interstate commerce has at times provided a more reliable handle than formulations about children's rights. Child labor reforms were initiated by efforts to restrict interstate commerce of products generated by the labor of children. Note that the Congressional committees on health fly under the protection of some banner other than health: in the House it is Energy and Commerce, and in the Senate it is Finance.

Financing represents the strongest federal role for influencing services on behalf of the MCH population. The historical development of the role has been tentative and inconsistent, sometimes putting federal government in direct relationship with health service providers and sometimes taking the form of grants to the states for development of their own programs. The first major MCH grants to the states (Sheppard-Towner, 1921-1929) were optional and many states declined the aid. The Social Security Act of 1935 under Title V established grants to the states with an obligation for them to provide matching funds and to develop a plan for MCH services. Standard setting, monitoring and review of the states' plans by federal agencies has been less than rigorous.

The Social Security Act of 1935 and its subsequent amendments provides to this day the strongest policy formulations forMCH. Burns provides an interesting analysis of the inconsistencies within the act.[12] The strongest force promoting passage of the act was old age security. It was established as a federal program. MCH, within the same act, was clearly a state program with federal financing. That position was modified in 1965 by establishment of the Children and Youth and Maternal and Infant Care Projects under Title V. They were federal programs until 1974, when they were tucked back under state authority.

The important health care financing amendments to the Social Security Act in 1965 illustrate entrenched confusion over federal-state roles. Title 18, Medicare, is essentially a national health insurance program for people over 65 years of age; it is administered under federal authority. Title 19, Medicine, passed by Congress at the same time, establishes partial federal financing for health care to the poor: it is a state administered program with wide variations in state determined eligibilities and benefits.

The potential is enormous for implementing uniform national MCH service entitlements through regulations that attach to federal financing. Title V provides an important mandate and an agency and service structure, but the major financial commitment is through Title 19, Medicaid. So far federal government has been disinclined to attach rigorous performance standards to Medicaid. The 1986 Medicaid revisions, which broke the previous obligatory linkage between Medicaid financing and state determined welfare eligibilities is an important policy development that could lead to greatly expanded benefits for previously underserved MCH populations. Those benefits are enabled by Congressional action, but implementation, as with many MCH services, requires state level initiative.

The provision of adequate supports and services in MCH has been removed from the arenas of partisan negotiation in most western countries. In the U.S., although the political will has been weak to expand society's commitment to the health of women and children, it bears an imperfect historical relationship to political orientation in other matters. For example, Herbert Hoover's Children's Charter stands as one of the nation's most enlightened pronouncements on the protection ofMCH. Hoover's Secretary of the Interior, Ray Lyman Wilbur, said these things when addressing the conference that developed the charter in 1930:

> In a word, parental responsibility is moving outward to include community responsibility. Every child is now our child. We have injected so many artificial conditions into our industrial civilization that the old normal relationships of mother and child, child and family, family and neighborhood have been changed. There is now a much less direct struggle with nature and her immediate forces than has ever been the situation before in our country. We have softened this struggle for man by all forms of protection — better houses, better clothing, more and better food supplies, and better preventive medicine and better medicine and sanitation in general. All of this has called for a delegation of functions, once performed by the individual in the home, to all sorts of outside dependencies. [13]

POLICY INFERENCES

Because public pronouncements about health policy bear so little relationship in actual practice, policy inferences need to be drawn from an analysis of how the ingredients of policy are distributed. Those ingredients are resources, largely money, and power. The following inferences are defensible: As a nation, we allocate resources as if medical care were the major determinant of health, contrary to the weight of epidemiologic evidence. Analysis of children's health suggest that greatest benefits would derive from emphasis on family planning, nutrition, improved housing, environmental protection, accident prevention, and income supplementation for poor families. Such interventions require public supports and regulations that run counter to some social values that are even more powerful than concern for children's health. The operative health policy appears to seek good health by means of medical care, even at great expense, rather than to engage in painful social reforms that would probably be more effective in terms of improved population-based health outcomes.

The political power associated with delivery of medical care has traditionally been entrusted to physician practitioners, and more recently to corporate structures such as hospitals, their suppliers, and insurance companies. MCH services make extensive use of mid-level practitioners. Neither they nor their clients participate appreciably in policy negotiations, requiring the participation of advocates on their behalf. Health services are predominantly distributed in a private economic market, traditionally on a fee for service basis, although corporate prepayments on a capitation basis are growing. They still involve a small proportion of the total population, and an even smaller proportion of poverty level households in which children are concentrated. Distribution of services in the private market is heavily subsidized and protected by government. Services left to public agencies are largely those that are not economically attractive, such as care for chronic illness, handicapping conditions, mental health, and the uninsured. Public agencies are also predominantly responsible for mass screenings and preventive procedures for which the private market has not been able to establish a stable population denominator.

A new emphasis in health policy begins to emerge suggesting that health-related resources and their regulation should be guided by attention to population based health status or outcome measures. The U.S. Department of Health and Human Services' program for Promoting Health, Preventing Diseases: Objectives for the Nation [14] is an example of such an emphasis. Another is Model Standards: A Guide for Community Preventive Health Services. [15] These measures enjoy only a status as guidelines, rather than as governmentally required objectives that might be attached to financing systems.

Many measures of health status suggest that MCH services are inadequate relative to need and that health status trends have become less favorable in recent years. [16] Programs that might correct these circumstances are for the most part well known: they are not costly when measured against overall health expenditures; their cost-effectiveness is well established. The nation's political will has not been strong to adopt corrective measures, but in the late 1980s the public conscience in relation to MCH appears to be stirring.

REFERENCES

1. Miller CA. Maternal Health and Infant Survival. Washington, D.C., National Center for Clinical Infant Programs, 1987.

2 Wald L. The House on Henry Street. Cited in Children and Youth in America, A Documentary History. Vol. II. edited by R.H. Bremner, Cambridge, Harvard Press, 1971, pp 757-758.

3. Takanishi R. Childhood as a social issue: Historical roots of contemporary child advocacy movements. Journal of Social Issues, 1978, 34, 8-28.

4. Heyburn WB. Senate debates on Children's Bureau. Congressional Record, 62 Cong., 2 Sess (1911-12), XLVIII, Pt 1, 189; Cited in Children and Youth in America. Edited by RH Bremner, Cambridge, Harvard Press, 1971, pp 764-765.

5. U.S. Statutes, 62 Cong., 2 Sess (1911-12), Pt. 1, Chap. 73, pp 79-80.

6. Caldwell BM. Balancing children's rights and parents' rights. Care and Education of Young Children in America: Policy, Politics, and Social Science. Norwood, NJ, Ablex, 1980.

7. Nixon R. Veto Message, Economic Opportunity Amendments of 1971. 92nd Congress, 1st Session, Senate Document 92-48, page 5.

8. Helfer RE. and Kempe CH: Child Abuse and Neglect: the Family and the Community. Cambridge, Ballinger, 1976, p 183.

9. Congressional Budget Office. Major Legislation Changes in Human Resources Programs since January, 1981. Washington, Congress of the United States, 1983.

10. Reagan R. 1983 radio broadcast cited by Moynihan DP, Family and Nation, New York, Harcourt Brace Jovanovich, 1986, p 69.

11. Grad FP. Public Health Law Manual. Washington American Public Health Association, 1975. pp 5-6.

12. Burns EM. Some Major Policy Decisions Facing the United States in the Financing and Organization of Health Care. Bull NY Acad Med, 42:1072-1088,1966.

13. Wilbur RL. White House Conference on Child Health and Protection, 1930, Addresses and Abstracts of Committee Reports (New York, 1931) cited in Children and Youth in Americas. Edited by RH Bremner, Cambridge, Harvard Pres, 1971, pp 1077-1080.

14. Department of Health and Human Services, Public Health Service. Promoting Health, Preventing Disease: Objectives for the Nation. DHHS Publication No. 017-001-00435-9. Washington, D.C., U.S. Government Printing Office, 1980.

15. Department of Health and Human Services, Centers for Disease Control. Model Standards: A Guide for Community Preventive Health Services. Second Edition, DHHS ISBN-0-87553-135-0 Government Printing Office, 1985.

16. Miller CA, Fine A, Adams-Taylor S, and Schorr LB. Monitoring Children's Health: Key Indicators. Washington, American Public Health Association, 1985.

THE CHANGING MATERNAL AND CHILD HEALTH POPULATION: DEMOGRAPHIC PARAMETERS* 3

Margaret W. Pratt

DEMOGRAPHIC PARAMETERS

In an earlier edition of this textbook, demographic analysis was referred to as a "numbers game." Major reasons for playing the numbers game are to identify problems or populations-at-risk, to define the dimensions of problems or groups in need of help and to measure the impact of efforts to deal with the problems.

The many efforts to impact problems affecting the MCH population are described elsewhere. This section will assess the most recent available information on the demographic characteristics of the MCH population, as it relates to various health status measures and will comment on trends which the data reflect.

The primary source of data on natality and mortality characteristics is material in Vital Statistics publications issued by the National Center for Health Statistics.

BIRTHS

Table 1 reviews the age distribution of the total U.S. population and the women of childbearing age. The 1980 figures show the "aging" of the baby-boom population after World War II. The current projections for the year 2000 reflect the

---

* There are a large number of tables in this chapter. They are placed at the end of the text in order to facilitate the ease of reading.

somewhat smaller proportions of the population expected in all age groups less than 25-years of age, following the lowered birthrates of the 1970s and early 1980s. Birth rates and fertility rates (Table 2) showed a low in 1975. These have stabilized well below the rates in the 1960s but have increased to a slightly higher level in the period from 1980 to 1986. This same pattern was seen in the white race birth and fertility rates, but is seen only for the Black race birth rate. The Black race fertility rate, after going up slightly from 1975 to 1980, dropped 6.7 percent by 1985 to 82.2.

In terms of births to mothers in the various age-groups (Table 3), a trend for decreases in birth and fertility rates for younger mothers (under 30 years) and increases (after 1975) in mothers 30-39 years is apparent in all race groups. The increase after 1975 is larger for the white race than for the "all other" races. There were slight decreases for birth rates of Black mothers in the older age groups. The birth rate for very young mothers (under 15 years) has remained essentially the same since 1980. The birth rate for mothers 40 years and older has been reduced slightly since 1975.

The median ages of women starting families (Table 4) has increased slightly from 1960 to 1985 with the increase in median age a bit larger for Black mothers than for white mothers. The same trend is seen for median ages of mothers for second-and third-order births. For fourth and higher birth orders, the median age is a bit lower from 1970 to 1985.

The percent distribution of births by birth order and race (Table 5) shows that the significant levels of decrease in proportions of higher birth-order births between 1960 and 1980 had slowed to a very small decrease between 1980 and 1985. The continued reduction was apparent, nevertheless, in all race groups.

Birth rates throughout the world (Table 6) also show most areas continue to reduce their birth rates. Exceptions in recent years are the USSR, Tunisia, Egypt, the Philippines Islands, Poland and West Germany. Even those countries' birth rates, with their slower rates of reduction, are significantly lower in 1983 or 1984 than they were in the 1950s and 1960s.

Estimates from studies by the National Center for Health Statistics indicate that about one-fifth of infants are born to "single" mothers. The Bureau of the Census estimates up to one-fourth of infants and young children (from the under-four year old group) live at or below poverty.

MATERNAL MORTALITY

While the U.S. maternal mortality rate for all race groups continues to be lowered, the differential between the rates for white race mothers, all other races' mothers and Black mothers has increased sharply between 1980 and 1985 (Table 7). The differential between the maternal death rates for white and Black races in 1985 is almost 1:4, favoring white mothers.

A new picture emerged in maternal death rates (Table 8). While age-specific death rates for all mothers and white race mothers were higher as the age of the mother increased, the "all other" races and Black mothers death rates for age groups 30-34 years and 35-39 years were significantly higher than for those mothers in these race groups 40 years and older. The leading causes of maternal deaths in 1985 were ectopic pregnancy (16.7 percent), complications of the puerperium (30.8 percent), hemorrhage of pregnancy and childbirth (13.9percent), toxemia of pregnancy, and spontaneous abortions (11.5 percent each). For the Black race mothers, ectopic pregnancy was the cause for 22.6 percent of the maternal deaths, spontaneous abortions caused 17.2 percent, complications of the puerperium caused 26 percent of the deaths, toxemia and hemorrhage caused 12.3 percent of the maternal deaths each.

INFANT MORTALITY

The Infant Mortality Rate (IMR) is the most often used measure of an area's health status. Simply described, it is the number of infants who died in a given period (usually a calendar year) per 1,000 infants born alive during the same period. It is useful because it is available annually on a uniform and generally comparable basis, is easily understood, and can be related to many characteristics: race, age-at-death, sex, causes of death, and geographic areas. There are also many characteristics of the mother and of the birth which can be related to the death—especially when there are files of matched birth and death records.

The IMR in the U.S. has continued to decline for the entire birth population as well as all race groups. However, the rate of decline has been sharply reduced. The average annual rate of decline for all deaths was only about three percent per year from 1980 to 1986. It is composed of about a 3.1 percent reduction per year (1980-1985) in white infant mortality rates and about a 3.0 percent reduction per year (1980-1985) in black infant mortality rates. The rates for races other-than-white-or-Black have had a slightly better rate of annual decline as the Oriental population, with its very good infant mortality rates in most nationality groups, increases in size.

The unfortunate part of the information on declining infant mortality rates is that the average annual rate of decline for infant mortality rates is essentially the same for white and Black infants. As a result, almost twice the proportion of Black infants per 1,000 Black live births continue to die during the first year of life as white infants.

The infant mortality levels continue to vary significantly among the various geographic areas of the U.S. (Table 9). The South Atlantic Region continues to have the highest proportion of neonatal deaths. The reduction of the IMR in the U.S. from 1980 to 1985 is reflected in all causes of infant death.

The most recent information on IMR for the 15 largest U.S. cities is 1983 (Table 10). Of these cities, only three (San Diego, San Antonio, and San Jose) had rates better than the U.S. 1983 IMR (11.2). San Francisco's rate was only slightly higher (11.3) than that of the U.S. as a whole. These city rates reflect primarily the size of the Black population as well as the Black infant mortality rate for that population. The urban population continues to have the greatest proportion of the U.S. infant mortality problem even though rates may be higher in some rural areas.

In comparison with the infant mortality rates in 20 selected countries, even showing the U.S. 1984 rate versus 1982 and 1983 rates in most other areas, the U.S. has lost relative position since the last edition of this book. It dropped from 12th to 18th on the list of selected countries ordered by their infant mortality rates.

BIRTHWEIGHT

The low birthweight (LBW) ratio is another long accepted measure of pregnancy outcome and health status. LBW has been related both to high mortality and morbidity levels. In the 1980s, persons concerned with MCH became increasingly concerned that various efforts which were reducing infant mortality levels were not reducing the proportions of low birthweight infants very much. The National Academy of Sciences prepared a major study entitled, "Preventing Low Birthweight," which presented the relative risk of a low birthweight infant for various characteristics of the mother and her prenatal care regimen (Table 11). In general, the results are as expected, e.g. young mothers and older mothers are at higher risk of having a low birthweight infant than mothers between 20 and 35 years of age. White mothers in the "at risk" age-groups were at greater risk than black mothers of producing a low weight infant. Unmarried mothers, mothers with lower education levels (probably related also to their age), those with late start or no prenatal care and mothers with a prior fetal loss were at higher risk of giving birth to a low-weight infant than others.

A number of studies now look not only at low birthweight ratios (under 2500 or 2501 grams) but at "very low" birthweight ratios. The survival rate of infants weighing 1500-2500 grams is now such that a very-low birthweight (VLBW) category (under 1500 grams) is now also analyzed (Table 12). The table shows that a number of countries also have lower (better) LBW ratios than the U.S. By the same token, while the U.S. LBW ratio was reduced from 7.9 to 6.8 between 1970 and 1980, virtually no decline occurred between 1980 and 1985. There was also almost no change in the VLBW ratio.

PRENATAL CARE AND HOSPITALIZATION

The picture of prenatal care—both the percent of women starting prenatal care in the first trimester (Table 13) and the percent of those receiving no prenatal care—improved for all categories of mothers (race, age groups and education level) between 1970 and 1980. Between 1980 and 1985, the picture in terms of proportions of mothers with start of care in the first trimester was unchanged for all race groups although there was a somewhat larger proportion of mothers 30 years of age and older initiating care early. Paradoxically, the proportion of mothers reporting no prenatal care increased in 1985 over 1980 for mothers in all race groups and for those mothers under 35 years of age. The proportions of mothers starting prenatal care in the first trimester increases with the education level while the proportion of mothers with no prenatal care is just the opposite. Even by 1985, only about one-third of mothers 15-19 years started prenatal care in the first trimester. In 1985, also, the proportion of mothers in the 20-24 year old age-group starting care in the first trimester is below the national average.

Since 1960, a very high proportion of all births have occurred in hospitals (96.6 percent) (Table 14). At that time, a significantly higher proportion of these were for white mothers (98.8 percent) than for other races mothers (85.0 percent). The same picture was seen in terms of births attended by physicians. By 1980 and again in 1985, almost all births (99 percent) were reported to have occurred in hospitals and almost 97 percent were attended by physicians.

DEATHS TO CHILDREN AND YOUTHS

The mortality levels for children once they are past the first year are significantly improved (Table 15). Instead of ten per 1,000 live births, the numbers are less than one per 1,000 population in the specified age-group. If it were not for accidents, the numbers of deaths and mortality rates would be very small indeed. The various campaigns to reduce accidents in the home and those to provide driving education and prevention of drunk driving have had major impact—reducing the death rate from accidents from 121.6/100,000 population 1-19 years in 1975 to 91.7/100,000 1-19 years in 1983. A notable problem is that for all deaths in the 15-19 year old group, suicides in 1983 were the second leading cause of death, replacing homicides. Homicides were still, in 1983, the leading cause of deaths for Blacks in the 15-19 year old group. The disadvantage of the Black-race children over the white races is seen in the 1-4, 5-9 and 10-14 year age groups. However, the rates for the two groups are about the same for the 15-19 year old group. Almost twice the proportion of white youths die in automobile accidents as Black youths and about twice the proportion of whites commit suicide as Blacks. However, three times the proportion of Black youths die of homicide or legal intervention than whites.

These natality and mortality measures of health status for mothers, infants, and children continue for the most part to show improvement. The problems stem from the fact that the improvement has slowed in a number of areas and certainly the relative position of the Black population compared to the white group has worsened. There appear to be various explanations for the slowing of rates of improvement and these relate initially to reductions in federal, state, and local monies to pay for health care and related services. Increasing levels of concern are also being expressed regarding lack of insurance coverage for prenatal, delivery, and postnatal care for mothers and for primary preventive care services for children in population groups not eligible for care from government programs. This relates both to persons without insurance and to those where the insurance coverage does not pay for these services. Another problem associated with the availability of care relates to the impact of rapidly rising costs of malpractice and liability insurance for physicians and hospitals. Many obstetricians are ceasing their maternity practice and many hospitals are no longer providing obstetrical (delivery) and nursery services. On the other hand, technical advances related to the practice of medicine continue to have a favorable impact on the health status measures.

HANDICAPS, CONGENITAL, OR FROM DISEASES AND INJURIES

The preceding sections have discussed what has been happening as a result of efforts which impact various health status measures related to natality and mortality characteristics of the population. The following materials will describe what health problems must be dealt with when the baby survives.

In recent years, a number of major efforts have sought to define more accurately the numbers and rates of handicapping conditions among children. The concern for having better information on handicapping conditions, as well as acute illnesses, relates to the need for a better basis for determining that they are receiving care and for estimating the need for providers and services, as well as assessing the potential cost benefits of prevention services, rehabilitation services, and services to ameliorate the conditions.

The data for this set of materials are usually from surveys either compiled by the National Center for Health Statistics, the National Centers for Disease Control, or special studies.

ACUTE AND CHRONIC ILLNESSES

One area of concern is the incidence of acute conditions in children with an indication of the proportion of these which are given medical attention. Table 16 indicates that there were about twice as many acute conditions reported in 1986 for the white children (an average of three per child) as were reported for Black children. Younger children (under five years) had more conditions than those over five years of age. There were fewer conditions reported in children in families with lower income levels. This probably is a reflection of problems in the reporting or perception of the seriousness of the problems and is not an indication of the true incidence of acute problems.

The information on prevalence for selected chronic conditions (Table 17) reflects significant increases in the mid-1980s over the period 1970-1971 for all conditions shown. It is not clear whether this is an artifact of changes in the reporting process or if the prevalence of chronic conditions in children is increasing.

Another perspective on the prevalence of chronic diseases in the population 0-20 years is shown in Table 18. In this material, a rate of 10 per 1,000 population under 21 years in 1980 was estimated to have moderate to severe asthma (as opposed to about 40 per 1,000 population under 18 years with any level of asthma), reported in Table 16. Over two percent of the child populations were estimated to have one of 11 categories of serious chronic diseases. As increasing proportions of this population survive to adulthood, new concerns about care needs must be considered in the planning for health care and services for these persons.

DISEASES, INJURIES, AND DISABILITY DAYS

The basic picture of notifiable childhood diseases (Table 19) continues to show the favorable impact of various interventions—immunizations, improved sanitation and more powerful antibiotics. The only problem which seems to be growing in the childhood diseases category is chicken pox ,where the 1984 rate is up about 40 percent over that in 1980.

The status of the sexually transmitted diseases of syphilis and gonorrhea in young people is shown in Table 20. In general, the data reflects a significant reduction in gonorrhea rates and a small reduction in the primary and secondary syphilis rates in 1985 over 1975. In fact, the 1985 rates for syphilis are down from highs in 1982 and 1983. The rates for the population 15-19 years are higher for both diseases than the rates for the total population. Females are reported to be at much higher risk than males for acquiring gonorrhea.

A new area of concern is the number of children and youth with Acquired Immune Deficiency Syndrome (AIDS). Children with the need for blood transfusions (e.g., those with hemophilia) or whose mothers have AIDS are at high risk, as well as those who may have sexual contact with persons with AIDS. The number of children with AIDS has increased from somewhat over 4,000 in 1984 to about 7,000 in January, 1988, according to the National Centers for Disease Control.

Information on newborn infants in short-stay hospitals is shown in Table 21. Sick infants, on average, have twice the average length of stay of well infants and almost 35 percent of discharged newborns have been defined as sick. The average length of stay is much shorter in the west than in other parts of the U.S.

The number of disability days is assessed as a measure of the health of children in Table 22. It is stated in terms of Restricted Activity and Bed Disability for children for children under five years and 5-17 years. For children 5-17, Loss of School Days is also shown. There appears to be no consistent trend in the changes and they may reflect the level of such factors as weather affecting respiratory problems and influenza levels.

Another way of looking at the need for health resources is the use of Special Education resources by the school age population. Table 23 shows the numbers using these resources, 1977-1985. The numbers served have increased about 17 percent. The total cost has increased 250 percent and the average cost per child has increased almost 200 percent. In terms of the distribution of the children with various categories of problems, there has been almost a 100 percent increase in the proportion of these children with learning disabilities, a 25 percent decrease in the proportion of those with reported speech impairment, and a 38 percent decrease in the proportion with reported mental retardation.

There have been improvements in the quality of the survey data and special study data on health status of mothers and children reflected in data from these sources. There are many more sets of information available for those who wish to look into a given area in more detail. There are also new efforts such as those stipulated under PL 99-457 which will provide even better information about children with handicaps and special health care needs. Efforts under PL 99-457 will, it is expected, identify these children and get them into a care system at the earliest possible time.

SUMMARY

This chapter has not repeated the background materials covered in the second edition of this publication. It has, instead, focused on changes in the characteristics and health status measures of the maternal and child population of the U.S. and on the changes in the amount and quality of data available for persons concerned with demography.

The following provides a summary of what has happened to the health status of mothers and children in recent years as reflected in the major data sources of this information:

- Birth rates and fertility rates in the mid-1980s are somewhat higher than the low of the mid-1970s, but are well below the rates in the 1960s when efforts to lower these rates were initiated. Both rates are substantially higher for the Black race than the white race. About one-fourth of infants are estimated to be born to families living in poverty. About one-fifth are born to "single" mothers.

- Mortality rates have continued to decline but the rate of decline has slowed in recent years despite the improvements in medical practice and technical advancements.

  - For deaths to mothers (related to their pregnancy), the most striking problem was the 4:1 disadvantage of Black mothers over white mothers in 1985. Older mothers (40 years and more) have 2-5 times the risk of younger mothers.

- For infants, the disadvantage of mortality rates for Black babies was about 2:1 over white babies, in 1985.

- The infant mortality rate in the U.S. has caused the U.S. to slip to 18th in 1984, from 12th in 1976, when compared to other selected nations.

- The threat of mortality in infants is significantly reduced after the first day of life and especially after the first 28 days of life. Roughly two-thirds of all infants who will die in the first year die by the end of the first month.

- After the first year, the threat of death to children is greatly reduced. About half of deaths to children after the first year of life in all age groups are caused by accidents. The disadvantage of Black children over white children is marked until the 15-19 year old group. At this point the deaths to Black children from homicide and legal intervention balances the deaths to white children from automobile accidents and suicide, so that the overall rates are very close.

• The health status measure defined by the proportion of children born with low birthweight has not been reduced to the same extent as infant mortality rates despite efforts to improve the picture of prenatal care. The risk of a Black low birthweight infant is greater than 2:1 over white infants.

• While the proportion of mothers starting care in the first trimester in 1985 is significantly improved over the picture in 1970, there has been little change since 1980. The proportion of mothers with no prenatal care in 1985 is lower than 1970 but is higher than in 1980, indicating a trend in the wrong direction.

• About one-two percent of all U.S. infants are born with a disabling condition. By age five years, around ten percent are believed to have some level of disabling condition.

• Because of the increasing size (in numbers) of the population at risk and somewhat better procedures for identifying the children with disabling conditions, the need for care to children with special health care needs stemming from these is growing in the U.S.

• Problems related to providing care and services for those with no insurance coverage include significant proportions of mothers and children who are not covered at all or have insurance that does not cover various elements of maternity care or preventive services, as well as the major levels of care required by persons with acute illnesses, chronic illness, or other handicaps.

- There are major problems related to availability of data to assist in detailed and explicit planning to deal with many of the health problems of mothers and children.

The most important insights gained in this update of the chapter prepared for the 1982 edition of this book are:

- Data are essential to effective planning and definition of priorities, goals, and objectives. However, data are of little value if programs are not appropriately defined, funded, and implemented. They can measure limited or no progress in dealing with the problems.
- There is increasing use of studies based on data with many limitations and constraints, from which general conclusions are drawn. This type of material is satisfactory as a start in problem definition. It is not satisfactory as a base for good program planning or measuring the impact of various interventions.

TABLE 1

UNITED STATES POPULATION AND WOMEN OF CHILBEARING AGE. a,b/

Age Group	1900 c/ Women Total	1900 c/ Women 15-44 yr	1950 c/ Women Total	1950 c/ Women 15-44 yr	1980 d/ Women Total	1980 d/ Women 15-44 yr	2000 d,e/ Women Total	2000 d,e/ Women 15-44 yr
Total number f/	76,094	17,795	151,868	34,341	227,255	53,074	267,432	57,542
Percent	100.0	100.0	100.0	100.0	100.0	100.0	100.0	100.0
Under 5	12.1		10.8		7.2		6.6	
5-9	11.7		8.8		7.3		7.0	
10-14	10.6		7.4		8.0		7.3	
15-19	9.9	21.4	7.0	15.4	9.3	19.6	7.0	16.1
20-24	9.7	21.0	7.7	17.1	9.4	20.1	6.3	14.6
25-34	15.9	33.1	15.8	35.6	16.5	35.6	13.3	31.3
35-44	12.2	24.5	14.3	31.8	11.4	24.8	16.2	38.0
45-54	8.5		11.5		10.0		13.9	
55-59	2.9		4.8		5.1		5.0	
60-64	2.4		4.0		4.5		3.9	
65-74	2.9		5.6		6.9		6.6	
75+	1.2		2.6		4.4		6.4	

SOURCES: White House Conference on Children: Profiles of Children. Bureau of the Census Population Division Report P-25, Nos. 704, 929, 952 and 1000. Data computed by ISRI.

a/ Excludes armed forces abroad.
b/ Percent distribution by age group.
c/ Forty-eight States and D.C.
d/ Fifty States and D.C.
e/ Projections.

TABLE 2

UNITED STATES BIRTH RATES AND FERTILITY RATES BY RACE

Year	Birth Rate Per 1,000 Population				Fertility Rate Per 1,000 Women 15-44 yr			
	Total	White	All Other		Total	White	All Other	
			Total	Black			Total	Black
1986 a/	15.5	—	—	—	64.9	—	—	—
1985	15.8	14.8	21.4	21.1	66.2	63.0	83.2	82.2
1984	15.5	14.5	21.2	20.8	65.4	62.2	82.5	81.4
1983	15.5	14.6	21.3	20.9	65.8	62.4	83.2	81.7
1982	15.9	14.9	21.9	21.4	67.3	63.9	85.5	84.1
1981	15.8	14.8	22.0	21.6	67.4	63.9	86.4	85.4
1980	15.9	14.9	22.5	22.1	68.4	64.7	88.6	88.1
1975	14.6	13.6	21.0	20.7	66.0	62.5	87.7	87.9
1970	18.4	17.4	25.1	25.3	87.9	84.1	113.0	115.4
1965	19.4	18.3	27.6	27.7	96.3	91.3	131.9	133.2

SOURCE: Monthly Vital Statistics Report, Advance Report of Final Natality Statistics, 1985, vol. 36, No. 4, Suppl., July 17, 1987, and Monthly Vital Statistics Report, Annual Summary of Births, Marriages, Divorces, and Deaths: United States, 1986, vol. 35, No. 13, August 24, 1987.

a/Provisional data; racial informational is not provided.

TABLE 3
BIRTH RATES a/ BY AGE OF MOTHER AND RACE

Race and Age of Mother	1985	1980	1975	1970
Total	15.8	15.9	14.6	18.4
10-14	1.2	1.1	1.3	1.2
15-17	31.1	32.5	36.1	38.8
18-19	80.8	82.1	85.0	114.7
20-24	108.9	115.1	113.0	167.8
25-29	110.5	112.9	108.2	145.1
30-34	68.5	61.9	52.3	73.3
35-39	23.9	19.8	19.5	31.7
40-44	4.0	3.9	4.6	8.1
45-49	0.2	0.2	0.3	0.5
White	14.8	14.9	13.6	17.4
10-14	0.6	0.6	0.6	0.5
15-17	24.0	25.2	28.0	29.2
18-19	70.1	72.1	74.0	101.5
20-24	102.8	109.5	108.2	163.4
25-29	110.0	112.4	108.1	145.9
30-34	68.1	60.4	51.3	71.9
35-39	22.7	18.5	18.2	30.0
40-44	3.6	3.4	4.2	7.5
45-49	0.2	0.2	0.2	0.4
All Other	21.4	22.5	21.0	25.1
10-14	3.8	3.9	4.7	4.8
15-17	62.9	68.3	80.5	95.2
18-19	128.7	133.2	146.1	195.4
20-24	138.5	145.0	141.0	196.8
25-29	113.5	115.5	108.7	140.1
30-34	70.3	70.8	58.8	82.5
35-39	30.5	27.9	27.6	42.2
40-44	5.9	6.5	7.5	12.6
45-49	0.4	0.4	0.5	0.9
Black	21.1	22.1	20.7	25.3
10-14	4.5	4.3	5.1	5.2
15-17	69.8	73.6	85.6	101.4
18-19	137.1	138.8	152.4	204.9
20-24	140.8	146.3	142.8	202.7
25-29	105.1	109.1	102.2	136.3
30-34	60.7	62.9	53.1	79.6
35-39	25.5	24.5	25.6	41.9
40-44	4.9	5.8	7.5	12.5
45-49	0.3	0.3	0.5	1.0

SOURCE: Monthly Vital Statistics Report, Advance Report of Final Natality Statistics, 1985, vol. 36, No. 4, Suppl., July 17, 1987.

a/ Rates per 1,000 population.

TABLE 4

**MEDIAN AGES a/ OF WOMEN IN UNITED STATES
STARTING FAMILIES AND BEARING SECOND,
THIRD, FOURTH, AND HIGHER-ORDER CHILDREN BY RACE**

Race and Birth Order	1985 b/	1980	1970	1960
Total	25.8	25.7	25.4	25.4
First Child	23.5	23.0	22.1	21.8
Second Child	26.3	26.1	24.7	24.0
Third Child	28.1	28.1	27.5	26.6
Fourth child and over	30.8	31.2 b/	31.4	30.2
White	26.1	25.9	25.6	25.5
First child	23.8	23.3	22.3	22.0
Second child	26.6	26.3	25.0	24.2
Third child	28.4	28.4	27.7	26.9
Fourth child and over	31.2	31.3 b/	31.7	30.6
All Other	25.0	24.6	24.3	24.9
First child	22.2	21.4	20.4	19.9
Second child	25.3	24.7	23.2	22.5
Third child	27.0	26.9	25.2	24.1
Fourth child and over	29.9	30.2 b/	30.3	29.2
Black	24.5	24.2	24.1	24.8
First child	21.4	20.7	20.0	19.6
Second child	23.6	24.2	22.9	22.3
Third child	26.6	26.6	24.8	24.0
Fourth child and over	29.6	30.0 b/	30.1 b/	c/

SOURCE: Vital Statistics of the U.S. 1970, 1980 vol. I, Natality, and Monthly Vital Statistics Report, Advance Report of Final Natality Statistics, 1985, vol. 36, No. 4, Suppl., July 17, 1987.

a/   Median age in years.
b/   Data computed by ISRI.
c/   Information not available for calculation.

TABLE 5

PERCENT DISTRIBUTION OF LIVE BIRTHS
BY LIVE BIRTH ORDER AND RACE

Race and Live Birth Order	1985 a/	1980	1970	1960 a/
Total	100.0	100.0	100.0	100.0
First Child	41.6	43.2	38.8	26.4
Second Child	33.2	32.0	27.5	24.7
Third Child	15.6	15.0	15.5	19.3
Fourth child	5.7	5.6	8.2	12.4
Fifth Child	2.1	2.2	4.3	7.1
Sixth and seventh child	1.3	1.5	3.7	6.5
Eighth child and over	0.4	0.6	2.0	3.7
White	100.0	100.0	100.0	100.0
First Child	42.1	43.9	39.1	27.2
Second Child	34.0	32.5	28.2	25.8
Third Child	15.4	14.7	15.8	20.0
Fourth child	5.3	5.2	8.1	12.4
Fifth Child	1.8	1.9	4.1	6.7
Sixth and seventh child	1.0	1.2	3.2	5.5
Eighth child and over	0.6	0.5	1.5	2.5
All Other	100.0	100.0	100.0	100.0
First Child	39.6	40.0	37.5	21.9
Second Child	30.2	29.6	23.8	19.1
Third Child	16.6	16.3	14.1	15.6
Fourth child	7.5	7.4	8.6	12.1
Fifth Child	3.3	3.3	5.5	9.2
Sixth and seventh child	2.2	2.4	5.9	12.0
Eighth child and over	0.7	1.0	4.7	10.2
Black	100.0	100.0	100.0	100.0
First Child	39.4	39.8	37.4	21.8
Second Child	29.8	29.2	23.5	19.2
Third Child	17.0	16.5	14.0	15.6
Fourth child	7.7	7.6	8.7	12.1
Fifth Child	3.3	3.4	5.5	9.2
Sixth and seventh child	2.1	2.4	6.1	12.0
Eighth child and over	0.7	1.0	4.9	10.2

SOURCE: Vital Statistics of the U.S., 1960, 1970 and 1980, vol. I, Natality and Monthly Vital Statistics Report, Advance Report of Final Natality Statistics, 1985, vol. 36, No. 4, Suppl., July 17, 1987.

a/ Data for 1985 and 1960 were computed by ISRI.

TABLE 6

BIRTH RATES a/ IN SELECTED COUNTRIES

Country	Rate	(Year)	1970-1974	1960-1964	1950-1954
North and South America					
United States	15.7	(1984)	16.2	22.4	24.4
Canada	15.0	(1983)	16.2	25.2	27.7
Cuba	16.6	(1984)	26.5	**	**
Mexico	33.9	(1980-85)	43.4	44.4	44.1
Panama	28.0	(1980-85)	34.9	40.6	37.5
Venezuela	35.2	(1980-85)	37.5	44.2	43.7
Europe					
Austria	11.7	(9184)	13.9	18.5	15.0
Belgium	11.9	(1983)	13.9	17.0	16.7
Czechoslovakia	14.7	(1984)	17.7	16.3	22.0
Denmark	10.1	(1984)	14.6	17.0	17.9
France	13.8	(1984)	16.5	18.0	19.5
Germany (East)	9.5	(1984)	12.1	17.3	18.7
Germany (West)	13.7	(1984)	11.6	18.3	16.1
Italy	10.3	(1984)	16.3	18.9	18.3
Netherlands	12.1	(1984)	16.0	20.9	22.1
Norway	12.1	(1984)	16.0	17.3	18.7
Poland	18.9	(1984)	17.5	20.0	30.1
Spain	13.4	(1982)	19.4	21.6	20.3
Sweden	11.3	(1984)	13.7	14.5	15.5
Switzerland	11.5	(1984)	14.5	18.5	17.3
United Kingdom	12.8	(1983)			
England and Wales	12.7	(1983)	14.7	17.9	15.5
Northern Ireland	17.3	(1983)	19.5	22.9	20.9
Scotland	12.6	(1983)	15.2	19.8	17.9
Yugoslavia	16.4	(1984)	18.1	22.0	28.8
Asia					
China	18.5	(1980-85)	26.9	**	**
India	33.3	(1982)	35.9	**	**
Israel	24.0	(1983)	27.9	25.5	32.5
Japan	12.7	(1983)	19.1	17.2	23.7
Philippines	32.3	(1980-85)	25.5	45.6	50.7
Africa					
Egypt	36.9	(1982)	34.9	**	**
Mauritius	19.7	(1984)	25.1	38.1	46.2
Tunisia	34.1	(1980-85)	35.7	44.2	30.8
Oceania					
Australia	15.5	(1984)	20.0	21.9	23.0
New Zealand	15.8	(1983)	21.3	25.8	25.7
U.S.S.R.	19.6	(1984)	17.7	22.4	26.4

SOURCE: United Nations: <u>Demographic Yearbook</u>, 1984. New York, 1986.

a/   Rates are per 1,000 population. "**" indicates no reported data.

TABLE 7

MATERNAL MORTALITY RATES a/ BY RACE
AND WHITE VERSUS OTHER DIFFERENTIAL

Year	Total	White	All Other Total	Black	Differentials Other Races /White	Black/ White
1985	7.8	5.2	18.1	20.4	3.48	3.92
1980	9.2	6.7	19.8	21.5	2.96	3.21
1970	21.5	14.4	55.9	**	3.88	**
1960	37.1	26.0	97.9	**	3.77	**
1950	83.3	61.1	221.6	**	3.63	**
1940	376.0	319.8	773.5	**	2.42	**
1930-34	636.0	575.4	1080.7	**	1.70	**

SOURCE: Vital Statistics of the U.S., 1980, vol. II, Mortality, Part A, and Monthly Vital Statistics Report, Advance Report of Final Mortality Statistics, 1985, vol. 36, No. 5, Suppl., August 28, 1987.

a/ Rates are per 100,000 live births. '**' indicates data not available.

TABLE 8

1983 MATERNAL DEATH RATES a/
BY AGE OF MOTHER AND RACE

Age Group	Total	White	All Other Other	Black
Under 20 Years	5.4	4.4	7.7	7.0
20-24	7.5	4.9	17.3	20.2
25-29	6.6	5.2	13.6	16.0
30-34	9.1	6.0	25.0	31.1
35-39	20.0	15.6	38.9	44.7
40-44	27.0	29.8	17.3	25.0
45-49	—	—	—	—
All Mothers	8.0	5.9	16.3	18.3

SOURCE: Vital Statistics of the U.S., 1983, vol. II, Mortality, Part A.

a/ Rates per 100,000 live births.

TABLE 9

**UNITED STATES AND REGIONAL INFANT AND
NEONATAL MORTALITY RATES a/ IN 1985**

Area	Infant	Neonatal
United States	10.6	7.0
New England	9.2	6.7
Middle Atlantic	10.8	7.4
East North Central	10.9	7.3
West North Central	9.5	5.9
South Atlantic	12.1	8.2
East South Central	12.1	7.9
West South Central	10.4	6.6
Mountain	9.8	5.7
Pacific	9.7	5.9

SOURCE: Monthly Vital Statistics Report, Advance Report of Final Mortality
Statistics, 1985, vol. 36, No. 5, Suppl., August 28, 1987.

a/   Rates per 100,000 live births.

TABLE 10
INFANT (BY RACE), NEONATAL, POSTNEONATAL, AND FETAL MORTALITY RATES a/ FOR THE FIFTEEN LARGEST U.S. CITIES, 1983

City	Infant Rates			Neonatal Rate	Postneonatal Rate	Fetal Rate
	Total	White	Black			
New York	13.6	11.8	17.3	9.0	4.6	11.3
Los Angeles	12.8	10.8	22.2	9.0	3.8	8.4
Chicago	17.7	11.2	24.9	11.2	6.5	10.0
Houston	13.0	12.0	17.1	8.6	4.4	8.3
Philadelphia	17.0	12.6	21.9	10.8	6.2	14.1
Detroit	19.8	11.4	23.1	14.2	5.6	6.7
Dallas	12.4	10.6	16.5	7.5	4.9	6.7
San Diego	10.4	9.8	20.2	6.9	3.5	8.5
Phoenix	13.7	12.6	25.7	8.5	5.2	7.1
San Antonio	10.7	10.7	10.6	6.2	4.5	6.9
Baltimore	17.5	11.1	20.9	11.6	5.9	13.0
San Francisco	11.3	13.2	17.7	7.7	3.6	7.2
Indianapolis	14.9	12.4	22.0	9.7	5.2	7.5
San Jose	10.1	10.3	13.0	5.4	4.7	6.3
Memphis	17.5	9.4	23.1	12.1	5.4	8.9

SOURCE: Health Planner's Handbook, ISRI, 1987.

a/ Rates per 1,000 live births.

TABLE 11

RELATIVE RISK OF LOW BIRTHWEIGHT (LBW) BY MATERNAL AGE, MARITAL STATUS, EDUCATION, START OF PRENATAL CARE, PREVIOUS PREGNANCY OUTCOME AND RACE

| | Relative Risk a/ | | | | | | | | Percent of Total Live Births (1981) | |
| | White | | | | Black | | | | | |
Characteristic	1971	1976	1981	1985 b/	1971	1976	1981	1985 b/	White	Black
LBW c/	6.6	6.1	5.7	5.6	13.4	13.0	12.5	12.4		
Maternal Age										
Under 15	1.95	1.91	1.84	1.86	1.43	1.31	1.33	1.19	0.1	0.9
15-19	1.26	1.32	1.36	1.36	1.13	1.17	1.12	1.07	12.7	24.4
15-17	—	—	1.54	1.48	—	—	1.17	1.12	4.2	10.5
18-19	—	—	1.27	1.29	—	—	1.09	1.04	8.6	13.9
20-24	0.93	0.98	1.02	1.02	0.96	0.97	1.00	0.97	33.3	35.4
25-29	0.91	0.86	0.88	0.89	0.88	0.87	0.91	0.96	32.5	23.7
30-34	0.98	0.94	0.88	0.92	0.89	0.89	0.90	1.00	4.0	3.4
35-39	1.20	1.14	1.10	1.07	1.02	1.01	0.99	1.02	4.0	3.4
40 or older	1.56	1.37	1.31	1.31	0.97	1.01	1.07	1.10	0.6	0.7
Marital Status										
Married	—	0.97	0.92	—	—	0.87	0.81	—	88.4	44.1
Unmarried	—	1.60	1.57	—	—	1.14	1.15	—	11.6	56.0

(Continued on next page)

Maternal Educational Attainment (years)

Q-8	1.35	1.39	1.46	—	1.08	1.14	1.17	—	3.7	4.7
9-11	1.32	1.35	1.47	—	1.10	1.12	1.18	—	15.8	30.1
12	0.94	0.96	—	0.92	0.92	0.95	—	44.0	41.5	—
13-15	0.80	0.82	0.81	—	0.81	0.85	0.83	—	18.9	15.5
16 or more	0.74	0.73	0.74	—	0.74	0.72	0.71	—	16.2	6.5

Start of Prenatal Care (month)

1st and 2nd	0.92	0.90	0.89	—	0.93	0.91	0.92	—	55.0	38.6
3rd	0.95	0.95	—	0.93	0.97	0.94	—	24.4	23.9	—
4th-6th	1.12	1.15	1.16	—	0.96	1.00	1.01	—	16.3	28.5
7th-9th	1.08	1.10	1.12	—	0.86	0.93	0.94	—	3.2	6.2
No care	2.75	2.69	2.88	—	2.13	2.22	2.21	—	1.1	2.87
7th or later or no care	1.42	1.48	1.56	—	1.24	1.31	1.35	—	4.3	9.1
4th or later or no care	1.17	1.20	1.23	—	1.04	1.06	1.09	—	20.6	37.6

Outcome of Prior Pregnancy

Live birth	0.95	0.94	0.92	—	0.95	0.94	0.95	—	75.6	72.6
Fetal death	1.31	1.32	1.21	—	1.32	1.28	1.11	—	17.8	17.0

SOURCE: National Academy Press: Preventing Low Birthweight, Washington, D.C., 1985; Vital Statistics of the U.S., vol. I, Natality; and Monthly Vital Statistics Report, Advance Report of Final Natality Statistics, 1985, vol. 36, No. 4, Suppl., July 17, 1987.

a/ Relative risk is the ratio of the low birthweight rate for each category to the overall low birthweight rate for the same specific race and year.
b/ Calculated by ISRI. '—' not available.
c/ Per 100 live births.

TABLE 12

PERCENTAGE OF VERY LOW BIRTHWEIGHT
AND LOW BIRTHWEIGHT LIVE BIRTHS IN SELECTED COUNTRIES,
AND IN SELECTED YEARS FOR THE UNITED STATES BY RACE

Country (Year)	Very Low Birthweight 1,500 grams or less	Low Birthweight 2,500 grams or less
Japan (1980)	0.4	5.2
Switzerland (1980)	0.5	5.1
Norway (1980)	0.6	3.3
New Zealand (1980)	0.7	5.3
Germany (East) (1980)	0.7	5.5
Denmark (1980)	0.7	6.0
Austria (1980)	0.8	5.7
Canada (1979)	0.8	6.1
Italy (1980)	0.8	6.1
Israel (1980)	1.0	7.2
United States		
1970 Total	1.1	7.9
White	0.9	6.8
All Other	2.2	13.3
Black	2.4	13.9
1975 Total	1.1	7.4
White	0.9	6.3
All Other	2.2	12.2
Black	2.4	13.1
1980 a/ Total	1.1	6.8
White	0.9	5.7
All Other	2.2	11.5
Black	2.4	12.5
1985 a/ Total	1.2	6.8
White	1.0	5.6
All Other	2.3	11.1
Black	2.7	12.4

SOURCE: United Nations: Demographic Yearbook, 1981. New York, 1983; Vital Statistics of the U.S., 1971, 1976, 1981, vol. I, Natality; and Monthly Vital Statistics Report, Advance Report of Final Natality Statistics, 1985, vol. 36, No. 4, Suppl, July 17, 1987.

a/ The definitions for very low birthweight and low birthweight live births are slightly different from the previous years; the very low birthweight births are those under 1,500 grams (excluding 1,500 grams) and low birthweight are those under 2,500 grams (excluding 2,500 grams).

TABLE 13

PERCENT a/ OF LIVE BIRTHS WITH PRENATAL CARE STARTED IN FIRST TRIMESTER AND NO CARE BY RACE, AGE AND EDUCATION OF MOTHER

Characteristic	1985 b/ Care in 1st trimester	No care	1980 Care in 1st trimester	No care	1970 c/ Care in 1st trimester	No care
Total	76.2	1.7	76.3	1.3	67.9	1.8
White	79.4	1.3	79.3	1.0	72.6	1.2
All Other	**	**	63.8	2.6	46.0	4.2
Black	61.8	3.4	62.7	2.7	44.1	4.5
Age in years						
Under 15	46.0	6.3	34.5	5.5	29.4	6.5
15-19	53.9	3.4	56.3	2.6	50.9	2.9
20-24	71.1	2.0	74.9	1.4	69.8	1.5
25-29	83.1	1.1	84.0	0.8	76.0	1.1
30-34	85.5	1.0	84.4	0.8	71.7	1.4
35-39	82.4	1.3	77.7	1.4	65.9	2.1
40 and over	72.9	2.5	66.5	2.5	59.2	2.6
Education in years						
0-8	**	**	54.4	3.9	45.2	4.5
9-11	**	**	59.7	2.7	53.4	2.7
12	**	**	78.9	0.9	72.4	0.9
13-15	**	**	85.1	0.5	78.1	0.5
16 or more	**	**	91.2	0.2	84.6	0.2

SOURCE: Vital Statistics of the U.S., 1970 and 1980, vol. I, Natality and Monthly Vital Statistics Report, Advance Report of Final Natality Statistics, 1985, vol. 36, No. 4, Suppl., July 17, 1987..

a/   '**' indicates no reported data.
b/   Computed by ISRI.
c/   Based on the sample of births in 39 reporting states and D.C.

TABLE 14

HOSPITAL BIRTHS AND BIRTHS ATTENDED BY PHYSICIANS AS A PERCENT OF ALL BIRTHS BY RACE

Characteristic	1985	1980	1960	1950	1940
Births in Hospital	99.0	99.0	96.6	88.0	55.8
White	98.9	99.0	98.8	92.8	59.9
All Other	99.3	99.2	85.0	57.9	26.7
Black	99.4	99.3	a	a	a
Births attended by physician	96.7	97.4	97.8	95.1	90.8
White	96.9	97.6	99.5	98.7	96.4
All Other	96.0	96.6	88.5	72.2	50.8
Black	96.2	96.9	a	a	a

SOURCE: Vital Statistics of the U.S., 1980, vol. I, Natality and Monthly Vital Statistics Report, Advance Report of Final Natality Statistics, 1985, vol. 36, No. 4, Suppl., July 17, 1987..

a/   No reported data.

TABLE 15

**RATES FOR LEADING CAUSES OF DEATH IN CHILDREN
AND YOUTHS BY 5-YEAR AGE GROUP AND RACE, 1983**

Age Group (Years)	Cause of Death	Death Rate a/		All Other	
		Total	White	Total	Black
1-4	All causes	55.9	50.8	78.5	85.3
	Accidents	21.8	20.2	28.9	31.8
	Congenital malformations	6.5	6.4	7.2	7.6
	Cancer	4.7	4.9	3.9	3.9
	Heart diseases	2.5	2.1	4.1	5.1
	Influenza and pneumonia	1.7	1.4	2.7	2.9
5-9	All causes	26.5	24.9	33.5	35.2
	Accidents	12.4	11.3	17.2	17.9
	Cancer	4.1	4.2	3.6	3.9
	Congenital malformations	1.5	1.5	1.8	2.0
	Heart diseases	1.0	0.9	1.4	1.4
	Influenza and pneumonia	0.3	0.3	0.4	0.4
10-14	All causes	27.2	26.1	31.9	33.9
	Accidents	13.0	12.9	13.4	14.3
	Cancer	3.6	3.6	3.8	3.9
	Congenital malformations	1.3	1.2	1.4	1.6
	Heart diseases	1.0	0.9	1.4	1.4
	Influenza and pneumonia	0.3	0.3	0.4	0.4
15-19	All causes	81.6	82.3	78.7	80.3
	Accidents	44.5	48.7	25.1	23.8
	Suicide	8.7	9.4	5.4	4.1
	Homicide & legal intervention	8.5	5.3	23.7	26.6
	Cancer	5.0	5.2	3.9	3.6
	Heart diseases	1.0	0.9	1.4	1.4

SOURCE: Vital Statistics of the U.S., 1983, vol. II, Mortality, Part A.

a/ Rate per 100,000 of specified population.

TABLE 16

INCIDENCE OF SELECTED ACUTE CONDITIONS PER 100 PERSONS PER YEAR
IN THE POPULATION CATEGORY AND PERCENT MEDICALLY ATTENDED FOR CHILDREN
UNDER 18 YEARS OF AGE, BY SELECTED DEMOGRAPHIC CHARACTERISTICS: UNITED STATES, 1986

Characteristic	Acute Conditions							
	All Acute Conditions		Infective/Parasitic Diseases		Respiratory Conditions		Injuries	
	Number	Percent Attended	Number	Percent Attended	Number	Percent Attended	Number	Percent Attended
Race								
White	313.5	58.4	49.4	65.3	161.6	41.1	33.8	93.9
Black	166.2	56.4	21.0	45.7*	93.2	45.9	21.0	88.7
Age-Sex								
Under 5 Years	360.4	74.5	55.5	74.5	177.9	61.2	23.4	93.5
Male	370.1	76.6	55.0	75.6	183.8	63.8	29.1	100.0
Female	350.2	72.1	56.1	73.4	171.8	58.2	17.5	82.2*
5-17 Years	260.0	49.1	39.9	57.4	139.5	32.0	34.5	93.5
Male	232.7	52.7	35.3	62.6	125.1	36.3	38.9	90.8
Female	288.7	46.0	44.6	53.0	154.4	28.2	29.9	97.3
Family Income								
Less than 10,000	227.1	63.0	25.8	65.8	111.9	48.9	26.6	90.5
10,000-19,999	263.8	53.1	42.4	57.9	148.5	38.7	23.4	82.5
20,000-34,999	322.7	57.3	60.0	60.9	169.1	42.2	32.1	98.5
35,000 and over	320.2	60.4	46.7	71.1	159.7	36.5	39.3	94.5

SOURCE: National Center for Health Statistics: Current Estimates from the National Health Interview Survey, United States, 1986. Vital and Health Statistics, Set 10, No. 164.

*   Estimates for which the numerator has a relative standard error of more than 30 percent.

TABLE 17

PREVALENCE OF SELECTED CHRONIC CONDITIONS REPORTED IN HEALTH INTERVIEWS FOR PERSONS UNDER 18 IN SELECTED YEARS: UNITED STATES

Year	Asthma	Chronic Bronchitis	Heart Conditions	Hearing Impairments	Vision Impairments
			Rate per 1,000 Persons		
1986	51.1	63.2	21.7	20.1	12.2
1985	47.8	55.5	21.2	19.2	10.8
1984	42.5	49.5	23.4	24.0	9.0
1983	45.2	59.3	19.4	18.8	10.3
1982	40.1	33.7	17.2	19.7	13.1
1979-1981 a/	37.9	37.5	19.6	16.7	9.6
1970-1972 a/	31.1	38.9	10.5	13.0	9.4

SOURCE: National Center for Health Statistics: Selected Reports from the Health Interview Survey. Vital and Health Statistics, Set 10, Nos. 84, 94, 99, 150, 154, 155, 156, and 164.

a/   Number per 1,000 persons under 17 years.

TABLE 18

ESTIMATED PREVALENCE FOR ELEVEN CHILDHOOD CHRONIC DISEASES, AGES 0-20, UNITED STATES, 1980

Disease	Estimated Proportion 1980 Prevalence Estimate per 1,000	Surviving to Age 20* (percent)**
Asthma (moderate and severe)	10.00	98
Congenital heart disease	7.00	65
Diabetes mellitus	1.80	95
Cleft lip/palate	1.50	92
Spina bifida	.40	50
Sickle cell anemia	.28	90
Cystic fibrosis	.20	60
Hemophilia	.15	90
Acute lymphocytic leukemia	.11	40
Chronic renal failure	.08	25
Muscular distrophy	.06	25
Estimated total (assuming no overlap)	21.58	

SOURCE: Gortmaker and Sappenfield, Pediatric Clinics of North America, 1984, 31:3-18.

*   Estimates are from population prevalence data or are defined from estimates of incidence (or prevalence at birth) and survival data.

**   Estimate refers to the survival expected of a birth cohort to age 20 given current treatments.

TABLE 19

REPORTED CASES AND RATES a OF SELECTED NOTIFIABLE DISEASES IN THE UNITED STATES

Disease	1984 Number	1984 Rate	1980 Number	1980 Rate	1970 Number	1970 Rate	1960 Number	1960 Rate
Diptheria	1	0.00	3	0.00	435	0.21	918	0.51
Poliomyelitis	8	0.00	9	0.00	33	0.02	3,190	1.77
Pertussis	2,276	1.10	1,730	0.76	4,249	2.08	14,809	8.23
Measles	2,587	1.10	13,506	5.96	47,351	23.23	441,703	245.42
Mumps	3,021	1.32	8,576	3.86	104,953	55.55	b	b
Chicken pox	221,983	138.44	190,894	96.69	b	b	b	b

SOURCE: Center for Disease Control: Final 1984 Reports of Notifiable Diseases, Morbidity and Mortality Weekly Report 34(54). Public Health Service, Atlanta, GA, December 1985.

a/   Rates are per 100,000 population; for rates greater than 0 but less than 0.005 are shown as 0.00.
b/   No reported data.

TABLE 20

MORBIDITY AND RATES FOR GONORRHEA AND SYPHILIS PER 100,000 POPULATION BY AGE-GROUP AND SEX, 1975 AND 1985

Disease	1985 Total	1985 Male	1985 Female	1975 Total	1975 Male	1975 Female
Gonorrhea						
All ages	384.3	457.5	315.8	467.7	574.9	367.6
0-9 years	6.5	3.6	9.5	8.2	4.5	12.1
10-14 years	47.7	23.8	72.9	46.7	20.9	73.6
15-19 years	1,189.9	930.5	1,445.1	1,275.1	1,103.9	1,446.4
Primary and Secondary Syphilis						
All ages	11.5	16.6	6.7	12.0	17.8	6.5
0-9 years	0.1	0.0	0.1	0.1	0.6	0.1
10-14 years	0.9	0.5	1.4	1.1	0.7	1.5
15-19 years	17.0	16.3	17.7	17.8	18.0	17.5

SOURCE: Center for Disease Control, Sexually Transmitted Diseases Statistics, 1985, Issue No. 135.

TABLE 21

NUMBER, PERCENT DISTRIBUTION AND AVERAGE
LENGTH OF STAY OF NEWBORN INFANTS
DISCHARGED FROM SHORT-STAY HOSPITALS BY
SELECTED CHARACTERISTICS, AND THE NUMBER OF
ALL-LISTED DIAGNOSES FOR SICK NEWBORN INFANTS
BY SELECTED DIAGNOSTIC CATEGORIES
AND SEX: UNITED STATES, 1985

Characteristic	Number of Discharges a/	Percent Distribution	Average Length of Stay in Days
All newborn	3,794	100.0	3.8
Well newborn	2,475	65.2	2.8
Sick newborn	1,319	34.8	5.9
Male	1,953	51.5	3.8
Female	1,841	48.5	3.8
Region			
Northeast	665	17.5	4.3
Midwest	909	24.0	4.2
South	1,364	35.9	3.9
West	856	22.6	2.9

Sick Newborn Diagnostic Category	Male Number of Discharges a/	Male Percent	Female Number of Discharges a/	Female Percent
All diagnoses b/	1,228	55.5	988	44.6
Congenital anomalies	102	58.9	72	41.6
Prematurity	112	54.1	95	45.9
Respiratory distress and other conditions	145	58.5	103	41.5
Hemolytic disease and other perinatal jaundice	321	55.2	261	44.8

SOURCE: National Center for Health Statistics: Utilization of Short-Stay Hospital, United States, 1985 Annual Summary. Vital and Health Statistics, Ser. 13, No. 91.

a/ Number in thousands.
b/ Includes data for diagnostic conditions not shown in table.

TABLE 22

SCHOOL-AGE POPULATION A/ USING SPECIAL EDUCATION RESOURCES, TOTAL APPROPRIATED FEDERAL FUNDS AND AVERAGE PER CAPITA EXPENDITURE, AND PERCENT DISTRIBUTION BY TYPE OF PROBLEM: UNITED STATES, 1977 TO 1985

Item	1985	1984	1983	1982	1981	1980	1979	1978	1977
Total Number (1,000)	4,315	4,298	4,255	4,198	4,142	4,005	3,889	3,751	3,692
Total Federal Funds ($1,000)	1,314,315	1,241,725	1,189,374	1,101,294	1,055,815	1,044,500	953,948	700,450	377,770
Per Capita Expenditure (in dollars) b/	304.6	288.9	279.5	262.3	254.9	260.8	245.3	186.7	102.3
Percent Distribution	100.0	100.0	100.0	100.0	100.0	100.0	100.0	100.0	100.0
Learning disability	42.4	42.0	40.9	38.6	35.3	31.9	29.1	25.7	21.5
Speech impairment	26.1	26.2	26.6	27.0	28.2	29.6	31.2	32.6	35.3
Mental retardation	16.1	16.9	17.8	18.7	20.0	21.7	23.2	24.9	26.0
Emotional disturbance	8.6	8.4	8.3	8.1	8.4	8.2	7.7	7.7	7.6
Hard of hearing and deaf	1.6	1.7	1.7	1.8	1.9	2.0	2.2	2.3	2.4
Multihandicaps	1.6	1.5	1.5	1.7	1.6	1.5	1.3	c	c
Other health impairments	1.6	1.2	1.2	1.9	2.4	2.6	2.7	3.6	3.8
Orthopedical handicap	1.3	1.3	1.3	1.4	1.4	1.6	1.8	2.3	2.3
Visual handicap	0.7	0.7	0.7	0.7	0.8	0.8	0.8	0.9	1.0
Deaf-blind	0.1	0.1	0.1	0.1	0.1	0.1	0.1	c	c

SOURCE: U.S. Department of Commerce, Bureau of the Census: Statistical Abstract of the U.S., 1987, 107th Edition.

a/ For persons 3 to 21 years of age.
b/ Obtained from dividing Total Federal Funds with Total Number of Population served.
c/ Not available.

TABLE 23

NUMBER OF DISABILITY DAYS PER PERSON PER YEAR FOR PERSONS UNDER 5 YEARS OF AGE AND FOR PERSONS AGES 5-17 YEARS, BY SELECTED DEMOGRAPHIC CHARACTERISTICS: UNITED STATES, 1986 AND 1983

Demographic Characteristic	Days per person under 5 years of age				Days per person ages 5-17 years					
	Restricted Activity		Bed Disability		Restricted Activity		Bed Disability		School Loss Days	
	1986	1983	1986	1983	1986	1983	1986	1983	1986	1983
Total	10.8	10.9	4.9	5.5	9.5	9.1	4.5	4.1	5.0	5.0
Sex										
Male	11.6	11.4	5.3	5.9	8.4	8.8	3.7	3.7	4.3	4.7
Female	10.1	10.4	4.5	5.0	10.5	9.4	5.3	4.5	5.8	5.4
Race										
White	11.1	11.8	4.9	5.7	10.0	9.5	4.7	4.4	5.3	5.2
Black	9.3	7.1	5.1	4.6	6.9	7.4	3.4	3.0	4.0	4.4
Family Income										
Under $10,000	10.5	14.2	5.7	8.3	10.5	11.1	4.3	4.9	5.8	6.3
10,000-19,999	11.9	9.4	6.0	4.9	8.3	8.6	4.4	3.8	4.5	4.9
20,000-34,999	12.0	10.3	4.9	4.4	10.5	8.6	4.5	3.8	5.1	4.6
35,000 or more	10.9	11.7	5.0	4.8	9.6	9.3	4.7	4.3	5.2	4.8

SOURCE: National Center for Health Statistics: Current Estimates from the National Health Interview Survey, United States, 1983 and 1986. Vital and Health Statistics, Ser. 10, Nos. 154 and 164.

RECOMMENDED READINGS

Publications of the Bureau of the Census based on the 1980 census and series P-25, No. 704,on population estimates, P-60 Series, City and County Data Book. U.S. Department of Commerce, Bureau of the Census.

Natality Volumes, Mortality Volumes (Pt. A), Vital and Health Statistics (monthly reports on vital statistics), and Studies from Health Interview Surveys and Health Examination Statistics. U.S. Department of Health and Human Services, Public Health Service, National Center for Health Statistics.

The Health Planner Handbook. Information Sciences Research Institute, Vienna, VA.

Congenital Malformations Surveillance Report (monthly) and Reported Morbidity, Annual Summary, other Surveillance Reports, U.S. Public Health Service, Centers for Disease Control.

Demographic Yearbook, 1984 and 1981, United Nations.

Preventing Low Birthweight, 1985, National Academy Press.

Infants Can't Wait—The Numbers, 1986, The National Center for Clinical Infant Programs, Washington, D.C.

Health: United States, Annual Report from the U.S. Department of Health and Human Services, Each Year.

Publications of the Children's Defense Fund, Washington, D.C.

THE CHANGING MATERNAL AND CHILD HEALTH POPULATION: SOCIOLOGICAL PARAMETERS

4

Ruth Sidel

In order to plan appropriately and effectively for MCH services, it is necessary to understand some of the key characteristics of the population to be served. It is particularly important to understand the social and economic forces that shape people's lives—and indeed often shape their health status as well. This chapter will attempt to describe some of these forces from a sociological perspective and will focus on those families in U.S. society who are the most deprived economically.

The vast majority of poor people in the U.S. today are women and children. According to the Census Bureau, in 1986, 13.6 percent of all American — 32.4 million people — lived below the poverty line. For female-headed households in 1986, the poverty rate was 34.6 percent, a rate nearly six times that for married-couple families. The poverty rate for white female-headed families was 28.2 percent, for Black female-headed families, 50.1 percent, and for Hispanic families headed by women, 51.2 percent. [1] Two out of every three poor adults are women.

The impact of women's poverty on the economic status of children is even more shocking. According to the Center on Budget and Policy Priorities, the number of poor families with children rose 35 percent since 1979 and one-third of that increase was due to a decline in the effectiveness of government anti-poverty programs. [2] Among children under 18, one out of five officially lived in poverty in 1986; 22 percent of all children under six-years old lived in poverty. For white children under six, the rate was 17.7 percent, among Black children 45.6 percent, and among Hispanic children 40.7 percent. [3]

What are the factors responsible for this "feminization of poverty?" In an era in which so many gains have been made by so many women, in a country as rich as the U.S., why do millions of women and their children live without adequate resources for food, clothing, and shelter? Before discussing these issues, let us first examine how poverty and the number of people living in poverty are officially determined.

In 1963, Mollie Orshansky and her colleagues at the Social Security Administration set the "official" poverty line by using, according to Michael Harrington, a "minimal diet—just sufficient to hold body and soul together—as the base."[4] Since U.S. Department of Agriculture studies in 1955 indicated that the average American family spent approximately one-third of its net income on food, Orshansky took a low-cost food budget prepared by the USDA, multiplied it by three, and came up with a "poverty line" for a family of four. And thus, the first U.S. poverty line was established in 1964 at $3,000.

Between 1965 and 1974, the cost of the USDA Economy Food Plan was used in determining the poverty line; since 1974, a new Thrifty Food Plan has been the standard. It is important to note, as one observer has stated, "The USDA does not consider the Thrifty Food Plan to be nutritionally adequate for long-term use, a fact that is simply ignored in setting the poverty line."[5] Today, the U.S. government poverty line still equals the cost of a Thrifty Food Plan for a family of four, multiplied by three, with adjustments for family size and for changes in the consumer price index. In 1986, the poverty line for a family of four was set at $11,203.

If we look closely at what the poverty line means for a family of four, we see that families at this level are barely surviving. If a family of four indeed spends one-third of its income on food, a family living at the 1986 poverty level of $11,203 would have $3,734 per year for food and $7,469 for everything else. This would mean that family members would have $71.00 a week, at $2.52 per-person per-day to spend on food. The remainder, $622.41 a month, would have to cover rent, utilities, transportation cost—including automobile maintenance—clothing, medical and dental bills, education expenses, entertainment, and taxes. As one analyst has stated, "In the real world, individuals who live at or below the poverty line live poorly, and they do so absolutely; they have considerable and persistent difficulty getting enough to eat, finding adequate shelter (with heat and light), securing appropriate clothing, and obtaining medical care."[5] Moreover, most poor families live well below the threshold of poverty. If an employed adult is paid the minimum wage of $3.35 an hour, he or she will only earn $6,969 a year, far below the poverty line.

But beyond the statistics, what is the meaning of poverty in an affluent society? What does it mean to be poor in a country as rich as the U.S.? When we think of poverty in poor countries, we think of emaciated or swollen-bellied children starving to death in Ethiopia, people dying by the side of the road in pre-revolutionary China, and large families huddling together in the squatters' settlements that exist in most Latin American cities.

But what are the images of poverty in America? Being poor in the U.S. means standing in line for food in soup kitchens; it means living in welfare hotels; it means a homeless woman sleeping in a doorway, her possessions all around her; it means people with no heat in the winter. These images are stark and real. This is absolute poverty. Absolute poverty means living below the official poverty line; absolute poverty is not having money for adequate food, clothing, and shelter. But relative poverty, particularly in an affluent society, is much more difficult to define. Is not having a telephone in this society relative poverty? Is not having a car in rural Vermont relative poverty? Are parents who are just getting by but know that their children are not getting their share of the American dream—are not getting adequate medical and dental care, are attending inferior schools, have no money for the extras that mean so much to children, particularly in a consumer society—living in relative poverty?

The feminization of poverty, or the pauperization of women, has been caused over the past 15 years by a convergence of several social and economic factors: the weakening of the traditional nuclear family; the rapid growth of female-headed families; the continuing existence of a dual-labor market that actively discriminates against female workers; a welfare system that seeks to maintain its recipients well below the poverty line; the time-consuming yet unpaid domestic responsibilities of women, particularly child care; and an administration in Washington that has, over the past seven years, systematically dismantled or reduced funds for programs that serve those who are most in need. Broader social, political and economic aspects of life in the U.S. in the waning days of the twentieth century, such as unemployment and under-employment; continuing discrimination on the basis of race, class, and age; and the changing nature of the economy also contribute to the increasing impoverishment of women and children.

One of the most significant social phenomena of the 1970s and 1980s has been the proliferation of female-headed families. Between 1970 and 1984, the number of families maintained by women mushroomed from 5.5 million in 1970 to 9.9 million in 1984, an increase of 80 percent. In 1984 single-parent families, 89 percent of which were headed by women, accounted for 26 percent of all families with children under 18.[6]

One of the reasons the number of female-headed families has grown so dramatically in recent years is that the divorce rate has soared. Nearly one out of every two marriages in the U.S. now ends in divorce, and the figures are even higher for teenage marriages. The impact of family disruption on the well-being of children is clear. Children who live in families that are disrupted by divorce or separation experience, according to one observer, "severe drops in economic well-being..."[7]

Furthermore, having and keeping a child outside of marriage has become far more acceptable during this period. During the 1970s, families headed by never-married mothers climbed to 3.4 million, an increase of 356 percent. [8]   In 1983, almost 70 percent of families headed by never-married mothers were poor. [9] Among female-headed families, those most likely to be living in poverty are those who began their child-bearing as teenagers and, as is well known, births to teenagers have risen explosively since the post-World War II period.

As significant as the increase in female-headed families is for the population at large, the implications for Black families are that much greater. While white female-headed families, with no spouse present and with children under the age of 18 increased from 8.9 percent of all white families with children under 18 in 1970 to 17.3 percent in 1984, Black female-headed families in the same circumstance increased from 33 percent to 55.9 percent. Over 50 percent of all Black families with children under 18 are headed by women. [6]

Similarly, the divorce rate for Blacks has soared in recent years. Between 1970 and 1981, the divorce rate for Hispanic women rose 80 percent, the white female divorce rate doubled, and the Black female divorce rate nearly tripled. The number of separated and divorced Black women, combined with the number of never-married Black mothers, substantially increases the risk of Black women and children living in poverty. Black children are three times more likely to live in poverty than white children, and black children living in female-headed families are far more likely to do so. In fact, in the early 1980s, 74.2 percent of all Black children under the age of six living in female-headed families lived below the poverty line.[10]

The wellbeing of children is affected by a variety of other factors. Millions of children in the U.S. have special needs that are, all too often, not being met. Homelessness, for example, has become a family issue. In New York City alone, on one day in November, 1987, 17,626 children and their parents were housed in shelters and hotels. [11] According to the Children's Defense Fund, a "typical" homeless family nationally is composed of a single-female head of household with more than one child, although over the past year or two there has been a noticeable increase in the number of two-parent families. [12] The brutality of life in some of the temporary shelters and hotels has been well-documented: constant violence, filth, drugs, hunger, and, above all, the knowledge that one is the ultimate outsider in an affluent society. [13] Moreover, many of the homeless children are not being educated. Schools are reluctant to accept them since they will be there only temporarily, and classes to educate them in the hotels are rare and, when they exist, are woefully inadequate.

The drop-out rate of young people is yet another serious problem afflicting individual students, their families, and the nation. According to a statement by the Research and Policy Committee of the Committee for Economic Development,[14]

"In 1987, nearly 1 million young people will leave the nation's public schools without graduating. Most of them will be deficient in basic skills, marginally literate, and virtually unemployable." The statement goes on to point out that "each year's class of dropouts will cost the nation more than $240 billion in lost earnings and forgone taxes over their lifetimes. This does not include the billions more for crime control and for welfare, health care, and other social services that this group will cost the nation."

Earlier in the age spectrum, families suffer with unmet day care and after-school care needs. During the past decade, mothers of young children have entered the work force in record numbers. In March 1984, 52 percent of women with children under six were working and almost 50 percent of women with children under three were in the labor force. [12] These families' massive needs for child care are being shockingly neglected. Due to federal cut-backs, many states which have the primary responsibility for establishing public child care programs spent less in 1984 than they did in 1981. It has been estimated, consequently, that seven million children ages 13 and under may be spending part of each day without adult supervision. [15]

A myriad of other problems face children and their families: the plight of children in foster care; the inadequate conditions and treatment facilities for juveniles in detention; the hopelessness of abused and neglected young people; and the several problems of drug and alcohol abuse.

These issues must be addressed if our children are to thrive. The U.S. is one of the few industrialized countries in the world without a family policy. Perhaps it is time to take stock of the special needs of families—particularly of women and children—and to develop a humane, comprehensive family policy for all Americans.

REFERENCES

1. US Bureau of the Census: Current Population Reports, Series P-60, No 157, *Money Income and Poverty Status of Families and Persons in the United States: 1986 (Advance Data from the March 1987 Current Population Survey)*, p 23, US Government Printing Office, Washington, DC, 1987.

2. "Poor Families With Children Rose 35% Since 1979, Analysis Finds," *The New York Times*, September 8, 1987.

3. Robert Pear. "Poverty Rate Dips as the Median Family Income Rises," *The New York Times*, July 31, 1987.

4. Michael Harrington, "The New Gradgrinds," *Dissent* ,31: 171-181, 1984

5. Leonard Beeghley. "Illusion and Reality in the Measurement of Poverty," *Social Problems* 31: 322-333, 1984.

6. US Bureau of the Census: Current Population Reports, Series P-20, No 398, *Household and Family Characteristics: March 1984*, US Government Printing Office, Washington, DC, 1983.

7. Greg J Duncan. *Years of Poverty, Years of Plenty: The Changing Economic Fortunes of American Works and Families.* Institute for Social Research, The University of Michigan, Ann Arbor, Michigan, 1984.

8. *A Growing Crisis: Disadvantaged Women and Their Children.* United States Commission on Civil Rights, Clearinghouse Publication 78, Washington, DC, 1983.

9. *Children in Poverty*: Prepared for the use of the Committee on Ways and Means by the Congressional Research Service and the Congressional Budget Office, US Government Printing Office, Washington, DC, 1985.

10. *A Dream Deferred: The Economic Status of Black Americans.* The Center for the Study of Social Policy, Washington, DC, 1983.

11. Josh Barbanel. "New York Shifts Debate on Homeless Problem," *The New York Times*, Nov 23, 1987.

12. *A Children's Defense Budget: An Analysis of the President's FY 1986 Budget and Children.* Children's Defense Fund, Washington, DC, 1985.

13. Jonathan Kozol. *Rachel and Her Children: Homeless Families in America* Crown, New York, 1988.

14. *Children in Need: Investment Strategies For The Educationally Disadvantaged*, A Statement by the Research and Policy Committee of the Committee for Economic Development. New York, 1987.

15. *A Children's Defense Budget: An Analysis of the President's FY 1984 Budget and Children.* Children's Defense Fund, Washington, DC, 1983.

PART I: ORGANIZATION AND PROVISION OF MAJOR PUBLIC PROGRAMS FOR MOTHERS, INFANTS, CHILDREN, AND YOUTH AND THEIR FAMILIES

5

Helen M. Wallace

It is essential that health workers in the maternal and child health (MCH) and crippled children (CC) field have a good working knowledge of both the organization of health services and the legislative base from which MCH and CC services stem. This knowledge makes it possible for MCH and CC health personnel to keep up to date on current thinking, planning, and trends; to know the place in an agency where consultation and advice are available; and to know where to apply for financial support. It is essential for local health workers to know the planning and demonstration projects currently under way because of the possibility that they may be able to adapt the programs to their own geographic locale. Furthermore, health workers in MCH and CC should play a significant role in proposing new legislation and in suggesting amendments of already existing legislation, regulations, and policies.

MATERNAL AND CHILD HEALTH

The organization of health services for mothers and children affects the planning, administration, and evaluation of the delivery of health care addressed to them. The administrative principle is that there be one official unit responsible for the health care of mothers and children at the national, regional, and state level, and in large cities and counties at the local level. The ministry of health in many countries has one unit for maternal and child health/family planning. In the U.S., there is currently major fragmentation of administrative responsibility for the health care of mothers and children among a number of units and agencies. For example, apart from the MCH unit, there are separate units for family planning, developmental disabilities, adolescent pregnancy, and operation of the special Medicaid program for children and youth (early and periodic screening, diagnosis and treatment). The U.S. Department of Education has some responsibilities for school health programs, including handicapped children and youth.

FUNCTIONS OF CENTRAL MCH ADMINISTRATIVE UNIT AT NATIONAL LEVEL[1]

The central MCH unit at national level is one of the primary advocates for the health care of mothers and children. It serves as the focal point for integrating and promoting information, policy, planning, and administration of health problems, needs, and services for mothers and children. It coordinates and guides related units in the national government, including those concerned with vital statistics, environmental health, education, mental health, and welfare. It collaborates closely with professional, educational, and community leaders and groups, as well as with voluntary agencies and programs.

The central MCH unit at national level is responsible for promoting and conducting studies related to MCH health problems, services, and needs by means of special surveys and the collection and analysis of reports, records, and other data. It is also responsible for stimulating, developing, financing, and coordinating MCH research projects and for making the results of research promptly available to MCH and other workers in the country.

Another important function of the central MCH unit is to seek and secure support for MCH service programs. It recommends and plays a vital role in national legislation relative to MCH. It prepares annual budgets and allocates grant-in-aid funds for regional, state, and local MCH services.

One of its responsibilities is to plan the development and extension of MCH activities and services throughout the country. It gives attention to the adequate distribution of services and to general coverage of mothers and children in the population, both urban and rural. It formulates plans for early case finding of high-risk mothers, infants, children, and youth, including the promotion of screening activities to identify special problem groups so that they can be provided with necessary services. It also establishes standards and performance norms, usually with the assistance of professional organization and advisory groups. It is responsible for the national planning for development and expansion of genetic services.

The central MCH unit is responsible for planning the program for health personnel, for formulating the training, for funding financial support to train personnel, and for planning the employment of personnel throughout the country to staff clinical and community health services for mothers and children. This is usually carried out with the advice and assistance of key university faculty members and professional organizations and societies.

The MCH unit is responsible for the development and use of mass media and other health educational materials in order to inform the general public about major health problems and needs in the health care of mothers and children and to inform parents, children, and youth about accepted practices of health care.

The central MCH unit at the national level should be responsible for special programs such as family planning, school health, adolescent health, and handicapped children and youth. It should also be responsible for the health care of children and youth in settings such as day-care and preschool programs, foster homes, residential facilities for children and youth, including the handicapped, juvenile detention facilities, and courts for adolescents.

ORGANIZATION OF SERVICES WITHIN THE U.S. FEDERAL GOVERNMENT

The executive branch of the U.S. government contains several departments responsible for major health programs. The U.S. State Department contains the Agency for International Development, which provides technical assistance and funds to developing countries, primarily in the fields of health (including nutrition, family planning, environmental health, MCH), education, agriculture, and economic development. The U.S. Department of Agriculture is responsible for the national school breakfast and lunch programs, food stamp programs, and Women, Infants, and Children (WIC) programs. The U.S. Department of Defense operates the program of providing medical and health care to armed service personnel and their dependents. In addition, the Veterans Administration operates its own system of health and hospital care. The U.S. Commerce Department contains the U.S. Bureau of the Census, which is responsible for the decennial census. The U.S. Department of Education operates many services related to the health care of children and youth.

The U.S. Department of Health and Human Services (HHS) is described below. It has four major units:

1. The Office of Human Development Services

    A. Administration For Children, Youth and Families
       Head Start
       Child Abuse and Neglect

    B. Administration for Public Services

    C. Administration for Native Americans

    D. Administration on Aging

    E. Rehabilitation Services Administration

Vocational Rehabilitation
Developmental Disabilities

2. Health Care Financing Administration
   A. Medicare (Title XVIII)
   B. Medicaid (Title XIX)
   C. Health Standards and Quality Bureau

3. Social Security Administration
   A. Social Security
   B. Aid to Families with Needy Children

4. Public Health Service
   A. Centers for Disease Control, Atlanta
   B. Food and Drug Administration
   C. Health Resources and Services
   D. National Institutes of Health
   E. Alcohol, Drug Abuse, and Mental Health Administration

Within the ten regional offices located in Boston, New York, Philadelphia, Atlanta, Chicago, Kansas City, Dallas, Denver, San Francisco, and Seattle, the U.S. Public Health Service is responsible for the health components that provide technical assistance and administrative functions to the states in each region.

CENTERS FOR DISEASE CONTROL, ATLANTA (CDC)

The CDC in Atlanta is responsible for monitoring communicable diseases in the U.S., for monitoring the abortion situation, for evaluating some family planning, for monitoring congenital malformations, for monitoring immunization status, AIDS, and other surveillance activities. It also has programs for venereal disease, lead screening, rat control, and laboratory standards.

THE NATIONAL INSTITUTES OF HEALTH (NIH)

The NIH is the primary research branch of the U.S. Government for the conduct and support of basic research in the health field. It encompasses institutes for child health and human development; cancer; heart, lung and blood; arthritis, and musculoskeletal and skin diseases; dental research; neurological and communicative disorders and stroke; allergy and infectious diseases; eye; environmental health sciences; aging, diabetes, digestive and kidney diseases.

ALCOHOL, DRUG ABUSE AND
MENTAL HEALTH ADMINISTRATION (ADAMHA)

The ADAMHA is responsible for services, training, and research in the fields of alcohol, drug abuse, and mental health.

HEALTH RESOURCES AND SERVICES ADMINISTRATION (HRSA)

HRSA includes the Office of International Health, the Indian Health Service, and the Bureau of Maternal and Child Health and Health Delivery.

ORGANIZATION OF SERVICES AT STATE LEVEL

Each state has a health department that contains the state unit on maternal and child health. The state MCH unit usually has a medical director, usually either a pediatrician or an obstetrician, and an interdisciplinary staff consisting of nurses, social workers, and nutrition consultants. The MCH units in larger states may have subdivisions, such as on perinatal care.

State MCH and CC units are responsible for administering federal funds from the Maternal and Child Health Block Grant.

Each state has a state department of welfare and/or social services, responsible for child welfare services-adoptions, foster home placement, institutions, and sometimes day care. The state welfare department is responsible for the administration of funds from Titles XX and IV of the Social Security Act.

Each state has a unit on developmental disabilities. This unit may be a separate department of state government or it may be located in the state department of health, mental retardation, mental health, vocational rehabilitation. This unit is responsible for administering funds from the federal developmental disabilities legislation.

Each state has a state department of education that is responsible for the administration of funds from the Elementary and Secondary Education Act. This Act provides state funds for programs for school health; health education; family life education, education regarding drugs, alcohol, smoking; mental health; teenage pregnancy. The state department of education also administers the federal school lunch program, the Education of the Handicapped Act (PL 94-142 and PL 99-457). Each state has an official unit responsible for administration of the federal Vocational Rehabilitation Act. This unit may be a separate department or may be located in another state agency, such as the State Department of Education. Each state has an official unit responsible for the administration of the Title XIX Medicaid program. This unit is most frequently located in the State Welfare Department.

FUNCTIONS OF THE STATE MATERNAL AND CHILD HEALTH AGENCY

Each state and territory of the U.S. has an official health department and within it a separate unit of maternal and child health. In many states, the MCH unit and the CC unit are combined under one state director of MCH and CC. Most state MCH units are also responsible for family planing. Most state MCH directors are either pediatricians or obstetricians. In addition, the state MCH staff usually includes consultants in nursing, nutrition, and social work. In some states, the state MCH unit may include dental health and the WIC program. Larger states may have MCH subdivisions for school health, maternal health, family planning, and crippled children.

A composite picture of the functions of state MCH units is as follows. Each state MCH unit serves as the advocate and focal point for health needs and health care of mothers, children, and youth in the state. It provides information and visible evidence about the needs of mothers, children, and youth to the public, the state legislature, the official state administrative agencies, and voluntary agencies in the state. The unit is also responsible for determining unmet needs in the health care of mothers, children, and youth in the state and for using such information for planning purposes. It proposes new legislation or suggests modifications in existing legislation in the state. The MCH unit is responsible for the promotion and development of standards for the health and medical services and for the health care of mothers, children, and youth in the state. The services include maternity and perinatal services, family planning services, abortion services, regional perinatal care, genetics services, child health services, pediatric services, day care institutions, foster homes, adoptions, neighborhood health centers. It promotes or conducts studies to evaluate services for mothers, children, and youth and participates in the promotion, planning, and conduct of maternal, perinatal, infant, and childhood mortality and morbidity studies.

The state MCH unit receives and administers federal funds allocated for state MCH services by the MCH Block Grant and matching state and local funds. It develops special services for high-risk mothers, infant, children, and youth, including methods of early identification of high-risk patients and provision of special services for them. It promotes the development of regional perinatal care, regional genetics diagnosis, counseling, and treatment services. The unit promotes the development of special laboratory services, for example, for Rh, inborn errors of metabolism, and genetics. It also provides advice and consultation to local communities to develop local MCH services. The state MCH unit promotes statewide immunization programs. It promotes and supervises family planning programs and is responsible for standards for abortion services, including licensure and supervision. It is responsible for the promotion of adolescent health services, including services to prevent and care for pregnancy in teenagers. It is responsible for promoting the development of prevention of child abuse and neglect and for the development of services for instances of abuse and neglect. It is responsible for developing and consulting with school health services in the state, usually with the State Department of Education. In some states, MCH administers school health services. It is responsible for improving the nutritional status of mothers, children and youth in the state.

The state MCH unit coordinates efforts and services with other state agencies such as education, welfare, mental health, agriculture, and with professional societies and voluntary agencies. It plays a role in education of the health professions, usually with professional schools or universities.

FUNCTIONS OF A LOCAL MATERNAL AND CHILD HEALTH UNIT

Some local health departments in the larger cities and counties in the U.S. have extensive programs providing a spectrum of direct services to large numbers of mothers and children. The MCH staff in a local health department may vary from none at all, to a one-person staff, to a highly developed staff in a very large local department. In the very large departments, there will usually be MCH subdivisions, such as maternal health and family planning, child health, school health, handicapped children.

The MCH functions in a local health department vary considerably, from a program largely consisting of public health nursing home visits and well child conferences to very highly developed local programs and services. A composite picture is as follows:

> The local MCH unit serves as advocate and speaker for improvement of health care of mothers and children in the local community. It is responsible for delivering some local, direct services to mothers and children, either alone or in partnership with hospitals, medical schools, voluntary agencies, or community groups. It works with such groups as neighborhood health centers, maternity and infant care projects, children and youth projects, well child conferences, prenatal clinics, family planning, diagnostic and treatment services for handicapped children and youth, day care, school health programs, adolescent health services, regional perinatal centers, care of children in foster homes and institutions, care of youth in detention centers, services for pregnant teenagers. The local MCH unit is responsible for setting and raising standards for maternity and newborn care, family planning, abortion counseling and services, hospital care of children, day care, foster homes, institutions, and services for handicapped children and youth.

> It works closely with related units of local government and with voluntary agencies, including education, welfare, housing, vocational rehabilitation, agencies for handicapped children, Head Start, and community health centers. It works with professional societies and with citizen and consumer groups. It conducts programs to educate the public and parents and participates in professional education.

PURPOSES OF FEDERAL GRANTS-IN-AID

The principle of U.S. federal or national grants-in-aid to the states (or to smaller political subdivision) is one used by many countries. The purposes are (1) to assist the states in developing services according to national needs and priorities, (2) to stimulate and assist the states; (3) to help the poorer states improve their services; (4) to upgrade the quality of personnel by use of the merit system, which in turn requires the establishment of qualifications of personnel. Federal grants-in-aid have had a long history in the U.S., beginning with land grants to the states in the 1800s to establish state colleges.

THE SOCIAL SECURITY ACT

Following the 1929 termination of the federal Sheppard-Towner Act (1921-1929), and because of the Great Depression, the president established the Committee on the Costs of Medical Care. This committee's activities resulted in the enactment of the Social Security Act in 1935. This Act has been amended a number of times, and currently it is one of the major pieces of federal legislation concerned with health, employment, and disability. It consists of the following sections or titles:

I	Grants to States for Old-Age Assistance and Medical Asstance for the Aged*
II	Federal Old-Age, Survivors, and Disability Insurance Benefits
III	Grants to States for Unemployment Compensation Administration
IV	Grants to States for Aid and Services to Needy Families with Children and for Child Welfare Services
V	Maternal and Child Health and Crippled Children's Services
VI	Repealed effective October 1, 1975*
VII	Administration
VIII	Taxes with Respect to Employment (Superseded by Chapter 21 of the Internal Revenue Code of 1954*
IX	Miscellaneous Provisions Relating to Employment Security
X	Grants to States for Aid to the Blind*
XI	General Provisions and Professional Standards Review
XII	Advances to State Unemployment Funds
XIII	Reconversion Unemployment Benefits for Seamen (the provisions of this title have expired)*
XIV	Grants to States for Aid to the Permanently and Totally Disabled*
XV	Repealed
XVI	Grants to States for Aid to the Aged, Blind, or Disabled, or for Such Aid and Medical Assistance for the Aged*
XVI	Supplemental Security Income for the Aged, Blind, and Disabled
XVII	Grants for Planning Comprehensive Action to Combat Mental Retardation
XVIII	Health Insurance for the Aged and Disabled
XIX	Grants to States for Medical Assistance Programs
XX	Grants to States for Services

---

* Repealed

Among the various titles, Titles IV, XI, XVII, XIX, and XX, in addition to Title V, affect the health and welfare of mothers and children.

TITLE V—MCH AND CC SERVICES

Title V is the major piece of federal legislation by which federal funds are allotted to the states for health services for mothers and children, including the support of research projects and training of personnel.

The total federal MCH appropriation for fiscal year 1987 is $478 million, equally divided into Funds A and B. Fund A, which is matched by the states, provides $70,000 to each state, plus an amount dependent upon the number of live births in the individual state—a rural birth counts twice as much as an urban birth. Fund B, which is unmatched, provides an amount to each state dependent upon the state's financial need. One-quarter of Fund B is used by the federal Bureau of Maternal and Child Health for special grants of regional or national significance.

The federal MCH appropriation for training of personnel consists of grants to universities for training of personnel for the health care of mothers and children. It includes support of programs of continuing education.

The federal MCH appropriation for research in MCH and CC consists of grants to public or other nonprofit universities, to MCH or CC agencies, or to public or nonprofit private agencies for studies, largely for program-operational studies.

THE MCH SERVICES BLOCK GRANT

In 1981, the federal Omnibus Budget Reconciliation Act consolidated 80 separate "categorical" programs into nine broader-based block grants, covering health and social services, education, community services and development, and energy assistance. These new block grants shifted much of the control and accountability from the federal to state governments. In general, more authority is given to the states, and the block grants entail fewer federal requirements. One objective of the block grants was to focus program responsibility and management accountability with the states. Block grants were expected to improve service delivery by promoting better integration of related federal and state programs. Some of the purposes of block grants were to promote management improvement and save fund.[2] A serious result of the new block grant mechanism is that there is less opportunity for federal oversight of state programs; for federal consultation to the states; for federal review of MCH/CC state plans; and for federal steps at standard setting and raising in the states.

MCH Services Block Grant

The new MCH Services Block Grant combined ten programs:

Crippled Children's Services

Maternal and Child Health Research
Maternal and Child Health Services
Maternal and Child Health Training
Childhood Lead Based Paint Poisoning Prevention
Sudden Infant Death Syndrome Information and Counseling
Comprehensive Hemophilia Diagnostic and Treatment Centers
Genetic Disease Testing and Counseling Services
Adolescent Pregnancy Prevention Services
Supplemental Security Income—Crippled Children Portion

Federal funding for the support of MCH services, training, and research has been as follows:

FY	AMOUNT	FY	AMOUNT
1980	$497 M	1984	$399 M
1981	331 M	1985	478 M
1982	373 M	1986	478 M
1983	373 M	1987	478 M

The new MCH Block Grant, as seen above, was accompanied by a substantial reduction in federal funds (approximately 30 percent) in a period of one fiscal year. There is little doubt that these two simultaneous events, conversion of funding for separate programs into a block and a significant reduction of funds, resulted in considerable negative reactions; this is particularly so, because of the constriction of MCH/CC programs and services and probably also because these steps occurred in a climate less favorable to human services at the national level.

Early Effects of MCH Block Grant Reported

A survey of the states conducted in the summer of 1982 indicated a number of early effects of the new MCH Services Block Grant. In the field of *maternal* health, these included reduction of screening and treatment of high risk patients, prenatal care, family planning, pregnancy testing, dental care, nutrition counseling, and amniocentesis. States also reported a decrease in the number of maternity patients served in these areas.

In the *child health* field, there was reported a similar loss of comparable preventive services—well child conferences, immunizations, nutrition services, safety and accident prevention, genetic services, dental care. The number of infants and children served decreased. There were similar decreases for children of school age and adolescents.

Services for handicapped children, with decreased federal funds, included case finding, diagnosis, treatment, rehabilitation, counseling, genetics and coordination.

**Review of the Experience with the MCH
Block Grant in Thirteen States by the General Accounting Office**[3]

A review by the General Accounting Office in 13 states (California, Colorado, Florida, Iowa, Kentucky, Massachusetts, Michigan, Mississippi, New York, Pennsylvania, Texas, Vermont, and Washington) concluded that the MCH Block gave more responsibility to the states. State programs became broader. The opinions of the states were that the administration was more flexible and desirable. However, the opinions of the special interests groups were that they liked the categorical approach more. As federal funds decreased, some states were able to assume more state responsibility, but others were not able to. These were decreases in MCH special projects, SIDS and lead activities. Some states moved to monitor the use of funds in their states more.

FAMILY PLANNING

Since 1970, the year of enactment of the Family Planning Services and Population Research Act, family planning education and services have developed considerably in the U.S. In 1983, 76 percent of the 3,135 counties in the U.S. were serviced by family planning services. Non-metropolitan counties are more likely to be without family planning clinics than metropolitan counties; there were 417,000 low-income women and 249,000 teenagers at risk of unintended pregnancy living in counties without family planning clinics. In 1983, a total of approximately five million women were served; health departments served two million; Planned Parenthood served 1.4 million; hospitals 0.5 million; the other million were served by other agencies and clinics. Of the five million women served, 1.6 million were under 20 years of age. The oral method was used by 68 percent of the women served; the IUD was used by five percent. [4]

In 1983, federal and state governments spent $340 million to provide contraceptive services. Title 10 of the Public Health Service Act accounted for $117 million (34 percent of all public expenditures). Title 19 of the Social Security Act expended $108 million (32 percent). Two block grant programs—Social Services and Maternal and Child Health—provided $38 million and $19 million, respectively. [5]

Under the present national administration, federal funding for family planning services was reduced beginning in 1981, principally in funding from Title 10 of the Public Health Service Act. This budgetary reduction has meant that some family planning clinics (six percent) were closed; patients were charged fees. There was an increased use of nurse practitioners, fewer physician hours spent in the clinic, and consolidation of individual clinics and agencies into larger ones.[6]

In addition to reduced federal funding for family planning services, there have been other intermittent federal actions to establish other constraints. One was the prohibition of use of federal funds for abortion counseling, referral, and services. Another was an effort to require teenagers under 18 years of age to secure written permission from the teenager's family, prior to receiving family planning services (This was declared unconstitutional).

In 1987, the Adolescent Family Life Act of 1981 was found unconstitutional.[7] The law had obliged applicants for funding to involve religious organizations in their activities and had encouraged religious organizations to become grantees. It had also permitted funding only to organizations that neither provided abortions nor referred clients to abortion facilities.

THE FIELD OF GENETICS AND ITS APPLICATION TO MCH

Extension of the field of genetics and its application began to receive support during the 1960s and considerable progress has been made. The field of genetics—genetic screening, diagnostic services, counseling, follow-up and case management—represents one of the specific measures of prevention in public health. Its role in the prevention of certain congenital malformations, inborn errors of metabolism, hemoglobinopathies, and mental retardation is specific.

The Sickle Cell Anemia Control Act of 1972 was the first federal legislation dealing with genetic disease. In addition to the mandate for increased research and treatment, the law provided for the establishment of voluntary sickle cell anemia screening and counseling programs, and for the development and dissemination of information and educational materials for health care providers. By 1975, there were 26 screening, testing and counseling clinics operating in 20 states.

The National Genetic Disease Act was enacted in 1976, and in 1978 provided funds for the establishment and operation of voluntary genetic testing and counseling programs, for the development of information and educational materials relating to genetic disease, and the dissemination of information and materials to health care providers, teachers and the general public. By 1978, genetic counseling programs had been established in virtually all major university medical centers in the U.S. In 1978, the first statewide genetic disease programs were funded. Funds were made available to support and strengthen statewide and regional genetic service delivery systems, which incorporated and strengthened existing service and education resources.

The federal Omnibus Reconciliation Act of 1981 replaced the National Genetic Disease Act and, by creating the Maternal and Child Health Services Block Grant, incorporated ten categorical programs, including genetics.[8]

In January 1984, an ad hoc advisory committee[9] to the federal Bureau of Maternal and Child Health recommended the following:

1. Methods to obtain third-party reimbursement for genetics services;
2. Expansion of regional genetic networks to encourage the sharing of laboratory facilities across state lines;
3. Establishment of standards for genetics services and providing technical assistance to states for meeting the standards;
4. Strengthen genetics educational efforts for primary health professional groups such as physicians, nurses and social workers;
5. Strengthen quality control in genetics laboratories;
6. Encourage the collection of minimum data on delivery of genetics services as a basis for documenting utilization of genetics programs;
7. Improve the delivery of comprehensive psychosocial services for individuals and families with genetic disorders.

A national conference in April 1987 established guidelines for newborn screening for sickle cell disease and other hemoglobinopathies. These guidelines have served as a basis for the beginning federal support of statewide newborn screening programs.

TITLE XVIII OF THE
SOCIAL SECURITY ACT—MEDICARE

Title XVIII, Health Insurance for the Aged, or Medicare, makes provision for individuals 65 years and over. Its provisions are in two parts: Part A provides hospitalization, nursing home care, outpatient diagnostic care, and home health care services. Part B provides supplementary medical insurance benefits, covers doctor's fees, and some additional health services.

Title XVIII is entirely federally funded. In fiscal year 1986, its budget amounted to $75.9 billion. It is administered by the Health Care Financing Administration of the U.S. Department of Health and Human Services.

TITLE XIX—GRANTS TO THE STATES FOR
MEDICAL ASSISTANCE PROGRAMS

MEDICAID

Title XIX makes provision for the indigent—those receiving public assistance, those receiving aid to families with needy children, the aged, the blind, and the permanently and totally disabled. In addition, Title XIX can also provide coverage for the medically indigent, with the level of medical indigency set by each state. Title XIX represents the largest program paying for the medical care of children. It is funded in part by federal funds and in part by state funds. The federal portion of the cost of Medicaid in fiscal year 1987 was $26.64 billion.

Early and Periodic Screening Diagnosis and Treatment (EPSDT)

As part of the 1967 amendments to the Social Security Act, EPSDT was enacted as part of Medicaid, to be implemented by July 1, 1969. The EPSDT Program is administered by the Health Care Financing Administration of the U.S. Department of Health and Human Services.

The purposes of EPSDT are: (1) to identify and diagnose health problems in children that need treatment; (2) to make arrangements for children to obtain the necessary treatment; (3) to encourage regular participation in the nation's health care system by children who have traditionally not been receiving adequate health care, with emphasis on preventive care. It is required that each state inform eligible families with children about the screening program. Each state must help families to use the program, and each state must identify and make arrangements with health care providers for screening, diagnosis, and treatment services. Services to be provided include assessment of the child's physical and mental health status; diagnostic services; treatment services, including corrective devices such as eyeglasses and hearing aids, other treatment for visual and hearing defects; and some dental care.

The EPSDT program is financed through the Title 19 Medicaid funds.

THE EPSDT program provides:

Outreach, recruiting, seeking out eligible children and their families, and informing them of both the benefits of prevention and the health services available;

Health Education, helping children and their families use health resources, effectively and efficiently;

Screening, assessing the child's health needs through initial and periodic examinations and evaluations; and

Case management, assuring that health problems found are diagnosed and treated early, before they become more complex and their treatment more costly.

In FY 1987, 30 percent of all eligible children received initial or periodic examinations and nine percent were enrolled in continuing care arrangements (a single source for screening, health supervision, treatment and case management).[10]

	Average Number of Eligibles	Continuing Care Enrollees		Initial/Periodic Examinations		
		Average #	%	Number Reported	Screening ratio (%)	w/health Problems
1985:	9,047,489	512,887	6	2,233,411	25	31
1986:	9,369,784	686,345	7	2,742,816	29	29
1987:	9,587,167	818,876	9	2,829,568	30	27

Medicaid and Maternity Care

Medicaid pays for over one-half million deliveries (about 15 percent of all women giving birth) at a cost of $1.2 billion maternity bill (about 10 percent of the Nation's $11.5 billion bill).

Medicaid Estimates—1984/85
Reported % of All Maternity Expenditures

Births	Births	Total	Per Birth
541,770	14.7	$1,190,355,000	$2,200

Provision of Medicaid for Pregnant Women and Children Under The Sixth Omnibus Budget Reconciliation Act (SOBRA)—1986 [11]

In October 1986, Congress broadened states' ability to provide Medicaid coverage to indigent pregnant women and young children, and enabled them to establish a program of presumptive eligibility (PE) for pregnant women, as part of the Sixth Omnibus Budget Reconciliation Act (SOBRA, P.L. 99-509). This legislation is a step in the coverage of low-income pregnant women and children by Medicaid. It should promote the provision of early and continuous prenatal and pediatric care. It is a step intended to modify restrictive financial eligibility standards, and to simplify complicated eligibility determination procedures. It liberalizes income standards, eliminates the assets test, makes continuous eligibility possible, allows states to establish presumptive eligibility. As of September 1987, 25 states had used SOBRA to raise income eligibility standards for pregnant women and children under age one year.

On an incremental basis, eligibility is to be extended to children up to age five years (up to age two in fiscal year 1988; age three in fiscal year 1989; age four in fiscal year 1990; and age five in 1991), if the children are in families whose income is below the federal poverty line but above the level needed to qualify for AFDC (Aid to Families With Dependent Children).

HEAD START [12]

The U.S. Head Start Program was begun in 1965 as part of the national effort to prevent and reduce poverty, and to interrupt the cycle of deprivation and poverty in disadvantaged families. In 1986, a total of 448,250 four-year-old children were cared for in Head Start. The federal budget in 1987 was $1305 billion.

Head Start provides a combination of preschool education for the child; health services and care for the child; socialization experience for the child; social services for the family; teaching parents, principally the mother about child care, growth and development, and parenting.

The effects of Head Start may be summarized as follows. Head Start produces substantial gain in children's cognitive and language development. The most needy children appear to benefit the most from Head Start—these include children of single parent families, children with low cognitive scores, and those whose mothers had a tenth grade education or less. Children showed almost twice the gains in racially mixed classrooms where the percentage of minority children was 26-89 percent, compared with classes composed almost totally of minority preschoolers. While Head Start children generally fared better in school than similar children who did not attend Head Start, the gains by Head Start children were not large enough to enable them to equal the performance of the average middle-class children in school or on standardized test.

In social development, Head Start children are found to be more aggressive and more attention seeking; also more sociable and assertive. Children generally improve in hemoglobin level, motor control, and physical development, compared to control-group children. Children are more likely to be of normal height and weight, to have fewer absences from school, and to perform better on physical tests.

Head Start has had a favorable effect on families. Parents volunteer in Head Start, serve as members of committees and councils, and generally report satisfaction with the program. Head Start also has provided jobs for parents and others in the community, and has increased parent participation in schools.

COMMUNITY HEALTH CENTERS

The community health centers in the United States are located in low-income areas in the central cities and in rural areas. They are designed to serve the underprivileged. The community health center movement began in 1965 as part of the Office of Economic Opportunity anti-poverty program. Some community health centers exist as part of general community services, including general counseling, welfare, housing, employment, and legal services. Others are more limited predominantly to the delivery of health care. It is intended that they provide care on a family basis. Most patients served are mothers and children; hence, they are largely MCH centers and represent an important MCH resource.The federal budget for community health centers in fiscal year 1987 is $400 million.

Concern has been expressed about the quality of care of mothers and children provided by some community health centers. A study by Morehead et. al.[13] comparing community health centers with Maternity and Infant (M&I) Care Projects and Children and Youth (C&I) Projects, based on a medical audit, found a considerably higher rating of M&I and C&Y over community health centers. There is a great need for MCH staff to work closely with community health centers to assist them in improving the quality of care.

THE NATIONAL HEALTH SERVICE CORPS

NHSC began in December 1970. The main purpose is to assign health personnel to unserved and underserved areas of high priority in the U.S. Another purpose is to encourage health personnel assigned to these high-priority areas, which have a personnel shortage, to decide to remain there on a permanent basis. The principles of assignment include that: (1) there will be community governance; that is, a community board be established and some community groups request it;

(2) there be cultural relevance, in regard to ethnic, cultural, and language needs; (3) there be outreach, through home visits, neighborhood clinics, transportation; (4) there be transfer of knowledge and skills through the use of local people to increase their capability. NHSC health personnel are being assigned to staff MCH services and projects in high priority areas, and, therefore, represent an important national resource in MCH.

In 1987, there were some 3,000 multidisciplinary health staff members assigned to medically underserved areas. The federal budget for this program for fiscal year 1986 was $55.8 million.

PROFESSIONAL SOCIETIES

Professional societies are of considerable assistance in a variety of ways for MCH and CC services. For example, they play an important role in professional education by conducting continuing education courses for which they provide continuing education credit. They may participate in setting and raising standards and quality through journals, publications, and technical statements on issues and subjects. They can influence legislation, budgets, and appropriations. Because of these multiple functions, it is essential that MCH and CC workers belong to and become active in these professional organizations. At the same time, leaders in the professional societies can be helpful to the MCH and CC services in assisting them M the quality of care.

VOLUNTARY AGENCIES

Voluntary agencies are of two types: (1) those founded by citizen groups and professional people; (2) those founded by parents. An example of the former is the American Heart Association. Examples of the latter are United Cerebral Palsy and Muscular Dystrophy Association. Regardless of the type, they usually perform the following functions: (1) provide direct services; (2) provide fellowships; (3) support research; (4) provide public education; (5) influence legislation and appropriations; (6) conduct demonstrations. Because of the very great assistance that voluntary agencies can be to MCH and CC services, it is important to establish close cooperative working relationships with them.

REFERENCES

1. World Health Organization: The Organization and Administration of Maternal and Child Health Services. Technical Report Series No. 428. Geneva, Switzerland. 1969.

2. U.S. General Accounting Office. Block Grants: Overview of Experiences to Date and Emerging Issues. Report to the Congress of the United States. April 3, 1985.

3. U.S. General Accounting Office. Maternal and Child Health Block Grant: Program Changes Emerging Under State Administration. Report to the Congress of the United States. May 7, 1984.

4. Torres A and Forrest JD. Family Planning Clinic Services in the United States, 1983. Family Planning Perspectives 17:30-35, January/February, 1985.

5. Gold RB and Nestor B. Public Funding of Contraceptive, Sterilization and Abortion Services, 1983. Family Planning Perspectives 17:25-30, January/February 1985.

6. Torres A. The Effects of Federal Funding Cuts on Family Planning Services, 1980-1983, Family Planning Perspectives 16:134-138, May/June 1984.

7. Adolescent Family Life Act of 1982 Found Unconstitutional. Family Planning Perspectives 19:134-136, May/June 1987.

8. Division of Maternal and Child Health, U.S. Department of Health and Human Services. Summary Report: Future Directions of the National Genetics Program Workshop. January 30-31, 1984. Rockville, MD, 18 pages.

9. National Institutes of Health: Newborn Screening for Sickle Cell Disease and Other Hemoglobinopathies. Consensus Development Conference Statement. Volume 6, Number 9. April 6-8, 1987. 22 pages. Bethesda, Maryland 20892.

10. Hiscock WM. Special Communication. September 4, 1987.

11. Rosenbaum S. Medicaid Eligibility for Pregnant Women: Reforms Contained in the Sixth Omnibus Budget Reconciliation Act (SOBRA). Children's Defense Fund, Washington, DC. April, 1987.

12. Collins RC and Deloria D. Head Start Research: A New Chapter. Children Today, July/August 1983, pages 15-19.

13. Morehead, MA, Donaldson, RS, Seravalli, MR. Comparisons Between OEO Neighborhood Health Centers and Other Health Care Providers of Ratings of The Quality of Health Care. American Journal of Public Health 61:1294-1306, 1971.

PART II: ORGANIZATION OF SERVICES FOR HANDICAPPED CHILDREN AND YOUTH (Children with Special Needs): Systems of Care for Handicapped Children and Youth in the United States

Helen M. Wallace

At present, there is not a comprehensive approach to the care, management, and assistance provided for handicapped children and youth and their families in the U.S.. Rather, there is a number of separate parallel systems of care. These include:

1. The official state Crippled Children's (CC) Programs;

2. The state education efforts at implementation of PL 94-142 and of PL 99-457, Education of All Handicapped Children;

3. The state Development Disabilities services and programs, serving children, youth, and adults with developmental disabilities;

4. The state programs to provide vocational rehabilitation services for disabled youth and adults; and

5. Head Start serving handicapped 3-5 year olds in Head Start.

Each of these state and local programs and services for handicapped children and youth is tied to specific federal legislation and appropriations.

There is need to pull together, coordinate and integrate these separately legislated/funded approaches to make it possible to provide a unified approach for the benefit of handicapped children, youth and their families.

THE OFFICIAL CRIPPLED CHILDREN'S PROGRAM [1]

The official CC Program is a partnership program between the federal and the state governments. It is designed to promote early identification of handicapped children and to provide evaluation, diagnosis, treatment, rehabilitation, continuing care, and case management services for handicapped children, youth, and their families.

The Legislative Base

Title V, Part 2 of the Social Security Act, enacted in 1935, established the federal authorization for the state Crippled Children's Programs, as follows:

To enable the states to extend and improve "services for locating crippled children and for medical, surgical, corrective, and other services and care for and facilities for diagnosis, hospitalization, and aftercare for children who are crippled or who are suffering from conditions leading to crippling."

Title V of the Social Security Act served as the federal legislative authority for the state CC Programs until 1981. In 1981, the Omnibus Budget Reconciliation Act established the Maternal and Child Health Block Grant. The MCH Block Grant continued the federal legislative authority, as reproduced above, and also added responsibility for disabled children under the Supplemental Security Income (SSI) Program, as follows: "Provide rehabilitative services for blind and disabled individuals under the age of 16 receiving benefits under Title XVI of this Act."

The MCH Block Grant became effective October 1, 1981. It gave the states greater discretion, within certain legislated limitations, to determine programmatic needs, set priorities, allocate funds, and establish oversight mechanisms. At the same time, it curtailed the opportunity of the federal funding agency to provide consultation and technical assistance to the states. It also reduced the requirement of accountability from the state CC Programs. [2]

Administration

The federal responsibility for the state CC Programs is located in the Bureau of Maternal and Child Health, U.S. Department of Health and Human Services, and in the ten federal Regional Offices.

Each state and territory has an official CC Program, which is administered by the state CC Agency. In 47 states, the CC Agency is located in the state health department. In the remaining 10, the CC Agency is located in other state agencies, such as the state university (3); the state welfare department (6); and the state education department (1).

Funding and Expenditures

The state CC Programs are funded primarily by a combination of federal and state funds. In 1981, the sources of funds expended by the state CC Programs were as follows:

Source	Amount	%
State	$224 Million	63
Federal*	103	29
Fees & Reimbursement	13	3.7
Local	6	1.6
Other	11	3.1
TOTAL	**$356 Million**	

* From both the MCH Block Grant and Supplemental Security

Federal funds for the support of state CC Programs are allocated to each state by a formula. Each state receives Fund A, which consists of a grant of $70,000, plus an additional amount determined by the number of children under 21 years of age; Fund A is matched by the state. Fund B, which is unmatched by the state, is determined by the financial needs of the state.

Under the MCH Block Grant, the state CC Programs have proportionately received a larger percentage of the available federal funds. The state CC Programs continue to have high priority. There has been a trend toward consolidating the SSI Program for disabled children into the state CC Program.[2]

Functions of The Official State Crippled Children's Program

These include:

- advocacy;
- promoting development, improvement for handicapped children and youth of all kinds and their families;
- expansion and extension of health and medical care services throughout all sections of the state;
- receiving and administering the federal funds for CC, from the MCH Block Grant;
- stimulating and improving earlier case finding of handicapped children and youth;
- promoting the development of and participation in the delivery of expert evaluation, diagnostic, treatment, and rehabilitative services for handicapped children and youth, using the interdisciplinary case management approach;

- promoting and providing demonstration services to demonstrate new patterns of delivery of comprehensive health care of handicapped children and youth;
- promoting and providing follow up and continuity of health care of handicapped children and youth, including case management;
- stimulating efforts to prevent the occurrence of handicapping conditions in children and youth (primary prevention), and to prevent the damaging effects of handicapping conditions (secondary prevention);
- evaluating health services provided to handicapped children and youth and their families;
- uncovering unmet needs and services for handicapped children and youth;
- conducting studies of needs and services for handicapped children and youth, collecting, analyzing, and disseminating data;
- participating in education of parents and the public;
- participating in education of members of the health professions;
- set and raise standards of health care for handicapped children and youth, and conducting quality assurance;
- drafting suggested legislation in regard to the health care of handicapped children and youth;
- working closely with other official, voluntary and private agencies and universities in order to coordinate care for handicapped children and youth, e.g. Education, Vocational Rehabilitation, voluntary agencies, various medical specialty groups, Developmental Disabilities;
- participating in evaluation of handicapped children and youth for special educational placement;
- referral and participating in evaluation of handicapped youth for vocational rehabilitation services;
- assisting the Department of Social Services in planning for the care of handicapped children;
- promoting the coordination of services for handicapped children and youth in the state;
- promote regional planning for services for handicapped children and youth;
- promote the development of genetic diagnostic and counseling services;
- plan and participate in third party payment from Title 19, Vocational Rehabilitation, Blue Cross, Blue Shield, and others; improve residential care of the handicapped; and
- administer the SSI Program for disabled children.

Quality of Care

The state CC Programs are one of the first attempts to enter the field of medical care. They have provided experience in the development and testing of new effective methods of planning, organizing, and implementing community programs designed to bring health services of high quality to vulnerable children and youth. There has been particular emphasis on quality of care.

Staff

The state CC agencies usually have a multidisciplinary staff. The staff consist of a director (usually a physician, a pediatrician), nurses, social workers, physical therapists, occupational therapists, psychologists, experts in the field of communicative disorders, nutritionists, and dentists. These staff members carry out the functions of the state CC Program listed above; a small core staff primarily carry administrative functions (planning, implementing, evaluating, coordinating); the majority primarily carry clinical functions in providing patient care (assessment, treatment, case management of patients and families).

Children Cared For In State CC Programs [1]

Each state determines the conditions for which the state CC Program will provide services. Each state establishes its own diagnostic and financial eligibility criteria. Thus, there is considerable variation in the number and types of children cared for. In general, the state CC caseloads include children requiring care throughout childhood and adolescence, and those with handicaps so incapacitating that the cost of care is beyond the resources of the family.

There have been changes in the types of children cared for in state CC Programs over the years; less children seen with conditions due to infections (osteomyelitis, tuberculosis, poliomyelitis) and to orthopedic conditions; more children with congenital defects, neurological conditions, multiple handicaps, and such conditions as cystic fibrosis, hemophilia, leukemia, and the mentally retarded who are also "crippled."

In 1984, 48 state crippled children's agencies (SCCAS) provided services to 627,699 children with handicapping conditions; 34 SCCAS reported a total of 2.2 million encounters for the children under their care, an average of 4.9 encounters per child. (An encounter is defined as a face-to-face contact between a patient and a provider of health care services who exercises independent judgment in the care and provision of health services to the patient.)

Demographic Characteristics

Of the total children seen in 1984, 34 percent were new patients, and 65 percent were return or carry-over patients. Thirty-five percent of all children served had been under SCCA care for more than three years.

The age distribution of children served by SCCAS in 1984 was as follows:

Age Group	Percent of Total
Less than age 1	7.6
1 - 4 Years	29.3
5 - 13 Years	39.8
14 - 19 Years	19.6
Over 19 Years	3.3
Age Unknown	0.4
TOTAL	**100.0**

The largest age group served during 1984 was that of children aged 5-13 years. One reason may be that the children may have been diagnosed upon entry into the school system (i.e., hearing, vision, and learning disorders). Another reason may be that treatment requires a certain level of development (i.e., cardiac, orthopedic, and orofacial conditions).

The distribution of children served by SCCAS in 1984, by family income status, is as follows:

Family Income Status	Percent of Total
At or below poverty level	52.6
Poverty level to 150% of poverty level	18.3
150-200% of poverty level	14.4
Over 200% of poverty level	10.4
Unknown	4.3
TOTAL	**100.0**

More than three-fourths of the children served were from families at or below 150 percent of the poverty level. This is in accord with the intent of the SCCAS to make services available to low income families or those with limited access to health services.

Diagnostic Conditions

Children served by the SCCAS in 1984 had the following diagnostic conditions:

Diagnostic Category	Percent of Children Served
Orthopedic	29.2
Hearing	19.8
Cardiac	11.0
Vision	8.5
Orofacial and Dental	6.0

Diagnostic Category	Percent of Children Served
Mental Retardation	4.0
Speech/Language	3.2
Learning Disorders	4.6
Emotional Disturbances	1.2
Chronic Medical	14.1
Other Neuropediatric-Development	13.2
Other medical/surgical	11.5
Unknown	9.4

The most frequently reported categories were orthopedic, hearing, cardiac, and vision.

Services Provided

All state CC Programs must provide diagnostic services without charge.The chronic nature of most handicapping conditions requires a multifaceted, multidisciplinary program of ongoing case management care. In addition to high quality evaluation, diagnostic, and treatment services, many handicapped children require long-term case management, and careful coordination of a broad range of health, social, educational, vocational, and rehabilitative services. These management programs include planning, individualized care, counseling, monitoring patient status, periodic reassessment, and coordinating services.

Funds of CC Programs are used to provide direct services in the following ways: (1) through state-operated and staffed clinics; (2) under contractual or fee-for-service arrangements with private practicing medical specialists; (3) a combination of full-time state staff and part-time private medical specialists working together in state-operated clinics. Regardless of the method used, all state CC Programs are designed to provide evaluation, diagnosis, treatment, and rehabilitative services to children with handicapping or chronic conditions. All use a multidisciplinary approach in care. The CC Programs assume responsibility for case management; they prepare an individualized service plan, arrange for the delivery of needed medical, health, and support services, and modify the plan as needed to reflect changes in the child's condition and development.

In addition to these patient care services, state CC programs also provide other broad services, which are listed below.

Other Services and Activities of State Crippled Children's Agencies

1. Direct Patient Services These include: laboratory, social work, speech therapy, physical therapy, hearing therapy, dental care, public health nursing, occupational therapy, outreach, transportation, nutrition, vision therapy, home health care, and case management.

2. Indirect Services SCCAS provide a wide variety of other types of services designed to expand, strengthen, and improve the delivery of care to handicapped children and youth and their families on a statewide basis. These include: coordination; technical assistance; education/counseling; planning; administration and management; collecting, recording, analyzing, and disseminating data; setting standards, evaluation of care and services; leadership; resource development and allocation; assessment of scope and nature of needs and problems; quality assurance; and research.

In 1984, SCCAS provided professional health care in an ambulatory setting to 76 percent of the children served. Eleven percent of the children served by SCCAS were hospitalized in 1984 for diagnosis and/or treatment. Other services most frequently provided were clinical management* (72 percent of children served) and case management** (59 percent)

Family counseling and training were provided to 31 percent of the children served. Special types of adaptive care (braces, prosthetics, and hearing aids) were provided to 15 percent, and family support services (home visits, homemaker services and transportation) to 11 percent of the children.

Eligibility

Eligibility criteria for care under state CC Programs represent a serious obstacle to reaching and providing care for all handicapped children and youth who need it. Each state sets its own eligibility criteria—both in diagnostic conditions and in financial eligibility. This not only prevents some children and youth from receiving the prompt necessary care; it also creates confusion in the understanding and utilization of state CC services because of serious inconsistencies from one state to another.

Unmet Needs

1. There is great need to broaden eligibility (both diagnostic and financial) so that state CC Programs may be able to provide the needed services for all handicapped children and youth who require them.

2. As a corollary, the financing of state CC Programs requires major expansion.

3. There is need for extension of state CC services to all sections of each state so that all handicapped children and youth will have equal access to quality services. There is need for more emphasis on statewide planning.

---

* Clinical management includes planning, arranging and coordination services related to the medical care and health of the child.

** Case management usually involves interdisciplinary coordination of all needed services, including medical, social, and educational; liaison and coordination of efforts among state and local agencies and professionals involved in the child's total care.

4. There is need for further development and use of a plan of regionalized care and services.

5. There is need for better planning, working together, and coordination of services with:

    The Developmental Disabilities Program
    The field of education and special education in the implementation of PL 94-142 and PL 99-457
    The Vocational Rehabilitation Program
    The Medicaid - EPSDT Program
    The state MCH Program
    The mental health programs
    Private agencies serving handicapped children and youth

6. There is need for a systematic planned evaluation of the component parts of state CC Programs.

THE SUPPLEMENTAL SECURITY INCOME DISABLED CHILDREN'S PROGRAM

In 1976, Congress established a separate categorical program to assist disabled children receiving SSI benefits. Under this program, the Social Security Administration refers blind and disabled children under 16 years of age, receiving SSI benefits, to state CC agencies for counseling and other services. For these children, the state CC agencies establishes individual service plans and provides referrals for services. In addition, they provide medical, social, developmental, and rehabilitative services mainly to children under seven years of age.

EDUCATION OF HANDICAPPED CHILDREN—PL 94-142

PL 94-142, the Education For All Handicapped Children Act, was enacted by Congress, in 1975, to make it possible for all handicapped children of school and preschool age to receive a free appropriate public education. The original Act of 1975 was landmark legislation, comparable in significance to the field of handicapped children and youth as Title V of the Social Security Act in 1935 was to the field of MCH.

At the time of enactment of PL 94-142, in 1975, there were more than eight million handicapped children in the U.S. and their special educational needs were not being fully met, as more than half did not receive appropriate education services. One million were excluded entirely from the public school system; many handicapped children were participating in regular school programs where handicaps were undetected; because of lack of adequate services within the public school system, families were often forced to find services outside the public school system, often at great distance from their residence and at their own expense. PL 94-142 is intended to assure that all handicapped children have available to them a free appropriate public education which emphasizes special education and related services to assure that the rights of handicapped children and their parents or guardians are protected, to assist states and localities to provide for the education of all handicapped children, and to assess and assure the effectiveness of efforts to educate handicapped children. The term "related services" means transportation, and such developmental, corrective, and other supportive services (including speech pathology and audiology, psychological services, physical and occupational therapy, recreation, and medical and counseling services) as may be required to assist a handicapped child to benefit from special education; it includes the early identification and assessment of handicapping conditions in children. PL 94-142 requires that handicapped children and youth receive their education in the least restrictive environment. It requires that an "individualized education program" be developed for each child, with annual goals. It provides federal funds to assist the states to implement the requirements of the Act. It provides procedural safeguards to protect the rights of the child and to assure the provision of appropriate education for each child, with right of appeal by the family.

Number and Type of Handicapped Children Served

In the school year 1983-84, slightly over four million children were served (Table 1), an increase over 1982-83. There were increases in all of the categories of handicapped children served.

Age

States in 1983-84 continue to report increases in the number of preschool handicapped children served, especially those aged three through five. Forty-two mandated services to at least some portion of the birth through age-five population and, where mandated, a larger population of this age group was served in 1983-84.

Secondary and Post-secondary Age

An expansion of services to secondary and post-secondary-age handicapped students has occurred, partly because of increased recognition of the importance of a successful transition from school to work and community life, and the need to preserve educational gains from earlier education. There was an increase in services for students aged 18 through 21, in 1983-84, over the previous year. All states have mandates to provide services to handicapped students through age 17, and 28 states have mandates to serve handicapped youths through the age of 21, if they have not graduated from high school. There is a growing trend toward expansion of vocational services and use of community resources to provide vocational training to this age group.

Least Restrictive Environment

Less than seven percent of all handicapped children are educated in either separate schools or separate environments. Of the more than 93 percent who are educated in regular schools, about two-thirds receive their education in the regular classroom with nonhandicapped peers. (Table 1)

Funding

States use a mixture of federal, state, and local funds to finance services for handicapped children and youth. For FY 1985, the following funds were appropriated by Congress for the education of the handicapped:

State Grants $1,135,000,000

Early Childhood 22,500,000

Secondary & Transitional Services...............................6,300,000

Post-secondary 5,300,000

Personnel Development...61,000,000

TABLE 1

NUMBER OF CHILDREN AGES 3-21 YEARS SERVED UNDER PL 94-142 BY HANDICAPPING CONDITIONS

Condition	School Year		
	1981-82	1982-83	1983-84
Learning Disabled	1,608,518	1,723,759	1,811,489
Speech Impaired	1,124,209	1,120,175	1,130,569
Mentally Retarded	698,429	678,054	750,634
Emotionally Disturbed	303,328	313,876	360,073
Multi-handicapped	58,753	50,367	67,537
Hard of Hearing and Deaf	50,275	49,119	74,279
Other Health Impaired	76,174	48,104	54,621
Orthopedically Impaired	48,438	46,459	56,209
Visually Handicapped	20,902	21,298	31,576
Deaf-Blind	1,410	1,383	2,512
All conditions	3,990,346	4,052,595	4,094,225

SOURCES:

1) For 1981-82 - U.S. Department of Education. Fifth Annual Report to Congress On The Implementation of Public Law 94-142: The Education For All Handicapped Children Act. Washington DC. 1983. 175 pages.

2) For 1982-83 - U.S. Department of Education. Sixth Annual Report To Congress On the Implementation Of Public Law 94-142: The Education For All Handicapped Children Act. Reported In Programs For The Handicapped, Number 5, Sept./Oct. 1984. Pages 7-9.

3) For 1983-84 - U.S. Department of Education. Seventh Annual Report To Congress On The Implementation Of The Education Of The Handicapped Act. Washington, DC. 1985. 299 pages.

Unmet Needs

Among the unmet needs are the following:

1. There is great need for Education, Developmental Disabilities, MCH and CC Programs, and Vocational Rehabilitation and services to work more closely together to provide comprehensive care for handicapped children and youth.

2. The term "related services," in the implementation of PL 94-142, needs to include all essential relevant services for each child, including medical and health participation.

3. The individualized education plan for each child needs to be comprehensive and able to be easily understood and interpreted by staff concerned and by parents.

4. Services and programs for the secondary and post-secondary age group need strengthening, so that the earlier gains made by the youth will not be lost. All states should mandate programs through age 21.

5. All states should mandate programs beginning at birth.

PL 99-457, THE EDUCATION OF THE HANDICAPPED AMENDMENTS OF 1986

PL 99-457, The Education of the Handicapped Amendments of 1986: (1) reauthorized the discretionary programs of the Education of the Handicapped Act (PL 94-142); (2) provides incentives to states to serve an estimated additional 70,000 handicapped children aged three through five who are currently not now being served (260,000 children are currently being provided services); and (3) creates a new discretionary program to address the special needs of handicapped infants and toddlers (birth through age two) and their families. The Act authorizes a total of $125 million for fiscal year 1987 and 1988 for the new birth-two year program. Congress has already appropriated $180 million for fiscal year 1987 for the three-five year program, more than a six-fold increase over FY 1986. (Table 2)

Under the Act, after four years, each state, if it wants continue receiving federal support under the birth-two and three-five programs, must have in place among other things a policy to provide appropriate early intervention services to all handicapped infants and toddlers in the state. The Act contains four parts.

Title 1 - Handicapped Infants and Toddlers Describes the requirements for the new program to serve infants, toddlers, and their families (birth-two). It defines early intervention services, and describes the infants and toddlers eligible for them. It specifies that case management services will be provided. It lists the elements of a statewide system, and requires an individualized family service plan. It requires a state interagency coordinating council. It specifies that this new source of funds prevents the state from reducing medical or other assistance available from Title 5 or Title 19 of the Social Security Act.

Title 2 - Handicapped Children Aged Three Through Five This Title establishes eligibility criteria. It is intended to supplement, not supplant. Interagency agreements, policies and procedures must be developed. States are already serving 260,000 children aged three through five.

Title 3 - Discretionary Programs This includes regional resource and federal centers; services for deaf-blind children and youth; early education for handicapped children; research, innovation, training, and dissemination of information concerning educational opportunities for the handicapped; research and demonstration projects in education of handicapped children; films and educational medial for handicapped persons; centers on technology, educational media, and materials for the handicapped.

TABLE 2

PL 99-457 FUNDING PROFILE

PART H: Handicapped Infants & Toddlery		1987 $60M	1988 $75M	1989 Funds as Needed
Section 619:	Preschool Grants	Funds	as	Needed
Section 621:	Regional Resource and Federal Centers	$ 6.7M	$ 7.1M	$ 7.5M
Section 622:	Deaf-Blind Children and Youth	$ 15.9M	$16.8M	$ 17.8M
Section 623:	Early Ed for Hand. Children	$24.47M	$ 25.87	$27.41M
Section 624:	Program for Severely Hand. Children	$ 5.3M	$ 5.6M	$ 5.9M
Section 625:	Postsecondary Ed.	$ 5.9M	$ 6.2M	$ 6.6M
Section 626:	Secondary Ed. & Transitional Services	$ 7.3M	$ 7.7M	$ 8.1M
Section 631: & 632	Grants for Personnel Training	$ 70.2M	$74.5M	$ 79M
Section 633:	Clearinghouse	$ 1.2M	$ 1.9M	$ 2.0M
Section 641:	Res. & Dem. Programs	$ 18M	$ 19M	$20.1M
Section 642:	Media & Captioned Films	$ 15M	$15.7M	$ 16.5M
PART G: Technology & Media		**$ 10M**	**$10.8M**	**$ 11.0M**
Section 618:	Evaluation	$ 3.8M	$ 4M	$ 4.2M

SOURCE: National Association of State Directors of Special Education. EHA Amendments of 1986 Becomes Law. In LIAISON Bulletin. Vol. 12, No. 12, October 22, 1986.

Title 4 - Miscellaneous This included removal of architectual barriers; an increase in funds for Native Americans; standards for personnel and evaluation of the program.

DEVELOPMENTAL DISABILITIES

History

In 1963, Congress enacted PL 88-164, the first federal categorical construction program for the mentally retarded. PL 88-164 provided federal funds to (1) build research centers for preventing and combating mental retardation; (2) construct public or nonprofit clinical facilities (i.e. university-affiliated facilities) which would provide inpatient/outpatient services, demonstrate how specialized services could be provided, and provide clinical training for physicians and others working with the retarded; and (3) encourage states to build community facilities for the retarded.

In 1970, Congress amended PL 88-164, which had expired, by the enactment of PL 91-517. The emphasis shifted from construction to planning and services. There was emphasis on developing a network of services for the disabled. The law broadened the target population to include cerebral palsy, epilepsy, and other neurological conditions closely related to mental retardation. A new term, *developmental disability* (DD), was adopted to describe this new target group.

In 1973, PL 94-103, the Developmentally Disabled Assistance and Bill of Rights Act, was enacted. This Act continued support of state grants and university-affiliated facilities (UAF's). Two new programs were added: a state Protection and Advocacy Program, and a Special Projects Program.

The state formula grants were for planning, administration, delivering services, and constructing facilities for the DD. *The state protection and advocacy program* was designed to establish and guard the rights of the DD and assure that they have quality services for maximum physical, psychological, and social development. *The university-affiliated facilities program* was to support the operation of demonstration facilities and provide interdisciplinary training to strengthen staff resources to serve the DD. The *special projects program* was to support the demonstration of new or improved techniques for delivering services and assist with meeting the special needs of the disadvantaged DD.

Administration of DD Program

Administration of the DD program is a shared responsibility among federal and state officials. At the *national* level, there is a DD office in the Office of Human Development of the U.S. Department of Health and Human Services, with a national advisory council. The federal Bureau of Maternal and Child Health also provides substantial support to the UAF program.

At the *state* level, each state has a state planning council. Each state has a state agency designated as responsible for administering the state DD program; this may be located in any one of a variety of state agencies—health, mental retardation, mental health, vocational rehabilitation, etc.

Definition of Developmental Disability

The term, *developmental disability,* means a severe, chronic disability of a person which:

A. Is attributable to a mental or physical impairment or combination of mental and physical impairments;

B. Is manifested before the person attains age 22;

C. Is likely to continue indefinitely;

D. Results in substantial functional limitations in three or more of the following areas of major life activity: (I) self-care; (II) receptive and expressive language; (III) learning; (IV) mobility; (V) self-direction; (VI) capacity for independent living; and (VII) economic self-sufficiency.

Current Legislation

On October 1987, Congress enacted the Developmental Disabilities Amendments of 1987. New priority area activities are as follows:

- Activities to increase the capacities and resources of public and private nonprofit entities and others to develop a system for providing specialized services or special adaptations of generic services or other assistance which responds to the needs and capabilities of persons with developmental disabilities and their families and to enhance coordination among entities;

- Demonstration of new ways to enhance the independence, productivity and integration into the community of persons with developmental disabilities;

- Conduct of studies and analyses; gathering of information; development of model policies and procedures; and presentation of information, models, findings, conclusions and recommendations;

- Outreach activities for persons with developmental disabilities to enable such persons to obtain assistance in Federal priority areas or a State priority area, including access to specialized services or special adaptations of generic services;

- Training of persons with developmental disabilities, family members, and personnel, including professionals, paraprofessionals, students and volunteers, to obtain access to, or to provide services and other assistance for persons with developmental disabilities and their families; and

- Activities designed to prevent developmental disabilities from occurring or to expand and enhance the independence, productivity and integration into the community of persons with developmental disabilities through the State on a comprehensive basis.

Federal priority areas are: community living activities, employment activities, child development activities, and case management activities. A State priority area is priority area activities in an area considered essential by the State Planning Council.

Present Federal Authorization and Funding

The Developmental Disabilities Act of 1984 which was enacted in September 1984, established the following *authorization* levels:

	FY 1985	FY 1986	FY 1987	FY 1988
State Grant Programs	$50.25 M	$53.4 M	$56.5 M	$62.2 M
Protection& Advocacy Sys.	13.75	14.6	15.4	20.0
University-Affiliated Fac.	9.0	9.6	10.2	13.9
Special Projects	2.7	2.9	3.1	3.65

University Affiliated Programs (UAPs)

UAPs comprise a network of 36 full-service programs and seven Satellite Centers, located in major universities and teaching hospitals throughout the U.S. which provide: (1) exemplary services at the community and regional level to persons with developmental disabilities and their families; (2) interdisciplinary training of professional personnel; (3) technical assistance to public and private agencies, associations and individuals; and (4) dissemination of applied research and promising practices in the field. The principal focus of UAPs is the training of physicians, pediatricians and allied professionals, ranging from occupational and physical therapists to speech pathologists, child psychologists and social workers. In FY 1986, this network served over 75,000 persons.

The new legislation authorizes appropriations of $13.9 million in FY 1988: $15.2 million for FY 1989; and $16.5 million in FY 1990 for grants to UAPs. The FY 1987 appropriation is $9.187 million. The 1987 amendments authorize the Secretary of Health and Human Services to make grants up to $35,000 to universities to study the feasibility of establishing new UAPs and satellite Centers in States which currently do not have them, and defines procedures for establishing new programs.

VOCATIONAL REHABILITATION

Administration

The federal unit responsible for the federal program of Vocational Rehabilitation, the Rehabilitation Services Administration, is located in the Office of Human Development of the U.S. Department of Health and Human Services. At state level, there is a state agency responsible for the administration of this program, either existing as a separate agency, or as a part of another state agency such as the state department of education.

Legislative Base

The basic legislation for the federal Vocational Rehabilitation Program is the *Rehabilitation Act of 1973, PL 93-112*. This legislation set forth the purpose to:

1. authorize programs to develop comprehensive and continuing state plans to meet the needs of funding vocational rehabilitation services to handicapped individuals;
2. evaluate the rehabilitation potential of handicapped individuals;
3. conduct a study to develop methods of providing rehabilitation services to meet the needs of handicapped individuals;
4. assist in construction and improvement of rehabilitation facilities;
5. develop new and innovative methods to apply the most advanced medical technology, scientific achievement, and psychological and social knowledge to solve rehabilitation problems;
6. initiate and expand services for those underserved;
7. conduct studies and experiments on long neglected problem areas;
8. promote and expand employment opportunities;
9. establish client assistance pilot projects;
10. provide assistance to increase the number of personnel through train ing;
11. evaluate approaches to architectural and transportation barriers.

The legislation established the Rehabilitation Services Administration in the U.S. Department of Health and Human Services.The legislation appropriated funds for the federal grants to the states for the support of basic state vocational rehabilitation services. It required an individualized written rehabilitation program, with annual review. It provided funds for innovation and expansion grants; for research and training; for construction of rehabilitation facilities. It established the National Center for Deaf-Blind Youths and Adults.

The *Rehabilitation Act Amendments of 1984* provide the following:

1. extends the state grant part of the Rehabilitation Act through FY 1986;
2. extends all other programs of the Act for three more years;
3. establishes a separate authority for the Helen Keller National Center for Deaf-Blind Youths and Adults;
4. establishes the National Council On The Handicapped as an independent agency;

5. requires the collection of individual client data for the annual report required of the RSA;

6. requires the development of standards for evaluation of existing independent living centers and projects with industry;

7. changes the client assistance program from a demonstration, discretionary program to a formal state grant program;

8. provides the Director of the National Institute of Handicapped Research with authority to test new concepts and innovative ideas;

9. continues authorization for the Architectural and Transportation Barriers Compliance Board for three years;

10. extends the DD Assistance and Bill of Rights Act.

Content

The Vocational Rehabilitation Program is intended to provide disabled teenagers and adults with a variety of services to assist them to become independent and productive in both living and work. Federal and state funds are used to cover the costs of providing rehabilitation services which include: diagnosis, comprehensive evaluation, counseling, training, reader services for the blind, interpreter services for the deaf, and employment placement. They also assist with payment for medical and related services, and prosthetic and orthotic devices, transportation to secure vocational rehabilitation services, maintenance during rehabilitation, tools, licenses, equipment, supplies, vending stands for handicapped persons including management and supervisory services, and assistance in the construction and establishment of rehabilitation facilities.

Funds are available for special projects, for projects and demonstrations which hold promise of expanding and improving services for groups of mentally and physically handicapped individuals. These may include client assistance, projects with industry, migrant workers, the severely disabled.

Funds are available to provide independent living services for severely handicapped individuals to assist them to function more independently in family and community settings or secure and maintain appropriate employment. Funds are used for attendant care, training in independent living skills, referral and more independently in family and community setup or secure and maintain appropriate employment. Funds are used for assistance in housing and transportation, peer counseling and advocacy.

Funds are also available to support training of personnel to increase the number and improve the skills and personnel trained to provide vocational rehabilitation services to handicapped individuals.

Significance

The age at which handicapped teenagers are eligible for the official Vocational Rehabilitation program varies from state to state. The significance of this is to be aware of the need of timing and referral of handicapped teenagers for evaluation, counseling, education, training, and vocational placement. There is need for close working and cooperation of CC programs and other agencies serving handicapped teenagers and vocational rehabilitation agencies for the full rehabilitation of handicapped teenagers.

The Rehabilitation Services Administration reported that for fiscal year 1980, the benefit/cost ratio of the federal-state vocational rehabilitation program is 10.4:1. This means that for every dollar spent on rehabilitation services, an estimated improvement of $10.40 in individual lifetime earings will result.

Funding

The federal appropriation for fiscal year 1985 for the Vocational Rehabilitation program is as follows:

Basic State Grants	$1,100.0	Evaluation	$2.0
Client Assist. Projects	6.3	Migrants/Indian Tribes	1.7
Severely Disabled	14.6	Helen Keller Center	4.2
Training	22.0	National Council On	
Projects with Industry	14.4	Handicapped	0.75
Recreation	2.1	National Institute for	
		Handicapped Research	0.39
Independent Living	27.0		

Clients Served

Data on clients served in the vocational rehabilitation program in FY 1982 are as follows: [3]

Of the 958,537 persons receiving rehabilitation services, 571,542 (59.2 percent) were severely disabled. Clients severely disabled who were rehabilitated in FY 1982 were 129,866 (57.2 percent of the total 225,924 rehabilitated).

Over 9,504 blind and 13,735 visually impaired individuals were rehabilitated in FY 1981.

In FY 1982, an estimated 18,736 persons with communication disabilities were rehabilitated.

There were 65 projects with industry in FY 1982 serving 11,000 disabled persons, most of whom were severely disabled.

Unmet Needs

1. There is need to promote the closer working relationship and coordination between efforts of the vocational rehabilitation agency and services with those of the official state CC Agencies, developmental disability services, and special education.

2. Adolescents who are handicapped need to be referred for vocational assistance services in their early adolescent years.

3. Vocational experts need to be allocated in secondary schools which disabled adolescents attend, in order to provide vocational assistance readily.

4. Vocational agencies need to provide a high quality of medical and health care to their clients, similar to that provided by state CC Agencies.

CARE OF HANDICAPPED CHILDREN IN HEAD START [4]

It is mandated than ten percent of the total number of enrollment opportunities in each state must be available for handicapped children. In 1984, there were 59,335 handicapped children enrolled in Head Start; in 1984, children professionally diagnosed as handicapped accounted for 12.5 percent of the total children enrolled. In 49 of the 50 states and the District of Columbia, children professionally diagnosed as handicapped accounted for at least ten percent of all Head Start enrollment.

The distribution of handicapped children in Head Start by primary handicapping condition is 61.5 speech impaired; 12.7 percent health impaired; 5.9 percent physically handicapped; 5.7 percent specific learning disabled; 5.1 percent mentally retarded; 4.6 percent seriously emotionally disturbed; 2.9 percent hearing impaired; 2.2 percent visually impaired; 0.3 percent deaf, and 0.2 percent blind.

In 1984, 17.2 percent of the handicapped children enrolled in Head Start had multiple handicapping conditions. Some 18.5 percent of the handicapped children served required almost constant special education or related services, 51.5 percent a fair amount, and 30 percent little or some of these services.

REFERENCES

1. Public Health Foundation. Services for Mothers and Children. Volume 3 of Public Health Agencies 1984. Washington DC. January, 1987.

2. General Accounting Office. Maternal & Child Health Block Grant: Program Changes Emerging Under State Administration. Report to the Congress of the United States by the Comptroller General. U.S. Government Printing Office, Washington, D.C. May 7, 1984.

3. Office of Special Education and Rehabilitative Services, U.S. Department of Health and Human Services. Programs for the Handicapped. Page 6, September-October, 1982, Washington, D.C.

4. Office of Human Development Services, U.S. Department of Health and Human Services. The Status of Handicapped Children In Head Start Programs. Twelfth Annual Report To The Congress. 1985. Washington, D.C.

MEDICAID AND MATERNAL AND CHILD HEALTH, AND PROGRAMS FOR CHILDREN WITH SPECIAL NEEDS

6

Stephen E. Saunders

OVERVIEW

In 1965 Congress passed legislation amending the Social Security Act to create the Medicaid program. Medicaid is financed jointly by federal and state funds and is mandated to provide health care for certain low income persons. It is administered independently by each state within broad federal guidelines. These guidelines specify certain basic services, the extent of coverage and certain administrative requirements. Beyond these guidelines states are given a great deal of flexibility. States must annually submit a State Plan to the Health Care Financing Administration describing services to be provided. Each state has the option to participate in the program; currently all states have a Medicaid program.

Medicaid could be described as a health care program in a welfare environment. The majority of persons eligible for Medicaid are on welfare and are receiving cash assistance to help the bills for food, housing and clothing. Historically, health care in America has been a two-track system; charity care for the poor and fee for service health care for those who could afford it. Medicaid became an avenue for the poor to move into the mainstream of medical care.

Medicaid covers only about 40 percent[1] of all persons defined as living below the federal poverty level. The percentage of the population with incomes below federal poverty who are eligible for Medicaid varies among the states from a low of 25 percent up to 100 percent. In excess of 22 million persons are recipients of Medicaid each year. About two-thirds of the Medicaid recipients are children and their parents, and 30percent of the recipients are elderly or disabled. The majority of recipients are female.

Medicaid has experienced dramatic growth in the number of recipients and total expenditures since its inception. The state contribution to this program is significant, as Medicaid program expenditures account for 10-15 percent [2] of individual state general operating funds. The federal government participation (matching) rate varies between 50 and 82 percent [3] of the total medical costs depending on certain affluence characteristics of the state. The expenditure patterns do not parallel utilization; the elderly and disabled constitute about 27 percent of the recipients; however, they consume in excess of 70 percent of all Medicaid expenditures. [2] (Figures 1 and 2, and Table 1). In fact, individuals in nursing homes are seven percent of the recipients but account for 44 percent of the overall expenditures.

The states control income eligibility levels for Medicaid. Because these eligibility levels vary among states, individuals residing in different states in identical financial situations may not both be eligible for Medicaid coverage. Not all poor people are Medicaid recipients, as income is not the only eligibility criteria. Eligibility categories are either mandatory or optional. Recipients in the mandatory eligibility category must meet income and resource considerations and be in one of the categorical groups—aged, blind, disabled (receiving Supplemental Security Income (SSI), or in a family with dependent children (AFDC). AFDC has two components; financial assistance and medical assistance. Recipients may receive medical assistance only.

The majority of states have elected to include optional eligibility groups and permit people with incomes above the state's welfare categorical level to become eligible for Medicaid. These are called the *medically needy* or *medically indigent*, i.e. they are needy or indigent in part because they are both poor and have higher medical costs than their income can pay. Medically needy persons must also fit the age, disability or dependency categories of AFDC and SSI, must not receive cash assistance, and have incomes that do not exceed 1331/3 percent of the maximum AFDC cash payment in that state. A standard medically needy program allows individuals to qualify once they incur large medical expenses ("spend down") which reduce their net income to welfare levels. Recent federal legislation has allowed additional optional eligibility for certain groups of pregnant women and children. The ranges of income eligibility vary widely among the states [4] — from $1,400 to $10,000 annual income for a family of three (Table 2). There are certain sub-populations of poor people who are not eligible for Medicaid, and these include some adults between the ages of 21 and 65 who are not disabled or pregnant, or poor persons with incomes above welfare levels of the state in which the state does not have a medically needy program.

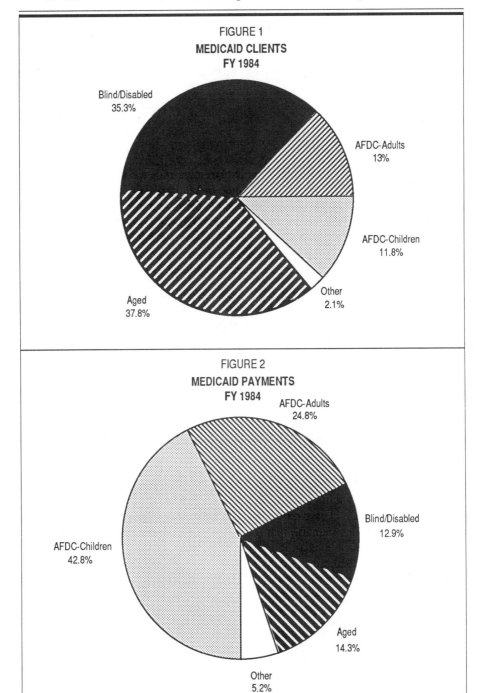

FIGURE 1
MEDICAID CLIENTS
FY 1984

Blind/Disabled
35.3%

AFDC-Adults
13%

AFDC-Children
11.8%

Other
2.1%

Aged
37.8%

FIGURE 2
MEDICAID PAYMENTS
FY 1984

AFDC-Adults
24.8%

Blind/Disabled
12.9%

AFDC-Children
42.8%

Aged
14.3%

Other
5.2%

As the eligibility levels vary, so do the benefits. Each state must cover a pre-scribed set of mandatory services, such as physician services, hospital care, skilled nursing services, and laboratory services. States are permitted to vary the scope and amount of these mandatory services and provide certain optional additional services. There are two ways to expand Medicaid benefits, options, and waivers. Options are federally legislated programs that states may adopt at any time by amending the State Plan. Waivers are arrangements which have legislative authorization and must be approved by the Secretary, Department of Health and Human Services. Both options and waivers are intended to expand a State's program flexibility and to target eligibility and services to specific recipients.

In conclusion, Medicaid consists of 50 separate programs that are administered by the states. Each state decides whether to participate, the eligibility criteria, who is medically needy, what services to cover, and the duration and amount of these services.

HISTORY

The Medicaid legislation was signed into law by President Johnson on July 30, 1965. The passage of this landmark legislation culminated a half-century of struggle for national health insurance. This legislation represented a substantial compromise of the goal of national health insurance. However, it was a major milestone in health care delivery to the poor.

TABLE 1

DISTRIBUTION OF MEDICAID RECIPIENTS, TOTAL PAYMENTS,
AND AVERAGE PAYMENT PER RECIPIENT,
BY ELIGIBILITY GROUP, FY 1984

Eligibility Group	Recipients (number in thousands)		Total Medicaid Payments (amount in millions)		Average Payment per Recipient
AFDC-related Children	9,681	42.8%	$3,979	11.8%	$ 411
AFDC-related Adults	5,599	24.8	4,420	13.0	789
Aged	3,238	14.3	12,819	37.8	3.959
Blind and Disabled	2,913	12.9	11,976	35.3	4,111
Other	1,186	5.2	699	2.1	589
TOTAL	22,617	100.0%	$33,895	100.0%	$1,569

SOURCE: HCFA, Office of the Actuary, 2082 data, FY 1984.

TABLE 2

ANNUALIZED MEDICAID ELIGIBILITY THRESHOLDS'

AFDC, MEDICALLY NEEDY - AS OF JULY 1987

	AFDC Family	Percent of Poverty (%)	Medically Needy Family of 3	Percent of Poverty (%)
Alabama	$1,416	15.2	$ —	—
Alaska	8,988	77.3	—	—
Arizona	3,516	37.8	—	—
Arkansas	2,424	26.1	3,000	35.5
California	7,596	81.7	10,200	109.7
Colorado	5,052	54.3	—	—
Connecticut	6,168	66.3	7,500	80.6
Delaware	3,720	40.0	—	—
District of Columbia	4,368	47.0	5,820	62.6
Florida	3,168	34.1	4,308	46.3
Georgia	3,156	33.9	4,200	45.2
Hawaii	5,892	55.1	5,892	55.1
Idaho	3,648	39.2	—	—
Illinois	4,104	44.1	5,496	59.1
Indiana	3,456	37.2	—	—
Iowa	4,572	49.2	6,096	65.5
Kansas	4,596	49.4	5,580	60.0
Kentucky	2,364	25.4	3,204	34.5
Louisiana	2,280	24.5	3,096	33.3
Maine	6,696	72.0	6,492	69.8
Maryland	4,308	46.3	5,004	53.8
Massachusetts	6,600	71.0	8.796	94.6
Michigan	6,480	69.7	6,444	69.3
Minnesota	6,384	68.6	8,508	91.5
Mississippi	4,416	47.5	—	—
Missouri	3,384	36.4	—	—
Montana	4,308	46.3	4,848	52.1
Nebraska	4,200	45.2	5,400	58.1
Nevada	3,420	36.8	—	—
New Hampshire	5,832	62.7	6,468	69.5
New Jersey	5,088	54.7	6,792	73.0
New Mexico	3,168	34.1	—	—
New York	5,964	64.1	7,400	79.6
North Carolina	3,108	33.4	4,200	45.2
North Dakota	4,452	47.9	5,220	56.1
Ohio	3,708	39.9	—	—
Oklahoma	3,720	40.0	5,004	53.8
Oregon	4,944	53.2	6,588	70.8
Pennsylvania	4,380	47.1	5,100	54.8
Rhode Island	6,036	64.9	7,896	84.9
South Carolina	4,656	50.1	—	—
South Dakota	4,392	47.2	—	—
Tennessee	4,236	45.5	2,604	28.0
Texas	2,208	23.7	3,204	34.5
Utah	8,316	89.4	6,012	64.6
Vermont	7,236	77.8	7,404	79.6
Virginia	3,492	37.5	4,300	46.2
Washington	5,904	63.5	6,804	73.2
West Virginia	2,988	32.1	3,480	37.4
Wisconsin	6,600	71.0	8,268	88.9
Wyoming	4,320	46.5	—	—
Average State	**$4,616**	**49.3%**	**$5,748**	**61.3%**

Efforts to establish a public health insurance system in the U.S. date back to the 1915-18 campaign of the American Association of Labor Legislation, but it was the later efforts during the 1930s to link health insurance to the Social Security Act that was the most important antecedent of the passage of the Medicaid bill. By 1940, President Roosevelt had abandoned the idea of linking health insurance to the Social Security Act because of strong opposition from a powerful medical profession.

During the 1940s, bills to establish a compulsory national health insurance program were regularly introduced into Congress and regularly defeated. In 1949, President Truman personally endorsed a national health insurance bill, the Wagner-Murray-Dingell Bill, that would have covered all medical, dental, hospital, and nursing services, and would have been financed by a payroll tax. Beneficiaries would have included all contributors and their dependents and certain categories of poor people. The American Medical Association conducted a massive public relations and lobbying campaign, which culminated in the defeat of this bill.

Following the defeat of Truman's national health insurance proposal, his chief advisors proposed a federal plan that would limit health insurance to the beneficiaries of the old age and survivors insurance programs, the social insurance part of the Social Security Act. They felt that tying the plan to the social security program would avoid the stigma of welfare and avoid political opposition. During the 1950s, this more limited approach to national health insurance, focusing on the elderly, was similarly unsuccessful.

During the 1960s, advocates continued to push for a program to help the elderly meet the high costs of health care. In 1965, a number of new proposals emerged. By focusing primarily on the needs of the elderly, Representative Wilbur Mills was successful in arriving at a compromise that was acceptable to both organized medicine and representatives from both political parties. This proposal included care for the elderly, as well as certain categorical populations of "deserving" poor. On July 30, 1965, President Johnson signed the bill amending the Social Security Act that created Medicare (a health care insurance program for the elderly) as Title XVIII, and Medicaid (a public assistance program) as Title XIX. Medicaid was envisioned as a lesser program than Medicare. It was intended to pay the cost for medical care for categorically indigent persons other than the elderly, and to supplement the Medicare program.

One of the greatest limitations of the Medicare and Medicaid legislation was the separation of the program of medical care for the poor from the program for the elderly.[4] As a social insurance program, Medicare is paid for by everyone, and ultimately benefits everyone as they reach retirement age. Medicaid is paid for by everyone but benefits only the poorest of society. Medicare has a broad base of political support while Medicaid's base is narrowed. A single social insurance program for the elderly and the poor would have made health care for the poor less vulnerable.

Enactment of the original Medicare and Medicaid legislation was followed by major changes in health care and improvements in the nation's health. In the next 15 years, visits to physicians by poor people rose by 40percent. Access to prenatal care rose dramatically, for example, in 1980, 63 percent [5] of Black women received care during the first trimester of pregnancy, as compared to 42 percent in 1969. Without question, Medicare and Medicaid have improved the access of the elderly and the poor to medical services.

EPSDT

The Early and Periodic Screening Diagnosis and Treatment program (EPSDT) was first proposed in 1965 on the basis of the health status and limited availability of medical care for poor children. In 1969, the concept of this preventive child health program was formally institutionalized with amendments to title XIX of the Social Security Act. Effective July 1, 1969, states were required to provide early and periodic screening diagnosis to Medicaid eligible children under age 21.

The focus of the EPSDT program is prevention and its goals include:[6] prevention of disease and disability; early identification of actual and potential health problems; provisions of early intervention and treatment; and provision of appropriate follow up.

The EPSDT program has several federal requirements. The program must contain an outreach component. All eligible persons must be effectively informed of the existence and nature of the program, as well as how and where services can be obtained. Screening services must be provided to all eligible recipients who request it. A schedule for rendering these services must be devised at the state level. The program must provide for diagnosis and treatment for problems identified as a result of screening, and follow up of these problems must be provided. Assistance with transportation and scheduling of appointments must be provided, if needed. All services must be free of charge.

EPSDT is a unique program within Medicaid. Many public health principles are inherent in the EPSDT program. The program mandates outreach, prevention, and the utilization of a periodicity schedule. EPSDT is now the largest Federal-State preventive child health program in the country. The program is not without problems, as it has a history of under-utilization (in FY 1986, 30 percent of eligible children received examinations) and wide state variation in periodicity schedules which rarely meet the Academy of Pediatrics' recommendations.

There are a number of policy options that states may consider to enhance service delivery to children:

    A. Expand the EPSDT benefit package and periodicity schedule to be consistent with the American Academy of Pediatrics' recommendations.

B. Design different EPSDT benefits package for high-risk populations, i.e. adolescents, chronically ill children, and children in foster care.

C. Develop targeted outreach strategies to specific high-risk populations to assure appropriate utilization of services.

MATERNITY CARE

Unlike EPSDT, there is no specific maternity care program in Medicaid. A growing population of childbearing-age women are entering the ranks of poverty and many will need publicly funded maternity care. Approximately 15 percent [7] of all deliveries are paid for by Medicaid, and it is anticipated this will increase in the next few years. There is a growing body of evidence to support that low-income adolescent and minority women are at greater risk of poor pregnancy outcomes; therefore, Medicaid's importance in maternity care cannot be overstated.

Recently, considerable attention has been directed to MCH care services within the scope of Medicaid. Congress has enacted various legislative reforms to increase the number of pregnant women eligible for Medicaid and to enhance the maternity component of the program. Since 1980, there have been a number of amendments of Title XIX which include:

A. The Deficit Reduction Act of 1984 (DEFRA)—This act mandated state Medicaid coverage to include all children under age five in two-parent families, whose family's incomes and resources meet the state's AFDC financial eligibility test. (Ribicoff children). In addition, any pregnant woman who would qualify for AFDC when her child was born and living with her would be eligible for Medicaid.

B. Consolidated Budget Reconciliation Act of 1985 (COBRA)—This act extended Medicaid coverage to all pregnant women (irrespective of family configuration) with family income levels to AFDC eligibility levels. It allowed states the option to offer pregnant women services that are not otherwise provided under the state plan—for example, nutritional assessment and counseling, psychosocial assessment and counseling, and health education. State's were also permitted to offer case management services. Case management services are defined as services that will assist eligible recipients "in gaining access to needed medical, social, educational, and other services."

C. Sixth Omnibus Budget Reconcilation Act (SOBRA) of 1986—This act provided states the option of extending Medicaid to pregnant women and children under age five, whose family incomes exceeded AFDC eligibility levels but are less than the federal poverty level, thus allowing state's to create a new "medically needy" category of pregnant women and children. Pregnant women in this new medically needy category are limited to pregnancy related services and the duration of coverage is during the pregnancy and 60 days postpartum. Additionally, states are allowed the option of waiving the resource test and initiating a presumptive eligibility process.

Legislation now establishes all poor pregnant women as eligible recipients of Medicaid, if they meet the state AFDC income and resource requirements. Family configurations and/or marital status can no longer affect eligibility. It seems clear that Congress intends that all poor women, regardless of family situation, will receive prenatal and postpartum care.

CHILDREN WITH SPECIAL HEALTH CARE NEEDS

There are a number of program options available to states that will impact on the availability and scope of services for children with special health care needs. The case management option under COBRA, and the potential for increasing eligibility levels up to federal poverty under SOBRA, are examples. States can also expand services available under EPSDT to include any treatment services prescribed by a physician for treatment or amelioration of a chronic condition identified through EPSDT.

In addition to expanding and improving services with program options, states may seek Home and Community Based Long Term care waivers.

A. Home and Community Based 2176 Waiver—The purpose of the section 2176 waiver program is to permit state Medicaid financing of home and community based long-term care services for recipients, who otherwise would require institutionalization. States are given permission to include ventilator dependent individuals. Under the regular 2176 waiver authority, a state also may expand eligibility by raising the income limits or waiving the usual deeming requirements. The basic condition for approval, under a 2176 waiver, is satisfactory documentation that home and community-based services will be less costly than institutional care. A state may provide any of the following services with the assurance that these services are not otherwise furnished under the state's Medicaid plan: home health-aide services, case-management services, personal-care services, adult day-health services, and respite-care services.

B. "Model" 2176 Waiver—This waiver is essentially the same as above but requires the states to waive the deeming requirement, applies to those living at home who would be eligible, if institutionalized, and can include no more than 50 people. This waiver applies in situations where children need hospital or skilled nursing care at home, but are considered ineligible for medical assistance because their family's incomes are above eligibility criteria.

TITLE V - TITLE XIX RELATIONSHIPS

The major publicly funded health programs to address the needs of low-income pregnant women and children, and children with special health care needs, are the Title XIX Medicaid Program and Title V Maternal and Child Health (MCH) Block Grant Program. Historically, Title V has financed a portion of the care for these families; however, it has never been adequately funded to properly address the need, and is not an entitlement program. Title V has financed a number of special projects, including maternal and infant care and children and youth projects. Programs funded under Title V have demonstrated various approaches to the delivery of health care, which have proven to be both effective and cost-effective. Title XIX is a state legislated entitlement program with resources to provide care to a significant number of the MCH population. Title XIX has extensive health care financing experience. Medicaid and MCH agencies are required by regulation to develop interagency coordination agreements that address mutual objectives and responsibilities. Title V and Title XIX agencies need to work cooperatively to maximize the expertise inherent in both agencies and thereby provide high quality preventive, primary, and rehabilitative care to low-income families.

There is no single list of approved roles for Medicaid and MCH agencies; however a number of creative projects and relationships have developed. Programs targeted to maternity care, child and adolescent preventive care, and for special-needs children have evolved.

In 1986, South Carolina initiated a Medicaid High-Risk Channeling Project. In this program all Medicaid maternity patients are risk-assessed and high-risk women are seen by obstetricians, case managed by health department staff, and must deliver in a level II or III hospital. These patients receive additional services, including nutritional assessment and psychosocial assessment. The Title V agency manages the project, provides case management and specialized services, and provides follow-up for one year after the pregnancy. High risk infants also receive specialized care.

In California, secondary to the success of the Obstetrical Access program,[8] Medicaid has adopted the Comprehensive Perinatal Services Program. In this program, Medicaid recipients are eligible to receive a full array of services, including obstetrical, nutritional, psychosocial, health education, and case management. The Title V agency developed the program and the standards, monitors the providers, and provides technical assistance.

Michigan has developed a Maternal Support Services Program. Prenatal care financed by Medicaid will include two types of services: a) medical and b) maternal support services—public health nursing, social work, and nutrition education and counseling. All maternity patients are screened and high-risk women are referred for support services. All maternal support services are provided by the Title V agency, with Medicaid reimbursement.

There are a number of cooperative EPSDT/Title V programs. Title V agencies are involved in outreach, case finding, follow-up and service delivery for EPSDT children. In Colorado, Medicaid contracts with the Title V agency to hire, train and monitor lay outreach workers to provide non-medical case-management services. In Kentucky, Medicaid has adopted standards developed by Title V for its child health program. In South Carolina, MCH is reimbursed by Medicaid for EPSDT case management and provides home visits. In Tennessee, the Title V agency assumes responsibility for follow-up of EPSDT recipients with referable conditions detected by an EPSDT screen. States have the option of providing a special EPSDT component/benefit package for adolescents, which can include targeted outreach and enhanced scope of services. The EPSDT program can also be used to finance creative programs. Minnesota uses EPSDT to help finance high school clinics that provide comprehensive health services for the school population. New York, in its "Child/Teen Health Plan," target children 13-and-older for special outreach, family planning, and pregnancy prevention services.

A number of states have cooperative programming arrangements between the Title XIX agency and the program for Children with Special Health Care Needs. These include the Title V agency developing case management systems, providing multidisciplinary health services to children with special health care needs, and developing programs for ventilator assisted children. In Iowa, the title V agency provides care coordination for all pediatric model waiver clients. Massachusetts has developed an early intervention program that targets high-risk infants at risk of developmental delay. This program is managed by the health department and is available to both Medicaid and non-Medicaid eligible infants.

CONCLUSION

Medicaid and MCH both have a long history of providing health care to mothers and children. Medicaid finances care for low-income, categorically eligible families, with a focus on primary and acute care. Title V has the responsibility to monitor the care of all mothers and children, and historically has had a preventive focus. Public health professionals must become aware of the Medicaid program in their state. An interest and a willingness to work with Medicaid administrators is necessary. By working collaboratively, it will be possible to further improve the accessibility and availability of high quality preventive, curative, and rehabilitative health care for low-income mothers and children.

REFERENCES

1. Myers BA. Social Policy and the Organization of Health Care, Public Health and Preventive Medicare. Edited by J. M. Last. Norwork, Appleton-Century-Crafts, 1986, p. 1659-1660.

2. US Public Health Service: First Six Months of Medicaid Data, Washington, DC, US Government Printing Office, 1986 p. 15-17.

3. Brown RE. Medicare and Medicaid: The Process, Value, and Limits of Health Care Reforms. J Public Health Policy 3(4):335-365, 1983.

4. Hill I. Medicaid Eligibility Threshold for Families and Pregnant Women Information Update. National Governors Association, 1987.

5. Hiatt HH. America Health in the Balance, New York, Harper and Row, 1987, p. 74-76.

6. Rers JS, Pliska SR, Hughes EF. A Synopsis of Federal-State Sponsored Preventive Child Health. J Community Health 9(3):222-239, 1984.

7. Kenney AT, Pittes N, Macros J. Medicaid Expenditure for Maternity Care and Newborn Care in America. Fam Plann Perspect 18(3):103-110, 1986.

8. Lennie AJ, Llun JR, Hausner T. Low Birth Weight Reduced by the Obstetrical Access Project. Health Care Financing Review 8(3):83-86, 1987.

7 CHANGING HEALTH CARE DELIVERY SYSTEMS

Patrick J. Sweeney

The system of health care delivery in the U.S. has changed so dramatically in recent years it is difficult to envision the problems which future providers will face. In fact, the rapidity with which these changes have taken place is part of the problem. Change always creates anxiety and resistance. In the past, major changes in health care delivery occurred gradually, permitting physicians and patients ample time to adjust. The transition from country doctors who primarily treated patients in their homes to office-based specialty practices concentrated in metropolitan areas passed almost imperceptibly through various intermediate stages. In contrast, there is perhaps no other major industry that has undergone the degree of reorganization which the U.S. health care industry has witnessed in the space of less than ten years. Patricelli states, "It is the economic equivalent of an ocean liner turning on a dime."[1] The exponential explosion of scientific and technical advances has been equally dramatic. Indeed, Smith, utilizing the analogy of radioactive decay, defines the half-life of a physician as "the number of years since graduation from medical school when half of the training and knowledge learned has lost its utility and application because of new developments in the field."[2]

Also, with rare exception the changes in medical practice and the scientific discoveries of the past shared two other characteristics which more recent changes have lacked. First, they were considered beneficial by both physicians and patients. For example, knowledge of antibiotics and blood replacement therapy dramatically saved lives which only a decade earlier would have been lost; and, although many patients undoubtedly mourned the loss of the "house call," most probably realized that an office-based practice allowed a physician to be more efficient and effective. In contrast, more recent developments in health care delivery have not been greeted with universal enthusiasm by patients, providers, hospitals, and insurance carriers.

Second, none of the early changes altered the traditional medical hierarchy. The physician remained in control—not only of his practice, but also of the hospital. The doctor's diagnosis was rarely questioned, consent to treatment was more "implied" than "informed," and malpractice was not a significant issue. Clearly this is no longer the case. Health care is big business; total costs for health care are now around $400 billion a year (11 percent of the gross national product).[3] Hospital administrators are usually not physicians, but individuals schooled in business administration and marketing. Even the independence of the private practitioner has been invaded by various regulatory agencies and third-party payers.

The spiraling cost of health care has been perhaps the greatest single factor in effecting change, since competition and the development of alternative delivery systems are among the best-known methods of cost control. Two 1985 articles reported that 80-94 percent of employers offered alternative delivery systems in their benefits packages, clearly indicating a market ripe for change.[4,5] However, health care is a service industry that for various reasons does not conform to general economic theory. The medical market does not respond predictably to such traditional forces as supply and demand, cost/price, competition, and advertising. In fact, Ginzberg believes that in the medical marketplace competition is an opponent, not an ally, of cost containment since it encourages the public to consume more services than necessary.[6]

Changes have occurred in both the public and the private health care systems. This chapter will discuss the advantages and disadvantages of these changes, including the possible implications for the future of maternal and child health.

PRIVATE SECTOR

Traditionally, health care for working-class Americans has been provided on a fee-for-service basis, supported in large part through private health insurance. While far from ideal, health insurance provided families with a certain level of protection against the financial burdens of accidents or illness.

Private health insurance has some advantages. Patients are free to chose their providers, and the premiums may be very reasonable, particularly if the insured is a member of a large group insurance plan, through employment or membership in an organization. Disadvantages include deductibles, co-payments, and a wide range of medical services which may not be covered—e.g. prescription drugs, eyeglasses, office visits, and dental care. Some physicians will not accept or file for direct insurance payment, requiring the patient to assume the full financial burden while awaiting reimbursement.

HEALTH MAINTENANCE ORGANIZATIONS (HMO)

An HMO is a prepaid health plan which provides its members with comprehensive medical care for a pre-established annual fee. Although the term, *health maintenance organization* ,was coined more recently, the concept is not new, having been proposed in the 1930s by the Commission on the Cost of Medical Care.[7] The rapid growth of HMOs was stimulated in 1973 by passage of the Health Maintenance Organization Act, which required employers to offer an HMO alternative to employees. By the end of 1985, 480 HMOs were serving over 21 million people.[8] With a current growth rate of 15 percent per year, membership is estimated to be 40 million by 1990.[9] Many health care economists and administrators, however, believe that HMO growth will soon reach its peak, and that future growth will be through consolidation, as larger HMOs purchase smaller organizations.[10]

Advantages

1. Comprehensive health care. The plan usually covers routine office visits, prescriptions, and diagnostic tests as well as hospitalization.

2. Predetermined fee. There are no deductibles or co-payments, thus eliminating the initial "out-of-pocket" expense for individual subscribers. Often these co-payments and deductibles are substantial. A 1983 survey of 143 large employers found that 80 percent had increased deductibles, 57 percent had increased co-payments, and 50 percent had mandated a second opinion prior to surgery.[11] Capitation payments also simplify budgeting for health care expenditures by employers.

3. Health promotion. Individuals are more likely to obtain routine, preventive health care if it is promoted and covered under the plan. Theoretically, the long-term benefit would be a healthier population which would ultimately decrease the need for more costly therapeutic services.

4. Decreased hospitalization. Due to the high cost of in-patient care, the number of procedures performed in ambulatory surgery centers has increased, permitting the patient to convalesce more comfortably at home barring some complication.

Disadvantages

1. Limited choice of provider. HMO subscribers are required to see physicians employed by the organization; similarly they must receive their in-patient care in the HMO's hospital or the facility with which the HMO contracts for hospital services. This disadvantage is much less significant for individuals whose jobs require them to move about since they are forced to seek new providers with each relocation. In fact, when moving to a new area, membership in a large HMO could provide a measure of reassurance, particularly for families which might require multi-specialty services.

2. Inconvenience. In order to provide services economically, it is important to avoid unnecessary duplication of services. Consequently, an HMO is likely to concentrate its diagnostic services in one facility, which may pose problems of

accessibility for some potential subscribers. On the other hand this, too, could be an advantage since all diagnostic and specialty services would be centralized, simplifying the process of referral and consultation.

Discussion

The HMO's capitation payment system is intended to lower the cost of medical care by providing the physicians with an incentive to be cost-conscious. Under the traditional insurance fee-for-service mechanism, physicians and hospitals are reimbursed independently; physicians receive their usual fees regardless of the cost of diagnostic and in-patient services. Prepaid health plans theoretically encourage their physicians to be frugal and efficient since the organization retains any excess capitation once the total expenses for medical care have been met. The physicians, being salaried employees of the organization, have an obvious vested interest in its financial success.

Initially, critics of prepaid health plans claimed that either by design or by default the poor and the elderly—two groups generally acknowledged as utilizing disproportionate amounts of medical care—were frequently excluded from membership. Although some HMOs now enroll medicaid patients, self-selection remains a significant problem with nearly all studies comparing HMOs with other providers.[12] Efforts to validate cost savings and evaluate quality of care concerns have been hampered by the lack of random patient assignment. HMOs have achieved a certain amount of success in decreasing costs for in-patient care—a success related primarily to fewer admissions and secondarily to shorter lengths of stay.[12,13] However, if HMO members are healthier than the general population, one would expect decreased hospitalization.

In an effort to minimize many of the biases inherent in studies comparing HMOs to fee-for-service programs, Arnould, Debrock, and Pollard [14] compared two groups of patients with respect to total hospital and doctor charges for four specific diagnoses (appendectomy, hysterectomy, cholecystectomy, and herniorraphy). Both groups of patients received their care from a medical staff that provided medical care to both HMO and fee-for-service patients, and the facilities used to provide medical care to both types of subscribers were identical. They found that for all four procedures, surgeon visits and laboratory fees were less for HMO patients and significantly less for two of the four diagnoses. Interestingly, they found no differences in length of stay between the two groups.

Although HMOs emphasize their ability to contain costs, employers frequently give more weight to other HMO advantages. A survey of Fortune 500 companies found that although 82 percent of the companies offered their employees an HMO, they assigned relatively little importance to the system's ability to lower health care costs.[4]

There is evidence to suggest that the presence of an HMO stimulates competition in areas other than premium costs. Conventional insurers may improve their coverage to maintain enrollment. Goldberg and Greenberg [15] have identified three areas in which coverage tends to be expanded when faced with competition from alternative health care systems—coverage for physician visits, hospitalization benefits, and extended maternity benefits.

PREFERRED PROVIDER ORGANIZATIONS (PPO)

Characterized by diversity, PPOs defy simple definition—a situation accurately summarized by a quote attributed to Max Fine, executive director of the American Association of Preferred Provider Organizations: "If you've seen one PPO, you've seen one PPO." [11]   Gabel and Erman provide a fairly general definition of a PPO as "a group of health care providers who agree to provide services to a specific group of patients on a discounted fee-for-service basis." [11]   A PPO may be classified as *limited* or *unlimited*, depending upon whether or not participation is open to all willing providers. The organizational structure of some PPOs has been investigated, and allegations of antitrust violations have already resulted in the dissolution of one California PPO. [9]

While the number of PPOs has increased from 33 in 1982 to 143 in December, 1984, [11] there is evidence that the rate of growth has decreased since that time. [16] The potential market share for PPOs remains speculative and controversial. PPOs currently serve less than 0.5 percent of the U.S. population [11] yet some predict that, by 1995, PPO enrollment will surpass that of HMOs in metropolitan communities. [9] Clearly, there are demographic and economic factors that play a determining role in whether or not an area is conducive for the establishment of a PPO. In 1984, 38 percent of all PPOs were in the State of California, with an additional 21 percent in the three states of Ohio, Colorado, and Florida. Perhaps related is the fact that two of these four states are among the nine states that have passed legislation permitting insurance companies to selectively contract with different providers at different reimbursement rates.

Advantages

1. Patients are not limited to the preferred providers but are encouraged to use them by means of economic incentives. For example, subscribers may have no out-of-pocket expense when utilizing preferred providers, but may only be covered for 80 percent of expenses when treated by non-preferred providers.

2. Patients benefit from the knowledge, bargaining power, and utilization review process of the PPO. Individual subscribers would never have the time or the resources with which to research the cost—much less the quality—of care rendered by local providers.

Disadvantage

PPOs reimburse providers on a "discounted" fee-for-service basis. Since the providers do not assume the financial risk of over-utilization, there is no incentive for individual practitioners to alter their style of practice. In fact, providers can compensate for discounted fees by increasing their patient volume.

Discussion

Although PPOs can be sponsored by various organizations, nearly 50 percent are provider sponsored. Not surprisingly, PPOs have been most successful in areas with excess physicians and hospitals, allowing the PPOs significant bargaining power. Due to the relative infancy of the PPO concept, which originated in California in 1982,[17] little empirical evidence exists to support the claims of either proponents or critics with respect to issues of cost and quality of care.

While the California Medicaid program reported significant savings following the first year of preferred provider contracting, others have found that savings from decreased hospitalization were more than offset by increases in outpatient care.[11] Numerous authors agree that utilization review mechanisms are much more important than price discounts in achieving cost savings.[11,16,18] Similar to the situation with HMOs, PPO evaluations have been criticized on the basis of biased enrollment—i.e. members of PPOs may be more likely to be young, healthy, and employed, and not truly representative of the general population.

INDEPENDENT PRACTICE ASSOCIATIONS (IPA)

The American Hospital Association defines an IPA as an "entity that provides for prepaid health care to subscribers through an arrangement with licensed physicians, dentists, osteopaths, or other health personnel to provide their services in accordance with a method of compensation established by the entity." [19] An IPA represents the solo-practice equivalent of a group practice HMO. IPAs may or may not include risk-sharing arrangements, but most require member physicians to adhere to a predetermined fee schedule.

IPAs also share some similarities with PPOs, in so far as individual providers establish contracts to provide services. IPA enrollees, however, do not have the option to use non-member physicians. This health care delivery hybrid has been studied even less than HMOs and PPOs making any meaningful discussion difficult and entirely subjective.

PUBLIC SECTOR

Just as many changes in the private sector have been economically inspired, public health providers have had to make adjustments in the delivery of MCH services, many of which are directly or indirectly related to issues of cost. With the advent of block grants, the individual states were given more flexibility and responsibility for allocating federal Title V funds among the various MCH programs. In recent years, public health departments have had to contend with budget cuts and employment freezes. Even when program funding levels remained unchanged, increased cost of living, increased cost of services and supplies, and the increased number of medically uninsured persons resulted in a net decrease in appropriations.

DIAGNOSIS RELATED GROUPS (DRG)

During the 1970s, the U.S. Congress realized that action was needed to stem the tide of rising medical care costs. As a result, the government replaced the existing retrospective reimbursement mechanism with a prospective payment system (PPS) for the in-patient care of those patients for whom the federal government was fiscally responsible. Previously, hospitals had been reimbursed on the basis of cost (hospital days, diagnostic tests, medications, supplies, etc.). Under the new scheme, the hospitals are paid a set fee for each diagnosis, the fee being determined by a set of formulas. Hospitals which can provide the service for less than the established rate can keep the excess; if the provision of services costs more than the established rate, the hospital must absorb the loss. The new payment system, based on diagnosis-related groups, became known as *DRGs*.

In 1976, New Jersey sponsored a statewide pilot project to study the feasibility and implementation of a prospective payment system utilizing DRGs. In 1980, 26 hospitals in New Jersey went on the system; an additional 35 hospitals followed one year later. In 1982, the New Jersey system was revamped to take into account variables such as complications and patient age. That same year, Congress passed the Tax Equity and Fiscal Responsibility Act (TEFRA), and on October 1, 1983, Medicare regulations for prospective payment went into effect nationally. Although originally targeted only for Medicare, at least seven state Medicaid programs have now instituted similar prospective payment programs. Other states are planning to do the same. [8]

Initially, 470 DRG categories were established. The U.S. was divided into nine regions, and separate rates were established for urban and rural hospitals within each region. Regional differences in rates were to apply only during the initial three-year phase-in, at which time a single, national rate would prevail.

DRGs are clinically based and, similar to prepaid plans, the predetermined reimbursement schedule should theoretically encourage efficiency. There are multiple problems, however:

1. Some provision must be made for the severity of illness, since some hospitals see more of the severely ill patients, resulting in longer lengths of stay and higher costs per DRG. Teaching hospitals frequently fall into this category.

2. The socio-economic impact on health care must be considered. For example, the medically indigent frequently have minimal (or nonexistent) preventive health programs and thus come to hospital emergency rooms when they are extremely ill. Many of these patients have no homes, and therefore cannot be discharged even though their acute problem has been resolved. The public general hospitals have traditionally been the source of much of the care of the poor.

3. Hospitals may want to attract clinicians who care for a desirable patient population, and be reluctant to give staff privileges to physicians who care for the poor, high-risk, more costly patients.

4. Hospitals may hesitate to cut costs, since their subsequent DRG rate schedule will be based on previous experiences.

5. The system invites discharge-readmission as a means to circumvent the shortened length of stay. Although safeguards are supposed to prevent such manipulation, it is interesting to note that from 1979 to 1982 the length of stay in New Jersey DRG-reimbursed hospitals decreased, whereas it increased in other U.S. hospitals. At the same time, the admission rate per 1000 population in the state increased at four times the national rate.[20]

MEDICARE/MEDICAID

Congress enacted the Medicare/Medicaid legislation in 1965 to help address the issue of access to care for the uninsured poor. The cost of these programs far exceeded original expectations and current estimates indicate that the Medicare Trust Fund will be depleted within ten years.[21] Since 1980, efforts to reduce federal health care expenditures have led many states to cut Medicaid eligibility, and there is evidence to suggest that in some areas health status indicators among the poor are declining. [22,23] Several efforts are currently underway to reverse the effects of these recent cutbacks.

Medicaid Changes

Some states have increased Medicaid payments to physicians in an effort to make Medicaid patients economically more attractive. Also, the Deficit Reduction Act (1984) extended Medicaid coverage to include prenatal care for (a) the woman who would normally be eligible for Medicaid following the birth of her child, and (b) pregnant women in two-parent families if the principal wage earner is unemployed. It has also been suggested that Medicaid eligibility should be independent of eligibility for Aid to Families with Dependent Children (AFDC), and, instead, be based solely on income.

Consolidated Omnibus Budget Reconciliation Act (COBRA)

The 1986 COBRA legislation required Medicare to selectively increase reimbursements to hospitals which cared for a disproportionate share of the medically indigent. This same legislation required employers with more than 20 employees to maintain group health insurance eligibility for the employee for 18 months following termination (three years for dependents, following death, divorce, or loss of dependent status). Finally COBRA established penalties for hospitals that transfer poor, uninsured persons because of their inability to pay—a process deserving the derogative term, *dumping*.

Malpractice

Indirectly, malpractice litigation is undermining long-established health care systems in some areas of the country. Across the nation, more and more family practitioners are giving up their obstetrical practices; their annual number of deliveries simply cannot justify the higher insurance premiums. In much of rural America, these family physicians have been a major source of obstetrical care. Now patients must drive to larger communities where they can seek care from specialists in obstetrics and gynecology. This seemingly simple arrangement poses several problems.

First, it adds or increases to the barrier of transportation. Patients without cars find it difficult to travel within their small communities, much less make monthly/weekly trips to distant cities. Second, obstetricians may not be willing or able to increase their maternity case load, particularly with patients whom they perceive as having significant medical or social risk factors. Third, the specialist's fee is likely to be higher than that of the local family practitioner. Last, if the patient is lucky enough to find a physician to accept her, if she can afford the fee, and if she can arrange transportation, she must also plan to deliver at the hospital where her physician has privileges, not her local community hospital. Small county hospitals which had maintained maternity units for the convenience of the local physicians and residents are happily closing their delivery suites in response to these changing physician practice patterns. In addition, in some areas of the country, some obstetrician-gynecologists are now limiting their practices to gynecology to lessen their risk of litigation.

The threat of malpractice has taken its toll on public health maternity programs in other ways, too. For years, public health providers have established good working relationships with the private physicians in their communities. Each recognized the important contribution of the other toward their common goal—quality health care for their community. Private physicians relied upon the health department to monitor the overall health status of the community and to provide preventive care and routine out-patient health services to the medically indigent. When the health department staff needed assistance—e.g. consultation or hospital admission for a patient—the private physicians willingly assumed responsibility. Recently, some physicians have been advised by their malpractice insurance carriers that they are subjecting themselves to an unacceptable level of risk by assuming responsibility for such patients in whose care they had not previously participated. Thus, nurse practitioners are left without local physician back-up.

MEDICAL EDUCATION

As the delivery of health care becomes increasingly driven by economic concerns, traditional methods of medical education will need to be revised. Hospital in-patients have always been a major teaching resource for medical students. The character of in-patients is likely to change as third-party payors and DRGs encourage fewer admissions and more outpatient surgery. The typical in-patient may be too ill for inexperienced students to be productively involved in their care. Some medical schools have already reported difficulty in finding adequate and appropriate patients for the teaching of history taking and physical diagnosis. [24]

In addition, teaching hospitals generally have higher perdiem costs than non-teaching institutions in the same locale. Unless some provision is made to subsidize the teaching centers, HMOs and PPOs will divert patients requiring hospitalization to lower cost facilities, removing yet another source of teaching material. One logical solution—namely to assign medical students to HMOs and ambulatory surgery centers—may not be feasible or desirable. First, teaching health professions students requires additional time, personnel, and space, and, consequently, additional money which would appear to be self-defeating to an organization established to contain costs. Second, there are not enough HMOs to accommodate all the students, and private practitioners are not likely to assume a greater role in medical education than they currently do. Third, as J.R. Folse points out, "the out-patient surgery setting provides an incomplete educational experience" since it is frequently impossible to arrange for the student to participate in the patient's preoperative evaluation or postoperative care.[25]

IMPLICATIONS

PRENATAL CARE

It is clear that early and adequate prenatal care can reduce the incidence of low birthweight and can improve the outcome of pregnancy, particularly for high-risk women. After a decade of steady improvement, the rate of early registration for prenatal care actually declined between 1981 and 1982, and has remained unchanged since that time. [23] The Institute of Medicine categorized the six major barriers to prenatal care as: [26]

1. Financial constraints
2. Lack of providers
3. Poor accessibility for certain high risk populations
4. Experience, attitudes, and beliefs of some women
5. Lack of transportation and child care
6. Inadequate outreach programs

Clearly, the changes in health care delivery systems discussed in this chapter address only the first two of these barriers, and only as they pertain to those women with some type of coverage. The new systems do not provide for improved access for the uninsured, a significant problem for MCH advocates since "maternity and maternity-related cost is the single most important contributor to the burden of unpaid hospital bills in the U.S. today." [23] As the demand for direct clinical services increases, public health agencies may find it difficult to support such activities as health education and outreach. Many health departments have increased their dependence upon fee income, and consequently have de-emphasized some of the non-reimbursable, preventive health programs. Miller[27] reported on the staffing and financing of several health departments and found that the minimal revenue derived from fees was not worth the expense of billing and time spent determining eligibility. The report states that the public health stance with relation to fees must be clarified or "we risk distorting health services in favor of whatever it is that third parties may be willing to reimburse, and neglecting some of the most critical interventions for achieving favorable health outcomes." [27] If economic considerations continue to be the driving force in health care decisions, emphasis must be placed upon the cost-benefit estimates of prenatal care and the potential savings which can be realized by decreased neonatal intensive care and lifetime rehabilitative services.

ADVOCACY

Public health professionals and administrators will have to assume an even greater advocacy role with respect to these new systems of care. As increasing numbers of HMOs and similar plans enroll Medicaid-eligible patients, some mechanism must be in place for evaluating the quality of care provided to these patients. Although reports to date are few, the available evidence indicates that the quality of care varies considerably. [27]

MALPRACTICE

Fears of litigation are severely limiting access to maternity services in some areas. In many cases, the impact is equally felt by the paying and non-paying patients. As more and more physicians stop seeing pregnant patients, those who continue to provide maternity care will not be able to absorb all of the additional patients. Logically, if a physician must limit his/her practice, the first group to be eliminated will be the uninsured. If the private sector cannot resolve the liability crisis, the government will have to impose some regulations and restrictions. Other alternatives would include: (a) government subsidies for malpractice premiums for those physicians providing care to the uninsured poor, (b) a federal malpractice insurance plan, or (c) immunity from litigation for physicians in cases involving federally funded patients (ethically, very questionable).

SUMMARY

Twenty-years ago we were concerned with access to health services to the poor. Medicare and Medicaid effectively addressed that issue, but proved to be expensive solutions. Now the emphasis is on cost containment, yet preliminary results following the first few years of prospective payment, HMOs, and PPOs suggest that successful cost-cutting may adversely affect access for the indigent.

Although hospitals and physicians enjoyed relative prosperity under the traditional fee-for-service system, they were also able to cross-subsidize and cover some of their losses due to unreimbursed care. As revenues decrease secondary to capitation and prospective payment, hospitals will no longer be able to subsidize charity care, resulting in ever-increasing numbers of uninsured patients being referred to tax-subsidized institutions. Concomitantly, the number of public community hospitals will decrease as they either close their doors or are purchased by large health care conglomerates. Competition in the health care marketplace has been credited with the potential to reduce costs and maintain quality. However, the competition is only for those who can pay—no one is competing for the poor!

Many discussions of recent health care changes concentrate on the problems and tend to be pessimistic. In addition, the rising cost of medical education, the predicted over-supply of physicians, the limitations on physician autonomy, and the liability crisis have led to a concern over the possibly decreased attractiveness of medicine as a career. Nevertheless we are living in exciting times, and those who choose to enter the health profession will doubtless be rewarded. The turn-of-the-century physician will have at his/her disposal diagnostic and therapeutic modalities which only a few years ago would have been considered science fiction. The real challenges of the future are for the private and public health care administrators—namely how to pay for the increased technology while maintaining quality of and access to health services for all segments of our society.

REFERENCES

1. Patricelli R. Musings of a blind man - reflections on the health care industry. Health Aff (Millwood) 5:128, 1986.

2. Smith EP. Measuring professional obsolescence: a half-life model for the physician. Academy of Management Review 3:915, 1978.

3. Guest DB. Health care policies in the United States. Can the American way succeed? Lancet 2:997, 1985.

4. Gardner SF, Kyzr-Sheeley BJ, and Sabatino F. Big business embraces alternate delivery. Hospitals 59:81, 1985.

5. Powills S. Business needs spur HMO, PPA growth. Hospitals 59:98, 1985.

6. Ginzberg E. Sounding board–the destablilization of health care. N Engl J Med 315:757, 1986.

7. Feldstein PJ. Health Care Economics, second edition. New York, John Wiley & Sons, 1983, p.327.

8. Gilman TA and Bucco CK. Alternative delivery systems: an overview. Top Health Care Finance 13:1, 1987.

9. Riffer J. PPO networking up; HMOs grow 15 percent. Hospitals 58:52, 1984.

10. Traska MR. HMOs: a shake-up (and shakeout) on the horizon? Hospitals 60:40, 1986.

11. Gabel J and Erman D. Preferred provider organizations: performance, problems, and promise. Health Aff (Millwood) 4:24, 1985.

12. Hornbrook MC and Berki SE. Practice mode and payment method - effects on use, costs, quality, and access. Med Care 23:484, 1985.

13. Frank RG and Welch WP. The competitive effects of HMOs: a review of the evidence. Inquiry 22:148, 1985.

14. Arnould RJ, Debrock LW, and Pollard JW. Do HMOs produce specific services more efficiently? Inquiry 21:243, 1984.

15. Goldberg LG and Greenberg W. The competitive response of Blue Cross and Blue Shield to the health maintenance organization in northern California and Hawaii. Med Care 17:1019, 1979.

16. Powills S and Weinberg W. PPAs: a new payment system evolves. Hospitals 59:43, 1985.

17. Sellers KG. To PPO or not to PPO? Hospitals 58:110, 1984.

18. Boland P. Questioning assumptions about preferred provider arrangements. Inquiry 22:132, 1985.

19. American Hospital Association: Hospital Administration Terminology, Second Edition. Ameri   can Hospital Publishing, 1986.

20. Stern RS and Epstein AM. Institutional responses to prospective payment based on diagnosis-related groups. N Engl J Med 312:621, 1985

21. Ginzberg E. The restructuring of U.S. health care. Inquiry 22:272, 1985.

22. Calkins DR. Assuring access in a changing health care system. Bull NY Acad Med 63:93, 1987.

23. Council on Maternal and Child Health: National Association for Public Health Policy: Background paper on universal maternity care. J Public Health Policy 7:105, 1986.

24. Egan RL. Recent events of special interest to medical education. JAMA 256:1549, 1986.

25. Folse JR. Changes in the health care system: implications for surgical education, Adapting Clinical Education to New Forms and Sites of Health Care Delivery. Edited by RF Jones. Washington, DC, American Association of Medical Colleges, 1987, p. 24.

26. Institute of Medicine: Preventing Low Birthweight. Washington, DC, National Academy Press, 1985, pp. 8-10.

27. Miller CA. An agenda for public health departments. J Public Health Policy 6:158, 1985.

CHANGING PROFESSIONALS IN MATERNAL AND CHILD HEALTH

8

George A. Little and Charlotte T. Houde

Philosophy and practice surrounding pregnancy, birth, and childcare have been passed down through centuries and generations. Historically, women prevailed as the keepers of this wisdom. Hippocrates instituted what is thought to be the first training program for midwives in the fifth century B.C. Until the 18th century, physicians played virtually no role in the conduct of normal labor and birth, being called upon only to assist with difficult situations, offering interventions that were often destructive to the fetus and aimed at saving the life of the mother. Issues of convention, acceptable behavior, and perhaps preference of women kept men out of the realm of women and infants.

The midwife in colonial America was a respected and valued member of the community. However, as formal medical education developed and women were deemed intellectually incapable of such study, the midwife was displaced by a more scientific and technical approach to childbearing. Childbirth was increasingly recognized as complex and potentially dangerous. More and more upper and middle-class American women sought out physician and hospital care. By 1930, the portion of deliveries done by midwives in the home had declined to 15 percent.[1,2] By 1987, these deliveries declined to one percent.[3]

This century has seen an ongoing effort in the professional and lay litera-ture to make the public aware of the significant needs of women and children. Provider roles were expanded or developed to support these efforts. For example, the Sheppard-Towner Act provided grants for the training of public health nurses and midwives.

149

During the 1950s and 1960s, sociologic trends competed with each other. Lamaze childbirth began its rise in New York City, while women in many major U.S. medical centers were being managed in labor by "twilight sleep" and amnesic sedation. Several influencing factors emerged in the 1960s and 1970s: the Feminist Movement, sensitizing women to their rights as women and mothers; and the consumer health care movement which, in addition to increased awareness of knowledge and technology, had four major concerns: a) the rising cost of health care, b) consumer activism, c) the demand for personalized care, and d) the childbirth education movement.

The convergence of these ideals led to many women seeking to claim autonomy over their bodies and their childbearing and childrearing experiences. Birth was to be a family affair, with sibling and extended family involvement. Further, some parents began to question the need for vaccines and innoculations and refused their children organized schooling, preferring to teach them at home.

In recent decades, federal funding and grant support from organizations such as the Robert Wood Johnson Foundation and the National Foundation-March of Dimes led to the education of nurses at advanced levels of clinical specialization, nurse midwives, pediatric nurse practitioners, family nurse practitioners, and clinical specialists. Master's level programs led to the preparation of nurses as clinical scholars. Concern about primary care also stimulated federal funding of physician residency programs having such an emphasis.[4,5]

OBSTETRICS AND GYNECOLOGY

The specialty status of obstetrics emerged in the 1800s during a series of advances and controversies. Puerperal sepsis was expounded upon by no less than Oliver Wendell Holmes in 1848, but the contagiousness theory remained subject to question and disregard for years. Anesthesia, developed in the U.S., received its seal of approval for childbirth when Queen Victoria inhaled chloroform during childbirth in 1853. Cesarean section with uterine suturing became more common. By 1876, an American Gynecologic Society had been founded and most American medical schools had a department of obstetrics.

The 1910 Flexner report on American medical education was not kind to obstetrics, and the subsequent report of John Whitridge Williams, later of textbook fame, was also critical. Too many students were seeing too few obstetrical patients and many professors were not competent in clinical procedures. Rapid change occurred, and by 1931 there were 83 residency programs and outside review was a matter of course. In 1988, there are 281 programs with approximately 4,550 residents of which 46 percent are women. The American Board of Obstetrics and Gynecology was founded in 1927 and incorporated in 1930 by the American Association of Obstetricians and Gynecologists and Abdominal Surgeons, the American

Gynecologic Society, and the Section of Obstetrics and Abdominal Surgery of the American Medical Association.

The American College of Obstetricians and Gynecologists (ACOG) can trace its direct roots to 1951, when it was organized as a national body of individual members. Indirect roots are represented by the many local and regional ob/gyn societies which began decades ago. The American Medical Association (AMA) Section on Obstetrics and Gynecology held its first meeting in 1860. ACOG began as an academy but changed its name in 1956 to a college by membership vote. A constitution states the organization's purposes as:

a. To establish and maintain the highest possible standards for obstetric and gynecologic education and postgraduate education in medical schools and hospitals, obstetric and gynecologic practice and research.

b. To perpetuate the history and best traditions of obstetric and gynecologic practice and ethics.

c. To maintain the dignity and efficiency of obstetric and gynecologic practice in its relationship to public welfare.

d. To promote publications and encourage contributions to medical and scientific literature pertaining to obstetrics and gynecology. [2]

The Nurses' Association of the College of Obstetricians and Gynecologists was organized in 1967 as an integral part of ACOG.

Maternal-Fetal Medicine

Three subspecialty divisions of the American Board of Ob/Gyn were formed in 1972: Gynecologic Oncology, Reproductive Endocrinology, and Maternal-Fetal Medicine. Maternal-fetal medicine is of special interest not only for its role in high-risk pregnancy but also for its role in regional perinatal care. The well-documented trend toward earlier, i.e. intrauterine, diagnosis of perinatal pathology suggests that the maternal-fetal medicine practitioner and investigator will be in considerable demand. Estimates suggest that approximately 500 maternal-fetal subspecialists will be available in 1990, and that needs will approximate 750.[6,7]

The Future

An AMA Council on Long Range Planning and Development has concluded that four major issues are presently not resolved: the professional liability crisis, medical practice competition, the feminization of poverty, and ethical issues.[8] Ob/gyn, with its unique involvement with the medical aspects of reproductive behavior, functions at the interface of social mores, application of knowledge, and changes in the role and perception of women. The specialty will be progressively feminized, as ACOG women fellows increase from about five percent of the total in 1975 to more than 20 percent in the 1990s. The years immediately ahead will undoubtedly see continued buffeting by medical, ethical, and socio-economic issues.

PEDIATRICS

Pediatrists, now called pediatricians, emerged in significant numbers toward the end of the nineteenth century. The AMA formed a Section on Pediatrics in 1880. The American Pediatric Society dates from 1888. By 1930, there were about 1,500 pediatricians seeing children exclusively and 2,000 other physicians with a chief interest in the field.

The first federal formula grant program, the maternal-infant targeted Sheppard-Towner Act of 1921, had a major impact on organized pediatrics. At a meeting in 1922, the AMA's pediatric section supported the act; the parent body vigorously opposed it. The open disagreement resulted in an AMA House of Delegates reprimand of the Society and an instruction that it deal only with social functions. Historians argue that, although it took eight years to occur, the organization of the American Academy of Pediatrics (AAP) in Detroit, in 1930, resulted in large part from that confrontation.

The American Board of Pediatrics was formed by action of the Executive Committee of the AAP, the American Pediatric Society, and the Section of Pediatrics of the AMA. Certification by the Board became a requirement for membership in the AAP, after 1937. In 1937, the Academy accepted two principles concerning health legislation:

1. Practicing pediatricians and organized pediatrics should be consulted when health legislation is proposed.
2. Public funds should be used to support maternal and child health services for those unable to pay.[9]

Membership in the AAP included 22,160 fellows in 1987. Women have always been better represented than in other specialties, and now exceed 1/3 of academy membership.

Neonatal-Perinatal Medicine

This subspecialty, commonly called *neonatology*, emerged in the 1960s and 1970s and has had a major influence on its parent specialty and upon perinatal care. In the late 1980s, it seems apparent that future decreases in perinatal mortality and morbidity statistics are more likely to result from prenatal care and obstetric management than neonatal intensive care. However, increased survival of very low-birthweight babies in particular, the presence of chronically ill babies, and the decreased involvement of pediatricians in the care of sick newborns at Level II hospitals has resulted in considerable demand for neonatologists. There were 1,509 neonatologists practicing in the U. S., in 1983, and there has probably been a steady increase since that time; considerable debate has taken place concerning what is an appropriate number.[10,11]

The Future

There is considerable debate about the present and future role of the pediatrician. The specialty has grown proportionately faster than many others, and is youthful. Eighty percent of patients are ten years of age or younger, although the specialty has recently emphasized its role with adolescents. By the year 2000, the number of patients per pediatrician is predicted to decrease to approximately half of the figure that it was in 1970. The so-called "new morbidity" reflects an increased emphasis on areas such as growth and development, adolescent medicine, school health, chronic and handicapping conditions. Changes in organization of health care and reimbursement have had and will continue to have a major impact on the practice of pediatrics, with the number of independent solo and small group practitioners predicted to continue to decrease. A fundamental determinant will be the degree of societal response and commitment to pediatric medical problems of diffuse organic and socio-economic causality.[12]

FAMILY AND GENERAL PRACTICE

Family and general practice are not synonomous. Family practice is said by its academy to be the "continuing and current expression of the historic medical practitioner and is uniquely defined within the family context." The American Academy of General Practice was founded in 1947, with a name change to American Academy of Family Practice (AAFP) occurring in 1971. The ABFP (American Board of Family Practice) was established in 1969 as the 20th medical specialty and the first to require periodic recertification.

The ratio of general to family practitioners in the U.S. approximates 4:2.5 (Table 1), while the ratio within the AAFP of family practice residency graduates

---

TABLE 1

FEDERAL AND NON-FEDERAL PHYSICIANS BY SPECIALTY

1985

Pediatrics 35,617

Obstetrics/Gynecology 30,867

Family Practice 40,021

General Practice 27,030

Physician Characteristics and Distribution in the U.S.,
1986, American Medical Association: Chicago.

to non-family practice graduates is 1:1. These ratios have changed, and will continue to change, rapidly as the age distribution curve of family practitioners is sharply skewed to the young. About 50 percent of graduates of residency programs include obstetrics in practice. Approximately nine percent of family practice office visits are represented by the under-15 years patient, a figure that is somewhat smaller (< 1 percent) than for other physicians. Routine prenatal examination ranked 6th and well-baby examinations 15th in the order of office visits reported by the AAFP for 1985 (derived from U.S. Dept. of Health and Human Services unpublished data).[13]

The Future

A number of issues related to the role of family/general practice in the health of women and children are active. There is some indication that while the AAFP aggressively asserts that obstetrics is a part of the specialty, the actual number of family practitioners attending deliveries may be decreasing. The liability insurance crisis appears to be impacting family practice in some locales, with significant numbers discontinuing involvement in hospital delivery if not prenatal care. Family practice and pediatrics seem to have competing roles in some areas, such as well-baby care. The specialty will continue to play an important role in MCH but that role may not increase proportionately.

NURSING

In recent decades, the nursing profession has seen, and probably will continue to see, more change in roles than in medicine. Concurrently, nursing has engaged in a more active policy and research role.

Traditionally, maternal and child nursing has focused on inpatient services, support of physicians in practice, and clinic and public health activites. The changes in maternity and neonatal nursing care in the last 25 years have impacted greatly on the role of the nurse. As technology has advanced in tandem with the demand for family-centered care, perinatal nurses are under increasing pressure to provide care and education in an environment valuing economic efficiency and decreased length of stay.[14,15] Inpatient pediatric nursing care is subject to similar pressures.

The nursing profession has been tapped to provide individuals with clinical and administrative skills who can function as nurse-coordinators with care teams and programs. The growth of numbers and diversity of these roles has benefited programs but contributed to the general shortage of nursing personnel.

Extended or Modified Nursing Roles

The rapid emergence of modified nursing roles in MCH is especially noteworthy. In the 1960s and 1970s physicians were considered to be in short supply and availability of primary care, especially in rural areas and among the disenfranchised, was a growing problem. Pediatric Nurse Practitioners (PNP) appeared in

1965 and a literature devoted to acceptance and efficacy followed. The neonatal nurse clinician/practitioner represents an example that functions in an intensive care environment.

Certification in maternal and child nursing is becoming routine for both the more traditional roles, as well as the extended or modified role. The Nurses Association of the American College of Obstetricians and Gynecologists (NAACOG) joined with The American Nurses' Association (ANA) in 1973 in a joint program which lasted until 1978, when the organizations parted company. Internal Revenue Service rulings that membership fees cannot be used to support certification led to a separate NAACOG Certification Corporation (NCC), which in 1988 was involved in certifying many roles. The ANA has a certification process for many fields, including several in MCH. (Table 2)

NURSE MIDWIFERY

Since the first school of nurse midwifery in the U. S., the number of educational programs has grown to 26 schools, preparing approximately 250 nurse midwives annually. There are currently 3000 certified nurse midwives, including about 15 males. The professional organization, the American College of Nurse Midwives (ACNM), was formed in 1955 as a formal governing body. It also functions as an accrediting and certifying agency.

A Certified Nurse Midwife (CNM) is an individual educated in the two disciplines of nursing and midwifery, who possesses evidence of certification according to the requirements of the ACNM. Practice includes the independent management of pregnancy-related care for normal women and newborns within a health care system which provides for medical consultation, collaborative management and referral.

TABLE 2

SELECTED CERTIFICATION EXAMINATIONS FOR MCH NURSE ROLES—1988

NAACOG Certification Corporation	American Nurses' Association
Inpatient Obstetric Nurse	Pediatric Nurse (Child and Adolescent)
Low Risk Neonatal Nurse	Maternal-Child Nurse*
Neonatal Intensive Care Nurse	High Risk Perinatal Nurse*
Ob/Gyn Nurse Practitioner	School Nurse
Neonatal Nurse Clinician/Practitioner	Pediatric Nurse Practitioner
	Family Nurse Practitioner
* to be redefined in 1989 as Perinatal Nurse	School Nurse Practitioner

The nurse midwife provides individualized care to low-risk women in a family-centered environment. Responsibilities include preconceptional and prenatal care, including nutrition education, evaluation of progress, management of labor and delivery, and evaluation and immediate care for the normal newborn. She helps the mother to care for herself and for her infant, to adjust the home situation with the new child, and to lay a healthful foundation for future pregnancies through family planning and gynecological services. The CNM remains with women during labor, providing continuous physical and emotional support and is prepared to teach, interpret, and provide support as an integral part of her service.

The practice of nurse midwifery has generated passionate consumer support within its clientele and heated debate in the professional realms. A body of research includes physician acceptance, patient acceptance, safety of practice, patterns of utilization, and cost-effectiveness. Issues of competition, collaboration, professional turf and role relationships create the framework for the developmental process of the profession.[16,1,6]

OTHER HEALTH CARE PROVIDERS

A number of other relatively new roles, including the Physician Assistant (PA) and the Child Health Associate (CHA), provide maternal and child health care. These individuals do not necessarily have nursing backgrounds. CHAs have three years of training after a minimum of two years of college, and have diagnostic and therapeutic responsibilities. There are approximately 7,000 PNPs and 200 CHAs practicing. A National Commission on Certification of Physician Assistants provides credentialing. CHAs also take an examination of the Colorado State Board of Medical Examiners.

Social workers are important providers of assistance and often are actively involved in counseling of MCH patients. Their role has also involved progressively more responsibility, including decision-making and interventions.

Lay midwives attend a portion of home deliveries. (Table 3) The number of lay midwives has decreased considerably since the earlier days of this century, as physicians and, to a lesser extent, CNMs have assumed responsibility for deliveries in the hospital. Interest in the role seems to remain at a relatively low but continuing level.

PUBLIC HEALTH AND ADMINISTRATION

Discussion of roles in MCH would be incomplete without acknowledgement of the importance of individuals with special interest and ability in program development, administration, and public health. The availability of graduate study in MCH, often leading to a Master of Public Health (MPH), has enhanced the sophistication of roles in this field. Entry to such study is commonly undertaken by individuals with backgrounds in medicine and nursing.

CHANGING PRACTICE ENVIRONMENT

Obstetric services have been impacted remarkably by the family-centered movement of the 1970s. The publication of *Family-Centered Maternity/Newborn Care in Hospitals,* in 1978, by ACOG, AAP, NAACOG, AMA, and NAPNAP (National Association of Pediatric Nurse Associates and Practitioners) represents a specific point in a long-term process. Hospital inpatient services have changed, and the roles of the professionals within them increasingly reflects a different attitude toward the birth experience.

Birth centers, in concept and form, reflect this attitudinal change and are seen in many hospitals. In 1975, The Maternity Center of New York pioneered a new concept, *The Childbearing Center,* as alternative to conventional care. A survey identified 93 centers and there continues to be interest in such alternatives. For the most part these centers are owned and operated by CNMs, but some were opened by obstetricians and included participation by CNMs and family practitioners.[17]

Planned home delivery now accounts for less than one percent of U. S. births. (Table 3) This very significant change in practice parallels an historic decrease in perinatal mortality and morbidity, and most authorities believe there is an association. Some, however, feel that home birth practice can be safe and appropriate. Advocates generally maintain that hospitals or birthing centers remain less than optimal because of loss of control, overuse of technology, and restriction on family involvement. There is some evidence that economic considerations and access to care are factors in out-of-hospital deliveries. For example, illegal aliens may account for a large portion.

TABLE 3

UNITED STATES BIRTHS OUTSIDE HOSPITALS

1940 — Approximately 44 percent of all births

1984 — Approximately 1 percent, or 38,900, of which:

- 9,300 M.D. attendant
- 17,100 "midwife" attendant
- 10,000 certified nurse midwife
- 7,000 lay midwife
- 12,500 "other" attendant (about 1/2 unplanned home delivery)

— **derived from**: Pearce, W. Parturition: Places and Priorities.
Am. J. Pub. Health 77:8, August 1987.17

Outpatient care is receiving the same emphasis in MCH as elsewhere and roles are being expanded and adjusted accordingly. Length-of-stay postpartum has been steadily decreasing, for example, necessitating specific attention to either home or office visits for the mother and neonate. Home care is emerging along the entire spectrum from prenatal management of high-risk pregnancy to home care for ventilator dependent children. The creation and reconfiguration of managed health care plans has changed the source of care for many patients, but as yet has not had a major impact on roles themselves.

The changes in non-physician roles have been both fostered and resisted by physicians. Some of the original impetus for expanded roles is no longer present as physicians are now not considered to be in short supply. Specific concerns, such as rural areas, seem to be experiencing relief through an influx of pediatricians and family practitioners. Availability of obstetric specialty care may remain problematic as availability may not approximate earlier predictors, as residency numbers are less than anticipated, and as obstetricians are pressured by liability concerns.

Involvement of the U. S. Office of Technology Assessment, in a report (1986)[18] directed toward quality and cost of care provided by NPs, PAs, and CNMs, is symbolic of the interest and importance of the subject. Considerable professional and patient experience and acceptance of collaborative practice models, such as obstetrician-midwife and pediatrician-pediatric nurse practitioner, suggest that these models will persist in the private and public sectors. Distribution of non-physician personnel in independent practice seems less likely to expand greatly.

REFERENCES

1. Tom S. The evolution of nurse midwifery, 1900-1960. J. Nurse Midwifery 27:4-12, 1982.

2. Speert H. Obstetrics and gynecology in America: a history. American College of Obstetricians and Gynecologists, 1980.

3. Pearce WH. Parturition: places and priorities. (Editorial) Am. J. Pub. Health 77:8, August 1987.

4. Diers DK. Preparation of practitioners, clinical specialists and clinicians. J Professional Nursing pp. 41-47, Jan-Feb 1985.

5. Lynaugh J, Gerrity P and Hogopian G. Patterns of practice: Master's prepared nurse practitioners. J Nursing Educ 24:291-295, Sept 1985.

6. Merrill JA. (Sub) specialization in obstetrics and gynecology: results of a survey by the American Board of Obstetrics and Gynecology. Am J Ob and Gyn 156:550-557, March 1987.

7. Pearce WH. Manpower in Obstetrics and Gynecology. Study Sets. Washington, American College of Obstetricians and Gynecologists, 1977-87.

8. Council on Long Range Planning and Development. The future of obstetrics and gynecology. JAMA 258:3547-3553, 1987.

9. Cone TE. History of American Pediatrics. Boston, Little, Brown and Company, 1979.

10. American Academy of Pediatrics, Committee on Fetus and Newborn: Needs in neonatal pediatrics. Pediatr 76:132-34, July 1985.

11. Merenstein GB, Rhodes PG and Little GA. Personnel in neonatal pediatrics: assessment of numbers and distribution. Pediatr 76: 454-456, September 1985.

12. Council on Long Range Planning and Development: The future of pediatrics. JAMA 258:240-245, 1987.

13. American Academy of Family Physicians: Facts About Family Practice. Kansas City, 1987.

14. Stolte K and Meyers ST. Nurses' responses to changes in maternity care. Part I. Family-centered changes and short hospitalization. Birth 14:82-86, 1987.

15. Stolte K and Meyers ST. Nurses' responses to changes in maternity care. Part II. Technological revolution, legal climate and economic changes. Birth 14:87-90, 1987.

16. Gatewood TS and Stewart RB. Obstetricians and nurse midwives: the team approach in private practice. Am J Ob/Gyn 111:111-118, 1971.

17. Rooks JB and Fischman SH. American nurse midwifery practice, 1976-1977: reflection of 50 years of growth and development. Am. J. Pub. Health 70:990-995, 1980.

18. US Congress, Office of Technology Assessment. Nurse practitioners, physicians' assistants and certified nurse midwives: policy analysis. Washington, DC, US Government Printing Office, Dec 1986.

|❚ PROFESSIONAL LIABILITY 9

Daniel K. Roberts and Elvoy Raines

INTRODUCTION

Maternal and child health (MCH) encompasses a variety of dynamic issues, causingthe field to be one in which change is commonplace. Such change has been quite positive, for the most part, reflecting advances in knowledge and technology, and the overall capacity of the field to deliver the very best of care in continually improved settings and circumstances. However, the process of evolution also has presented painful dilemmas, ranging from unprecedented ethical challenges to questions of resource allocation. Perhaps the most difficult of issues to arise in recent years concerns the professional liability of physicians.

Health care professionals in MCH should be accountable for their performance, and every indicator suggests that they are, indeed, engaged daily in objectively evaluating their ongoing performance as part of quality assurance, peer review, and credentialing activities. Unfortunately, as the professional liability system has affected health care professionals in recent years, the consequence is not the positive product that those systems seek.

The history of medical professional liability suggests previous periods of concern and sudden changes in the impact of the law upon medicine, yet the 1970s and 1980s have revealed a new propensity to litigate differences, resulting in significant increases in the frequency and severity of claims. Evidence suggests that the result has been a measurable impact upon the availability and accessibility of

MCH care, and upon its quality and cost. Health care policy makers have now joined physicians and other professionals in calling for reform, both internally and externally.

A HISTORY OF MEDICAL PROFESSIONAL LIABILITY

ORIGINS OF THE CONCEPT AND EARLY LITIGATION

The concept of holding health care providers—specifically physicians—legally accountable for their acts is not new. [1] The first recorded case in English common law alleging medical malpractice occurred in 1375. [2] Medical malpractice litigation was common enough by 1518 to warrant inclusion of disciplinary provisions for malpractice in the charter of incorporation of the College of Physicians of London. [3]

In the U.S., the first case arose in 1794 [4] and there have been recurring periods of sharp increases in litigation. Between 1900 and 1940, for example, there were 1,296 medical malpractice cases filed, and nearly 40 percent of those cases occurred between 1930 and 1940. [3] During those earlier periods of litigation fervor, explanations for the steep increases were several that today sound familiar: increased patient expectations, improvements in diagnostic procedures, and erosion of the physician-patient relationship, especially in large urban centers.

THE CRISIS OF THE 1970s

After World War II, there began a gradual increase in claims against physicians. By 1974, there was a sudden increase in the frequency of claims, catching many insurers unprepared and ultimately driving them from the market. The result was the first medical malpractice insurance "crisis," a "crisis of availability." [5] Suddenly, physicians found it difficult to obtain professional liability insurance coverage *at any price*; it simply was not available.

Because of the obvious public health impact, states responded quickly, passing more than 300 state statutes in an attempt (1) to curb the rise in claims and size of awards, and thereby reduce the cost of insurance; (2) to assure the availability of insurance by creation of Joint Underwriting Associations and patient compensation funds; and (3) to enable new entrants into the insurance market, including physician-owned or sponsored insurance companies. [6]

Many existing commercial companies converted their policies from occurrence to claims made, to allow for more certain annual confirmation of losses. [6] Physicians and their medical societies also entered the insurance market, and more than 30 physician-owned or sponsored companies were established. [6]

Coincidental to all this activity, a brief lull in litigation against physicians occurred between 1975 and 1978, causing many to assume that the reforms and new programs had effectively "solved" the medical malpractice crisis.

THE CRISIS OF THE 1980s

The crisis returned in the 1980s, as frequency and severity (size) of claims once again began to increase. This time, it was not a crisis of availability, but rather a "crisis of affordability."[7] Both commercial insurers and physician-owned companies experienced unprecedented losses, causing them to raise their rates more frequently, and by larger increments. [8] Between 1982 and 1985, the cost of professional liability insurance for all physicians rose 81 percent; for obstetrician-gynecologists, 113 percent. [9]

The total amount physicians spent on professional liability insurance premiums increased from $2.4 billion in 1983 to $3.8 billion in 1985. [3] Average premiums skyrocketed, increasing for Ob-Gyn's from an average $10,900 to $23,300 per year. [10] In some states, the figures were substantially higher: in Florida, for example, the average reached $92,830 for Ob-Gyn's. [11]

CURRENT TRENDS IN FREQUENCY AND SEVERITY OF LITIGATION AGAINST PHYSICIANS

Frequency

Claims filed against physicians more than doubled between 1967 and 1975.[12] After the lull of 1975-78, the increase was renewed. Since 1978, the upward trend has continued for all physicians, with special impact upon Ob-Gyn's, as illustrated in Table 1.[12]

TABLE 1

**FREQUENCY OF CLAIMS AGAINST PHYSICIANS, 1978 - 1985.
CLAIMS PER 100 PHYSICIANS PER YEAR.**

Time Period	All Physicians	Ob-Gyn's
Prior to 1981	3.2	7.1
1981-1984	8.2	20.6
1985	10.1	26.6

Physicians were not alone as targets of litigation. Hospitals experienced more than a doubling of claims frequency between 1980 and 1985, from 2.1 to 4.3 claims per 100 occupied beds.[13]

Severity

Not only were there more and more claims filed, but the amounts of claims, awards and settlements also grew. In the 1970s and 1980s, the severity of claims increased faster than inflation, at an average annual growth rate of 25 percent.[14] The average paid per claim increased approximately 54 percent between 1982 and 1985; during the same period, the Consumer Price Index increased only 11 percent, and the Medical Care Price Index increased 23 percent.[15]

In 1984, there were 73,000 claims "closed," or resolved, with only 43 percent resulting in payments to claimants.[16] The total indemnity paid for the 32,000 claims which resulted in payments amounted to $2.57 billion.[16]

IMPACT UPON OBSTETRIC AND GYNECOLOGIC CARE: AVAILABILITY, ACCESSIBILITY, QUALITY, AND COST

For MCH, the consequences of the continuing professional liability problem amount to more than dollars and cents. There is a clear and immediate impact upon the scope and cost of services, their accessibility to the full range of patients in need, and, arguably, the quality of what remains available. For these reasons, resolution of the problem is demanded more for public health and welfare, than for economic stability.

Availability

The American College of Obstetricians and Gynecologists has twice surveyed its Fellows, seeking information about the impact of litigation and high insurance rates upon the scope and manner of practice.[17] In the most recent study, 35 percent of the respondents reported modification of their practice as a direct result of these pressures.[17] They report having reduced the number of deliveries performed (14 percent) and the amount of high risk obstetrical care provided (23 percent). Twelve percent have discontinued obstetrical practice altogether.

In a similar study in 1984, the American Academy of Family Physicians found that 21 percent of their respondents had restricted their obstetrical practice rather than pay higher insurance fees.[3]

If the number of high-risk pregnancies or obstetrical cases were declining, such restrictions might not have such an impact, but with steady demand, restriction of practice only limits availability of needed care.

Accessibility

Access to care is further restricted as physicians either become more selective as to who they will treat, or treat only those patients able to pay fees high enough to absorb rising overhead costs associated with increasing insurance premiums. As a result, low-income patients, including Medicaid recipients, state and local public health department patients, and the medically indigent, are hardest hit. They are also most likely to be in need of high-risk care, because of their socio-economic and environmental circumstances.

Quality

It is difficult to assess at this point the degree to which restriction of the scope of practice has affected quality. Theoretically, however, it appears inevitable that quality will decline. If board-certified Ob-Gyn's are driven from the health care marketplace, and their family practice colleagues follow, surely nurse-midwives, nurse practitioners and others will experience the same pressures. As each successive layer of available expertise is reduced, quality will suffer accordingly.

Cost

The first and most apparent impact upon cost of health care comes in the direct costs associated with increases in insurance premiums. To the extent that they can, physicians pass through the increased costs in the form of increased fees. Professional liability insurance added $3.02 per inpatient day to the cost of hospitalization in 1983; by 1985, the figure had risen to $5.60. The average annual cost per bed for professional liability insurance rose from $1,000 in 1983 to $1,784 in 1985. [13]

Perhaps a greater impact is felt in indirect cost consequences, as physicians alter their practice behaviors by adoption of "defensive medical practices," those "practice changes in response to increased claims risk." [18] It has been established that the indirect cost of defensive medicine amounts to more than $10 billion per year. [19]

Prospects for Change

Reform is gradually occurring, both within the health care system and in the tort law arena. In the medical profession, strengthening of credentialing and licensure procedures is complemented by risk management, quality assurance, and peer review activities. Improved primary and continuing medical education for risk identification and reduction is becoming more widespread. All are targeted at reducing the risk of actual compensable injury.

Tort reform efforts are also continuing, as well as investigation of alternatives to litigation for resolution of disputes. It is clear to health care policy makers that the existing systems cannot continue to bear the burden of alleging and proving "fault" in order to achieve effective and efficient compensation for injuries and deterrence of substandard practice.

CONCLUSION

Professional liability introduces a destabilizing influence upon MCH which is not unprecedented, but is complicated in its consequences. Physicians and other health care professionals must and will be held accountable for their performance, but the system applied in the past is one which must evolve as dynamically as the specialty it affects, in order to keep up with the needs and interests of both providers and patients.

As the frequency and severity of litigation continue to increase, the reaction of health care providers will continue to include those behavior modifications which result in a restriction of the availability and accessibility of care; ultimately quality will suffer; and in the course of such changes, the cost of MCH care will be unnecessarily inflated. For these reasons, improvements both internal and external to the systems are desperately needed.

REFERENCES

1. See Reed. Understanding tort law: The historic basis of medical legal liability. J Legal Med, Oct 1977; Amundsen: The liability of the physician in classical Greek legal theory and practice. J Hist Med, April 1977.

2. Stratton v. Swanlond, Y.B. 48 Edw. 3, f. 6, pl. 11 (1375); see generally Chapman: Stratton v. Swanlond: The fourteenth century ancestor of the law of malpractice. Pharos, Fall 1982.

3. United States Department of Health and Human Services: Report of the Task Force on Medical Liability and Malpractice, GPO 190-412/70133, August 1987.

4. Cross v. Guthrie, 2 Root 90 (Conn. 1794).

5. United States Department of Health, Education, and Welfare: Medical Malpractice: Report of the Secretary's Commission on Medical Malpractice, DHEW Pub No (OS) 73-88, Jan 16, 1973.

6. Danzon. Medical Malpractice: Theory, Evidence, and Public Policy. Cambridge, MA, Harvard University Press, 1985.

7. Raines. Professional liability in perspective. J Obstet Gynecol 63(6):839-845, June 1984.

8. American Medical Association: Professional Liability in the '80s: Report 1. AMA Special Task Force on Professional Liability and Insurance, October 1984.

9. United States General Accounting Office: Medical Malpractice Insurance Costs, GAO/HRD-86-112, August 1987.

10. American Medical Association: Socioeconomic Monitoring System Surveys, Chicago, IL, 1984-1986.

11. American Medical Association: Socioeconomic Monitoring System Surveys, Chicago, IL 1986.

10. American Medical Association: Socioeconomic Monitoring System Surveys, Chicago, IL, 1984-1986.

11. American Medical Association: Socioeconomic Monitoring System Surveys, Chicago, IL 1986.

12. American Medical Association: Socioeconomic Characteristics of Medical Practice, Chicago, IL 1986.

13. United States General Accounting Office: Medical Malpractice: Insurance Costs Increased but Varied Among Physicians and Hospitals, 1986.

14. Danzon. New Evidence on the Frequency and Severity of Medical Malpractice Claims, 1986.

15. Bureau of Labor Statistics, United States Department of Labor, Consumer Price Index cited in National Center for Health Statistics, Public Health Service, Department of Health and Human Services, Health: United States 1986.

16. United States General Accounting Office: Medical Malpractice: Characteristics of Claims Closed in 1984, April 1987.

17. American College of Obstetricians and Gynecologists: Professional Liability Insurance and Its Effects: Report of a Survey of ACOG's Membership, Washington, DC, 1983 and 1985.

18. Hershey. The defensive practice of medicine: myth or reality. Milbank Mem Q 50:69-97, 1972.

19. Reynolds, Rizzo, Gonzalez. The cost of medical professional liability. JAMA 257:2776, 1987.

ETHICAL ISSUES IN MATERNAL AND CHILD HEALTH

10

Thomas E. Elkins

This chapter outlines many of the concepts and theories that form a base for biomedical ethic considerations in maternal and child health (MCH). Rather than consider one or two issues in detail, a construct is presented of ethics and its relationship to medical decision-making and development of health care policy in MCH.

In the spring of 1985, the Committee on Bioethics for the American College of Obstetricians and Gynecologists was asked to list their three major areas of concern in biomedical ethics for the coming decade. The three areas mentioned were:

1. Maternal-fetal rights (including abortion, genetic counseling, prenatal care guidelines, fetal therapy, fetal surveillance, controversies in labor and delivery, etc.);

2. New reproductive technologies that allow childbirth without traditional family arrangements or intimacy (including surrogate parenting, artificial insemination, in-vitro fertilization, embryo transfer, basic infertility management, etc);

3. Factors involved in the contemporary allocation and availability of health care resources (including health care for the indigent, marketing of medicine, government financial constraints, pre-payment health care plans, the malpractice crisis, the international concern about maternal mortality in the third world, etc.).

This chapter will briefly describe a framework of ethical analysis that may be of help in using theories of ethical thinking to address ethical concerns in contemporary health care. This chapter discusses the following aspects:

I.   Principles of Biomedical Ethics
II. Influencing Factors
III. Normative Guidelines
IV. The Recognition of Ethical Issues
V.   Individual Physician Responsibilities

I. PRINCIPLES OF BIOMEDICAL ETHICS

Principles of biomedical ethics remain important in medical decision-making in MCH today. Those principles include (at least): (1) autonomy, (2) non-maleficence, (3) beneficence, and (4) justice. Because of the brevity of this chapter, it will not be possible to describe these principles in detail but some explanation about them should be included.

1. Autonomy

Autonomy is a form of personal liberty of action where the individual determines his or her own course of action in accordance with a plan chosen by himself or herself.[1] Autonomy is also a basic concept of political freedom. Since the 1960s, autonomy has become a forceful term in biomedical ethics that has fostered such documents as the American Hospital Association's statement of patients rights.[2] Autonomy is also seen as the basis for the contemporary emphasis on informed consent in medicine. Multiple case precedents in Anglo-American law have defined a doctrine of informed consent intended to protect bodily integrity, privacy, and individual autonomy. The elements of informed consent generally include:

a. the ability of patients to act voluntarily;
b. the provision of information in simple language about the risks of procedure or treatment, the proposed benefits,the alternative to the treatment the chances of failure if not treated;
c. the mental capacity of patients to understand;
d. evidence that the patient understands the information given; and
e. evidence that the patient actually made a decision regarding the treatment proposed.[3]

2. Non-Maleficence

The second principle, that of non-maleficence, is defined as being generally related to the maxim, *primum-non-nocere*, above all, do no harm." The principle of non-maleficence has been notable since at least the age of the Hippocratic Oath, i.e., "I will use treatment to help the sick according to my ability and judgment, but I will never use it to injure or wrong them."[1] The principle of non-maleficence is involved in discussions of such issues as euthanasia, both active and passive, and involves terminology as "optional" versus "obligatory" treatment, "ordinary" versus "extraordinary" care, and "killing" versus "letting die." The question of whether or not to provide long-term intensive and invasive nursery care for a non-responsive but living infant is another such issue in MCH.

3. Beneficence

The principle of beneficence means very simply "wishing the good for another." Throughout time, physicians have been identified for their compassionate approach to patient care. The principle of beneficence also has limitations. In contemporary MCH, the wide availability of technological advances may foster the temptation to provide technological assistance even when it would be hopeless in terms of improving a clinical condition. These considerations always lead to cost-benefit analysis on the part of some ethical advisors, or to quality-of-life discussions by others. For example, the gynecologic infertility specialist who feels led by a patient's desperation to offer repetitive pelvic infertility surgery, even when the chance of success is extremely minimal, is experiencing one inherent difficulty in attempting to practice solely by the principle of beneficence.

4. Justice

The principle of justice is best defined in terms of fairness, and may be separated into categories which relate to individual justice or distributive justice, that refers more to the proper distribution of social benefits and burdens.[1] Certainly one of the major ethical problems facing MCH today is the provision of care that is equitable, or even available, to all segments of society, including the medically indigent. A recent issue involving this principle is the unnecessary transfer of indigent patients to public hospitals from more profit-oriented institutions.[4]

Each of these principles may become problematic if assumed to be absolute. In most medical decision-making, different bioethical principles can be shown to be in conflict.[5] Decision-making occasionally becomes a matter of balancing the value of different principles and understanding the controversial aspects and limitations inherent to each principle.

II. INFLUENCES

Multiple external influencing factors are not considered by physicians in almost every medical decision. Contemporary medical decision-making is being influenced by a wide range of factors that may also shape the ethical analysis being considered in a given situation. Some of these influences are briefly described below with mention given to their effect in MCH.

1. Technology Rapidly changing technology has been the trademark of MCH over the past 20 years. However, some advances have created new ethical concerns, as well. An example is the development of fetal surveillance methods that have greatly elevated the status of the fetus as a patient during the same era in which a concern for women's rights has seen abortion made legal. Changing limits of fetal viability and technology that now offer documentation of fetal heart rates, fetal breathing movements, and amniotic fluid volumes have all brought ethical concerns for the fetus into greater prominence.

2. Societal Input During the past several years, since the value of ethics committees was suggested in a courtroom during the Karen Quinlan case, society has been requesting and receiving more input into medical decision-making. The Federal Register recently suggested infant care review committees that included non-medically trained persons. Such individuals are thought to be able to more accurately reflect the societal viewpoint, and give insights into coping mechanisms and capacities that may be overlooked in the objective assessment of a medical problem by medical professionals. However, it represents the most direct attempt to date to interject societal opinion into the arena of medical decision-making. The sudden rise of ethics committees in our society makes it almost certain that they will be much more in evidence in the future.[6,7]

3. Cultural Influences The concern for rights of women has created a notable change in consumer-oriented MCH care. The physician especially concerned about such influences may be more likely to provide care that is heavily weighted on the side of total autonomy. The extent to which patient demands are followed by physicians may create ethical dilemmas in patient care. For the concerned physician, performance of cesarean section on request may be as problematic as performance of a cesarean section against a mother's will. This is only one example of the many ways in which changing cultural viewpoints may result in ethical concerns in medical decision-making.

4. Religious Factors Whenever religious factors are discussed, the obstetrician and pediatrician offer the example of Jehovah's Witness patients. While most would agree that deep religious convictions should be respected in almost every situation, in the case of the Jehovah's Witness patient competing values exist among physicians responsible for their care. Their commitment to the Hebraic Maxim "to save a life" is in direct conflict with the willingness of the devout Jehovah's Witness to die rather than accept blood transfusions. Religion will remain a controversial ethical topic in medicine when it results in competing understandings of personal autonomy.

5. Economic Factors Physicians today are under great pressure to provide marketing that will allow their practices to thrive in a consumer-oriented society. One of the major ethical debates in medicine over the past ten years has been whether or not health care professionals should publicly advertise.[8] Another economic factor frequently debated has been "should medical professionals form unions?"[9] New physician payment plans that promote non-hospitalization and still demand quality health care represent yet another economic factor influencing ethical decision-making.[10]

6. Governmental Factors   The advent of DRG's (diagnostic related groups) and the increasing number of federal regulations dealing with health care potentially interfere with the physician's ability to provide that care he or she thinks best for their patients. The ethical issue of the rights of the individual, when in conflict with the rights of society, to husband its resources is as yet unresolved.

7. Legal Parameters and Precedence   During the past 20 years, state legislators and case law experts have become extremely interested in medical decision-making. A physician training in a field related to MCH must be prepared with knowledge of key legal decisions. Certainly the controversial Roe vs. Wade decision governing much of our abortion and maternal/fetal rights dilemmas must be understood. Others, however, are becoming equally important. The recent Conroy case in the New Jersey Supreme Court defines new precedents about the right to die for an individual.[11] The ongoing discussion in numerous states about sterilization of persons who are mentally handicapped defines more clearly the issues involved in sterilization when no informed consent is possible, but such a procedure seems to be desirable to family and health care providers.[12] The Infant Doe legislation helps to clarify those situations in which euthanasia might still be permissible in the neonatal nursery in our society, although still leaving much of the burden on the physician's reasonable judgment.[13] The list of important legal concepts includes a thorough understanding of malpractice tort laws and the concepts of contract responsibility and negligence. These would appear to be essential features in training of the contemporary health care professional and have a marked influence on bioethical decision-making in medicine.

8. Ethics, Codes, and Statements   In 1980, the American Medical Association revised its *Principles of Medical Ethics* to create a document that recognized the importance both of patients' rights and community responsibility. The principles clearly defined that a physician had a responsibility not only to patients, but to society, to other health professionals, and to self, enhancing a need for conscience and integrity in actions. Even more recently, the President's Commission for the Study of Ethical Problems in Medicine and Biomedical and Behavioral Research published, in 1982 and 1983, insights into ethical dilemmas that directly affect MCH policies. The American College of Obstetricians and Gynecologists has now published policy statements concerning the ethical issues involved in: commercial ventures in medicine, surrogate motherhood, informed consent, pregnancy counseling, new techniques in fertilization, sterilization, induced abortion, and perinatal research. These stand alongside the Ethical Considerations in the Practice of Obstetrics and Gynecology found in the handbook of Standards for Obstetric-Gynecologic Services.[14] For the health care provider to function in coming years it will probably be imperative that some introduction be provided to the concepts in these documents. They provide some of the history of the "traditions and events that shaped people's behavior and attitudes in and out of medicine." Moral problems arising out of health care policy for indigent care, treatment of the handicapped newborn infant, or in-vitro fertilization cannot be truly understood or even intelligently approached without a sense of this history. Any ethical analysis that neglects prior human experience is bound to be superficial or abstract.[15]

III. NORMATIVE GUIDELINES

Normative guidelines are concepts to be considered in medical decision-making. These include:

1. Burdens vs. Benefits A consideration of Burdens vs. Benefits resulting from any medical decision is an appealing method of analysis. "Burdens" may include physical harm, financial costs, family stress, the need for societal support, and the availability of care for any given patient. "Benefits" would be a similar list of positive effects. This method of analysis may also be problematic. For example, although such reasoning can be fairly clear in discussions of risks and benefits for some emergency surgical procedures, it becomes very uncertain when an issue such as the withdrawing or withholding of life sustaining treatment is in question, since the calculation of the benefit of human life is rarely clear.[16]

2. Sanctity of Life vs. Quality of Life Normative Thinking This normative guideline has become extremely controversial in the past decade in America. The extreme sanctity of life norm is based on the religious conviction that man, valued as one created in the image and likeness of God, must be preserved in any state and at any cost. It is a norm usually associated with the pro-life, anti-abortion movement. The converse position is that life without quality is life without value. However, attempts to quantify quality of life predictions have been controversial. The compromise legislation in the Infant Doe rulings of 1986 overruled the sanctity of life viewpoint by adding terminology that allowed non-treatment of patients when, in the reasonable medical judgment of the physician, such treatment would be inhumane.[13] However, such legislation did not include an option to make critical care decisions solely on the basis of predictions of future quality of life.

3. The Best Interest of the Patient Norm This guideline was championed as a guide to decision-making by the American Academy of Pediatrics throughout the 1982-85 series of court hearings and debates over federal regulations regarding withdrawing or withholding life-sustaining treatment in neonatal nurseries.[17] It served a purpose in clarifying family, physician, health care institution, government, and societal interests as being distinctly different on occasion from the interests of the newborn.

Other normative guidelines, such as *The Golden Rule*, treating others as one would like to be treated, although enhancing compassion and responsibility could still be problematic in a pluralistic society.[18] Ethics by consensus, or seeking to further define a "reasonableness standard" seem equally non-exact pathways to decision-making.[19] All of these guidelines for thinking are dependent upon accurate medical information. It will be essential for the physician of the future to seek adequate consultation in order to provide patients, families, and society with information that is technically accurate and ethically appropriate.

IV. A RECOGNITION OF ETHICAL ISSUES

Perhaps the most important task of any study of biomedical ethics in maternal and child health is to identify the issues of ethical concern. [20] In a recent pilot curriculum program, a lecture series covering major issues was supplemented by frequent conferences concerning ethical issues pertinent to particular patient management situations. However, when an ethicist was present for routine patient rounds, it became obvious that almost every medical issue had ethical components as well. Routine counseling for spontaneous abortions suddenly became a concern because of the lack of emphasis placed upon the recognition of a grief response. Contraceptive counseling for an early adolescent flared the controversy between paternalism and autonomy. The indigent patient requesting infertility surgery, the sexually abused child, the single parent requesting artificial insemination, the pregnant patient refusing to stop smoking, the alarming rate of maternal mortality in developing countries, the laboring patient refusing fetal monitoring...all become objects of ethical concern. Therefore, in MCH, the study of medical ethics is essential, although it will never be simple, or easy.

An understanding of ethics in MCH does not provide a road map to a "right answer," but provides an adequate framework for reflection that will insure thoughtful, reasonable medical decisions and health care policies, even in the face of controversial issues.

V. CONCLUSIONS:
INDIVIDUAL PHYSICIAN RESPONSIBILITIES

In the final analysis, the above principles and guidelines, with all their presumptive powers, do not remove the physician from a central position as a responsible, moral agent in health care. Although philosophers have debated the extent of the physician's role as a moral agent, rather than as a technician, few would eliminate such a role entirely in favor of society and/or individual patient autonomy.[21]

In an era of increasing concern about biomedical ethics, the physician of the future will become more involved in such dilemmas. A new emphasis in medical education must address the gap in knowledge and understanding that most practicing physicians feel when faced with biomedical ethics issues in order that the physician will be able to use ethical principles and norms, and knowledge of other influences as resources for decision-making.

REFERENCES

1. Beauchamp TL, Childress JF. Principles of Biomedical Ethics. New York, Oxford University Press, 1979.

2. Annas G J. The Rights of the Hospital Patients: The Basic ACLU Guide to a Hospital Patient's Rights. New York, Avon Books, 1975.

3. Meisel A, Roth L, Lidz CW. Toward a Model of the Legal Doctrine of Informed Consent. Am J Psychiatry 134(3):285-289.

4. Schiff RL, et al. Transfers to a Public Hospital: A Prospective Study of 467 Patients. N Eng J Med 314(9):552-7, Feb. 27, 1986.

5. Chervenak FA, McCullough LB. Perinatal Ethics: A Practical Method of Analysis of Obligations to Mother and Fetus. Obstet Gynecol 66(3):440-446, 1985.

6. Cranford RE, Doudera AE. The Emergence of Institutional Ethics Committees. Law, Medicine, and Health Care, Feb. 1984, pp 13-20.

7. Rosner F. Hospital Medical Ethics Committees: A Review of Their Development. JAMA 253 (18):2693-5, 1985.

8. Veatch RM. Ethics. JAMA 245(21):2187-9, 1981.

9. Marcus SA. Trade Unionism for Doctors. N Eng J Med 311(23):1509-11, 1984.

10. Showstack JA, Stone MH, Schroeder SA. The Role of Changing Clinical Practices in the Rising Costs of Hospital Care. N. Eng J Med 313(19):1201-1207, 1985.

11. In the Matter of Clarie C. Conroy, 98 N J 3211, 486A 1209 (1985).

12. Haavik SF, Menninger KA. Sexuality, Law and the Developmentally Disabled Person. Baltimore, Paul H. Brookes Publishing Co., 1981, pp 105-150.

13. Child Abuse Prevention and Treatment Act and Child Abuse Prevention and Treatment and Adoption Reform Act Amendment of 1984, Pub L No 42, 98-457 (October 9, 1984).

14. American College of Obstetricians and Gynecologists: Standards for Obstetric-Gynecologic Services, Sixth Edition, Washington, D.C., pp 98-100.

15. Ryan KJ. Ethics in Obstetrics and Gynecology. Am J Obstet Gynecol 151(7):840-843, 1985.

16. Gerry MH. The Civil Rights of Handicapped Infants: An Oklahoma Experiment. Issues in Law and Medicine. 1(1):15-68(23-24), 1985.

17. American Medical Association. Physicians Opinion on Health Care Issues: 1984. Chicago: Survey and Opinion Research, September, 1984.

18. Clements CD, Sider RC. Medical Ethics' Assault Upon Medical Values. JAMA 250(15):2011, 1983.

19. Englehardt HT. Current Controversies in Obstetrics: Wrongful Life and Forced Surgical Procedures. Am J. Obstet Gynecol 151(3):313-318, 1985.

20. Weil WB. Issues Associated with Treatment and Non-Treatment Decisions. AJDC 138:519-522, 1984.

21. Englehardt HT. The Physicians as Moral Agent: Closing Reflections in Philosophical Medical Ethics: Its Nature and Significance. Edited by Stuart F. Spicker and H. Tristram Englehardt, Jr, Boston: D. Reidel Publishing Co, 1977 p. 245.

❚❙ THE CONCEPT OF RISK $\quad$ 11

Donald A. Cornely

INTRODUCTION

Developing classifications of subgroups within a population is a frequent and useful task in public health. The parameter chosen as the basis for a classification permits discriminating among subgroups of the population in relation to one or more conditions, diseases or health status. Many simple (uni-dimensional) classifications, especially those using demographic characteristics of a population, have multiple applications. As classifications become more complex, either by using multiple parameters or based on specific biological or behavioral characteristics, they are intended to reflect a specific association with a stated condition.

Risk refers to an increase in the probability of developing a disease, disorder, or diminished health status associated with the presence of attributes or qualities of individuals or their environment. These characteristics, known as *risk factors*, vary in their distribution within a population and may also vary in the level or strength of their association with a stated condition. Risk factors operate to change the equilibrium among forces which produce the condition and are not themselves the etiologic basis of the condition. When the risk factors are aggregated for an individual or groups in a population, they generate a range or scale of vulnerability from low to high. While any one risk factor may have a meaningful association with several distinct conditions or disorders, the nature and level of association will vary by the condition under discussion.

A single risk factor may have an independent influence on the occurrence of a condition. Risk factors, however, usually interact to exert their influence and thus call for a multifactorial form of analysis to assign a risk rating to an individual or population in relation to a stated condition. Implicit in the concept of risk factors and risk ratings is the understanding that there exist other factors having the effect of lowering the vulnerability or probability of developing a condition. The latter attributes or qualities, sometimes called *protective factors*, may operate simply by competing with risk factors, or could function by modifying risk factors directly. Indeed, one of the common purposes of risk determination is to identify individuals to receive targeted therapeutic interventions which, when effective, can lessen or remove the risk associated with the factors prior to therapy. It follows that in drawing inferences about the association of risk factors to a condition, the effect of subsequent care or management must be considered. While some risk factors are themselves immutable, e.g. age, gender, race, socio-economic status; others are amenable to being changed, e.g. hemoglobin levels, blood lead levels. The immutable risk factors, however, are susceptible to having their association with the condition modified.

CONCEPTUAL BASIS OF RISK

Many risk factors are initially identified through clinical observation, and require an appropriately controlled population based study to establish the legitimacy of their association with the stated condition. Frequently, the mechanism by which a risk factor exerts its influence on a condition is not understood. Some risk factors are viewed as pre-disorder states, e.g. elevated blood cholesterol in relation to cardiovascular disease.

Two concepts underlie the development and use of risk, correlation between an attribute and a condition or disorder, and predictive validity. Correlation refers to the level and direction of association between two variables, in the case of risk, one variable would be the risk factor and the other variable being the stated condition. Correlation coefficients are indexes both of the strength and direction of an association. A risk factor would always require that the correlation coefficient is positive, while a negative correlation could represent a protective factor. Having demonstrated a significantly high and positive correlation between a quality or attribute and a condition, it is necessary to develop a classification which stratifies the population along the dimensions of the risk factor, i.e. either its presence or absence, or by the quantitative level or dose of the risk factor. Should the condition under discussion itself have implicit levels or degrees, it is possible that the correlational analysis must examine levels of the risk factor against levels of the condition. If obesity is understood as a risk factor for the development of hypertension, it is possible that levels or stages of obesity are associated not simply with the presence or absence of hypertension but with levels of the latter.

The second concept of importance in considering risk factors and risk ratings is that of predictive validity. Sattler [1] in referring to predictive validity, indicates it addresses the question whether a test score or attribute of an individual accurately predicts future performance on a stated criterion. An essential feature of predictive validity is the time interval between the identification of the attribute, test score or quality present in an individual and later performance. Time, with the many possible influences that could intervene between risk status identification and the later condition of interest, represents an important dimension in the application of the risk concept. Establishing factors as risk factors for a condition not expected to appear until much later in time requires attention to the intervening circumstances which could have the effect of modifying the association. Again, therapeutic interventions are examples of circumstances influencing the basic association between a risk factor and a condition. Other examples, not necessarily involving therapy as intervening, are risk status early in pregnancy changing as pregnancy proceeds, relating obesity in childhood to development of hypertension in later years. In both examples, other risk factors could develop apart from therapy and change the association. The need for multifactorial analyses is again made evident.

A particularly important consideration with reference to children is the concept of *tracking*. Some biological traits found in young children maintain a consistency of presence over long periods of time, extending into adult ages, and some such traits are risk factors for conditions found in adult life. Tracking is defined by Webber et al. [2] as the tendency for an individual to retain a consistent rank on a trait in relation to his peer group over time. Tracking has been demonstrated in children for cardiovascular risk factors (anthropometric measures, blood pressure and serum lipid values) in relation to the development of atherosclerosis and hypertension several decades later. [3] The importance of the observations on tracking in children is the awareness that many useful risk factors are easily accessible and measurable (anthropometry, blood pressure), and the potential for intervention to reduce the probability of conditions not anticipated to appear, perhaps, for several decades later.

EXPRESSING RISK STATUS

Associations between one or more risk factors and a stated condition are most commonly expressed using correlational statistical methods. Simple linear relationships can be identified using the correlation coefficient where values above the .35-.50 level indicate a fair to moderate relationship. [4] At times, *Odds Ratio* and *Relative Risk* are used to distinguish risk in a group having exposure to the risk factor compared to a group without exposure to the risk factor.

Because individuals and groups in a population possess multiple risk factors in relation to a given condition, and because the relationship among these factors is not always simply additive, multivariate techniques are necessary to demonstrate important variables or to delineate groups by the clustering of risk factors associated with respective groups. Factor analysis or principle component analysis are techniques used for reducing multiple risk factors whose association with the condition in question are interdependent. Where multiple risk factors are not interdependent, the association of the respective factors could be demonstrated using a stepwise multiple regression technique. [5]

Once one or more risk factors have been identified as having an important level of association with a condition, there remains the problem of applying that information in clinical and administrative programmatic activities. Creating an index to capture in a summative manner, the total risk represented by all risk factors present in an individual, is frequently employed. Rules of evidence for declaring an association between one or more risk factors and the condition must be kept in mind to avoid spurious associations and to assist in drawing inferences. Ibrahim [6] offers useful guidelines to avoid such problems and also provides several examples using risk concepts in developing health policy.

In developing an index which utilizes several risk factors to achieve a single summary score, the issue of differential weighting for individual risk factors must be considered. Commonly, clinical experience and judgment are initially utilized to assign a weight to various risk factors anticipated to occur in an individual or in a group of patients in association with a specific condition. Hobel [7], for example, developed a risk rating for pregnant women which has intended to discriminate among a population of pregnant women as to their risk of specific pregnancy outcomes. Hobel used a dichotomous weighting scheme in which some risk factors carried twice the weight of other risk factors in arriving at an overall risk rating of pregnant women during prepartum and intrapartum periods. His initial assignment of weights for each risk factor was drawn from clinical experience. Guidance in assigning different weights to each of several risk factors would be available by using a multivariate technique. Occasionally, an established risk index is modified either in the clinical setting or in administrative programmatic activities by substituting risk factors for those in the established index, or by adding new risk factors. These improvisations jeopardize inferences from such data since interrelationships among risk factors can change the level of prediction or association with the condition under question. Again, attention to rules of evidence for associations among variables (risk factors) is important to ensure legitimacy of associations.

USE OF RISK CONCEPT IN MCH

The concept of risk and the use of risk factors and risk ratings are important considerations in MCH because of the long association of this field of public health with personal health services and continuing efforts to define vulnerable subgroups within the population of children and childbearing age women. Since risk involves an association with a condition separated by time, the powerful influence of physical growth and developmental functions unique to fetal, infant and adolescent age groups on the association must be carefully assessed. Changes unassociated with disease or therapy and representing the unfolding of normal inherent capacities could modify an association between a risk factor and a stated condition. The need to have a longitudinal perspective, awareness of the range of normality as growth and development proceeds, and appreciation of the measures used to characterize risk factors at differing stages of growth and development are considerations which can influence the inferences drawn from what otherwise appears as a simple association between risk factors and the condition under study.

Colton[4] calls attention to the exceptional opportunities to identify risk factors and to develop risk profiles by using vital statistical data. Vital statistical data are one of the most commonly used information sources in MCH. These data present abundant opportunities in birth and death certificates, for example, to examine factors in pregnant women associated with various pregnancy outcomes, such as abortions, fetal deaths, live births, preterm and low-birthweight newborns. Such data provide salient characteristics of newborns and relationships to guide clinical management of pregnant women and newborn infants. Combining live birth and infant death certificate data adds appreciable useful information associating neonatal and postneonatal mortalities with risk factors present in the mothers of such infants and in the circumstances surrounding the early period of life. Williams,[8] for example, has utilized vital statistical data to develop perinatal rates for California hospitals, in which observed rates can be compared to expected rates with adjustments for several known risk factors associated with perinatal mortality. He offers such an analysis as a means of utilizing risk profiles to assess aspects of effectiveness of perinatal programs.

The application of risk factors and risk assessment to pregnant women during the period of prenatal care requires special attention to changes in risk ratings as pregnancy proceeds. These changes in risk ratings could occur either because some risk factors do not appear until the later stages of pregnancy or earlier identified risk factors are modified by therapy. Prenatal care itself is a broad intervention in that it extends over a long period of time and includes several forms of intervention. These circumstances make it necessary to be circumspect in interpreting risk associations in pregnancy. Distinguishing pregnancy outcomes by risk status of the pregnant women cannot ignore either the time risk was identified or specific therapeutic interventions which could influence the association of risk and outcome.

Klerman and Rosenbach[9] describe several applications of risk factors in the efforts by program administrators to distinguish need among communities and population groups. Need assessments performed by state program directors are used to guide assignment and allocation of resources to counties and other population groups, and incorporate a variety of risk factors, some as single measures, but most in a composite form. This use of risk factors is adopted because of the capacity to arrive at a quantitative score enabling communities to be ranked on the basis of need, i.e. having greater or lesser risk factors present. While scientific evidence exists to justify that a factor present does represent a risk, administrative judgment is utilized in selecting the combination of risk factors expected to discriminate among communities. It is not always possible to have demonstrated before the fact that such a basis for ranking communities does represent a relevant difference in need for resources or that assigning resources on this basis results in differences in later health status. The risk factors chosen are associated with specific conditions whereas need is frequently represented by several conditions of interest. Multifactorial analyses help in assigning relative weights to the chosen risk factors, but the efficacy of using known risk factors to reduce need and thereby improve health status remains to be established.

REFERENCES

1. Sattler JS. Assessment of Children's Intelligence and Special Abilities. Second Edition 1982, Allyn and Bacon, Inc.

2. Webber LS, et al. Tracking of cardiovascular disease risk factor variables in school-age children. Journal of Chronic Diseases 36:(640-660), 1983.

3. Harsha DW, et al. Tracking of body composition variables. Pediatrics (Supplement) 80:5:2 (779-783) Nov. 1987.

4. Colton T. Statistics in Medicine, Little Brown and Co., 1974, pp. 207-214.

5. Feinstein AR. Clinical Biostatistics, C.V. Mosby Co., 1977, pp. 378-379.

6. Ibrahim MA. Epidemiology and Health Policy, Aspen Systems Corp., 1985.

7. Hobel CJ, et al. Prenatal and intrapartum high-risk screening. American Journal of Obstetrics and Gynecology 117(1):1-9, 1973.

8. Williams RL. Measuring the effectiveness of perinatal medical care, Medical Care, 1979, 17(2), 95-111.

9. Klerman LV and Rosenbach M. Needs indicators in maternal and child health planning, 1984. Brandeis University.

ENVIRONMENTAL HEALTH RISKS* 12

Carl W. Tyler, Jr. and Lowell E. Sever

At a time when an estimated 70,000 chemicals are in everyday use and 500 to 1,000 new ones are synthesized each year,[1] it is reasonable to ask what this change in our environment means to the health of pregnant women and their children—both unborn and newborn. Moreover, exposure to chemicals is not the only reason this question is important. Exposure of women to health risks in the workplace has new importance as the number of women in the workforce has increased from 54.6 million in 1955 to 82.3 million in 1985.[2] Clearly, the role of the environment in MCH has attained a new level of importance.

But what do we mean by environment? It is no longer sufficient to simply classify the causes of human health problems as genetic or environmental. Health professionals must now be able to specifically categorize the components of the environment and the physical and chemical exposures associated with each. Only then can we offer practical advice on preventing or avoiding these exposures.

The term environmental has been used both broadly and narrowly. In the broadest sense, environmental refers to all those factors that originate outside the individual. In this context, then, environmental exposure would include such things as the use of drugs, smoking, use of alcohol, poisonings, and injuries. More narrowly, environmental indicates exposures through such pathways in the ambient

_____

* This chapter is excluded from the copyright of this book because it is "a work of the United States Government".

environment as air, water, and soil, as well as such physical agents external to the individual as radiation, heat, and high altitude. All these exposures have the potential for adverse effects on the health of women and their children.

This chapter uses the broader of the two concepts of environment. It has two major sections. The first emphasizes general concepts about environmental exposures and their effects on the health of mothers and children. The second discusses the exposures which we judge to be the most important in terms of 1) maternal risks, 2) risks to the fetus and newborn, and 3) risks to children.

GENERAL CONCERNS ABOUT ENVIRONMENTAL EXPOSURES AND MCH

There are several key issues associated with children's health and the environment. Clearly they are complex and involve concerns similar to those related to adult health, plus those unique to the embryo/fetus and the growing child. For example, one is the concern regarding the effects of air pollution on respiratory function in both children and adults. Another—the fact that growth is much more rapid during in utero development and childhood—also makes the developing child more susceptible to environmental insults. The rate of cellular turnover is greater during this period, increasing sensitivity to adverse influences. A third concern is any behavior that results in a unique relationship between children and their environments. This includes eating habits, such as pica and oral exploration of toys and other objects, that may result in lead exposure. Finally, we must address such unique physiological relationships with the environment such as nourishment by the mother—initially through the placenta and subsequently through breast milk.

Studies of chemical-production facilities, metal smelters, environmental contamination, and hazardous-waste sites have suggested that exposure of pregnant women to such situations is sometimes associated with adverse reproductive effects. The adverse outcomes observed have included spontaneous abortions, congenital malformations, low birthweight, developmental disabilities, and infant mortality.[3] One of the major problems with such studies is a frequent inability to adequately characterize exposure.

When we look at the potential effects of environmental exposures on the child, we find evidence that a variety of agents generate adverse health outcomes. For example, increased levels of pollutants in ambient air have been associated with exacerbation of chronic respiratory diseases such as asthma.[4] Pollutants, such as NO_2 from gas ranges and pollutants from cigarette smoke indoors, have been associated with increased rates of respiratory symptoms and chronic respiratory disease in exposed children.[5]

At present, one of the greatest areas of concern is the potential association between childhood leukemias, as well as other types of cancer, and environmental exposures. Exposures in this category involve both chemical and physical agents. Situations involving chemicals have been associated with chemical-production facilities, hazardous-waste sites, [6] and parental occupational exposures.[7] Situations involving physical agents have been associated with electric fields [8] and in utero exposure to ionizing radiation. [9]

Prevention of environmental health risks requires that the level of risk be identified and that the subsequent exposure be removed or at least reduced. A key issue is the ability to determine what risks may be associated with prolonged low levels of exposure. Another issue is the ability to recognize potential human risks before people are exposed. In regulatory arenas, considerable emphasis is placed on the use of animal data to estimate human risks. It is logical to assume that the most appropriate use for such animal data is in predicting human risks before human exposures occur. When human exposures do occur, the strongest evidence for human risk comes from well-designed epidemiologic studies. The prevention of environmentally related human disease requires more complete knowledge of risks, as determined through analysis of appropriate human and animal data.

DETERMINANTS OF ADVERSE HEALTH EFFECTS IN PREGNANCY AND EARLY CHILDHOOD

Health professionals and pregnant women should recognize that the risks from environmental agents—e.g., tobacco smoking, alcohol misuse, and the inappropriate taking of drugs—are often transmitted to the fetus and newborn. Moreover, pregnancy does not protect a woman from these risks.

The embryo/fetus is particularly sensitive to effects of environmental agents. While the data suggesting a major role of the ambient environment in abnormal development are far from compelling, there are reasons for concern. Substances such as pesticides, heavy metals, and organic solvents have been shown to have developmental effects in animals. [10] Data for humans are more limited, but the example of Minamata disease, associated with exposure to organic mercury, serves as a reminder of the potentially devastating effects of environmental contamination.[11] Table 1 indicates the relative role of environmental causes in human developmental defects.

ENVIRONMENTAL EXPOSURES AND HEALTH EFFECTS: MATERNAL RISKS

Tobacco Smoking

Maternal smoking has its most profound effect on the fetus and newborn. Smoking accounts for an estimated 4,600 perinatal deaths each year.[12] Women who smoke while pregnant substantially increase (an increase of 36 percent-47 percent) the likelihood that their offspring will weigh less at birth (about 300 gms less) than the infants born to women who do not smoke. Moreover, a woman who smokes during pregnancy is also more likely to have a child who has less vitality at birth, as measured by the Apgar score, than a woman who does not smoke. Passive smoking has a similarly adverse effect on the fetus.[12]

Smoking by adults influences the health of young children, but it is not clear whether the effects begin during pregnancy or reflect continued smoking by adults, with its attendant involuntary health effects on their children. The occurrence of lower respiratory infections as measured in terms of visits to the doctor and hospitalization is more prevalent for the children of smoking parents. Neurological and intellectual effects measured in terms of overall cerebral dysfunction for a group of children age 61/2 years of age also indicate an association with maternal smoking.[13]

The key to preventing these effects is clear: pregnant women should not smoke if they wish to optimize their health and that of their offspring. The same can be said of parents whose children will be exposed involuntarily to the effects of the tobacco those parents smoke. Smoking intervention can be effective during pregnancy and should be accepted as the responsibility of every health professional, mother, and prospective parent.

Alcohol

Alcohol misuse can adversely influence the ability of a woman to carry a pregnancy to term successfully and can affect the offspring for a lifetime. Alcohol is a proven teratogen (Table 2). Moreover, the fetal alcohol syndrome (FAS) (a

---

TABLE 1

CAUSES OF DEVELOPMENTAL DEFECTS IN HUMANS

Cause	Percentage
Genetic transmission (Mendelian)	20
Chromosomal abnormalities	5
Environmental causes	
Drugs and environmental chemicals	4-6
Ionizing radiation	1-2
Infectious agents	1-2
Maternal metabolic imbalances	1-2
Interactions/combinations	?
Unknown, including polygenic/multifactorial	65-70

SOURCE: Mortensen ML, Sever LE, Oakley Jr GP: Teratology and the epidemiology of birth
defects, Obstetrics: Normal and problem pregnancies. Edited by SG Gabbe, JR
Niebyl, JL Simpson. New York, Churchill Livingstone, 1986.

condition characterized by decreased weight, height, and head circumference; impaired motor and intellectual function; and distinctive abnormalities of the face and head) affects one-two neonates per 1,000 births and is the most serious result of maternal alcohol misuse associated with pregnancy. As many as 23-29 infants per 1,000 births may have fetal alcohol syndrome if their mothers are problem alcohol drinkers.[14]

The prospects for preventing alcohol-related problems for mothers and their children are promising. Married women, 55 percent of whom drink before pregnancy, often stop drinking alcohol after they become pregnant; more than 60 percent say they abstain.[15] In addition, a community education program directed at obstetricians showed that these physicians modified their approach to prenatal education after being informed of the importance of FAS.[16] The importance of planning pregnancy, however, cannot be overlooked. The changes found in children with fetal alcohol syndrome are consistent with their having been exposed to alcohol in the first trimester of pregnancy.

Diethylstilbestrol

In 1971, Herbst, Ulfelder, and Poskanzer reported a cluster of an unusual form of vaginal cancer in women exposed to diethylstilbestrol (DES).[17] What made

---

TABLE 2
KNOWN AND SUSPECTED HUMAN TERATOGENS

PHYSICAL AGENTS —	DRUGS AND CHEMICALS —
Hyperthemia	Alcohol
Ionizing radiation	Aminopterin, Methylaminopterin (folate antagonists)
	Androgenic hormones
	Bulsulfan (alkylating agents)
	Coumarin anticoagulants
	Diethylstibesterol (DES)
	Isotretinoin
INFECTIOUS AGENTS —	Lead
Cytomegalovirus	Organic mercury compounds
Herpes hominis type II virus	Phenytoin
Rubella virus	Polybrominated biphenyls (PBBs)
Toxoplasma gondii	Polychlorinated biphenyls (PCBs)
Treponema palliidum	Tetracyclines
Varicella virus	Thalidomide
	Trimethadione
	Valpronic acis

SOURCE: Shepard TH: Catalog of teratongenic agents. Fifth edition. Baltimore: The Johns Hopkins University Press, 1986.

this cluster important was that all of the women affected had been exposed to DES while they were still in utero. Their mothers had taken DES as treatment for infertility. Instead, the drug crossed the placenta and caused their children to have cancer—when they were, on average, 19 years old.

More recently, women exposed to DES in utero have been found to conceive normally, but then to have difficulty carrying pregnancies to term. Women whose mothers took DES during pregnancy may have structural abnormalities of the uterus and hypoplastic changes in the cervix.[18] Some are more likely to complete a term pregnancy if they undergo surgery to encircle the cervix with the material that prevents dilation.[19]

ENVIRONMENTAL EXPOSURES AND HEALTH EFFECTS:
RISKS TO THE FETUS AND NEWBORN TERATOGENESIS

Teratogenesis

A *teratogen* is a substance, organism, or physical agent capable of causing abnormal development. Traditionally, identification and definition of teratogenic agents were based on an agent's ability to produce structural defects. More recently, the concept of teratogenesis has been expanded to include agents that act during embryonic or fetal development to produce deviations from normal morphology, function, or both. With this expanded view, the outcomes of teratogenic exposure are thought to include not only structural defects but functional abnormalities, growth retardation, and death of the organism.[11]

The number of known and suspected human teratogens is limited (Table 2). The best known examples are the rubella virus, thalidomide, and alcohol. Two of the drugs listed, isotretinoin [20] and valproic acid, [21] were recently introduced, and their teratogenicity for humans has only been established within the last five years. The interested reader is referred to the current edition of Dr. Thomas Shepard's *Catalog of Teratogenic Agents* for up-to-date information on recognized and suggested teratogens.[22]

Other drugs are also considered to have potential adverse effects on intrauterine growth or postnatal function. Important among these are narcotics associated with respiratory depression and addiction at birth and such drugs as aspirin that interfere with blood clotting. A number of books are available with clinically useful data on the use of drugs during pregnancy, for example, Niebyl's *Drug Use in Pregnancy.* [23]

Preventing or reducing occupational and environmental exposures to agents suspected of leading to adverse reproductive effects is important. Considerable attention has been paid to the necessity of preventing adverse exposures of pregnant women, while at the same time protecting employment rights. This is a complex issue, well beyond the scope of this discussion, but the reader should be cognizant of some of the considerations. Table 3 shows some recent guidelines regarding exposures during pregnancy. While the scientific basis for some of these recommendations is not firmly established, the reader should note that these kinds of guidelines are often proposed.

Breast Feeding

Environmental contamination with such substances as DDT, Heptachlor, PBBs, and PCBs has led to concerns regarding the toxicity of breast milk for infants whose mothers have ingested the chemicals through the food chain. In some instances, the levels of contaminants in breast milk have exceeded levels allowed in marketed food products.[24] Developmental effects in infants have been demonstrated following exposure to PCBs through breast milk. Breast milk contamination is of particular importance in developing countries where breast feeding is being strongly encouraged for nutritional reasons and where the use of pesticides is often widespread and poorly controlled. The possibility has also been raised that adverse effects can result from the passing of workplace chemicals to nursing infants. [25]

TABLE 3

EXAMPLES OF GUIDELINES REGARDING EXPOSURE TO OCCUPATIONAL AGENTS SUSPECTED OF BEING HAZARDOUS TO REPRODUCTION FOR WOMEN WHO ARE PREGNANT OR PLANNING PREGNANCY

EXPOSURE	RECOMMENDATIONS
Anesthetic gases on a daily basis if fully effective scavenging system is not in place	Mandatory transfer
Lead if blood level has been greater than 30 ug/dl	Mandatory transfer
Radiation exposure potentially greater than 0.5 rem for the duration of the pregnancy	Mandatory transfer
Direct mixing of cytotoxic drugs without protective clothing and a hood	Mandatory transfer
Other organic solvents	Transfer or job modification to minimize exposure
PCBs, PBBs, organochlorines, pesticides, and defoliants	Job transfer or rigorous exposure controls

SOURCE: Rosenstock L, Cullen MR: Endocrine and reproductive disorders, clinical occupational medicine. Philadelphia: WB Saunders Company, 1986.

ENVIRONMENTAL AND
HEALTH EFFECTS: RISKS TO CHILDREN

Poisonings and injuries

Today, unintentional and intentional or violent injuries are the prime causes of early death among children and adolescents. Although the death rate for injuries among children continued to drop throughout the period 1967-1979, it dropped only half as much as the death rate from all other causes combined (9 percent versus 22 percent). Thus, injuries have become the leading cause of death for children and adolescents.

The prevention of poisonings and injuries is an important area of public health concern. Notable achievements have been made in some areas. For example, the frequency of poisonings involving children has been markedly reduced as a result of the introduction of child-proof caps on containers for aspirin and other medication. It has been estimated that child-resistant closures prevented nearly 86,000 ingestions between 1973 and 1985. Burn-treatment units experienced a dramatic decline in sleepwear-associated flame burns after the enactment of the Flammable Fabrics Act. The development and enhancement of injury-control procedures is under way in many state and local health developments. An important theme is that injuries are not accidents and, thus, can be prevented.

Lead

The identification and prevention of lead poisoning, both clinical and sub-clinical, have been major public health activities for a number of years. A broad array of adverse effects in children—ranging from acute toxicity to IQ and other neurobehavioral alterations—are potentially associated with lead exposure. In the past, lead-based paints and lead from automobile emissions released into air and soil were major sources of lead exposure. With lead-abatement programs, aimed at eliminating exposure to lead-based paint, and with the replacement of leaded with unleaded gasolines, the frequency of elevated blood-lead levels among children tested in lead screening programs has declined. [26] In some areas, however, high blood-lead levels continue to be a problem. The currently acceptable blood-lead level is 25 ug/dl, [27] but there is concern about the possible harmful effects of even lower levels. For example, prenatal lead exposure, represented by cord blood-lead levels well below 25 ug/dl, has been linked with lowering of cognitive development scores at age six months. [28] Research continues to be directed at improving the level of knowledge about the possible subtle effects of lead exposure and at reducing further exposures and concomitant blood-lead levels.

AN UNRESOLVED ISSUE—
THE WORKPLACE AND ITS RELATIONSHIP TO PREGNANCY

Unfortunately, the epidemiologic basis for minimizing risks for the pregnant working woman is not as strong as one would hope. Moreover, some of the agents with established risks influence pregnancies at their very early stages (Table 4), so that only those working women planning to conceive can manage their risks thoughtfully. [11]

The effect of physical activity on pregnancy outcome is less clear than the effect of exposure to specific chemical agents. While some investigators state that arduous physical activity at work is associated with prematurity, their comparisons have been confined to the workplace, and their recommendations are directed at efforts to change policies regarding maternity leave. Others indicate that the risk of prematurity is greater for unemployed than for employed women. A well-referenced appraisal of the problem is found in the work by Saurel-Cubizolles and Kaminski. [29]

TABLE 4

OCCUPATIONAL AND ENVIRONMENTAL AGENTS BELIEVED TO BE ASSOCIATED WITH ADVERSE REPRODUCTIVE OUTCOMES IN HUMANS

AGENT	OUTCOME
Anesthetic gases	Spontaneous abortion Birth defects
Lead/arsenic	Spontaneous abortion Low birth weight Birth defects
Methylmercury	Mental retardation Cerebral palsy Seizures
Ionizing radiation (chronic low dose or exposure before pregnancy)	Down syndrome
Antineoplastic (cytotoxic) drugs	Spontaneous abortion
Ethylene oxide	Spontaneous abortion
Organic solvents	CNS congenital malformations Orofacial clefts
Polychlorinated biphenyls	Lower birth weight Smaller head circumference
Polybrominated biphenyls	Low birth weight Developmental disability

SOURCE: Mortensen ML, Sever LE, Oakley Jr GP: Teratology and the epidemiology of birth defects, Obstetrics: Normal and problem pregnancies. Edited by SG Gabbe, JR Niebyl, JL Simpson. New York, Churchill Livingstone, 1986.

The most rational approach to managing risk during pregnancy for the working woman can be stated in the form of just two rules:

1. Plan each pregnancy before it occurs so that exposure to chemicals known to cause birth defects and abortion can be avoided.
2. Limit or, better, totally avoid exposure by any route (direct contact, respiratory, or oral) to known teratogens.

More specifically, we agree with the recommendations of Rosenstock and Cullen, [30] which are modified slightly and shown in Table 4.

REFERENCES

1. Postel S. Defusing the toxics threat: Controlling pesticides and industrial waste. Washington, DC: Worldwatch Institute, 1987.
2. US Bureau of Census: Money income of households, families, and persons in the United States: 1985. Washington, DC: US Govt Printing Office, 1987; Current Population Reports no. 156.
3. Sever LE, Hessol NA. Overall design considerations in male and female occupational reproductive studies. Prog Clin Biol Res 160:15, 1984.
4. Shy CM, Goldsmith JR, Hackney JD, et al. Health Effects of Air Pollution. New York, American Thoracic Society, Medical Section of the American Lung Association, 1978.
5. Lebowitz MD. Health effects of indoor pollutants. Ann Rev Public Health 4:203, 1983.
6. Lagakos SW, Wessen BG, Zelen M. An analysis of contaminated well water and health effects in Woburn, Massachusetts. J Amer Statist Assoc 81:583, 1986.
7. Savitz DA. Childhood cancer. Occup Med: State of the Art Rev 1:415, 1986.
8. Wertheimer N, Leeper E. Electrical wiring configurations and childhood cancer. Am J Epidemiol 109:273, 1979.
9. Brent RL. The effects of embryonic and fetal exposure to x-ray, microwaves, and ultrasound. Clinics in Perinatology 13:615, 1986.
10. Clement Associates, Inc. Chemical hazards to human reproduction. Washington, DC, US Government Printing Office, 1981.
11. Mortensen ML, Sever LE, Oakley Jr GP. Teratology and the epidemiology of birth defects, Obstetrics: Normal and problem pregnancies. Edited by SG Gabbe, JR Niebyl, JL Simpson. New York, Churchill Livingstone, 1986, pp 183-209.
12. Sachs, BP. Sharing the cigarette: The effects of smoking in pregnancy, smoking and reproductive health. Edited by M Rosenberg. Littleton, Massachusetts, PSG Publishing Company, Inc, 1987, pp 134-149.
13. US Dept of Health and Human Services: Pregnancy and infant health. In: The health consequences of smoking for women. A Report of the Surgeon General. Office of the Assistant Secretary for Health, 1980, pp 189-249.
14. Spiegler D, Malin H, Kaelber et al. Fetal alcohol syndrome: public awareness week. MMWR 33:1-2, 1984.

15. Prager K, Malin H, Spiegler et al. Smoking and drinking behavior before and during pregnancy of married mothers of live-born infants and stillborn infants. Obstet 99:117, 1984.

16. Little RE, Streissguth P, Guzinski et al. Change in obstetrician advice following a two-year community educational program on alcohol use and pregnancy. Am J Obstet Gynecol 146:23, 1983.

17. Herbst AL, Ulfelder H, Poskanzer DC. Adenocarcinoma of the vagina: association of maternal stilbestrol therapy with tumor appearance in young women. N Engl J Med 284:878, 1971.

18. Kaufman RH, Adam E, Noller K et al. Upper genital tract changes and infertility in diethylstilbestrol-exposed women. Am J Obstet Gynecol 154:1312, 1986.

19. Ludmir J, Landon MB, Gabbe SG et al. Management of the diethylstilbestrol-exposed pregnant patient: a prospective study. Am J Obstet Gynecol 157:665, 1987.

20. Lammer EJ, Chen DT, Hoar RM et al. Retinoic acid embryopathy. New Engl J Med 313:837, 1985.

21. Lammer EJ, Sever LE, Oakley Jr GP: Teratogen update: valproic acid. Teratology 35:465, 1987.

22. Shepard TH. Catalog of teratogenic agents. Fifth edition. Baltimore: The Johns Hopkins University Press, 1986.

23. Niebyl JR. Drug use in pregnancy. Philadelphia: Lea & Febiger, 1982.

24. Rogan WJ, Gladen BC, McKinney JD et al. Polychlorinated biphenyls (PCBs) and dichlorodiphenyl dichloroethene (DDE) in human milk: effects of maternal factors and previous lactation. Am J Public Health 76:172, 1986.

25. Rogan WJ. Breastfeeding in the workplace. Occup Med: State of the Art Rev 1:411, 1986.

26. Annest JL, Pirkle JL, Makue D et al. Chronological trend in blood lead levels between 1976 and 1980. New Engl J Med 308:1373, 1983.

27. Centers for Disease Control: Preventing lead poisoning in young children. Atlanta: US Dept of Health and Human Services, 1985.

28. Bellinger D, Leviton A, Waternaux C, et al. Longitudinal analyses of prenatal and postnatal lead exposure and early cognitive development. New Engl J Med 316:1037, 1987.

29. Saurel-Cubizolles and Kaminski M. Work in pregnancy: its evolving relationship with perinatal outcome (a review). Soc Sci Med 22:431, 1986.

30. Rosenstock L, Cullen MR. Endocrine and reproductive disorders, clinical occupational medicine. Philadelphia: WB Saunders Company, 1986, pp 103-118.

13 | EVALUATION OF MCH/CC PROGRAMS

Mary D. Peoples-Sheps

INTRODUCTION

Program evaluation is inextricably linked to needs assessment and program monitoring. Evaluation is a process which involves systematic comparisons between actual program activities and outcomes, on the one hand, and program objectives or standards, on the other. The purpose of program evaluation is to make a judgment about the value of the program, based upon specified criteria.

In Maternal and Child Health (MCH), program evaluations have been extremely useful for planning and managing programs, allocating and accounting for the use of resources, and promoting promising intervention strategies. In some cases, they have contributed substantially to the MCH knowledge base.

While the results of MCH evaluations can be of great benefit to program managers and directors, in addition to other interested parties, the conduct of evaluation is often difficult, complex, and expensive. In this chapter, some basic evaluation concepts are explored. Special emphasis is given to the evaluation of program effectiveness.

TYPES OF EVALUATIONS

Evaluations of effort, effectiveness and adequacy [1] are particularly useful to MCH programs. Effort evaluation involves an assessment of the quantity of activity that takes place within a program. Included under the category of effort are measures of 1) the resources required to get the project off the ground 2) the number and type of services provided, and 3) the number and type of clients who received the services. When values on these measures are compared with target values in corresponding program objectives, a judgment can be made regarding whether or not the program is functioning in the way it was designed.

To explain the different types of evaluation,[1] Suchman used various attributes of a bird. The question to which effort evaluation is responsive is, "How many times did the bird flap its wings?" Effort evaluation is often called monitoring of program operations.

Evaluation of effectiveness refers to the results (outcomes) of the effort; that is, the relative success of a program in achieving its desired results. Effectiveness evaluation assesses the degree to which changes in knowledge, behavior, medical conditions, and health status in the recipient population, have occurred. It responds to the question, "Given that the bird has flapped his wings, how far has it flown?"

An evaluation of adequacy attempts to determine the degree to which program activities and effects are adequate in relation to the total amount of need. A ratio is required to measure adequacy. It may be derived either from an indicator of effort or one of effectiveness. In terms of effort or coverage, for example, if approximately 500 women were in need of prenatal care each year in a community, an assessment of adequacy would involve comparing the number actually served to that total amount of need. Whether the result is adequate depends on criteria set by the program or other interested parties, such as the community or legislature.

It is often more informative to use a measure of effectiveness as the numerator in an adequacy ratio. For example, a program for children with special needs can measure its effectiveness by the number of clients whose cleft lips and/or palates are repaired. If the program served 300 children with this condition and 200 of them had their malformations repaired, the program might be considered very effective, with a 67 percent surgical repair rate. However, if it is estimated that 700 children with cleft lip and/or palates are eligible for the program, the adequacy of the program would be 200/700, or 28 percent, when compared with the amount of need.

With regard to Suchman's bird, this type of evaluation addresses the distance the bird has flown in terms of how far it has to go.

EVALUATION METHODS

EVALUATION RESEARCH

As indicated, the primary focus of this chapter is on evaluation of effectiveness. Program effectiveness can be assessed by comparing the actual health outcomes of enrollees to the intended outcomes as expressed in the program objectives.

In a family planning program, for example, the actual percent of women who postponed pregnancy for more than one year could be compared to the percent of women for whom the program expected to do so. The result of this comparison would indicate progress towards achievement of a program objective. However, it would not provide evidence that the program caused any pregnancies to be postponed.

Evaluation research is an area of social science that is devoted to the discovery of cause-effect relationships between programs and their outcomes.[2] If a program has a logical hypothesis (i.e., accomplishment of one objective is expected to contribute to accomplishment of another one, until the anticipated improvement in health status is reached), and the substantive elements of its objectives (e.g., program activities, client behaviors, health status) can be measured, it can be subjected to evaluation research methods to investigate whether program activities "caused" the observed effects.

PRINCIPLES OF DESIGN

Basically, three conditions must be met in order to demonstrate that a program influenced an outcome.[2] First, a change in the outcome must correspond to a change in the program. To know whether changes in both elements have occurred, outcomes of individuals or groups who received the program must be compared with outcomes of those who did not receive the intervention. This can be accomplished by comparing a group that received the services, to itself before the services were available, and/or to a concurrent group that did not receive the services.

The second condition is that the intervention must precede the change in the outcome. This condition can only be assured if a measure of the intended outcome is taken before the intervention is applied. For example, assume that a group of children was exposed to an intervention designed to reduce the prevalence of iron deficiency anemia. After the program was in operation for a period of time, blood tests for iron were taken on enrollees. The program could be suspected of being the cause of any positive results only if baseline values on the tests were obtained before the services were received by the children. Without baseline measures, the evaluators could not know whether the children had the same levels of iron before the services were received as they did afterwards.

The third condition for causality is that alternative explanations for the findings must be ruled out. The health problems of mothers and children are often influenced by a complex array of factors, many of which are not well understood. Health services are only one set of factors. Others include environment, socioeconomic circumstances, general health status, and genetic endowment. The most effective way of controlling for these and other potentially confounding factors is to use an experimental research design.

An experimental design involves selecting a group of subjects and applying a pretest to measure the characteristics that the program is intended to change. Next, the subjects are randomly assigned to two or more groups. One group receives the intervention while the others do not. Finally, a post-test to measure any change in the characteristics of interest is administered to all subjects. The basic principle underlying this framework is that any potentially biasing factors will be distributed evenly across the groups so they will not influence the findings for one group more extensively than they do for another.

Even with an experimental design, eliminating alternative explanations may be difficult. Measures of the potentially confounding factors (e.g., age) should be taken on each group to be sure that the random assignment process indeed distributed those factors evenly across the groups. Stratified designs and large sample sizes can help to improve the distribution and multivariate statistical procedures can provide additional control for the effects of measurable confounders.[3]

Unfortunately, many MCH programs cannot be evaluated in this ideal fashion. To randomly assign subjects to groups, the evaluation must be a part of the program plan and ongoing activities which, of course, means that it must be prospective. Often, program managers are trying to determine the effectiveness of programs that have been operating for some time; this often means that they must develop retrospective designs for their studies. Ethical and political factors may also inhibit random allocation even when prospective data collection is possible. For these and other reasons, MCH program managers are usually faced with the challenging task of building a quasi-experimental evaluation design that will approximate the control of an experiment.

In situations where experimental designs are not possible, identification and measurement of confounding factors are critical. The factors, or variables, are used in quasi-experimental designs to create one or more comparison groups that are as similar as possible to the experimental group, except that the comparison groups do not receive the services that are being evaluated. There are many standard quasi-experimental evaluation designs described in evaluation texts.[4,5] The challenge to the evaluator is to determine which of the many options is most appropriate for the situation at hand. Very often the evaluator must construct, rather than select from a textbook, a quasi-experimental design that is appropriate to the circumstances of the program and its recipients. Again, the purpose is to develop a framework that will allow alternative explanations for the findings of the evaluation to be eliminated.

MEASUREMENT ISSUES

Another challenge to MCH program evaluators is selecting appropriate measures for an evaluation. The measures, or indicators, should represent characteristics of the recipient population or a larger community that are expected to change as a result of the program. They should, therefore, correspond directly to the health problems to which the program is addressed and the corresponding objectives that have been specified for the program. There may be several levels of measures. For example, a program may be intended to reduce the rate of preterm birth. Among other activities, it may include a risk-assessment strategy to identify women who are more likely to have preterm deliveries, an educational component to inform those at risk of danger signs and what to do if those signs occur, and health care system components that should be activated in the event that preterm labor occurs. An evaluation of this program should include enumerations of enrollees who experience preterm births and those who do not. But measures of the intervening events should also be taken to provide greater depth to the findings. For example, if the study finds that women have been assessed for risk, they know what to do when signs of preterm labor appear, and they receive appropriate treatment by the health care system, but the rate of preterm births is not reduced, the theoretical basis of the program may be faulty. On the other hand, if the same end results occur and the study further documents that many of the women at risk did not know what to do when danger signs appeared, the theoretical basis may be very sound but one link in the chain of events (education) may require attention. The above interpretations cannot be made unless measures of the effectiveness of each major program activity are taken.

Typical indicators of MCH program effectiveness would include biochemical measures (e.g., hematocrit), indicators of levels of knowledge, behavioral measures (e.g., smoking, drug use), health service measures (e.g., low birthweight, functional ability). When selecting measures, it is helpful to become familiar with the ones that have been used in evaluations of other programs with similar objectives. Also, consultation with researchers who have experience constructing, collecting and analyzing measures of interest may save valuable time and contribute substantially to the quality of the evaluation. Selected references which include frequently used indicators of MCH services and health status are listed at the end of this chapter.

Options for data collection must be considered when measures are being selected. If the data can be collected through pre-existing information systems, they may be readily and inexpensively obtained. Most MCH and CC (Crippled Children's) programs now have information systems that include selected socio-demographic, health care, biochemical, and diagnostic data. Usually the systems have been developed for routine program monitoring. They generally include some, but often do not include all, indicators of interest in evaluations of effectiveness. The information included in these data systems can be greatly enhanced if they can be linked to birth and death registration systems, Medicaid data files, and the data systems of other relevant programs, such as the special supplemental programs for Women, Infants and Children (WIC).

For many MCH program evaluations, however, the necessary measures are not routinely collected. If the required data are not available, new data collection systems may have to be imposed, and it may be necessary to train or hire personnel specifically to collect the data. Requirements such as these increase the costs of the evaluation, particularly when new data must be collected from a comparison group as well as the recipient group.

ADDITIONAL CONSIDERATIONS

Evaluation research requires substantial resources. It may take, for example, two or three years to design the study, collect and analyze the data, and then prepare a report. During that time, the services of highly qualified individuals with skills in research design, data collection, and data analysis may be required. Moreover, the management of an evaluation research project must be taken into account. It may demand a great deal of time and financial resources, especially if a comparison group outside the purview of the program is needed.

Because of the demands that evaluation research can place on a program's resources, it should not be undertaken without careful consideration. The most compelling argument for a research approach to evaluation is that the effectiveness of many interventions, particularly new ones, has not been demonstrated. Future decisions may benefit from knowing whether a previously untested intervention was indeed effective. Even in that case, though, it may not be necessary to use research methods in the evaluation of every demonstration of the same intervention.

It is recommended that new programs be implemented on a demonstration basis, and then evaluated for effectiveness before statewide implementation. An evaluation of a demonstration project is much less expensive and logistically manageable than a larger scale study. Moreover, if the intervention is found to be ineffective, widespread human and financial investments may be averted. This can only occur, however, if the timing of the evaluation corresponds to the timing of a major decision about program continuation or expansion. Even the results of the most careful evaluations can remain unused if they become available after an important decision about the program must be made.

CONCLUSION

The results of evaluations of program effectiveness can stand alone and they can be used in conjunction with other information to inform programmatic decisions. They can be used with cost data to construct cost-effectiveness ratios which, in turn, can be compared with cost-effectiveness ratios of other programs with the same objectives to determine the least expensive approach to achieving those objectives. As previously noted, results of effectiveness studies may also be compared with measures of the extent of need in the community to estimate the adequacy of the program.

With a firm grasp of the basic principles of program evaluation, managers and administrators of MCH programs can begin the difficult but challenging process. Expert consultation with regard to design, measurement, data collection, and data analysis should be sought and used wisely. Evaluations that are conducted with care will contribute to progress in the field of MCH and, ultimately, to the health of the constituents of MCH services: mothers, infants, and children of all ages and with all types of needs.

REFERENCES

1. Suchman EA: Evaluative Research. New York: Russell Sage Foundation, 1967.
2. Langbein LI: Discovering Whether Programs Work: A Guide to Statistical Methods for Program Evaluation. Santa Monica, CA: Goodyear Publishing Company, 1980.
3. Reicken HW, Baruch RF (Eds): Social Experimentation: A Method for Planning and Evaluating Social Intervention. New York: Academic Press, 1974.
4. Shortell SM, Richardson WC: Health Program Evaluation. St Louis: CV Mosby Company, 1978.
5. Cook TD, Campbell DT: Quasi-Experimentation: Design and Analysis Issues in Field Settings. Chicago: Rand McNally College Publishing Company, 1979.

ADVOCACY FOR WOMEN AND CHILDREN

14

Kay Johnson, Dana Hughes, and Sara Rosenbaum

INTRODUCTION

This chapter reviews maternal and child health (MCH) advocacy in the U.S. Under the broadest definition, child advocacy can include any intervention on a child's behalf that does not involve direct provision of a service. Child health advocacy encompasses a broad spectrum of activities ranging from individual case advocacy, in which a single child is assisted obtaining services, to class advocacy, in which reforms or services are sought or protected for a group of children. The subject of this chapter is *class advocacy*.

THE NEED FOR CHILD ADVOCACY

Despite enormous advances in medicine and technology, thousands of infants in the U.S. die needlessly each year. In 1985, more than 40,000 babies died before their first birthday.[1] Of these deaths, at least 2,100 could have been prevented simply if their mothers received early and continuous prenatal care during pregnancy.[2] In 1985, when more than 17 percent of all infants were not fully immunized against preventable childhood diseases, the incidence of preventable childhood disease increased, especially among low income and minority children who were the least likely to be immunized.[3]

In 1985, more than 11 million uninsured children[4] and 500,000 pregnant women risked serious delays, or outright denials, in access to necessary health care.[5] Two-thirds of the uninsured had family income below 200 percent of the federal poverty level and were thus without out-of-pocket resources to pay for care.[6]

Despite voluminous evidence of the value of preventive health care and extensive documentation of the immense difficulties that uninsured Americans face in obtaining any health care, these circumstances persist, in large part, because the health care delivery system in this country is not designed to respond to the needs of those without health insurance. However, because they cannot vote and have no national policy or program to protect them, children are especially vulnerable to these inequitites and rarely benefit from reforms. Thus, children need strong advocates—persons who can raise a voice on their behalf, shape policies to respond to their needs, and secure for children and their families basic services and supports.

TYPES OF ADVOCACY

Improved health care for children is not achieved by any single approach. Policy reforms may be achieved through structural changes in laws, improved administration of existing programs by regulatory agencies, increased funding levels for key program, or changes in political bodies to include policymakers concerned about child health. Specific activities identified by Alfred Kahn include:

> Affirming new concepts of legal entitlements; offering needed services in areas where none existed; persisting in the provision of services where more conventional programs dropped cases; assuring access to entitlementsand help; mediating between children or families and institutions such as schools, health facilities, and courts; and facilitating self organization among deprived community groups, adolescents, or parents....[7]

Just as effective child advocacy involves different activities, it also involves different individuals, organizations, and bodies who, by virtue of their placement, expertise, and power, perform different types of advocacy activities. The four primary types of advocacy are: advocacy by government; advocacy by trade associations; advocacy by religious and other voluntary groups; and advocacy by representational groups. All four types of advocacy are highly related and dependent on one another.

Advocacy by Government

Kahn defines advocacy as "a planning, coordinating, and monitoring system on each level of government to assert priorities on behalf of children.[7] With its unique authority and access to information, governmental bodies have provided, and continue to provide, an essential child advocacy role. The first federal-level governmental agency that met Kahn's criteria was the Children's Bureau, established in 1912. Charged to "investigate and report on all the matters pertaining to the welfare of children and child life among all classes of our people,"[8] the Children's Bureau used its investigative power to study the causes of infant mortality and establish the need for federal funds for maternal and healthy services, primarily by making a link between infant mortality and poverty. The Children's Bureau also contributed to the field of child health advocacy through its successful use of data collection and statistical analysis to advance the cause of child health.

The Children's Bureau is an example of a government agency performing classic governmental functions by using an internal agency of government to study and report on problems. Governmental advocacy can also involve the creation by elected officials of independent, executive, and non-executive entities to investigate and report on major problems. Three contemporary examples of effective governmental advocacy by external groups include: the President's Commission for the Study of Ethical Problems in Medicine and Biomedical and Behavioral Research, which was formed in 1980 and charged with reporting, among other matters, on the "differences in the availability of health services" among various U.S. populations;[9] the Select Panel for the Promotion of Child Health, which was created by Congress in 1978 and which produced, in 1981, a comprehensive analysis of, and recommendations for, the nation's child health care system;[10] and the U.S. House of Representatives' Select Committee on Children, Youth and Families. Established in 1983, the Select Committee has responsibility for studying and reporting on all issues affecting children.

Whether established by a President or by Congress to perform advocacy activities, these bodies can have tremendous influence because of their sponsors and their official imprimatur. Yet, because of their independence, such external bodies can make more far-reaching recommendations than entities within the government. Thus, these independent bodies are often established by elected and non-governmental child advocates to do what they cannot.

Advocacy by Trade Associations

The new national focus on the needs of children, led by the Children's Bureau at the turn of the century, eventually gave rise to child health activism among groups formerly dedicated exclusively to the wellbeing of their profession or trade. In 1929, physicians in support of the renewal of the Sheppard-Towner Act, which had authorized grants to states for MCH services since 1921, broke from the American Medical Society to form the American Academy of Pediatrics (AAP).[8] Today, AAP is one of the most effective trade associations that advocates on behalf of children. Other trade associations active in child health advocacy include the Child Welfare League, the National Association of Children's Hospital and Related Institutions, the Association of Maternal and Child Health Directors, (made up of state directors of Maternal and Child Health agencies); the American Public Health Association; and the National Association of Community Health Centers.

Trade associations bring much to child advocacy. As providers and administrators, they have first-hand knowledge about the problems faced by poor uninsured children in obtaining quality health care and therefore can identify a needed remedy, whether it is additional funding, improved program design, or technical changes in the law or its regulations. Trade associations also may have access to important data on outstanding need, the efficacy of programs and the cost-effectiveness of services. Finally, because trade associations are often made up of respected professionals, they have credibility and influence which can greatly advance an advocacy effort.

Using their unique knowledge, access to data and influence, trade associations can be especially effective lobbyists. In Washington, D.C., and in state capitols, they provide testimony, convene policymakers, and educate legislators on behalf of children. However, while generally effective as child health advocates, trade associations, like governmental bodies, sometimes face conflicts between the needs of children and the organizations' agenda to support and promote its membership or governmental priorities.

Advocacy by Religious and Voluntary Associations

Many religious and voluntary groups, as a part of their mission and goals, are child health advocates. Examples of such groups are the National Council of Churches, Catholic Charities, and the March of Dimes. Their work involves organizing and education of their memberships on a local level, and lobbying legislators and other policymakers on the state and federal level. Among the qualities of religious and voluntary associations that make them effective advocates are their large memberships. When such an organization issues a statement, it does so on behalf of a large number of voters. When a letter writing campaign is launched, policymakers receive vast numbers of letters.

For religious and voluntary organizations, child health advocacy is usually a product of their overall mission or agenda. Most religious organizations involved in child health advocacy, for example, regard improved access to quality care as a moral and ethical issue. Voluntary organizations like the March of Dimes recognize that achieving their overall goal—the prevention of birth defects—requires that all children receive needed health care, and therefore advocate on behalf of children without access to care. However, because the primary function of religious and voluntary associations is not specifically child health advocacy, organizational priorities may occasionally shift away from child health to other issues.

Advocacy by Representational Groups

The fourth type of child health advocacy can be called *representational advocacy*. By representational advocacy we mean entities and organizations whose mission is solely their representation of an affected consumer population group. These representational organizations include Legal Service programs that represent children as part of their mission to represent the poor, and other organizations such as the Children's Defense Fund and numerous state and local advocacy groups, which represent only children. What distinquishes representational advocates from others is that the work of these organizations is propelled and defined exclusively by the needs of the client population.

THE ELEMENTS OF ADVOCACY

Despite the diversity in the types of advocates and advocacy activities, effective child health advocates share an understanding of the key elements of advocacy.

- Effective advocacy is specialized. Issues to be addressed are carefully and narrowly defined. Large, comprehensive projectsare broken down into manageable pieces.
- Effective advocacy involves issues affecting large numbers of people for the broadest impact.
- Effective advocates involve the greatest number of advocates and supporters possible. This requires that other groups and individuals with potential interest be identified and included.
- Effective advocates build a strong base of support from non-traditional allies, such as corporate leaders and key legislators not normally involved in their issues. This requires making an issue attractive by popularizing the subject and appealing to others interests, such as sharing that a desired goal is not only good but cost effective, as well.
- Effective advocates recognize that there is no one way to change. There are a variety of strategies which can be used in advocacy, and reform can be sought at all levels of government.
- Effective advocates move when the time is right, not when it is merely convenient or easy.
- Effective advocates know when to pass an issue on to others and when to maintain control, to avoid co-optation.
- Effective advocates are patient and persistent.
- Effective advocates are the best in their field—not just the best advocates, but respected experts.

AN EXAMPLE OF CHILD HEALTH ADVOCACY

How these elements of advocacy are actually applied is best illustrated through example. The brief example presented there—adoption of the Medicaid Child Health Assurance Program (CHAP) as part of the Deficit Reduction Act of 1984 [11]—was selected because it demonstrates the multifaceted and dynamic nature of advocacy. This review is also important because it illustrates the basic tenents of effective advocacy and the common barriers that advocates face.

CHAP refers to sweeping Medicaid reforms enacted in 1984. Enacted as part of the Deficit Reduction Act of 1984, CHAP effectively ended Medicaid's linkage to AFDC (Aid for Dependent Children) by mandating coverage of children under age five on the basis of financial need alone. Subsequent laws expanding this guarantee to pregnant women and liberalizing the test by which financial need is measured all were made possible as a result of these 1984 reforms.[12] With CHAP, an additional 400,000 children and 200,000 pregnant women became newly eligible for the Medicaid program. Yet the importance of CHAP goes beyond its direct impact on the children and pregnant women provided Medicaid coverage. The process of winning approval for CHAP taught advocates several important lessons. These lessons, and the momentum created by CHAP's success, led to additional Medicaid reforms in 1986[13] and 1987,[14] and to countless reforms on the state and local level.

The success of CHAP was not achieved overnight but was the result of eight years of long and difficult work. Indeed, a prior, and more expansive, version of CHAP failed to pass in the 95th Congress (1977-78) and in the 96th Congress (1978-79). While this first bill never suffered from lack of justification, as its supporters and others knew, it did fail to meet several tenets of successful advocacy. Specifically:

1. **The original bill had too many objectives.** In the face of multiple barriers to care for poor children, the framers of the original CHAP bill sought to achieve several results: increase eligibility; expand benefits; strengthen provider qualifications; and improve reimbursement rates. While admirable in its intent, the approach proved too confusing and cumbersome for legislators and for a sufficiently range of advocates to understand, absorb, and develop consensus around. For some, the effort to address multiple barriers created reasons for opposing the bill; for others, it prohibited themfrom lending their support.

2. **The health care needs of uninsured children was not sufficiently popularized in the mid-1970s.** Very few policymakers understood the need for improved access to health care and the vital role of Medicaid in addressing child health needs before the campaign for CHAP began. For most, the children CHAP sought to reach were faceless, their problems foreign, and the social and economic implications of failing to meet health care needs were unknown. As a result, few policymakers recognized the importance of the measure or the need to enact it.

3. **Essential allies were not recruited and potential opponents were not recognized.** Key groups, such as the American Public Welfare Association and the American Academy of Pediatrics, were not enthusiastic about the bills' administration and provider qualification provisions.The Right to Life congressional block, just emerging as a potent force, had

not yet included in its position a call for expanded maternity and pediatric care and instead viewed the bill only as a vehicle for Medicaid anti-abortion efforts.

4. **Key leadership was lacking.** CHAP literally was an after-thought for the Carter Administration, which was primarily focused on national health insurance and cost containment. While the House Leadership was deeply committed, the key subcommittee chairman, Paul Rogers, retired in 1978, and the then-new subcommittee chairman, Henry Waxman, was not yet the major policymaker he has subsequently become. In the Senate, the key leader, Russell Long, simply had no interest in the bill.

Forces then began to move toward changes in the political base, public awareness, and consensus. First, the mid-term election of 1982 created a small but significant shift in Congress and a new willingness to consider social reforms. The persistence of advocates who had bided their time became all-important in recognizing that the shift had occurred. Second, the deep recession of the early 1980s made social action not only palatable but essential in the eyes of many. Third, advocates had become much more sophisticated about popularizing the problem of child health and virtually deluged the press with information about the health needs of children. They did their homework and presented their findings in a startling and thorough manner. Fourth, government advocates had become far more powerful and sophisticated. Several key Congressmen, such as Henry Waxman of California and John Dingell of Michigan, had literally saved Medicaid from destruction in 1981. They had built extensive reputations and power-bases. Also, creation of the Select Committee for Children, Youth and Families in 1983 gave children's advocates an organized group of key lawmakers willing to work for children. Several of these members were pro-life, and an extremely effective job of public education by religious advocacy groups persuaded them that support for MCH improvements was a moral obligation. Fifth, advocates learned how to make cost-effectiveness arguments in an era of economic constraint. These arguments ultimately gained the attention of even conservative lawmakers.

Finally, and perhaps more importantly, advocates were more experienced and thus far smarter about the process of legislation. Indeed, they turned the chief weapon of the Reagan Administration to their own use by incorporating the CHAP bill into the fiscal 1984 Budget Reconciliation Act, in the same manner in which the Administration had cut programs in 1981.[15] So eager was the administration to achieve a budget by the 1984 election that it agreed to accept CHAP. Thus, all of the elements of effective advocacy came together in 1984. This process has been repeated in subsequent years at both the federal and state levels.

TOOLS FOR EFFECTIVE ADVOCACY

There exists a diverse set of tools which can be used by advocates to organize reform efforts. Among these tools are: coalitions, grassroots networks, printed materials with facts and statistics, lobbying, and the media. The selection of tools for advocacy is dependent on the problem and the strategy, and multiple strategies are generally used in combination to expedite the advocacy effort. The CHAP example can be used to illustrate how these tools might be used.

The most widely recognized advocacy tool is lobbying. Lobbying efforts are most often used when the strategy is focused on reform of a law or policy. It is important to remember, however, that advocates can lobby for or against legislative proposals. The work of a lobbyist consists of the following: gathering and using facts to develop arguments for or against legislation, developing policy positions or legislative proposals on the basis of the facts, educating policymakers regarding the positions formulated, monitoring progress of legislative proposals, and using other tools such as coalitions, grassroots networks, or media as needed to ensure successful passage or defeat of a proposal.

In efforts to pass CHAP, lobbying was a critical tool. However, there was also a period during which no actions were taken to move the initiative. After having been defeated in the 1976-77 and 1978-79 Congressional sessions, advocates stopped legislative activity for two years. This time was used to develop a stronger political base, to increase public awareness of the problem, and reshape the initiative to allow for future success.

Another common tool which has long been used to advocates is coalition building. Whether a temporary or "ad hoc" coalition or a permanent, chartered coalition is developed, a coalition can have more power and greater effectiveness in many situations than a single advocacy organization. Coalitions may be built around a single issue or be joined together by commitment to one program or a set of ideals. There also are disadvantages to using coalitions. In some cases, the structure of a coalition may be too cumbersome to allow decisions to be made quickly or the disparate views of coalition members may rule out pursuit of certain remedies. Under those circumstances, individual members of a coalition may need to act independently, thus potentially negating the value of the coalition's work.

As discussed above, the early CHAP efforts were unsuccessful in part because the bill was too large to allow for effective coalition building. Key groups who would support the later CHAP initiative could not support the bill as structured in the late 1970s. By 1984, a more specific agenda had been defined, which allowed for more successful coalition building. Coalitions were built which included both liberal and conservative organizations (most notably, pro-life groups who had actively worked in opposition to the early CHAP bills).

Another tool available to advocates, which is similar to a coalition, is a grassroots network. A grassroots network is composed of a variety of individuals across a state or the country who care enough about a particular issue to support related advocacy efforts. It differs from a coalition in that its members rarely, if ever, meet, and generally it is made up of individual citizens, rather than groups, acting out of concern. The value of a grassroots network is that policy makers, particularly those who are elected, weigh differently the opinions of individuals and those of trade associations or representational groups (who may be viewed as "special interest groups"). Another positive feature of a grassroots network is that it can be quite large and thus generate substantial support for a proposed reform.

In order to build a broad-based grassroots network, an issue must be widely understood and recognized as important. By 1984, the CHAP bill was supported across the country as a result of public information efforts by advocates. The problem of lack of access to health care services by poor mothers and children, as well as the cost-effectiveness of preventive health services, such as prenatal care, were much more widely understood by the mid-1980s than they had been in the late 1970s.

Facts are another important tool in advocacy. Research and statistics are an important part of the process, frequently used for problem definition, for public education, and in building arguments in favor of proposed remedies. Few issues are so compelling or intuitive that policy makers naturally support them, even motherhood. Policy makers must be convinced that there is a problem and that the proposed remedy will be both effective and cost-effective.

One other important tool is media. In recent years, media coverage of political issues has become increasingly sophisticated, and advocates have developed a greater understanding of ways in which the media might be used. Some advocates have made extensive use of the media through development of advertisements or public service announcements which serve to educate the public and policy makers about key issues. However, more modest efforts can be effective. For example, making statistics regarding program use or health status available to the press can generate important stories. Advocates can write letters to the editor which broaden awareness of an issue, and they might use press releases to inform local media of the publication of statistics and reports or the passage of key legislation.

Media efforts were used in the 1984 CHAP advocacy effort. For example, near the time of a critical Congressional vote in 1984, the Children's Defense Fund placed large and targeted advertisements in key newspapers. This ad highlighted both the provisions of the bill and the type of information which had moved the initiative toward success, such as the cost-effectiveness of prenatal care, the problems caused by lack of access to preventive care, and the growing unmet need for MCH services.

CONCLUSIONS

This chapter has discussed the key elements of effective MCH advocacy. Since the 1970s, more MCH advocates have become involved in the battles to maintain and improve such key programs as Medicaid, the Childhood Immunization program, and the Title V MCH Block Grant. While battles were lost in some cases, increasingly effective advocacy efforts have allowed for substantial improvements in access to health care services for children and pregnant women in other cases. The passage of the Medicaid improvements, known as *CHAP*, is but one example. Similarly, dramatic reforms have been enacted in such states as Texas and Mississippi. Yet much remains to be done. Hundreds of thousands of low-income pregnant women and millions of low-income children continue to lack access to prenatal care. As in the past, further improvements will depend on the efforts of advocates across the country, working both inside and outside of the government. Such advocacy is essential because, as one child advocate expressed it at the turn of the century, "It is easier to form than reform. To cure is the voice of the past; to prevent, the divine whisper of today."[16]

REFERENCES

1. National Center for Health Statistics: Advance Report of Final Mortality Statistics, 1985. Monthly Vital Statistics Report, 36:5, Supplement, U.S Department of Health and Human Services, 1987, p 7.

2. Hughes D, Johnson K, Rosenbaum S, et al: The Health of America's Children: Maternal and Child Health Data Book, Washington, D.C., Children's Defense Fund, 1987.

3. Johnson K: Who is Watching Our Children's Health? The Immunization Status of American Children, Washington, D.C., Children's Defense Fund, 1987.

4. Employee Benefits Research Institute: A Profile of the Nonelderly Population without Health Insurance. Issue Brief, No.66, Washington, D.C., 1987, p 2.

5. Gold RB, Kenney AM: Paying for Maternity Care. Fam Plan Perspect 17:103, 1985.

6. Sulvetta M, Swartz K: Chartbook of the Uninsured, Washington, D.C., Urban Institute, 1986, p 8.

7. Kahn AJ, Kamerman SB, McGowan BG: Child Advocacy: Report of a National Baseline Study, Washington, D.C., US Government Printing Office, 1973, p 9.

8. Takanishi R: Childhood as a Social Issue: Historical Roots of Contemporary Child Advocacy Movements. Jour of Social issues, 34:22, 1978.

9. President's Commission for the Study of Ethical Problems in Medicine and Biomedical and Behavioral Research: Securing Access to Health Care. A Report on the Ethical Implications of Differences in the Availability of Health Services. Washington, D.C. US Government Printing Office, 1983.

10. Select Panel for the Promotion of Child Health: Better Health for Our Children: A National Strategy. Vol. 2. Analysis and Recommendations for Selected Federal Programs. US Department of Health and Human Services, 1981.

11. Public Law 96-396: Deficit Reduction Act of 1984.

12. Public Law 99-272: Consolidated Omnibus Reconciliation Act of 1986.

13. Public Law 99-509: Omnibus Budget Reconciliation Act of 1986.

14. Public Law 100-203: Omnibus Budget Reconciliation Act of 1987.

15. Public Law 97-35: Omnibus Budget Reconciliation Act of 1981.

16. Wiggin KD: Children's Rights, Boston, Houghton Mifflin and Co., 1892.

SECTION II

BASIC SERVICES IN MATERNAL AND CHILD HEALTH

PREVENTIVE SERVICES IN MATERNAL AND CHILD HEALTH

15

Paul H. Wise and Julius B. Richmond

THE SIGNIFICANCE OF PREVENTION

Much of modern history has been shaped by the struggle to improve the quality of life. Basic to a better life is good health, representing both a central objective and common prerequisite of life improvement. This fundamental linkage of health and social progress inextricably ties the processes of disease prevention with those of social change.

A common illustration of the interweaving of health promotion and social transformation is the profound decline in mortality from tuberculosis in the U.S. Falling from a mortality rate of 195 per 100,000 in 1900 to fewer than 1 per 100,000 today, the largest portion of this decline occurred prior to the common availability of relevant chemotherapy. The major preventive forces were the profound improvements in living conditions during this period, including gains in nutrition and housing.[1,2] Even immunizations provide insight into the linkage of disease prevention and societal activity. The ability to prevent many diseases by enhancing host immunity remains one of the most impressive and practical achievements of modern science. However, a large portion of the world's children remain unimmunized in 1988.

Technical innovations depend on society's action for their implementation. It is therefore somewhat artificial to stratify the preventive accomplishments of the past century into those due to social progress and those due to medical innovation.

Widespread public improvements in sanitation depended upon both technical advances in engineering and microbiology and the political commitment to assure their common implementation. Clearly, the prevention of disease requires knowledge; it requires the knowledge to interfere with the processes causing disease even if we do not fully understand all dimensions of causation. For example, we know cigarette smoking causes lung cancer even though we do not know the quantities of the specific ingredients of the smoke which cause the disease. However, prevention also requires the social strategy which shapes a policy's social purpose and practical context. Last, prevention policy requires action. For virtually all preventive interventions, this action is the product of political debate and, in the end, the political will that generates the resources available for programs. The interaction of knowledge, social strategy, and political will in shaping prevention policy is depicted in Figure 1.

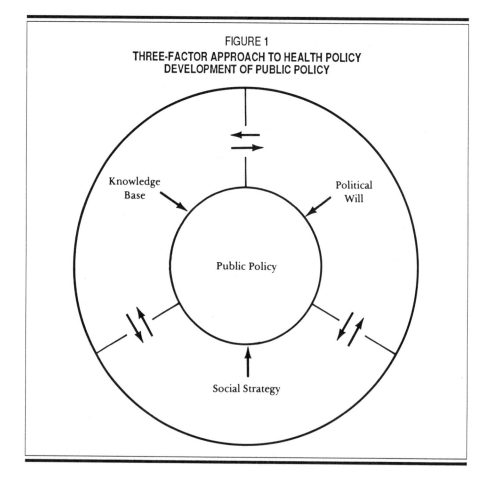

FIGURE 1
THREE-FACTOR APPROACH TO HEALTH POLICY
DEVELOPMENT OF PUBLIC POLICY

Knowledge Base

Political Will

Public Policy

Social Strategy

LEVELS OF PREVENTION

Preventive services can be categorized in a variety of ways. Depending on the reason for scrutiny, preventive services may be assessed on the basis of the nature of the services rendered, the populations to be served, or mechanisms of delivery. However, it is conceptually useful to relate preventive interventions to the point in the cascade of disease causation the preventive intervention acts. This is helpful because prevention implies the alteration of cause and causal interaction.[3]

PRIMARY PREVENTION

Primary prevention represents endeavors which prevent the initiation of a pathologic process. For disease to occur, a set of requisite causes must exist. Primary prevention implies a capacity to block these causes from becoming sufficient to generate a disease process. A classic example of primary prevention is immunization for measles. In order for the clinical disease of measles to occur, the child must be exposed to the measles virus and lack immunity to it. The measles immunization induces effective immunity to the virus, thereby preventing the coupling of causes sufficient to induce disease.

SECONDARY PREVENTION

Secondary prevention is directed toward altering the impact of a pathologic condition after it has begun but prior to its actual expression as recognized symptoms. Here, causation was sufficient, but the human impact of such causation remains open to modulation. An example of secondary prevention is newborn screening for phenylketonuria (PKU). The most serious manifestation of this genetic disorder is mental retardation, caused by the abnormal metabolism of phenylalanine, found ubiquitously in normal dietary proteins. Mental retardation can be prevented by the early restriction of dietary phenylalanine. This requires the identification of newborns who possess the genetic defect and abnormal accumulations of phenylalanine, but have not yet experienced its devastating symptoms.

TERTIARY PREVENTION

Tertiary prevention confronts the failures of primary and secondary prevention. It is directed at limiting the disability and suffering associated with the human expression of chronic illness. Here, the pathologic process has produced symptoms, and the task becomes the reduction of suffering and the promotion of adaptation. An example of tertiary prevention is the comprehensive physical therapy programs designed to prevent contractures and optimize mobility for children with spastic cerebral palsy.

THE DETERMINATION OF RISK IN RELATION TO PREVENTION

Prevention depends on the reduction of risk or the alteration of risk's relationship to outcome. This places the identification of risk squarely in the center of efforts to prevent disease. Once the components of elevated risk are elucidated, they are usually termed *risk factors*, and can then become the focus of efforts to reduce their prevalence, severity, or impact on health. However, because risk is a product of the profound biologic and social diversity in a society, risk is not likely to be randomly distributed. The term *high risk* is generally used to describe individuals or populations in which risk factors are concentrated. Therefore, the identification of risk provides the basis for two important mechanisms of prevention: the reduction of specific risk factors in a total population, and the targeting of preventive efforts toward individuals or populations considered at high risk for the disease in question.

Evidence that a particular factor elevates the risk of a particular disease is usually derived from some estimate of relative risk: the rate of disease occurrence in those exposed to the factor in question relative to the rate of disease in those not exposed. The attributable proportion (often termed *attributable risk percent* or *etiologic fraction*) accounts for the frequency of exposure and represents a measure of the portion of disease occurrence in the total population that would be eliminated if the exposed group had the same disease rate as the unexposed group.[3] Both relative risk and attributable proportion represent quantitative insights into the true health-related impact of a particular risk factor and, therefore, may have important implications for the development of preventive policies.

In developing preventive policies, relative risk and attributable proportion should not be confused. High relative risk may be observed for risk factors that are, in the real world, relatively rare. Major public initiatives directed at such factors, therefore, may be misplaced. Risks associated with lower relative risks may be so common that preventive strategies may be indicated. On the other hand, if attributable proportion dominates preventive strategy development, population groups with attributes conveying high relative risk but of relatively small numbers, could be ignored. Because risk is not randomly distributed in the community, strict attributable proportion analyses could discount the great suffering of a minority population.

Risk-reduction activities may be more efficient if targeted at individuals deemed at high risk for disease. The search for such individuals is often termed *screening*. Screening can be primary in nature, designed to identify undiseased individuals at elevated risk for disease, as well as secondary, designed to identify asymptomatic diseased individuals.

Screening methods may be directed to singular risks (eg. phenylalanine in newborn blood samples) or multiple risks (eg. pregnancy risk for premature birth).

The utility of screening depends upon the characteristics of the methodology or test used to identify high risk individuals. The sensitivity of a test is defined as the portion of the truly diseased or high-risk population correctly identified by the test as diseased or high risk. The specificity of a test is defined as the portion of the truly undiseased or low-risk population correctly identified by the test as undiseased or low risk.[4] Shifting the value defining a positive test to increase sensitivity will capture more of the truly high-risk group, the true positives; however, it will also likely increase the number of misidentified low-risk cases, the false positives. Shifting the value of a positive test to improve specificity will increase the number of undiseased or low-risk cases correctly identified as such, the true negatives; however, it will also tend to reduce the correct identification of truly high-risk individuals. Also critical to the utility of a test is the prevalence of the health outcome in question. If the outcome is very rare, then the number of false positive tests will be relatively high and the predictive value of a positive test will be low. If the outcome is more common, then the likelihood that identified high-risk cases will truly be at high risk is increased substantially, and the predictive value of a positive case will be relatively high.[4]

Preventive policy must transform these quantitative assessments into human judgements. If the outcome is appreciated to be particularly tragic or severe and the potential to prevent it is significant, then a relatively high false positive rate may be acceptable. If the outcome is relatively mild or the efficacy of prevention poor, then a high false positive rate may prove prohibitive.

FINANCING PREVENTIVE SERVICES

Because the nature and mechanics of preventive interventions are so varied, the means of financing preventive MCH services in the U.S. are quite heterogeneous. Those services delivered through direct clinical care tend to be linked with clinical financing mechanisms. Those delivered via social welfare programs are often tied to these programs, while broad public health programs, including dental caries prevention and nutritional supplementation programs, are financed through still other means; while still other preventive interventions take root in the private sector or larger popular culture. Regardless of the ultimate source of financing, the costs of prevention, like those of therapy, are both complex and ultimately borne if their associated benefits are deemed profound.

ASSESSING PREVENTION'S COSTS AND BENEFITS

All preventive interventions have associated costs and, presumably, associated benefits. Determination of whether a proposed preventive service is to be adopted must, in some measure, reflect an assessment of how potential benefits relate to estimated costs. This process may be informal and intuitive. However, in recent years, more formal analytic methods have been developed which attempt to quantify the relationship between cost and modified health outcome.

Cost-benefit analysis translates all costs and all benefits into standard numerical units, principally dollars. In this way, net cost or net savings can be estimated directly. Cost-effectiveness analysis, on the other hand, is expressed in units derived from the field under scrutiny. For prevention, units commonly take the form of *years of life extended* or *years of disease-free life*. Cost-benefit analysis estimates the bottom line, while cost-effectiveness helps assess the relative impact of competing programs. [5]

Unquestionably, the most powerful issue currently reshaping health policy in the U.S. is the containment of health care costs. Not surprisingly, much of the current enthusiasm for prevention stems from the notion that preventive services save money. Deficiencies in study design and methods have plagued efforts to quantify this assertion, in large measure due to the difficulties in quantifying present costs, intervention effectiveness, and the worth of benefits occurring some time in the future. Nevertheless, prevention holds the potential to reduce costs if its capacity to prevent disability or conditions requiring costly therapeutic care is significant.

COST AND BENEFIT IN THE PUBLIC ARENA

The real issue in determining whether a preventive measure is implemented is less the assessment of absolute cost and benefit than it is the judgment as to whose cost and whose benefit is at stake. Private costs and benefits may differ significantly from social costs and benefits. The social benefit of a screening test may be defined as the savings associated with early diagnosis; however, the private benefit may relate to the comfort of certainty associated with a negative finding. Similarly, a health maintenance organization (HMO) may hesitate at instituting a preventive intervention advanced by the public sector, but whose impact is not likely to affect health costs for many years to come.

Of greater consequence for public policy is the conflict over how cost and benefit relate to the concentration of need, and therefore potential benefit, in one sector of the population, but whose cost must be borne by all. Here, public resources of the many may be committed to preventive strategies for the few. This is most likely to be successful where the disease in question could strike anyone (eg. newborn hypothyroidism), can affect those not suffering from the condition (eg. drunk driving), or represents a social good relevant to concerns of social justice (eg. food stamps).

When a preventive intervention is effective, then equity of access to the intervention becomes crucial. Consequently, assurance that access will be provided to all those in need, regardless of their independent ability to afford its cost, becomes an important element of policy. Equity remains an enduring touchstone in our society, and in no small measure shapes directly the debate over public financing of preventive services. Perhaps too often, in the desperation of unending advocacy, preventive measures are cast fundamentally as cost savers. In the political reality of restricted public spending, this may be a necessary tactic. However, this approach runs the risk of being undermined by a paucity of data substantiating such claims, or by unconvincing evaluative data resulting from the limits of our current evaluative techniques. In addition, caution should be exercised in coupling spending on prevention with reductions in required medical care. For many reasons, including long lag times between intervention and effect, the impact of preventive interventions may not be fully reflected in a reduced need for medical care. The need for therapeutic services is real and, at present, inadequately met. The objective must be to recognize the inherent linkages between prevention and therapy and integrate more fully the effective delivery of both preventive and therapeutic services. At some point, the prevention of disease must be embraced for what it truly is—not necessarily a mechanism to cut costs, but inherently a human endeavor to enrich life. We must be careful not to fight humanitarian battles with financial arguments.[6]

UNMET NEEDS

Evidence of unmet needs for prevention fills our clinics and hospitals. Potentially, preventive strategies could be developed for all morbidity and mortality not mandated by the ultimate limits of human longevity. However, certain conditions of importance to MCH are of particular concern because of their impact, potential impact, or persistence as causes of ill health despite the availability of highly efficacious preventive interventions.

Conditions affecting the health of the newborn, including prematurity, intrauterine growth retardation, and congenital anomalies, represent an important arena for prevention.[7] The early identification of high-risk conditions in pregnancy remains an area of intense investigation. This issue must include the state of women's health in general and not merely direct attention to health post-conception. The emerging challenge of the Acquired Immunodeficiency Syndrome (AIDS) makes this point all the more telling. Services to infants afflicted with the sequelae of serious conditions occurring in the newborn period present a new range of preventive opportunities for the health care and education systems.[8] In turn, the broad struggle to provide the optimal social and educational environment for physically and developmentally disabled school-aged children has ushered in new challenges for prevention.[9] The early identification of learning disabilities and constructive intervention to reduce their devastating impact also represent arenas for preventive innovation.[10] The challenges of preventing significant mental health disorders, particularly in adolescence, have deservedly attracted considerable recent attention.[11]

The prevention of injuries in childhood remains a major issue for the MCH community.[12] The implementation of public strategies to reduce motor vehicle occupant injuries, fire and scald injuries, and consumer product-related injuries, have all reduced the tragic toll inflicted by catastrophic traumatic events. However, it is clear that more needs to be done, both in preventing fatal injuries as well as less serious injuries, including those occurring at school. Both risk identification and intervention development and delivery remain important areas for research and evaluation.

With the deeper understanding of the risks associated with the major causes of adult morbidity and mortality, particularly heart disease and cancer, preventive strategies beginning in childhood have been proposed.[13] The development of health-related behaviors often begins in childhood, thereby creating opportunities for prevention. Alterations in diet, patterns of exercise, and substance abuse all represent possible vehicles for intervention. However, in the end, the greatest unmet need relates to our current failure to provide all children in our society with a social environment that is compatible with healthy growth and development. The impact on adult health and well-being is profound, and the human tragedy of its inherent injustice of exposure to preventable risks remains immeasurable.

Prevention policy, therefore, must integrate evidence of the role that specific risk factors play in shaping patterns of disease with evidence that these risks can be both identified and altered. This is the domain of the *knowledge base*. However, prevention policies are also invariably shaped by its place within the broader context of prescribed societal action. This is the domain of *social strategy*. And ultimately, the implementation of preventive policies depends on the energy, resources, and directed compassion of the public. This is the domain of *political will*. All three aspects of policy development will help shape the nature and dimensions of preventive interventions. But more important, it will always determine its relative success. The public perception of human suffering provides those who care for the health of women and children with a substrate of preventive sentiment. But it is the public appreciation of this suffering's causation and the power to prevent it that will ultimately transform sentiments into purposeful societal action.

REFERENCES

1. McKeown T. The Role of Medicine: Dream Mirage or Nemisis? London, Nuffield Provincial Trust, 1976.

2. Kass E. Infectious diseases and social change. J Infect Dis 123:110-114, 1971.

3. Rothman K. Causal inference in epidemiology, Modern Epidemiology. Boston, Little, Brown and Company, 1986.

4. Ahlbom A, Norell S. Sensitivity and specificity, Introduction to Modern Epidemiology. Chestnu Hill, MA, 1984.

5. Banta HD, Luce BR. Assessing the cost-effectiveness of prevention. J of Comm Health 9:145-165, 1983.

6. Eisenberg L. Preventive pediatrics: The promise and the peril. Pediatrics 80:415-422, 1987.

7. Wise P, Kotelchuck M, Wilson M, Mill, M. Racial and socioeconomic disparities in childhood mortality in Boston. New Engl J Med 313:360-6, 1986.

8. Taeusch HW, Yogman MW (ed). Follow-up Management of the High-Risk Infant. Boston, Little, Brown and Company, 1987.

9. Gortmaker S, Sappenfield W. Chronic childhood disorders: Prevalence and in pact. Pediatr Clin North Am 31:3-18, 1984.

10. Levine MD, Brooks R, Shonkoff F. A Pediatric Approach to Learning Disorders. New York, John Wiley and Sons, Inc., 1980.

11. Gruenberg EM. The strategy of preventive trials, Suicide and Depression Among Adolescents and Young Adults. Edited by G. Klerman. Washington, DC, American Psychiatric Press, Inc, 1986, pp 317-334.

12. Rivara FP. Traumatic deaths of children in the United States: Currently available prevention strategies. Pediatrics 75:456-462, 1985.

13. Richmond JB, Kotelchuck M. Personal health maintenance for children. West J Med 141:816-823, 1984.

PREVENTIVE DENTAL HEALTH FOR WOMEN AND CHILDREN

16

Kenneth C. Troutman

Dental diseases are painful, debilitating, and expensive health problems that require the concern and efforts of everyone interested in the total health of children or adults. Although we know that dental diseases are preventable, most preventive efforts are not directed toward preventing the disease from occurring but toward preventing their recurrence. Primary prevention and early intervention are of the utmost importance in controlling dental diseases. The challenge of today is to disseminate and use current information maximally to effect better dental health.

DENTAL HEALTH NEEDS

DENTAL CARIES

Dental diseases are recognized as a major public health problem. The dental disease which causes the most concern, results in the most pain, and requires the greatest expense to treat is tooth decay or dental caries. Therefore, one of the truly significant developments in the field of dental health has been the well-documented 20-50 percent decline in caries during the past decade.[1,2] The reduced susceptibility to dental caries, particularly among children and young adults, is altering the oral health status of the population, not only in the U.S. but in many nations of the world.

Etiology

A unique group of streptococci is believed to be primarily responsible for dental caries [3] facilitating extracellular synthesis of long-chain dextran polymers. The extracellular enzyme system responsible for dextran synthesis can function only with sucrose as its substrate. The disaccharide molecule is split, with the glucose components being added to a dextran chain and the fructose being intracellularly phospholated and used for energy production or stored for future use. Through the synthesis of long-chain dextrans, an insoluble gummy mass, called *plaque*, is produced which is capable of forming a matrix for colonization by organisms on tooth surfaces. Coating of dental enamel by the dextran plaque establishes a unique local environment between the organism-laden plaque and the tooth surface. The production of acids as a consequence of energy metabolism by the bacteria lowers the pH of this environment past the critical level at which decalcification occurs; this organic destruction leads to the cavitation of the enamel surface.

Prevalence

Comparing the National Health Examination Surveys of the 1960s, [4,5] the early 1970s, [6] and the 1980s, [7,8,9] a higher percentage of children were caries free or had low Decayed Missing & Filled Teeth (DMFT) scores in the more recent survey. In the 1979-80 Decayed Missing & Filled Surfaces (NDCPS), [9] 37 percent of the five to 17-year olds were caries free in their permanent dentition, and another 40 percent had Decayed Missing & Filled Surfaces (DMFS) scores of four or less. (Table 1). This represents a 32 percent decline in caries prevalence from the 1971-74 levels.

The decline in caries in the permanent dentition has not occurred equally across all tooth surfaces. Smooth proximal surfaces have exhibited the greatest percent reduction in disease (Table 2). The mean decrease from 1.7 to 0.8 DMFS was a 53 percent decline.

Treatment Needs

The most gratifying outcome related to declining caries experience in children is the marked reduction in the extraction of permanent teeth. The M (missing) component, as a proportion of the DMFS scores, declined from 18.1 to 7.1 percent between the 1971-74 Health and Nutrition Examination Survey (HANES) [6] study and the 1979-80 NDCPS survey. [7,8] In addition, need for treatment has decreased, as evidenced by the decline in the relative proportion of decayed teeth from 29.9 to 16.8 percent, with a concomitant increase in the percent of filled surfaces. [8,9]

The percent of U.S. Children needing restorative dental treatment in 1980 is depicted in Table 3.

GINGIVAL AND PERIODONTAL DISEASE

Gingivitis

An early, reversible stage of periodontal disease, gingivitis, is confined to the gum. Inflamed gums, irritated by plaque buildup, may look red and puffy, feel tender, and bleed easily when brushed. Pockets form between gums and teeth and accumulate plaque. In addition, a cement-like substance, called *tartar* (or *calculus*), forms on teeth, trapping even more plaque. Tartar cannot be removed by brushing; it must be scraped off by a dentist or dental hygienist.

Unless gingivitis is intercepted, a vicious cycle develops: plaque and continued tartar build-up cause deepening of tissue pockets, which in turn trap more plaque. If left untreated, gingivitis may progress to periodontitis.

Periodontitis

This more severe stage of periodontal disease involves progressive destruction of the gums, bones, and tooth-supporting tissues. As bone deteriorates, teeth may loosen and fall out or may need to be extracted.

TABLE 1
MEAN DMFS FOR U.S. CHILDREN AGED 5-17

Age	HANES 1971-74[6] Mean DMFS	NDCPS 1979-80[7,8] Mean DMFS
5	0.15	0.11
6	0.41	0.20
7	0.69	0.58
8	1.86	1.25
9	3.59	1.90
10	4.14	2.60
11	4.58	3.00
12	6.36	4.18
13	8.67	5.41
14	9.60	6.53
15	11.67	8.07
16	15.12	9.58
17	16.90	11.04
All Ages	**7.06**	**4.77**

Etiology

Almost every adult suffers from periodontal disease to varying degrees. This destruction of the dental supporting structures is the leading cause of tooth loss in people over 35-years of age, and by age 45, 97 percent of the U.S. population is affected by some form of periodontal disease. [10,11,12] The course of the disease seems to be established during childhood. Missing teeth, malocclusions, and habitual patterns of poor oral hygiene all contribute to it. Although all factors associated with the etiology of this condition are still not completely understood, the principle cause is thought to be bacteria.

The clinical signs of periodontal disease usually do not appear until puberty. Prior to puberty, the principle expression of an irritation in the dental supporting

---

TABLE 2

MEAN DMFS BY SURFACE TYPE, AGE 5-17

	HANES 1971-74 [6]	NDCPS1979-80 [7,8]
Occlusal	3.5 - 49%	2.6 - 54%
Proximal	1.7 - 24%	0.8 - 17%
Buccal-lingual[1]	1.9 - 26%	1.4 - 29%
All surfaces	**7.1 - 100%**	**4.8 - 100%**

TABLE 3

PERCENT OF UNITED STATES CHILDREN NEEDING TREATMENT IN THE PERMANENT OR PRIMARY DENTITION BY RACE [9]

	Permanent Dentition		Primary Dentition	
	Whites	Blacks & All Others	Whites	Blacks & All Others
Restorations	24	33	30	40
Extractions	1	4	6	8
Crowns	2	5	6	8
Replacements	2	6	–	–
Pulpal Treatment	1	4	–	–

structures is gingival inflammation at the marginal areas. Except in conjunction with systemic diseases, this inflammation is usually due to local causes, especially poor oral hygiene.

The form of gingivitis seen in young children generally occurs at the gingival margin and is characterized by prominent bulbous interproximal papillae, in contrast to the absence of papillae seen in adult Vincent's-type periodontal infections.

The conditions associated with gingival enlargement in children may be relatively transient, as during eruption of the primary teeth in infancy, at times of primary herpetic infections, during puberty, following the use of many of the drugs used in the treatment of leukemia, during times of severe Vitamin-C deficiency, and during the period of the mixed dentition (primary and permanent teeth present at the same time) when the teeth are in various stages of exfoliation and eruption.

Prevalence

The 1979-1980 NDCPS [9] indicates that 92 percent of all U.S. school children (approximately 44 million) have mild or moderate gingival inflammation, indicating that these children would benefit from improved oral hygiene procedures at home and regular visits to the dental office for routine oral prophylaxis. An additional three percent (1.4 million children) have severe gingival conditions which warrant treatment by a dentist or periodontist.

Based on the National Survey data, there appears to have been a significant decrease in oral hygiene scores and a significant drop in the prevalence of gingivitis in the American population in recent years. [13] Approximately one-half of all Americans appear to be free of any form of inflammatory peridontal disease.

Although bacterial plaque is the primary cause of periodontal disease, other factors may contribute to its severity or to one's susceptibility to it. Physical stress, a faulty bite, misaligned teeth, defective fillings, or poorly fitting partial dentures can be destructive to oral tissues. Metabolic disease such as diabetes and some blood disorders lower the body's overall resistance to infection. Hormonal changes during puberty and pregnancy, certain anti-epilepsy drugs, steroids, oral contraceptives, and anti-cancer drugs affect gingival tissue. Some researchers are currently investigating the theory that susceptibility to periodontal disease is hereditary.

Treatment of Periodontal Disease

The only treatments necessary in the early stage of gum disease may be scaling (removal of plaque and tartar), root planing (smoothing the root surface of the tooth), and possible curettage (removal of diseased soft tissues lining the gum pockets). In more advanced cases, a consultation with a periodontist (a specialist in treating periodontal disease) and possible surgery might be appropriate. Meticulous daily plaque removal by the patient is the most significant prerequisite to successful periodontal disease treatment.

PRENATAL CARE

It has been suggested that endocrine changes related to pregnancy modify the already present etiological factors of periodontal disease; and that the incidence of gingivitis is high during pregnancy and decreases following delivery. [14,15,16] There is no evidence that pregnancy aggravates dental caries, [17] although only 22 percent of the women in a Chicago study were found to be caries free (32 percent in the 12-16 years of age group; this decreased to 21 percent in the 17-20 years of age group). [14]

TOTAL FINDINGS IN 2,200 PREGNANT WOMEN EXAMINED [14]

Missing Teeth 4,895

Periodontal Disease 373

Carious Teeth 5,711

Extraction Indicated 1,032

There has been little dental education as a part of classical prenatal services. What the mother ignores or is not aware of will not be taught to her children and family. Physiologic changes of the oral cavity should be discussed with these women as part of prenatal education. At the same time, instruction in dental disease prophylaxis should be provided. Oral and dental pathology discovered during pregnancy should be treated as in the nonpregnant state. If there is a need for radiographic studies, a leaded apron should be employed. Extractions, fillings or bridges are not contraindicated, nor is the use of a local anesthesia.

INFANT ORAL HEALTH CARE

The primary infant oral health goal is the development and maintenance of optimum oral health in children that can be carried into adulthood. To achieve this goal, it is desirable to begin preventive dental care at a very early age. The success of a preventive program depends on the timeliness of beginning preventive procedures. Based upon the following two factors, a rationale for a preventive dentistry program for newborn children can be developed:

1. Prevention must begin early enough to prevent dental diseases in every child. Some children under one year of age already have dental caries. Many of these lesions can be prevented.
2. For optimum caries preventive effect, fluoride must be present in the diet within a few months following birth.

Infant oral health care should begin with dental health counseling for the parent with the newborn child and should include a dental office visit for preventive oral health counseling no later than 12 months of age. If one begins before the onset of dental diseases, successful primary prevention is possible. A child's oral health should not be ignored or neglected until three years of age, as is frequently recommended.

MALOCCLUSION

Dental malocclusions usually do not interfere with biologic survival. A malocclusion is usually a problem only if it bothers the patient. Many occlusions are inherited growth deviations, and are not pathologic conditions but represent a cultural definition of deviation from socially defined esthetic standards.

In a 1973 assessment of children 6-11 years of age, approximately 75 percent of the children and 89 percent of the youth had some degree of occlusal disharmony. Only 8.7 percent of the children and 13 percent of the youth had what was considered a severe handicapping malocclusion for which treatment was highly desirable, and 5.5 percent of the children and 16 percent of the youth had a very severe handicapping malocclusion that required mandatory treatment. [18]

The early loss of primary teeth and the reduction in tooth size and function due to the breakdown of tooth structure as a result of caries are additional causes of malocclusion. If a primary tooth must be extracted, a space maintaining appliance should be inserted to prevent the adjacent teeth from drifting into the space, thereby blocking the eruption of the permanent succedaneous tooth which is developing underneath the primary tooth space.

Over five million children are currently receiving or have completed orthodontic treatment. [18] The increasing success of fluoridation programs and other measures for the prevention of dental caries should yield significant progress in reducing the incidence of malocclusion due to tooth destruction by dental caries.

PREVENTIVE MEASURES

FLUORIDE

Fluoride represents the single most significant factor contributing to the decline of caries prevalence among children and young adults. Investigation of the anticaries effects of fluoride has shown its primary function to be a consequence of replacement of the hydroxyl ions in the hydroxyapatite crystal of tooth enamel by fluoride ion, creating fluorapatite. The function of fluoride in forming apatite is that it appears to induce formation of larger, more stable enamel crystals which are less susceptible to attack by acid. In addition, fluoride has been found to be effective at the enamel surface. The presence of fluoride appears to increase the percentage of calcium and phosphate incorporated into the surface hydroxyapatite and fluorapatite and in this way, is thought to aid in the remineralization of demineralized surface enamel.

FLUORIDATION

About 56 percent of the U.S. population, having access to public water systems, now have the tooth decay prevention benefits of natural or adjusted fluoridation. [19] Scientific evidence clearly documents the safety and efficacy of drinking water fluoridation as a public health measure for preventing tooth decay.

The incidence of dental caries has been found to be from 48 to 70 percent lower, among groups of 12 to 14-year old children on optimally fluoridated water from birth, than among children of the same ages on fluoride-deficient water. Of even greater significance is the decrease in the number of missing teeth, ranging from 65 to 89 percent, among children in the same group on fluoridated versus nonfluoridated water. [20]

SYSTEMIC FLUORIDE THERAPY

Fluoridation of municipal water supplies has dramatically reduced caries in the U.S.; however, many communities have not been fluoridated because they are either not served by a central water supply or because they have not implemented this preventive procedure. Systemic fluoride supplements should be considered for all individuals residing in areas with water supplies deficient in this micronutrient.

Prescribing Fluoride Supplements for Home Use

Early initiation of treatment with fluoride supplements produces the best caries protective results. When preschoolers receive dietary fluoride supplements, their tooth decay rate is lowered 50 percent to 70 percent. When a fluoride supplement program is started at six years of age, the decay is reduced 20 to 45 percent. [21]

For fluoride supplements to provide optimal anticaries protection, prescriptions must be tailored to the specific needs of the individual patient. This requires:

1. Establishing the fluoride content of the patient's water supply.
2. Determining the proper dosage by age.
3. Selecting the appropriate type of supplement.
4. Teaching the patient and parents how to properly use the supplement.

The fluoride concentration in drinking water is the most important factor to consider when writing a prescription for a fluoride supplement. When the fluoride content of the home or school water supply is unknown, samples must be analyzed. Because of daily variations in some public water supplies, the collection and testing of water samples on two or three separate dates produce the most accurate measurements.

Prenatal Fluoride Supplements

In 1966, because of a paucity of clinical data, the U.S. Food and Drug Administration banned pharmaceutical companies from advertising that prenatal fluoride supplements inhibit dental caries. [22]   The clinical efficacy of prenatal fluorides and how they might impart cariostasis is unclear. Unknown as yet is the fetal fluoride plasma level for optimal dental therapeutic benefits. Nor is it known whether fluoride incorporated into the organic matrix of the developing tooth is beneficial or whether the principal clinical effect is derived from the incorporation of fluoride into the calcifying enamel. If the latter is true, it indicates that prenatal fluoride supplementation is unnecessary, since the most caries-susceptible areas of the teeth calcify after birth.

Selecting the Appropriate Type of Supplement

Several vehicles for delivering sodium fluoride may be used for systemic supplementation. Solutions which dispense 0.125 mg fluoride per drop are convenient formulations for infants since the dose can be easily adjusted. Tablets that contain 0.25 or 0.5 mg fluoride can replace the solution in children older than three years, if the child prefers and can properly chew and swallow a chewable tablet. Full strength tablets, or a fluoride rinse (5 cc = 1.0 mg F ion), can be prescribed at the appropriate age, usually after three years. The patient's age and degree of development and cooperation are the main factors to consider when determining which type of supplement to prescribe. To prevent toxic effects of accidental overdoses, one should prescribe no more than 120 mg F ion at any one time.

Fluoride Dose Levels for Specific Ages

DIETARY FLUORIDE SUPPLEMENTATION DOSE SCHEDULE*
IN MILLIGRAMS OF FLUORIDE PER DAY[+]
FLUORIDE CONTENT OF WATER

Age (years)	Less than 0.3 ppm	0.3 to 0.7 ppm	Greater than 0.7 ppm
Birth to 2	0.25 mg F	0 mg F	0 mg F
2-3	0.50 mg F	0.25 mg F	0 mg F
3-13	1.00 mg F	0.50 mg F	0 mg F

*   Recommended by the American Dental Association and the American Academy of Pediatric Dentistry
+   2 .2 mg of Sodium Fluoride provides 1 mg fluoride

School Water Fluoridation

In areas where community water fluoridation is not possible, fluoridation of school water supplies is an effective method of improving the dental health of children, reducing caries by about 40 percent. [23] There are several notable differences between the fluoridation of a school water supply. Since school-age children spend only about 20 to 25 percent of their waking hours in school, the fluoride content of the water supply in the school is adjusted to a level of 4.5 times the optimum indicated for community fluoridation in a particular geographical area. Thus, where the geographical area would indicate a level of fluoride ion of 1 ppm for community fluoridation, the school water supply in the same area would be adjusted to contain 4.5 ppm of fluoride.

TOPICAL FLUORIDE THERAPY

Self-Applied Fluoride Mouth Rinsing Programs in Schools

For the past three decades, considerable research has been conducted on the use of fluoride tablets or fluoride mouth rinses in schools. [24] Because children attend school regularly and because schools operate on a more rigid schedule than do individual families, schools are a logical place for administering self-applied topical fluoride to children. Results of studies show that tooth decay can be reduced by 20 to 50 percent by once-a-week fluoride mouth rinsing, and by 20 to 35 percent by the daily use of a fluoride tablet in school. [24] These results are based on the use of the respective agent only during the school year.

It is recommended that, in geographical areas with low fluoride levels, school-based fluoride mouth rinsing programs be initiated using dilute, unflavored solutions of neutral fluoride. Two options are available as to the concentration of fluoride to use for such programs. For daily mouth rinsing, a 0.05 percent solution of sodium fluoride is recommended; for one weekly rinsing, a 0.02 percent solution of sodium fluoride should be used.

Professionally Applied Topical Fluorides

The protective benefits of topical fluoride treatments are an important key to dental health, particularly for people living in nonfluoridated communities. Topical fluoride is also important to people in fluoridated areas, especially to individuals who continue to show a high susceptibility to dental caries in spite of optimal fluoride levels in their drinking water or appropriate systemic supplementation.

In most dental offices, topical fluoride in the form of 1.23 percent acidulated phosphate fluoride (APF) is applied using a paste, a gel, or a solution. Generally two applications a year, coinciding with the usual six-month dental recall schedule, are adequate. In highly susceptible patients, it is advisable for the application to be repeated three or four times a year. As a single caries preventive program, however, professionally applied topical fluorides are not very cost-effective.

Toothbrushing and Fluoride Toothpaste

There is presently no worthwhile evidence indicating that toothbrushing, per se, will reduce dental caries. However, brushing with the aid of fluoride toothpaste has been shown to reduce dental caries by the topical effect of the fluoride. [25]

The fluoride component of a dentifrice reacts with surface enamel to form fluorapatite, which chemically increases the enamel's resistance to acid demineralization. When this interaction involves sound enamel, new carious lesions are prevented.

Enamel that is already partially demineralized has a propensity for greater uptake of fluoride ions from the dentifrice. This effect inhibits incipient lesions from progressing to a higher state of demineralization.

The frequency of use of fluoride dentifrices, rather than the efficacy of any single formulation, may be a principal factor in achieving the caries reduction observed in clinical studies.

Dentifrice Swallowing by Young Children

Dentifrices, as applied topically to the teeth with the toothbrush, are generally rinsed and expectorated. Nevertheless, it is not uncommon that small amounts of the dentifrice will be retained in the mouth after brushing and swallowed. This is more common in children younger than five years of age. It has been reported that children aged two to four may ingest as much as 35 percent of the dentifrice applied to the toothbrush and this may result in the daily ingestion of 0.2 mg F, an amount equivalent to 20 percent of a systemic fluoride table (2.2 mg NaF). [26, 27, 28]

Although several studies have failed to show a relationship between enamel fluorosis and the early use of fluoride dentifrices and a history of dentifrice ingestion, [29,30,31] parents should be instructed to take precautions to prevent preschool children from inadvertently swallowing large amounts of fluoride dentifrice. Dentifrice precautions should include:

1. place a "pea-size" amount of dentifrice on the bristles of the toothbrush (Figure 1) rather than the one inch strip frequently shown in dentifrice advertisements;

2. have children rinse thoroughly and expectorate after brushing; and

3. supervise a child's brushing to ensure that the dentifrice-saliva mix-ture is expectorated and not swallowed.

FLOSSING

Research has revealed a significant reduction in proximal caries when children's teeth were flossed in school; [32,33] but studies also indicate that, in periodontally healthy subjects, the toothbrush is more effective than floss for removing observable plaque. Proper flossing technique is extremely difficult to learn, and parental assistance is required for children under eight years. A concentrated instruction effort is required for 8 year old children and annual reinforcement is necessary. [34]

NURSING CARIES

When children are kept on demand feeding beyond 18 months of life and are permitted to go to bed with a propped bottle, the milk curds formed in the acid media of the mouth are broken down and cause etching of the enamel. Similar effects have been observed in children who are breast-fed and who sleep with their mothers and are demand fed throughout the night. This condition, known as *nursing caries*, has received considerable attention in the past several years. This type of decay has a very specific pattern. Usually the maxillary incisors and canines are affected first, exhibiting white, decalcified areas (Figure 2).

The relationship between prolonged bottle and breast feeding and dental caries is related not only to milk but to fruit juices as well. The American Academy

FIGURE 1

PEA-SIZED AMOUNT OF FLUORIDE DENTIFRICE
RECOMMENDED FOR PRESCHOOL CHILDREN

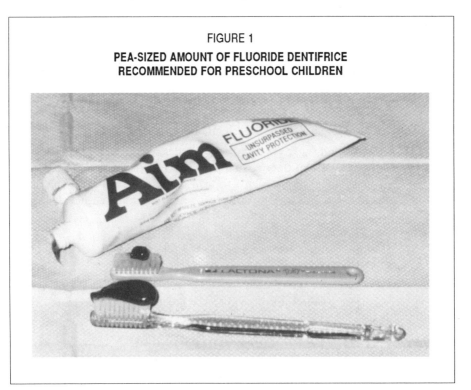

of Pediatrics and the American Academy of Pediatric Dentistry have made a joint statement on "Juices in Bottles Causing Dental Decay." [35] The marketing of juices in ready-to-use nursing bottles may tend to prolong bottle feeding and encourage the use of the bottle as a pacifier, both of which promote dental caries. The use of juices from a bottle should be discouraged and infants should be offered juice from a cup as soon as possible."

ADHESIVE SEALANTS

The high susceptibility of the pits and fissures of the occlusal surfaces of molars and premolars to dental caries has long been a major dental problem (Figure 3A to 3B). Although the occlusal (chewing) surfaces account for only 12.5 percent of the total dental surfaces, they currently account for about 54 percent of the permanent tooth caries activity in children. [7] (Table 2) Even in communities with optimally fluoridated drinking water, occlusal decay remains a serious problem, as the occlusal surfaces are not protected by fluoridate as well as the smooth surfaces of the teeth.

FIGURE 2

NURSING CARIES
AREAS OF DECALCIFICATION EVIDENT
IN PRIMARY MAXILLARY INCISORS AND CANINES

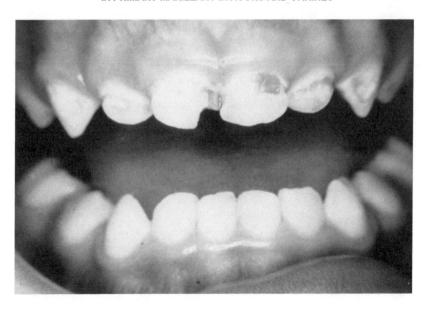

Recently, plastic sealing agents have been developed to help protect these vulnerable occlusal areas (Figure 4). These agents, in effect, act as a physical barrier to prevent oral bacteria and food debris from accumulating in the pits and fissures and setting up the favorable conditions necessary for dental caries initiation. Promising results have been reported, particularly on recently erupted permanent teeth in children. [36]

Sealants are designed mostly for children up to the age of 15. As teeth develop, grooves and ridges form on the chewing surface of the enamel and food particles and bacteria collect there and promote decay.

The effectiveness of sealants has been shown to vary and to be related to several factors, such as age, the combination of preventive methods used, and re-application and retention of the sealant. Their cost effectiveness is reduced if sealants are applied in a non-fluoridated community where proximal caries are likely to develop and involve sealed teeth. Sealants, properly applied usually last five

FIGURE 3A

VIEW OF OCCLUSAL FISSURES
IN A PERMANENT MANDIBULAR FIRST MOLAR

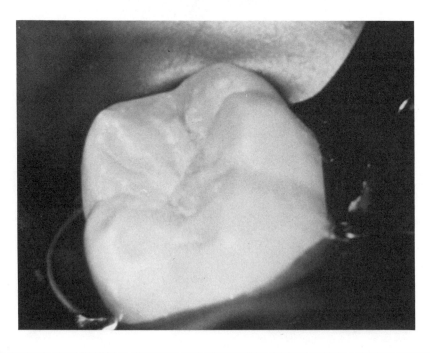

years or longer.   Even if a tiny cavity is already forming, the plastic seal protects the tooth from further bacterial damage. [36]

SUMMARY

Despite the high quality of dental care Americans receive, a high degree of need still exists. High caries levels have endured for so long that, by comparison, the current caries decline in permanent teeth appears attractive. There is a danger in becoming complacent about a disease whose prevalence and economic impact remain significant.

There is a dire need to support the inclusion of dental health services in comprehensive health programs for pregnant women and all children. The close cooperation of the dental, medical, and nursing professions is mandatory in any comprehensive health program, especially in programs for children.

FIGURE 3B

ELECTRON MICROSCOPE VIEW OF
OCCLUSAL FISSURES IN A PERMANENT MANDIBULAR FIRST MOLAR.

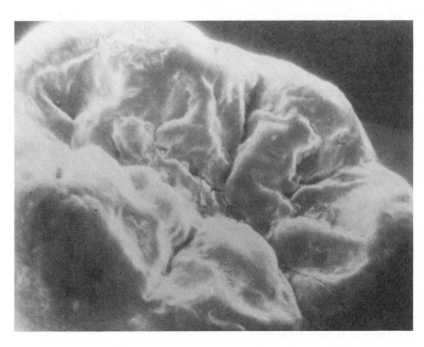

If the caries-free generation is to become a reality, oral health evaluation and counseling should be a part of all prenatal, infant, child, and youth health care programs. All children should be referred to a dentist by the age of one year with an explanation to the parents as to the reasons and significance of dental referral. All children with clinical evidence of dental decay, gingival disease, or orthodontic problems should be referred immediately for dental care, with follow-up to ascertain that appropriate care is received. Dental screening should be a part of all school health screening programs and well-child care programs. This can be accomplished by general health care providers (physicians and nurses) with appropriate training, and should include referral to a dentist and followup.

COST AND PAYMENT OF DENTAL SERVICES

Current annual expenditures for dental care in the U.S. amount to about $10 billion or about $45.41 per capita.[37] This amounts to approximately eight percent of the total U.S. health care expenditures.[38] Preventive dental services account for about eight percent of these dental expenditures, basic dental restorations (silver

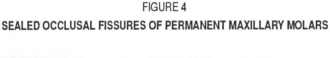

FIGURE 4

SEALED OCCLUSAL FISSURES OF PERMANENT MAXILLARY MOLARS

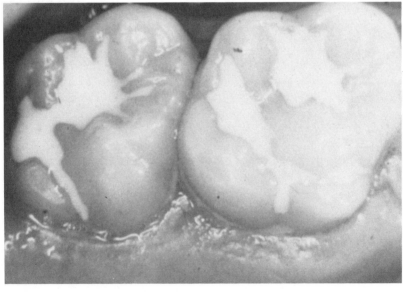

amalgam fillings) account for 49 percent, and reconstructive, esthetic, and prosthetic dental services account for about 43 percent, of which three percent is for orthodontic treatment.

Traditionally dental services have been paid on a fee-for-service basis by direct out-of-pocket consumer payments. This method is still by far the predominant method of payment of dental services. For instance, in 1977, direct consumer payments for dental services amounted to nearly eight billion dollars. This converts to $35.10 out of the total $45.41 per capita expenditure for dental services.[37] As a comparison, dental services represent 39 percent of about $92.74 per capita spent annually for out-of-pocket payments for both medical and dental care. This direct payment for dental services may help explain some of the dynamics of the dental care market. People seem to think they are paying high amounts for dental care because they pay directly out of their pocket. This explains the reason why among "poor children," 85 out of every 100 decayed teeth go unfilled.[39]

Third-Party Payment

Dental insurance plans have been very slow to follow medical care coverage, most likely due in part to the need to afford the average citizen some protection for hospital and medical costs before focusing on dental costs. But, with an expanding economy and the political acceptance of health care as a right, third-party payments in dentistry grew from insignificant prior to the 1950s to about 65 million people who have some dental care coverage today.[38,40] In 1977, private dental insurance paid $2.055 billion of the nation's dental bills, representing 15.5 percent of the total expenditures for dental care[37] and today there are more than 140 carriers in the dental prepayment field.[41]

Publicly Financed Dental Care

Federal, state, and local government expenditures account for about five percent of the nation's dental bill. The largest portion of federal funds are paid through Medicaid, about $225 million; followed by the Veteran's Administration, $63 million; and MCH Care, $10 million. State and local expenditures for dental care amount to about $190 million, of which about $173 million is paid through state Medicaid programs and about four million dollars through state MCH Care Programs. [37,38]

REFERENCES

1. Graves RC, Stramm JW. Oral health status in the United States: Prevalence of dental caries. J Dent Ed 49:341-351, 1985.

2. Stookey GK, et al. Prevalence of dental caries in Indiana school children: results of 1982 survey. Ped Dent 7:8-13, 1985.

3. Tanzer JM. Essential dependence of smooth surface caries on, and augmentation of fissure caries by, sucrose and Streptococcus mutans infection. Infect. Immun 25:526-531, 1979.

4. Kelly JE, Scanlon, JV. U.S. Public Health Service, National Center for Health Statistics. Decayed, Missing, and Filled Teeth Among Children, United States. DHEW Publication No. (HSM) 72-1003-Ser. 11-NO. 106. Washington, D.C. Government Printing Office, 1971.

5. Kelly JE and Scanlon, JV. U.S. Public Health Service, National Center for Health Statistics. Decayed, Missing, and Filled Teeth Among Persons 12-17 Years, United States. DHEW Publication No. (HRA) 75-1626 Ser. 11-No. 144. Washington, D.C: Government Printing Office, 1974.

6. Harvey CR, and Kelly JE. U.S. Public Health Service, National Center for Health Statistics. Decayed, Missing, and Filled Teeth Among Youths 1-17 Years, United States 1971-74. DHHS Publication No. (PHS) 81-1678-Ser. 11-No. 223. Washington, D.C.: Government Printing Office, 1981.

7. Brunelle JA, Carlos JP. Changes in the prevalence of dental caries in U.S. school children, 1961-1980. J Dent Res 61 (Spec Iss) 1346-51, 1982.

8. U.S. Department of Health and Human Services: The Prevalence of DentalCaries in United States Children, The National Dental Caries Prevalence Survey, NIH Publication No 82-2245, December 1981.

9. U.S. Department of Health and Human Services: Dental Treatment Needs of United States Children, The National Dental Caries Prevalence Survey, NIH Publication No. 83-2246, December 1982.

10. Belting, C, Massler M, and Scheur I. Prevalence and incidence of alveolar bone disease in men. JADA, 47:190, 1953.

11. Day CD, et al: Periodontal disease: Prevalence and incidence. J Periodont.26:185,1955.

12. Pelton WJ, et al: Tooth mortality experience of adults. JADA, 49:439, 1954.

13. Page RC: Oral health status in the United States: Prevalence of inflammatory periodontal disease. J Dent Ed 49:354-363, 1985.

14. Poma PA, et al. Oral cavity evaluation: A part of prenatal care. Ill Med J 155:85, 1979.

15. Loe H. Periodontal changes in pregnancy, J Periodontol. 26:209-217, 1975.

16. Cohen DW, et al:. "A Longitudinal Investigation of Periodontal Changes During Pregnancy," J Periodontol. 40:563-570, 1969.

17. James JD. Dental caries in pregnancy, J Amer Dental Assoc. 28:1857-1862, 1941.

18. Kelly JE, et al. An assessment of the occlusion of teeth of children 6-11 years, United States. Data from the National Health Survey, Vital Health Stat., Ser. 11, No. 130, DHEW Publication No. (HRA) 74-1612, 1973.

19. U.S. Department of Health and Human Services: USPHS, Fluoridation Census 1980. Atlanta, GA: Centers for Disease Control, 1984.

20. Douglas BL, et al. The impact of fluoridation on patterns of dental treatment. J Pub Health Dent. 31:225-40, 1971.

21. Parkins FM. Prescribing fluorides for home use, in Fluorides: An Update for Dental Practice. New York, Medcom, Inc, 1976.

22. Food and Drug Administration: Statements of general policy or interpretation,oral

prenatal drugs containing fluorides for human use. Federal Register, October 20, 1966.

23. Horowitz HS, Heifetz SB, and Law F.E. Effect of school water fluoridation on dental caries: final results in Elk Lake Pennsylvania after 12 years. JADA 84:832-38, 1972.

24. U.S. Department of Health, Education and Welfare: National Institute for Dental Research, Preventing Tooth Decay - A Guide for Implementing Self-Applied Fluoride in Schools, DHEW No. (NIH) 77-1196, 2-3, 1977.

25. Forward GC. Action and Interaction of fluoride in dentifrices. Community Dent. Oral Epidemiol. 8:527-566, 1980.

26. Baxter PM. Toothpaste ingestion during toothbrushing by school children. Br Dent J, 148:125-128, 1980.

27. Barnhart WE, Hiller LK, Leonard, GJ, et al. Dentifrice usage and ingestion among four age groups. J Dent Res. 53:1317-1322, 1974.

28. Ericsson Y and Forsman B. Fluoride retained from mouthrinses and dentifrices in preschool children. Caries Res 3:290-299, 1969.

29. Driscoll WS, Heifetz SB, Horowitz HS, et al. Prevalence of dental caries and fluorosis in areas with optimal and above-optimal water fluoride concentrations. JADA 107:42-47, 1983.

30. Soparkar PM and DePaola PF. History of fluoride ingestion among children diagnosed with and without fluorosis (Abst. #459). J Dent Res (Abstracts): 226, 1985.

31. Houwink B and Wagg BJ. Effect of fluoride dentifrice usage during infancy upon enamel mottling of the permanent teeth. Caries Res 13:231-237, 1979.

32. Bohannon HM, Ochsenbein C, and Saxe SR. Preventive periodontics. Dent Clin North Am 9:7, 1965.

33. Horowitz AM, et al. Effect of supervised daily plaque removal by children. Results afterthe third and final year. J Dent Res 56:185, 1977.

34. Terhune JA. Predicting the readiness of elementary school children to learn an effective dental flossing technique. J Am Dent Assoc 86:1332, 1972.

35. News and Comments. A Joint statement from the American Academy of Pediatrics and the American Academy of Pediatric Dentistry. Pediatric Den 29:1:29, 1979.

36. Horowitz HS, Heifetz SB and Paulson S. Retention and effectiveness of a single application of an adhesive sealant in preventing occlusal caries; final report after five years of a study in Kalispell, Montana. JADA 95:1133-1139, 1977.

37. Gibson RM, CR Fisher. National Health Expenditures, Fiscal Year 1977, Soc Sec Bull 41(7):3-20, July, 1978.

38. Douglass CW, Day JM. Cost and payment of dental services in the UnitedStates. J Dent Ed, 43:330-348, 1979.

39. Greene JC. Dental health needs of the nation. J Am Dent Assoc, 84:1073-1075, May, 1972.

40. Feldstein PJ, Roehrig CS, Hall J. An Econometric Model of the Dental Sector. Boston, Mass. Policy Analysis, Inc., June, 1977.

41. Wei SHY. Diet and dental caries. In Stewart et. al. (ed.): Pediatric Dentistry Scientific Foundations and Clinical Practice. St. Louis, The C.V. Mosby Co., 1982, p. 576.

PRIMARY HEALTH CARE FOR CHILDREN AND YOUTH 17

Joel J. Alpert

Primary health care for children and youth in the U.S. remains a story of high aims and important but incomplete achievements. Few would disagree with the wisdom of investing in the health of society's future citizens, but often, when that investment is made, it is found uneven in its commitment. The thesis of this chapter is that achievement and failure are two important characteristics of primary health care for children and youth in the U.S. Achievement may be seen in the excellent primary care received by many children. Failure is seen in our inability to organize and to finance primary care services so that all children benefit effectively and equally. Perhaps as many as 75-80 percent of U.S. children are fully immunized, enjoy the personal services of a well-trained and competent physician, and are protected through private insurance against minor and major medical costs. However, the remainder may be inadequately immunized and incompletely serviced, and at times underinsured or totally exposed to the expenses generated by child health supervision, minor illness, let alone catastrophic events.

This chapter will (1) describe and define primary health care for children; (2) review the content of these primary care services; discuss the (3) personnel, (4) settings, and (5) education necessary to provide primary care; (6) review current primary care standards; (7) identify continuing deterrents to delivery; and (8) close with a prescription for primary care services for children and youth for the future.

DEFINITION OF PRIMARY CARE

The term, *primary care*, is now an established part of our medical vocabulary.[1] Primary care for children focuses upon the needs of children and families. Primary care is part of a system of services which includes secondary and tertiary care services. *Secondary care* means referral care, usually in a physician's office or in a hospital outpatient department. It may mean less complicated hospital care, such as might be delivered in a community hospital. *Tertiary care* is care that takes place in a hospital bed dealing with the most complicated of medical care problems. Tertiary care in many minds is equated with care delivered in an academic medical center, but many community hospitals provide excellent tertiary care services whatever their location or academic affiliations.

There are four anchoring points in the definition of primary care. These are first contact, longitudinal responsibility, integration of services, and a family and community orientation.

Primary care is first contact care, which means access to care. However, first contact cannot be equated solely with access. The decision for a child to seek out and to continue with medical care is influenced by a large number of important social and individual factors. Those in greatest need may not seek care appropriately and, also, may not follow advice adequately. First contact must include outreach especially targeted at categories of children at risk.

Primary care means assuming longitudinal responsibility for the child regardless of the presence or absence of disease. Primary care physicians, such as pediatricians and family practitioners, hold the contract for providing personal child health services. The primary care physician with his or her colleagues is available continuously, provides continuity of care in the office, hospital, or patient's home, and provides important elements of secondary and tertiary care. The physician assuming responsibility for care in the hospital is a feature which distinguishes pediatric care in the U.S. from many other countries where primary care is largely delivered in the physician's office or health center.

Primary care means acting as the integrationist for the child. When other health resources are involved, the primary care physician has the responsibility of managing to the limit of his or her capability the physical, psychological, and social aspects of patient care. Preventive and curative services are provided by the same physician.

Family and community are the final part of the definition. Awareness of the family is a major part of primary care child services since the family is the largest determinant of how medical services are sought and used. A functioning family is a resource for the child and positively influences outcome and compliance. Similarly, a malfunctioning or absent family can produce negative outcomes and poor compliance. Primary care for children recognizes that since families are the unit of living in society, the family is also the unit of health and illness.

The community also influences personal health. The primary care practitioner, both in professional and personal activities, should care for individual patients with knowledge of the community from which the patient comes. A pregnant adolescent comes from a community that may need better family planning services. Similarly, a poor inner-city community requires different primary care than a more advantaged suburban one, and an under-immunized community may be at risk for a preventable disease. While the primary care physician is most concerned with the needs of individual patients, the practice of primary care pediatrics needs to occur with an epidemiological awareness and knowledge about effective community interventions. The term, *community -oriented primary care,* has been proposed as a model for the delivery of these services. [2]

CONTENT OF PRIMARY CARE

The major reason that primary health care has assumed greater importance for children has been the changing and evolving nature of childhood health and disease. In the 1950s, there was considerable discussion about the new pediatrics, which, at that time, referred to the changing content of pediatric practice. [3] Because of the rapid improvements in child health (immunizations, antibiotics, better nutrition), pediatrics had become an ambulatory specialty, and pediatricians were being asked to develop expertise in problems with an increasing psychosocial content. In the 1960s, this new pattern of practice was described as the new pediatric morbidity. [4] The issues for pediatrics were no longer life-threatening diseases but common and high prevalence issues, such as health maintenance, care of common infections, behavior disorders, and concerns about growth and development. Pediatricians in the 1970s were expected to see more and more children for reasons of health and common illness, as opposed to serious illness which had become increasingly unusual. This was not to say that children no longer experienced serious life-threatening diseases but, rather, that these serious problems affected fewer children and that most children could anticipate a childhood free of life-threatening infections. Poliomyelitis had yielded to injuries, and gross malnutrition to obesity and unhealthy lifestyles.

In the 1970s, there was a need to shift from a pure biomedical model to a biopsychosocial one in addressing children's primary health needs. Management of acute illness, of course, was part of the physician's job, including caring for the unusual. Physicians who care for children need to be aware of such illlnesses as mycoplasma, chlamydia, group B strep, AIDS, new hazards and injuries (skateboards, trampolines, all terrain vehicles), and new therapeutic agents with unanticipated side effects (especially antibiotics) that require updated professional expertise and knowledge. Common diseases could be associated with uncommon complications, the prescription of powerful agents produced iatrogenic diseases, and new environmental hazards produced injury risks. Technological advances in such areas as newborn intensive care increased survival and minimized handicaps, but survivors were also children with chronic and handicapping conditions.

Adolescents in the 1980s experienced rising mortality due to violent events, such as injuries, suicide, and homicide. Sexually transmitted disease and disturbances of learning and eating were increasingly brought to the attention of the responsible primary care physician. An informed public, in the 1980s, worried about sudden infant death, a toxic environment, and preventive nutrition.

There is an inescapable social dimension to primary care services. Unhealthy lifestyles, including drug and alcohol abuse, dangerous driving practices, and lack of exercise are childhood antecedents of adult disease. The fastest growing part of child health care is the area of behavioral pediatrics, especially learning disorders and other school problems. All of these issues contribute to primary care child health practice.

PERSONNEL TO DELIVER PRIMARY CARE SERVICE

There is a number of professional models proposed for the delivery of primary care services to children. These professionals can work in a number of distinctly different organizations. These organizations may be in the public or private sector, urban or rural, and require different mixes of staffing and teams depending upon whether the patients are affluent or poor.

The manner in which primary care is delivered reflects the strengths and weaknesses of our society. The possible models provide a pluralistic approach, which can be imaginative and exciting. However, the pluralism also produces uneven, inadequate, and, often poor quality services. Striking evidence of this is the failure to provide even basic immunization to all children, let alone to address the psychosocial needs of a stressed child population and the presence of major areas in the U.S., both urban and rural, which are medically underserved.

A standard by which all primary care professionals must be judged is a career commitment to the care of children. Whether the practitioner is a pediatrician or family practitioner, there must be a major, if not full-time, commitment to the care of children. The major accomplishment of separating the needs of children from those of adults must not be lost as larger and different numbers of child-health caretakers appear.

The pediatrician model is one standard of comparison. No matter what the organization, there is ample evidence that the pediatrician is readily accepted by families, is committed to children, and is most thoroughly educated in the care of children. Most pediatricians consider themselves as providers of primary care. Unfortunately, pediatricians are concentrated geographically in large urban areas and highly populated states, and there are major areas of the U.S. which continue without these services.

Primary care can be carried out by at least two kinds of pediatricians: those who are specifically trained for primary care; and those who are trained as subspecialists. Primary care pediatricians are largely office-based and may work in solo practice, small groups, or large multispecialty groups. Single-specialty groups are generally composed of a smaller number of physicians. The single-specialty model has the advantage of small size, and patients can have a feeling of personal identification with their physician.

Pediatric subspecialists can also provide a significant amount of primary care. While some satisfaction can be taken from the fact that subspecialists see more primary care patients than previously judged, serious questions must be raised as to whether these services are delivered well. If primary care pediatricians were asked to deliver subspecialty care without specific training, quality would suffer. The reverse is also true and it is preferable having well-trained family physicians delivering primary care to children if the alternative is the pediatric subspecialist.

Because of the geographic maldistribution of pediatricians, family practitioners can be expected to deliver considerable primary care to children. This is especially likely in rural settings. The family practitioner offers knowledge in breadth about the family but at some sacrifice in depth of knowledge about children.

Much of the discussion about family practitioners, compared with pediatricians, as primary care professionals would diminish if family practice would increase the amount of pediatric learning during training. But more important is whether family practitioners make a career commitment to the care of children. As physicians age, so do their practices, and only those family practitioners who actively recruit infants and children to their practices can be expected to remain competent in the field of child care.

As pediatricians expand their knowledge about families, and were family practitioners (at least some) to expand their knowledge about children, there would be little difference in the described models. The future holds the exciting promise that out of pediatrics and family medicine may come the development of a generalist for younger and developing families.

Health professionals other than the physician accept increased responsibility for the delivery of child primary care services. Numerous studies have shown that trained nurse practitioners successfully provide many of the services provided by primary care pediatricians. As many as 80-90 percent of health care decisions can be made by a nurse practitioner, and possibly at a lower cost. [5]

Especially in areas of high risk, such as the inner city, no one profession can provide all of the needed health services. Not only are different skills needed, but no single individual can be available all of the time. It seems reasonable, therefore, to assume a future of team, as opposed to single profession, practice especially with at-risk populations.

There are different methods of organizing primary care. It may be more important to provide vigorous outreach in the inner city than in the suburbs, and the private pediatrician model may require modification and different team composition, depending upon the geographic area and patient needs.

An unanswered question for primary care is the relationship between physicians and other health professionals. The question is answered in part by the system in the U.S., namely that physicians who care for patients outside of the hospital also have a responsibility for secondary and tertiary care services. The role of the physician will increase as the increased numbers of students in the 1980s become the physician surplus of the 1990s.

Much of the discussion surrounding the different models of primary care for children occurs because there is little evidence that clearly favors one model over another. Data suggest that continuity of care can be associated with decreased and shorter hospitalizations, increased satisfaction, fewer operations, lower costs (because of decreased use of laboratory and hospital admissions), and fewer illness visits. [6] In these studies, there was no evidence of morbidity differences. Moreover, comparative studies of different models of care (hospital, prepaid group practice, private practice, health center) indicate no outcome differences for selected tracer conditions. While the available studies may be imperfect, the fact remains that those who prefer one model over another must temper their judgment because of the lack of hard data. While the pediatrician model is one standard, absolute evidence for that position is lacking.

Whatever the professional model for primary care delivery, the manner in which care is paid for influences the services provided. In a private practice fee-for-service setting, the services provided are largely determined by the patient and physician. In health maintenance organizations, services may be determined after more complex negotiations. In the prepaid setting, generalist physicians, whether pediatricians or family physicians, appear to be the preferred care giver.

Group practice, either single-specialty or multispecialty is the dominant model for physicians delivering primary care services. The size, combination of physicians, and mix of other health professionals in each group is usually determined by the setting and the physician's training.

The notion of a single source and a regular source of primary care are major issues whatever the economics or geography of the community. People use more than one source of care, and the provision of a new source often adds just one more site for care to a family's use pattern. Multiple facility use for a given child appears to be a more common pattern for inner city families, as opposed to the suburban affluent or rural poor, although there is some evidence that the use of the suburban community hospital as a source for emergency and off-hours care is increasing, and multiple physicians for one family is a common pattern for the suburban family.

Multiple use is not haphazard but is developed after families carefully and logically explore alternatives.

Available data support the notion that families use a widely dispersed system of primary care, with a substantial split between the private and public sectors and between preventive and acute care professionals. The primary care system for the poor remains largely separate from the system for the affluent. The poor are more apt to use public and hospital-based care, while the affluent are more likely to use private office-based pediatrician care. For affluent suburban children, except in the case of an emergency, a private pediatrician is most likely to provide most basic primary health services. However, increasing emphasis upon managed care, which will limit choice, is likely to effect the utilization of both the affluent and the poor.

SETTINGS FOR PRIMARY CARE SERVICES

The physician's private office remains the site where most primary health care for children is provided. Unlike other countries, this setting in the U.S. combines curative and preventive services. The changing nature of pediatrics has seen most private practitioners confronted with the new morbidity. In 1987, there are about 40,000 pediatricians, most of whom practice in this setting and this number is expected to increase.

The community or neighborhood health center has become an important source of health care for inner city residents. The center concept takes its origins in the milk stations of large cities, especially in Boston and New York, around the beginning of this century. These centers, which for over 75 years provided largely preventive services, took on a new significance with the rediscovery of poverty in the 1960s and were an essential part of the health initiatives as part of the "War on Poverty." These centers, as are all facilities caring for the poor, continue to experience a stormy time due to inadequate third-party reimbursements, especially Medicaid, and their dependence upon grant support. There has been difficulty in attracting physicians over time and these physicians have not yet made long-term career commitments. The National Health Service Corps assigns physicians to these underserved inner city areas, and graduates of new training programs in primary care have chosen careers in these settings. [7]

Health centers have in most cases been the first new services brought to inner-city neighborhoods to replace the pre-World War II general practitioner. Their acceptance has been enhanced by their broad community support. They have been associated with decreased use of hospitals. [8]

The hospital's ambulatory services continue to be an important source of primary care services, especially the emergency room. There continues to be evidence that hospital use is both appropriate (for emergencies and because families view the hospital as their physician) and inappropriate (because the usual source, the neighborhood health center, was bypassed, or families came because of convenience, or a non-emergency reason). Many inner-city hospitals stimulated by inappropriate use of the emergency room, and also for training objectives, have developed group practices or reorganized their outpatient department services with mixed results since the hospital was not designed to be supportive of the delivery of primary care services.

For the older child, the school is a source of primary care services. Screening and health education can take place in this setting. Concern about teenage pregnancy, sexually transmitted diseases and the unmet health needs of young adolescents prompted increased interest in school health clinics. Over 60 clinics were operational in the late 1980s and have provoked both support and opposition with the opposition focusing on and opposing the delivery in the school of contraceptive and family planning services. Even if widely established, these clinics would fall short of needs since studies have confirmed the large number of school dropouts and school absentees. [9] Most school health clinics have concentrated on middle and high-school students but a similar effort emphasizing education and prevention, would be appropriate in the elementary school. It is likely that these services will increase, especially stimulated by the need to educate about, and prevent, AIDS, which has forced the health education issue to the forefront. In developing these services, care should be taken not to duplicate already available services, such as those provided by practicing pediatricians, family physicians, and neighborhood health centers. Neighborhood health centers can be linked with schools, as can private practitioners.

Settings which deliver largely first-contact care, such as the emergency room and free standing walk-in clinics, deliver considerable acute care services. Free-standing clinics largely exist because of the inappropriateness of the emergency room but, while more efficient, do not meet the standard required to achieve primary care, as has been previously defined.

EDUCATION FOR PRIMARY CARE

Education for primary care has changed and considerable attention is being paid to the education of a large range of health professionals for primary care.

Physician education is especially important because it is the medical model that dominates the delivery of primary care. All of the health professionals involved in primary care delivery (pediatricians, internists, family practitioners, nurses, and others) have had programs developed emphasizing primary care content. In general, this means concentrating upon activities in the ambulatory setting that occur commonly and have a large psychosocial content. The Task Force for Pediatric Education, in its 1978 report, summarized many of these recommendations. [10] The

Task Force's recommendations included increased ambulatory experiences, increased psychosocial content, and increased emphasis on allergy, dermatology, management of behavior disorders, orthopedics, child development, and adolescent services. The American Board of Pediatrics also required three years of general pediatric training for board certification, that no more than 11 months of the three year training be in the subspecialties, and that no more than six months be in any one subspecialty. The official review body (the Residency Review Committee in Pediatrics), in 1987, implemented revised requirements for the subspecialties, which limited program directors to a specified list of subspecialties which share in common their status as subboards of the American Academy of Pediatrics. These revisions may be justified both for setting standards for marginal programs and also to emphasize the role of the pediatrician as a consultant. However, the list (cardiology, endocrinology, critical care, pulmonary, nephrology, and hematology/oncology) omits such specialties as gastroenterology, genetics, infectious disease, neurology, and allergy and immunology. There is no formal list which includes child development, adolescent medicine, and behavioral pediatrics. These educational issues reflect the tension which exists in pediatric education regarding the primary and secondary/tertiary care role.

Since 1974, the federal government has provided targeted training funds for physician education by supporting both family practice and pediatric primary care residencies, using the term *general pediatrics*. [11] Federal support for primary care requires increased ambulatory and continuity experience to qualify for funding, as well as development of model practices and a clinical and non-clinical curriculum in primary care. This curriculum includes child development, adolescent care, behavioral pediatrics, practice management, and social science topics relevant to primary care for children.

The distinguishing features of primary care education appear to be continuity, experience, and psychosocial content, in addition to usual pediatric training. There is, as of yet, no evidence that training a physician differently results in different practice patterns or content. Such data are needed, and investigation in this area should take place.

STANDARDS OF PRIMARY CARE

Acceptable standards of primary care for children are also subject to re-evaluation and revision. It has been possible to develop criteria for individual tracer conditions, and standards have been described for record keeping. The effort by the Joint Committee for Quality Assurance to define quality in office practice largely documented the inadequate state of patient records in pediatric office practices.[12]

Standards for primary care include emphasis upon prevention and has physical, biomedical, social, emotional, and cognitive content. Child development content is a major part of these standards. The American Academy of Pediatrics has established standards of health promotion and has made an important and valuable contribution to standard setting. [13]

In establishing standards for primary care for children, it must be realized that not even the most effective model presently provides every necessary service. For example, while neighborhood health centers may have effective outreach programs, the center may not be successful in delivering continuity. Similarly, the private practice model does not usually include effective outreach but does provide continuity.

What then should be considered as optimal standards? In developing optimum services, the goal is to define specific content. Moreover, quality also has to be defined and, when defined, measured.

There must be effective access to care. This is accomplished by outreach, appropriate location of services, and available transportation. There is telephone access 24-hours a day, seven days a week, as well as a specified time when families can consult with their physicians. There are appointment systems that are designed to promote continuity of care.

Preventive health care is central to the services children receive. These preventive services include prevention of catastrophes (sudden infant death, injuries, homicide, suicide) and the development of unhealthy lifestyles (smoking, substance abuse). There is effective screening.

There should be periodic evaluation of the child's health status. There has been considerable discussion about decreasing the frequency of periodic health visits. However, some circumstances require additional contacts. These include: (1) first born, adopted children, or those not with natural parents; (2) parents with a particular need for education and guidance; (3) disadvantaged social or economic environment; (4) the presence or possibility of perinatal disorders, such as low birth weight, congenital defects, or familial disease; (5) acquired illness, or previously identified health-related problems.

Appropriate care of the child during illness can be provided by telephone, in the office, in the hospital, and in the patient's home. These services include taking a history, physical examination, using the laboratory, and providing appropriate intervention that includes supportive and symptomatic therapy, as well as those requiring prescription. Chronic illness and handicapping conditions require special services, including not only expert knowledge but also the coordination and integration of the many services required.

Office facilities should be adequate and all equipment functional. This includes not only location but attention to patient flow with appropriate means of achieving isolation. Office furnishings should be consistent with a setting that is a special place for children. By designing a safe office, by insisting upon no smoking, by providing toys and literature that promote health education, the medical office setting can promote primary care health goals. Adequate and readable medical records are important. Records should provide a pediatric data base, allow retrieval information, and chart review.

The major goal of these recommendations is the development of a long-term parent-child-physician relationship. The goals of periodic assessment go beyond the act of providing preventive services. The outcome of this program should be a child about whom there is a complete data base; regular physical, cognitive, and emotional assessments; effective sensory screening; full immunization, and dental care. Every child should have a medical home that would provide a full range of primary care services.

DETERRENTS TO PRIMARY CARE

The major deterrent to successful delivery of primary care services is financial. Unlike other countries, the U.S. has not decided as policy that primary care services are important. Reimbursements for primary care services are inadequate. The fact that the near poor are not insured makes this group even more vulnerable to financial barriers.

Attitudes and personalities of professionals are also a deterrent. The existence of a separate system for minorities, the poor, and the middle class is a barrier. The pluralistic system that has previously been noted to be an opportunity is a deterrent to rational planning and prevents fundamental decisions from being made.

Medicine's complete commitment to a biomedical model is also a barrier. While there have been major achievements, primary care has historically not been assigned equal importance.

Medical education has been a deterrent. The separation of preventive from curative services (schools of medicine, schools of public health) has been reinforced by the excessive reliance upon the hospital as the major educational setting to learn about medical practice. Even if medical education were totally supportive, there are only limited means to pay for educational programs in ambulatory settings, especially outside of the hospital, suggesting the need for targeted support far beyond that presently provided for education in and out of hospital settings.

FUTURE

For future planning, it is important to realize that predictions are based upon variables that are not fixed and are subject to change. Whether the birth rate decreases or increases will have a great deal to say about needed primary care services. The new emphasis upon self-help may impact upon the health use and outcomes of the next generation. In an important experiment with elementary school children, it was demonstrated that by third grade, 15 percent of the children were using 50 percent of the services offered. [14] Children were shown to be able to initiate their own need for health services. The real significance of the study will be measured in the long run, when we can assess childhood learning and the manner in which adult health services are used. This study suggested that while high users were not affected, a large number of students felt that they could participate in decisions regarding treatment of their medical concerns, and there was greater reliance on self-seeking care.

One future goal will be to put together the various components of a primary care system, recognizing that the present system, while capable of high quality, is fundamentally fragmented. For the decades following World War II, we have spoken of the U.S. having the highest quality of medical care available, setting a world standard. It is not enough to say the U.S. is the best if the the 20 percent at risk because of financial barriers do not benefit.

The driving force for restructuring must be a national health insurance program. Removing the financial barrier will be the giant step towards overcoming the present major shortcomings of the U.S. system as it exists in the 1980s.

Primary care pediatrics, as it now stands, involves the care of children with largely ambulatory needs. The professional currently in the best position to offer and to organize these personal services is the pediatrician. There are many attempts to offer as less important the highly personal relationship of the child, family, and physician. This highly individual role between the physician and the individual patient is as important today as it ever was and is fundamental to the delivery of primary care.

REFERENCES

1. Alpert JJ, Charney E. The education of physicians for primary care. DHEW No (HRA) 74-3113, 1973.

2. Nutting P. Community oriented primary care: A practice assessment. Volume 1: The Committee Report (National Academy Press), 1984.

3. May C. Can the new pediatrics be practiced. Pediatrics 23:253, 1959.

4. Pless IB. The changing face of primary pediatrics. Pediatr Clin North America 21:223, 1974.

5. Charney E, Kitzman H. The child health nurse (pediatric nurse practitioner) in private practice: A Controlled Trial. New Eng J Med 285:1353, 1971.

6. Alpert JJ, Robertson LS, Kosa J, et al. Delivery of health care for children: Report of an experiment. Pediatrics 57:917, 1976.

7. Shelov S, Alpert JJ, Rayman F, et al. Primary care training programs and pediatric careers. Am J Dis Child 141:65, 1987.

8. Hochheiser L, Woodward K, Charney E. The effect of a neighborhood health center of pediatric emergency room use. New Eng J Med 285:148, 1971.

9. Weitzman M, Alpert JJ, Klerman L, et al. The case of excessive school absence. Pediatrics 78:313, 1986.

10. American Academy of Pediatrics Task Force on Pediatric Education: The future of pediatric education, Evanston, IL, 1978.

11. Mathieu O, Alpert JJ. Residency training in general pediatrics: The role of federal funding. Am J Dis Child 141:754, 1987.

12. Osborn EE, Thompson HE. Criteria for evaluation of child health care by chart audit. Pediatrics (suppl) 56:625, 1975.

13. American Academy of Pediatrics: Management of pediatric practice, Elk Grove Village, IL, 1986.

14. Lewis CE, Lewis MA, Lorimer A, et al. Child initiated care: The use of school nursing services by children in an "adult free system." Pediatrics 60:499, 1977.

NUTRITION SERVICES

18

Johanna T. Dwyer and Judith Freedland

INTRODUCTION

TYPES OF MALNUTRITION

Nutrition services must deal with six different forms of malnutrition and under-nutrition. Three of these are more common among the poor: starvation, under-nutrition and dietary-deficiency diseases of vitamins and minerals. In contrast, obesity, nutrient imbalances, and toxicities of alcohol, vitamins, and minerals are especially common among the affluent in well-to-do countries. In the U.S. today, all of these forms of malnutrition exist and changes in them must be monitored.

SIZE AND EXTENT OF THE PROBLEM

The problems involved in assuring that women, infants, and children receive adequate nutrition services are well-reviewed in the Surgeon General's Report on Nutrition and Health.[1]

HISTORICAL CHANGES IN RELEVANT NUTRITIONAL PROBLEMS

The nutritional problems afflicting mothers and children have changed dramatically since 1900. Early in the century, the major problems were under-nutrition, the classical dietary-deficiency diseases, and malnutrition due to infectious diseases. Real gains have been made since then in the prevention of nutrition problems, and several vitamin-deficiency diseases have all but disappeared. However, much remains to be done.

Today, while problems of dietary inadequacy and poverty-related malnutrition continue to plague the less fortunate members of our population, nutritional problems associated with affluence, such as over-nutrition and imbalances in nutrients, are more common. Nutritional problems secondary to chronic degenerative diseases and handicapping conditions also must be dealt with.[2]

SOCIETAL CONDITIONS AND NUTRITIONAL RISK FACTORS

The nutritional health of most mothers and children depends far more on societal and environmental influences than it does on heredity. Thus, changes in the larger society influence nutritional health profoundly. The factors which have influenced MCH policies over the past few decades are summarized elsewhere.[3] Also important are changes in health care technologies and reimbursement mechanisms.

Of particular concern in the nutrition area are changes in family structures, which affect food-related activities and often nutritional status. These have both positive and negative effects on familial foodways and child feeding. The number of single-parent families, working mothers, and unsupervised children are greater today than formerly. The traditional nutrition-related service provider within families, the mother, is often no longer available or willing to perform all the food getting, preparation, cooking, feeding, and cleanup functions her mother or grandmother did.

More equitable divisions of labor between parents and other sibs to cover food getting, food preparation, and food provision often leave gaps in these functions within the household.[4,5] The nutrition of dependents may suffer as a result.

In the past several decades, the food supply and consumption of food outside of the home have also changed dramatically, but not always in positive directions beneficial to health. More and more people lack the time, skills, or inclination to cook for themselves or to use meals as family social occasions. Prepared, "fast" or "convenience" foods are often costly and sometimes imbalanced in nutrients, with excessive amounts of calories, fat, salt, and sugar.

While few American children fail to be provided with sufficient food as a result of these trends, nutrition-related guidance and food-related socialization within the home may be in short supply. Institutions outside of the home have not yet filled this gap. Public health nutrition services need to fill these lacunae by developing nutrition-related health services and education.

ORGANIZATION OF NUTRITION SERVICES

NUTRITION AS PART OF COMPREHENSIVE CARE

Nutrition is part of the entire life cycle and also of the whole comprehensive care cycle, involving primary (prevention and risk reduction), secondary (control and curative), or tertiary (rehabilitation) prevention measures. It follows that the nutrition component of health services must be integrated with all aspects of preventive, curative, and rehabilitative services.

ROLE OF NUTRITION AT VARIOUS AGES AND STAGES OF LIFE

Table 1 documents the nutritional factors promoting and enhancing MCH at various times during the life cycle.

PLANNING OF NUTRITION SERVICES

Planning nutrition services involves a series of steps. First, the health problems and unmet needs of the target population are identified. Such an analysis includes consideration of nutrition-related morbidity and mortality, and related socio-economic circumstances. The size and nature of the problem must be considered. Issues include what the problem is, how may people are affected, the seriousness of the problem, the consequences of doing nothing, the adequacy of resources involving staff and of funds to address the problem, and the likely effect of the intervention in preventing or reducing the problem.

Second, available and potential resources are assessed. Third, objectives are established and consideration is given to various alternatives and their consequences. Sound objectives for nutrition services must set forth specifically what is to be accomplished—measurable results related to ultimate outcomes. They must be feasible (consistent with the known range of available resources) and specify the time frame or target date for their accomplishment. The objectives should be ranked in order of priority. Fourth, necessary administrative actions are taken to achieve program goals. Fifth, and finally, results are assessed and evaluated. The evaluation process is most effective when it is built in as part of the services delivery system and done continually as a part of quality assurance. [6,7,8]

THE NUTRITION SERVICES
MASTER PLAN AS PART OF THE STATE PLAN

The ultimate goal of nutrition services is to maintain or improve the nutritional status and general health of mothers and children. Such a goal should be included in the state's MCH Plan. If no such plan exists, much useful material may be available for creating one from the plan for spending block-grant funds. The state

TABLE 1

FACTORS ENHANCING NUTRITIONAL STATUS AT VARIOUS TIMES OF LIFE

PRECONCEPTIONAL PERIOD
- Achieve desirable weight prior to pregnancy by diet and physical activity.
- Select a variety of foods from all the food groups to provide amount of essential nutrients, balance and moderation in energy yielding nutrients.
- Attain or maintain desirable weight.
- Encourage smoking cessation before pregnancy and abstinence or moderation in alcohol, over the counter and prescription drugs.
- Consult a physician if medical conditions exist that may complicate pregnancy (diabetes, hypertension, etc.)
- Correct nutritional anemia if present.

PREGNANCY:
- Consume 36 cal/kg pregnancy body weight and not less than 30 cal/kg.
- Monitor weight gain to achieve 10-12 kg on the average at term.
- Avoid weight reduction during pregnancy; weight control may be called for if gains are excessive.
- Increase diet quality by increasing intakes of protective nutrients relative to energy to met the elevated needs of pregnancy.
- Supplement with 30-60 mg of elemental iron and 300-800 ug of folic acid per day.
- Treat iron deficiency anemia if present with therapeutic doses (up to 200 mg) of elemental iron.
- Provide guidance to cope with therapeutic diets or other complex problems (vegetarian, alcohol or drug abuse, adolescent pregnancy, diabetes, kidney disease, etc.).
- Cease or reduce tobacco use and treat or refer smokers to self-help group.
- Abstain or moderate alcohol use. (Total abstinence is best.).
- Abstain from non prescribed over the counter drugs or illicit drugs.
- Enroll in relevant food programs (WIC, food stamps) and MCH programs if eligible.
- Submit to screening for glucose intolerance; adjust diet and if necessary insulin as needed.

LACTATION:
- Learn breast feeding techniques prenatally.
- Increase energy intakes by about 500 calories per day over non pregnancy needs.
- Assure fluid intakes are adequate.
- Avoid or moderate alcohol use.
- Use supplements of 30-60 mg elemental iron for 2-3 months postpartum.
- Attain desirable weight.
- Maintain high diet quality.

INTERCONCEPTIONAL PERIOD:
- Maintain high dietary quality and adequate nutrient intakes.
- Attain or maintain desirable weight.
- Recoup and replenish iron stores if depleted in pregnancy by use of iron supplements.
- Consider family planning to maximize good outcomes of pregnancy by birth spacing, correction of weight and health problems prior to pregnancy especially among women at high risk.
- Moderate or abstain from alcohol and tobacco.

MENOPAUSE:
- Attain or maintain desirable weights.
- Increase calcium intakes (1200-1500 mg).

(Continued on next page)

(TABLE 1 – Continued)

- Consider estrogen replacement therapy (ERT) to relieve the symptoms and signs of menopause, such as hot flashes, night sweats, vaginal dryness, involutional bone loss and possible high serum cholesterol values. (5).
- Attain or maintain normal serum cholesterol, blood pressure and hyperclycemia by diet or other means.

EARLY INFANCY: (0-6 months)
- Breast feed until 4-6 months of age.
- If breast milk is not provided, feed a hygienic, nutritionally adequate source of heat-treated formula until 4-6 months of age.
- Supplement with vitamin D and iron if these are not provided in the formula or if the infant is solely breast fed for the first six months of life.
- Supplement with fluorides if water or formula are devoid of the nutrient.
- Avoid unsuitable feedings (solids, cow's milk, skim milk).
- Assure that the infant receives enough food by monitoring growth.
- Use proper feeding techniques to avoid gas, aspiration, and other problems.
- Delay introduction of solid foods until 4-6 months, when the infant is developmentally ready to deal with them.
- Avoid foods commonly causing allergies, intolerances, or hypersensitivities.
- Assure that water intakes are adequate.
- If family resources are inadequate, obtain assistance from federally sponsored food programs for infants and children (WIC, CCFP, food stamps.).
- Obtain relevant anticipatory guidance on feeding and health.

LATER INFANCY: (6-12 months)
- Use iron fortified formulas, iron supplements and iron fortified cereals.
- Assure gradual transition to family diets rather than attempting to wean suddenly.
- Introduce solid foods sequentially after four to six months when child is developmentally ready and needs supplementary feedings.
- Take common problems in stride. Temporary refusals of solid foods at weaning and failures to switch over from pureed or baby foods to foods which must be chewed are normal setbacks.
- Consult health providers if feeding problems persist.
- Help and encourage self feeding.
- Realize that some decrease in appetite in late infancy is to be expected as growth slows, and that it is no cause for alarm.
- Avoid struggles and battles of will with the child about food.
- Keep environments safe (especially with respect to lead and common household chemicals which are poisons) and begin to teach child to shun mouthing and eating non-food objects.

PRESCHOOL YEARS:
- Assure that levels of physical activity and rest suffice to maintain normal growth and development and a good appetite.
- Provide nutritious food in the home and in other settings in which the child eats to encourage good food choices.
- Teach the child to choose and eat nutritious foods for meals and snacks.
- Avoid sticky sugary snacks and encourage oral hygiene practices to promote good dental health.
- Foster appropriate eating behaviors by providing suitable role models, by permitting the child to choose food portions, by giving some latitude in food preferences, by exposing him/her to new foods, by fostering table manners appropriate to his/her development, and by keeping meals as times for social interchange.

(Continued on next page)

Plan's nutrition portion then becomes the master plan for state public health nutrition service activities in maternal and child health.

Figure 1 illustrates the necessary components of the nutrition services master plan. The master plan should include the plan's goals and objectives and outline the means by which they will be reached. All relevant health care professionals should

---

(TABLE 1 – Continued)

- Recognize and deal with feeding problems early before they become well established.
- Handle struggles over food reasonably to avoid the development of feeding problems.
- Feed and hydrate children appropriately during illness.
- Help the child grow out of fatness by encouraging physical activity.
- Assure that iron needs are met by wise food choices (red meat, fish, poultry, iron fortified cereals, vitamin C sources, etc.).
- Assure that the child learns to distinguish food and non food objects.

SCHOOL YEARS:
- Monitor growth in height to assure that nutritional status is satisfactory.
- Provide good examples and guidance to instill healthy habits and attitudes about foods and eating. (Develop regular eating patterns; eat nutritious snacks as well as meals; use moderation in providing food rewards, especially sweets; encourage the child to eat breakfast; and help the child become a sophisticated and responsible food consumer.).
- Establish consistent guidelines and follow them to assure that the child's diet is nutritionally adequate.
- Promote eating and physical activity habits which will foster normal body fatness.
- If excessive fatness is a problem, encourage child to increase physical activity and help him/her to cut energy intakes slightly so that the child can grow out of his/her fatness.
- Assure that diet-related risks of dental caries are minimized.
- Help the child to distinguish between reliable sources of information on food choices and promotional messages which may be unreliable.
- Assure dietary moderation with respect to dietary fat, cholesterol, sugar and sodium.
- Assure that diets are adequate in fiber.
- Assure that iron needs are met by wise food choices.

ADOLESCENTS:
- Maintain desirable weights. Avoid obesity and eating disorders by healthful attitudes toward food, appropriate energy intakes, and a physically active life-style.
- Abstain from self induced vomiting, bulimia and laxative abuse.
- Eat a variety of foods to ensure dietary sufficiency of protective nutrients, including protein, vitamins, and minerals.
- Avoid dietary imbalances, stressing moderation with respect to fat, saturated fat, cholesterol, sugar, and salt by moderation in intakes of foods high in these and low in protective nutrients.
- Find ways to eat that fulfill the teenager's individual needs, philosophies, wants, and schedules, without doing violence to nutritional status.
- identify and alter eating habits that are not conducive to good nutrition, including long standing poor dietary intakes, irregular or unplanned food intakes, and excessive intakes of fat, cholesterol, sodium and sugar.
- Avoid alcohol use.
- Provide assistance for special problems (teenage pregnancy, diet for athletes, diets for those with allergies, disease, etc.).

contribute to its development. This includes many disciplines and representatives of both the public health and primary care services. The nutrition plan must be flexible so it can be modified in response to changing needs, priorities, and resources. [9]

PUBLIC HEALTH NUTRITION SERVICES

Figure 2 shows that the betterment of MCH is the focus of both the public health and individual primary care services delivery systems in nutrition. The outer circle, entitled program management planning, includes indirect public health services, such as administrative, supervision, consultation, and training. Program

---

FIGURE 1
COMPONENTS OF A NUTRITION PLAN

1. DOCUMENTATION OF NEED:
- Broad health goals.
- Food and nutrition needs and problems of the target population, including quantitative estimates.
- Nutrition services presently available from public or voluntary health agencies to meet needs.
- Gaps.

2 NUTRITION GOALS AND OBJECTIVES:
- What is to be accomplished.
- Measurable results.
- Feasibility.

3 RESOURCES REQUIRED:
- Nutrition professionals and other personnel to achieve objectives.
- Space, equipment, and supplies.
- Money and budget

4. IMPLEMENTATION PLAN:
- Time table for achieving objectives.
- Activities needed.

5. POLICIES AND PROCEDURES FOR IMPLEMENTATION:
- Standards for nutritional care.
- Nutrition screening and assessment procedures.
- Referral criteria for nutrition counseling 1) within program 2) to outside agencies.
- Records and methods for recording and retrieving nutrition data.
- Communication and coordination within the project, within the agency, within the community.
- Staff development including continuing eduction in nutrition

6. EVALUATION METHODS TO BE USED:
- Internal self assessment, external assessment using State, regional or private consultant, cost effectiveness studies, etc.

Adapted from: Guide for developing Nutrition services in Communities U.S. Department of Health, Education and Welfare. DHEW Publ. no (HSA) 78-5103.

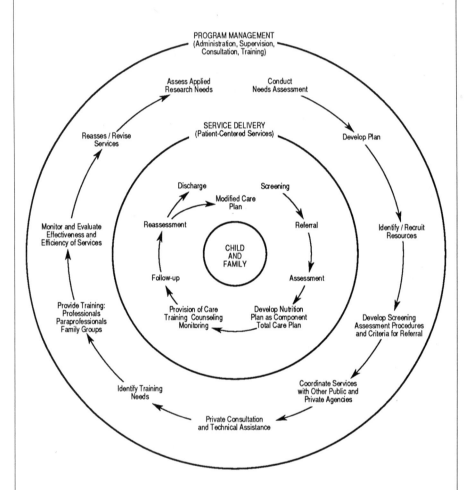

FIGURE 2

SYSTEM FOR NUTRITION SERVICES*

*Adapted from Managing Nutrition Service Needs of Clients,
of Crippled Childrens Services and Supplemented Security Income Disabled Children's
Programs, Ohio State University 1980.

management activities at the indirect service level provide the policies and tools which are necessary for patient-centered primary care and for service delivery to occur smoothly. These include the development of screening and assessment tools, policies for programs, standards of care, and training materials. Direct service providers usually have too little time, too little access to other providers, and insufficient expertise to produce such materials themselves. Therefore, it is essential for the public health nutrition services to assist primary care providers and to carry out many of these indirect supportive functions, if those in both service sectors are to relate closely to each other. [8]

Primary Care Services in Nutrition

The inner circle in Figure 2 shows primary care services in nutrition. Direct primary care services at the primary level include nutrition assessment, development of the nutrition care components as part of total health care intervention plans, the actual provision of care, related educational activities, followup (including monitoring, reassessment, and modification of care plans), and finally discharge.[8]

Direct patient care services are most efficient and effective on a population basis when they are carried out in a coordinated fashion with support and consultation from specialists and providers of indirect services, within the context of the nutrition service master plan mentioned above.

ALTERNATIVES FOR PROVIDING CARE IN DIFFERENT SETTINGS

The characteristics and settings in which care is provided determine what nutrition services will be offered, how the nutrition intervention plan will be carried out, and, when referral is necessary, how best to accomplish it. Nutritionists are not available in all settings. Most private-practice settings are too small to justify fulltime nutrition personnel on the premises. Thus routine nutritional screening, assessment, and counseling must be carried out by appropriately trained physicians and nurses who are knowledgeable about food composition and clinical nutrition, in consultation with a nutritionist-dietitian backup. Patients who are at especially high risk from the nutritional standpoint, and who have multiple and complex problems (such as acute conditions affecting food intake or metabolism, chronic degenerative diseases, or inborn errors of metabolism), should be referred to a nutritionist in another setting for treatment.

In larger care settings, where nutrition services are available on a more fulltime basis, wise utilization demands that the nutritionists deal first with the most difficult and complex cases. They can furnish backup and consultation services to other professionals for problems which are more simple, straightforward, and common.[10] They can also provide consultation and parttime staffing to smaller settings.

Coordination and Referral Systems

Close working relationships between nutrition providers in various programs are helpful for sharing information, for coordinating goals, and for developing objectives, standards, and criteria for services. Of special concern to mothers and children is the need to coordinate services between MCH sponsored clinics, WIC programs, and other child health and welfare programs.[11] Assuring that nutrition services are provided requires cooperation, coordination, and referral between professionals at various levels within the health care services. Referrals may also be in order to other institutions in the community, especially those involving health, public and social welfare, education, and the food system.[13]

STAFFING FOR THE PROVISION OF NUTRITION SERVICES

The best staffing patterns for providing nutrition services depend on the type and size of the population to be served, the type of service product that the agency produces (e.g., supportive or direct services), the availability of nutrition services elsewhere in the community, and the expectations of the public and health care providers. Below are descriptions of the personnel commonly involved in services planning and delivery.[13]

Public Health Nutrition Services Administrator

The administrator is often also a direct care provider unless the service is so large that management is fulltime. The administrator supports efforts to define the extent and nature of the target population, assists in mobilizing the resources required to solve identified problems, facilitates services organization, develops nutrition plans and strategies, and provides the continuous support required for a responsible and dynamic nutrition program. In order to do this, the administrator must be aware of the role of nutrition in health and be capable of gaining support for nutrition services within the bureaucracy, as well as from legislative and community leaders.[13,14]

Public Health Nutritionists

The public health nutritionist should preferably be a registered dietitian with a masters degree in public health nutrition. The nutritionist works with the administrator to plan, organize, and manage public-health nutrition services and provides necessary nutrition consultation and continuing education in nutrition for health care staff who are providing direct services to patients. Other duties may include dietary counseling to patients, and organization and implementation of relevant nutrition education activities. [13,14]

Direct Health Care Providers of Nutrition Services

Nutrition is everybody's business in health care services delivery. It is vital that appropriate identification and referral systems be developed for complex and difficult nutrition problems. This is especially true if several providers are to take partial responsibility for nutrition services. Otherwise, instead of similar nutrition messages being reinforced by each health services provider, nutrition can become nobody's business, and patients will suffer as a result.

Nutritionists and dietitians are specialists trained at the baccalaureate level or higher, who are experts in the provision of food and nutrition-related services. Many are also public health nutritionists. Unlike certain of the other health professions, licensure is not universal and no legal definition of the title *nutritionist* exists. Therefore, individuals with varying degrees of competence and expertise may claim to be nutritionist, including some who have little, no, or inappropriate scientific training or experience to deal with nutrition related issues. The title of *registered dietitian* (R.D.) is somewhat clearer. It is restricted to individuals who have been certified as competent after appropriate academic preparation (at least a baccalaureate), clinical or community training under supervision, and successful completion of national examination.

Dietitians and nutritionists provide specific nutritional counseling to patients to prevent, control, cure, or ameliorate various diet-related diseases and conditions over the life cycle. They also provide advice on life-cycle related nutritional modifications, as in infancy, childhood, adolescence, pregnancy, lactation, and during family planning. [15,16] In some settings, they may provide general nutrition advice and plan educational programs as well.

Physicians provide medical direction and should participate in establishing standards, criteria, and policies for nutrition services. They are responsible for the assessment of nutritional status, diagnosis, and for making appropriate referrals for dietary counseling.[13] If they choose to provide nutrition services directly, it is vital that they receive training in addition to that usually required to obtain a license to practice medicine.

Nursing professionals can also be helpful in nutritional assessment, provision of education, counseling, and general nutrition information. Appropriate training is essential if nurses are to take on these tasks. Existing nutrition training, in most nursing schools, is inadequate. The nurse is an underutilized resource in nutrition.[13]

Social workers contribute to the mobilization of community resources and social services needed to support nutritional wellbeing. They assist in developing referral mechanisms and in counseling patients whose nutritional problems are complicated by poverty, social, and emotional factors. [13] They need to be knowledgeable about food programs and other services, such as patient self-help groups which may be needed by patients.

Physical therapists, occupational therapists, dentists, dental hygienists, and those in other health disciplines can also be helpful in dealing with patients who have nutritional problems touching their areas of expertise.[13]

NUTRITION SERVICES PROVISION MODEL

The major components of nutrition services are problem identification (involving screening and assessment); intervention (which includes curative treatment for disease, control, and rehabilitation); and follow up (for monitoring and evaluation purposes). Completion and accurate documentation of the provision of each component maintains communications, provides useful management information, assures quality, enhances continuity of care, and helps meet regulatory requirements. [10]

PROBLEM IDENTIFICATION: SCREENING

Every patient should be screened for the presence of characteristics which are known to be associated with nutritional problems. The main purpose of screening is to identify individuals in the target population who are potentially at highest nutritional risk. To serve this purpose, screening criteria must be simple, relatively straightforward, and easy to administer. Screening is also helpful in establishing priorities for the most efficient use of the time and money that are available.

PROBLEM IDENTIFICATION: ASSESSMENT

Individuals whose characteristics at screening suggest nutritional high risk (that is, the presence of complex and involved problems touching on nutrition) require a more detailed investigation by a nutritionist of diet, eating habits, food resources, and household management, as well as any disease-related issues which may affect nutritional status. Further examination involves not only dietary assessment, [17] but a review of biochemical, anthropometric, clinical, and dietary history information available on the patient.[10] After such a review, definitive conclusions on the nature of the problem can be made. It is a poor use of resources to give patients who are screened, and exhibit a low probability of potential problems, the same thorough examination as those who exhibit many risk factors.[10]

INTERVENTION: HEALTH PROMOTION

Factors promoting and enhancing nutritional health in mothers and children are provided in Table 1. Note that the actions which can be taken to promote nutritional health are largely informational and educational in nature. All health care providers can be helpful in reinforcing these messages.

INTERVENTION: RISK REDUCTION (PRIMARY PREVENTION)

The *Dietary Guidelines for Americans* have been widely publicized over the past decade. These guidelines assure adequacy of diet, while helping to reduce risks for diet-related chronic degenerative diseases in adults. In brief, they counsel maintaining or achieving desirable weights, decreasing intakes of total fat, cholesterol, sodium, and sugar, increasing intakes of starch and fiber, and moderation in the use of alcohol. [18] For infants, children, adolescents, pregnant, and lactating women, special care in interpreting such guidelines is necessary. The reason for this is that during periods of growth, pregnancy, and lactation, nutrient needs rise. Thus, preventively oriented dietary advice for adults must be adapted before it is appropriate for these groups. References are available for designing menus to do this.[19] Popular books and magazines provide advice of varying quality on such dietary adjustments. Medically authoritative guidelines, such as those published by state and federal health services and professional associations, are to be preferred.

INTERVENTION: DISEASE TREATMENT
AND CONTROL (SECONDARY PREVENTION)

Dietary measures can also help to control disease and to alleviate signs and symptoms of some conditions after patients fall ill. For example, therapeutic diets incorporated into the context of total health care for the hyperlipidemias, diabetes mellitus, Crohn's disease, and the inborn errors of metabolism have measurable benefits in reducing morbidity and mortality.

INTERVENTION: REHABILITATION (TERTIARY PREVENTION)

Nutrition is also a vital part of tertiary prevention. In addition to primary and secondary prevention, nutrition care plans must include attention to rehabilitation. This is especially important in dealing with handicapped children and other children with special long-term developmental and health needs.

Table 2 lists the prevalence of certain handicapping conditions and common nutritional problems for them.[20,21] For children born with some handicapping conditions, special nutritional support measures are essential. Measures include therapeutic diets, nutritional counseling on drug diet interactions, feeding positioning, feeding behavior problems, and related issues. For all handicapped children, general nutritional advice tailored to their disability must be provided.

NEW DIRECTIONS FOR PUBLIC HEALTH NUTRITION SERVICES

Primary and secondary prevention activities to reduce dietary risks of chronic degenerative diseases in childhood and adolescence are now well-accepted. Community-based interventions are being used to do this, providing new challenges and opportunities to public health workers in monitoring and operating large scale products.

Public health nutrition services are (or should be if they are not) also expanding beyond their traditional focus on primary prevention into secondary and tertiary prevention, as home and ambulatory care for acute, serious chronic conditions,

TABLE 2

PREVALENCE OF CERTAIN HANDICAPPING CONDITIONS WITH ASSOCIATED NUTRITION RELATED PROBLEMS

DISORDER	PREVALENCE ESTIMATES PER 1,000 (AND RANGE)	EXAMPLE OF NUTRITION PROBLEMS AND FACTORS CONTRIBUTING TO HIGH NUTRITIONAL RISK													
		Child-related										Caregiver-related		
		Altered nutrient needs	Altered energy needs/intake	Problems with oral cavity	Nutrient deficiencies	Constipation/diarrhea	Poor appetite	Delayed feeding skills	Malabsorption	Nutrient-drug interactions	Maladaptive behaviors	Lack of knowledge	Difficulty understanding diet	Does not limit intake	Inappropriate feeding practices
Asthma	38 (20-53)	●	●							●		●			
Moderate to severe	10 (8-15)														
Visual Impairment	30 (20-35)														
Impaired Visual Activity	20														
Blind	0.6 (0.5-1)														
Mental Retardation	25 (20-30)	●	●	●	●	●	●	●			●	●			●
Hearing Impairment	16														
Deafness	0.1 (0.6-1.5)														
Congenital Heart Disease	7 (2-7)	●	●		●	●	●		●	●	●				
Severe Congenital disease	0.5		●				●			●				●	
Seizure Disorder	3.5 (2.6-4.6)	●	●							●	●	●	●		●
Cerebral Palsy	2.5 (1.4-5.1)	●	●	●	●	●	●					●			●
Arthritis	2.2 (1-3)	●	●	●	●		●				●	●	●		●
Paralysis	2.1 (2-2.3)	●	●		●	●	●				●	●			
Diabetes Mellitus	1.8 (1.2-2.0)	●	●				●				●	●	●	●	●
Cleft Lip/Palate	1.5 (1.3-2.0)	●	●		●			●				●		●	
Down's Syndrome	1.1	●	●		●		●	●							
Sickle Cell Disease	<1.0	●													
Neural Tube Defect	<1.0							●							
Autism	<1.0				●						●	●			
Cystic Fibrosis	<1.0	●			●	●			●	●		●			●
Hemophilia	<1.0						●						●		●
Acute Lymphocytic Leukemia	<1.0	●	●	●	●	●				●		●		●	
Phenylketonuria	<1.0	●	●	●		●						●	●	●	●
Chronic Renal Failure	<1.0	●	●		●	●				●	●	●			

and rehabilitation become more common. More and more complex care is now being rendered outside of hospital settings, as institutional boundaries between preventive and curative medical services break down. Special parenteral (intravenous) and enteral (nasogastric or intragastric) feeding techniques and formulations are now available for sustaining mothers and children at home who formerly required long-term hospitalization. [22] However, these therapies can be extremely labor intensive and may severely strain family emotional, physical, temporal, and financial resources. They also stress the public health system. Therefore, public health nutritionists are faced with both new problems and opportunities and old difficulties involving insufficient resources to meet unmet needs. Thus careful planning is mandatory.

COMPONENTS OF NUTRITIONAL CARE AND MANAGEMENT

After problems are identified they must be managed. Food and nutrition-related dimensions of care are the special province of the nutritionist or dietitian.

A nutrition care plan must be formulated—not only at the public health level but also for each patient. The plan describes what the problems are and how needs for counseling, nutrition education, help with home and money management, food assistance, and community resources will be implemented. These intervention measures may be necessary for health promotion, primary, secondary, and tertiary prevention.

Counseling

The goal of nutrition counseling is to make the fewest changes necessary in the patient's eating habits and to meet health objectives. When changes are needed, it is best to focus first on specific eating behaviors for which reasonable success is anticipated by both the patient and counselor, since successful accomplishment engenders future success.

The nature of a nutrition-related problem and its likely solution determine who should do the counseling. The related types of nutritional interventions which are likely to be necessary include: therapeutic diets with accompanying counseling; lengthy nutritional planning of a special nature to solve food-related problems, such as needs for food assistance, home and money management, and special education for managing difficult home situations; and nutritional advice of a more generalized nature. [10]

Those who are at especially high risk from the nutritional standpoint and who have multiple and complex problems, such as acute conditions affecting food intake or metabolism, chronic degenerative diseases, or inborn errors of metabolism should be referred to a nutritionist or specially trained physician. If no one is available, they should be referred to such a professional in another setting for treatment. At the very least, a consult is called for with such an individual.

Multiple or extremely complex problems involving therapeutic diets or special nutrition support routes (either parental or enteral) usually require the services of a registered dietitian and/or a nutritionist with a masters degree in dietetics, nutritional science, or public health. Such counseling is also possible by some other individual who has extensive expertise in both food and nutrition, such as a highly specialized baccalaureate-level registered dietitian or physician, who has successfully completed his or her subspecialty boards in nutrition and requirements for membership in the American Society for Clinical Nutrition, the American College of Nutrition, or the American Society for Parental and Enteral Nutrition.

Lengthy nutritional advice of a special nature can be handled by a registered dietitian or by others if they have been trained to deal with these problems. Simple delegation, without training of ancillary personnel, accomplishes nothing and wastes resources, as outcome-oriented chart reviews will quickly reveal.

General nutritional advice can be coped with by most professional staff after suitable inservice training. This advice should be reinforced with audiovisual and print materials.

Education

Only some patients need lengthy nutrition counseling. But all patients should need general nutrition and health education in line with their beliefs and lifestyles, and which relates to the presenting problem, to dispel many of the harmful nutritional myths which adversely influence eating behaviors.[10]

Help with Management of Food and Other Resources

Some patients lack knowledge about meal planning, preparation, purchasing, and access to food programs for themselves or their children. Others lack the time and resources to manage food wisely. The combination of these lacks, social, and medical problems, and the need to cater to special dietary constraints may be insuperable for some patients, without a nutritionist's help. Such food and nutrition-related problems are not confined to the poor. Many high-income, dependent people have also never learned to use food, monetary, and time resources wisely, to shop or to cook, and they too require counseling at times of nutritional stress. Those with emotional problems—the mentally ill, the retarded, teenagers who are pregnant, and others, such as those with unusual eating styles or cultural backgrounds—also present particularly difficult problems in management. [10]

Food Assistance

Food assistance programs must be routinely utilized in coordination with health care, if some patients are to remedy their nutrition-related problems. Four current federal programs providing food assistance include the National School Lunch and Breakfast Program; Child Care Food Program; Supplemental Food Program for Women, Infants and Children (WIC); and the Food Stamp Program.

The National School Lunch and Breakfast Program offers free or reduced-priced nutritious school lunches or breakfasts to children from households with incomes at or below 185 percent or 130 percent of the poverty line, respectively. Other children from families at higher-income levels also can receive food, but pay more. The school lunch meal pattern provides a minimum of one-third the age-appropriate Recommended Dietary Allowances for key nutrients. It includes a serving of meat or a meat alternative, fruit and/or vegetables, bread or a suitable equivalent, and milk. The school breakfast pattern includes a serving of bread or cereal, fruit or fruit juice or vegetable juice, milk, and a meat or a meat alternative as often as possible. [23]

The Child Care Food Program provides low-cost meals to non-residential public and nonprofit private institutions and group activities for children in facilities, such as day care centers, summer day camps, and other recreational programs. The Head Start program often is combined with this program. Centers can provide up to two meals and one snack a day at either free or reduced prices for families with income levels at or below 185 percent or 130 percent of the federal poverty line, respectively. Children from more affluent families pay more. [23]

The WIC Program provides specified foods and nutrition education to low-income pregnant and postpartum women, lactating mothers, infants, and children up to five- years old, who are determined to be at nutritional risk by WIC criteria. Monthly vouchers are provided that can be exchanged at participating grocery stores for iron, protein, calcium, and Vitamin-C rich foods, such as eggs, iron-fortified cereals, 100 percent fruit juices, milk, cheese, dried beans, peanut butter, and infant formula. Special nutrition education is provided. Referrals to other resources, such as day-care centers, the food-stamp program, and MCH services, may be offered when indicated.[23]

The Food Stamp Program enables low-income individuals and families to buy more food than their income levels would normally permit. Food stamps and vouchers can be used like cash to buy food at most grocery stores. Alcohol, tobacco, or non-food items, such as soap and paper goods, cannot be purchased with the stamps. Monthly allotments of food stamps are based on the household's size and net monthly income.[23]

FOLLOW UP

The final step in the nutrition care process is to review what has been accomplished and to link it to outcome measurements. Quality assurance, process evaluation, monitoring, and surveillance are all important activities which are helpful in following up on the quality of services provided.

Quality Assurance Nutritional standards of care help assure that the quality of services provided can be measured and changes can be made, if quality slips.

Recent references focusing upon quality assurance in nutrition services are now available. [24,25] They provide specific care plans for a variety of conditions. Informal and formal continuing-education efforts for staff are also helpful in assuring quality. These educational activities include professional consultation, collaborative work with health care providers who have special expertise in problem areas, consultation with professional organizations, and attendance at courses sponsored by educational or professional institutions which are involved in community service.

Process Evaluation   The most successful types of process evaluation are built into the entire nutrition services planning process, from the onset. Measurable end-points permit the utility of the services which are provided to be documented. Increasingly, ethical, legal, and fiscal requirements are such that accurate records must be kept which document all services provided. Meaningful process evaluation, including aspects addressing administrative, professional, and consumer perspectives, enhances the problem identification and management process. [27] Evaluations based on morbidity, mortality, growth, and other "hard" outcomes are long- term, complex research undertakings. They require a highly trained, specialized, and stable staff and are beyond the capacity of most MCH nutrition service units. Instead, such units should concentrate on the delivery of high quality nutrition services already known to be beneficial in an efficient and effective manner. [10]

Monitoring and Surveillance   Monitoring is the periodic measurement of factors which indicate changes in nutritional status in specific groups of interest or in the general population. It is analogous to screening at the clinical level. Surveillance is continuous and regular data collection is compiled to detect warning signs of problems at the community level early enough to provide feedback that planners and managers can use.

The purpose of nutrition monitoring and surveillance is to provide continuous, reliable information on the target group's nutritional status and factors that influence it for the purpose of acting to improve them. Monitoring and surveillance can take place at many levels of aggregation and within various time frames. They are especially helpful when environmental conditions change drastically.

At the federal level today, nutrition monitoring and surveillance are conducted by several different government agencies. Within the Department of Health and Human Services, the National Center for Health Statistics conducts the Health and Nutrition Examination Survey (HANES). HANES is a periodic population-based survey providing national data on specific health-status measures, include dietary intakes, eating habits, biochemical, and anthropometric indices related to nutrition. HANES surveys are done at least once a decade, but the number of children and adolescents surveyed is small and not all relevant problems can be examined in each survey.

The Food and Drug Administration (FDA) also conducts continuing surveys on the regulatory impact of actions involving food products. For example, in the late 1970s, when formulas were sold which were deficient in chloride, the FDA surveyed the marketplace and determined use of these products. The Centers for Disease Control conducts ongoing nutritional monitoring activities based on indices various states provide to them, consisting of data collected on children and pregnant women enrolled in health department clinics, WIC, and Head Start programs. The Food and Nutrition Service of the U.S. Department of Agriculture conducts its National Food Consumption Survey at least once a decade, which also provides such useful data on food consumption. [27]

Today's federal efforts are far superior to those of two decades ago, yet major problems still exist. These include lack of coordination between departments, lack of timeliness in issuing reports, inclusion of insufficient information to evaluate program efforts, and lack of target group specificity. Of the many problems of mothers, infants, and children, only a few are covered in the monitoring and surveillance systems which exist today. State and local-level efforts are far more limited and need to be further developed so that decision makers who must plan, justify, and implement programs at these levels have better and firmer data on which to base and evaluate their programs. [27]

NUTRITIONAL RISK: CURRENT STATUS OF PUBLIC HEALTH MANAGEMENT EFFORTS

Table 3 lists some of the preventable problems which were singled out in the document, *Promoting Health, Preventing Disease, Objectives for the Nation*, issued by the Department of Health and Human Services [28] in 1980, to provide health goals to be reached by 1990 or beyond. It discussed their progress to date. Additional goals of current interest are also included.

CONCLUSION

Nutrition services involve a combination of interventions involving health, food, education, social, and public welfare measures. Planning for them is critical at the public health level if they are not to be neglected at the services delivery level.

(References follow Table 3)

TABLE 3
PROGRESS TOWARD ACHIEVING NATIONAL NUTRITIONAL HEALTH GOALS

OBJECTIVE TO BE ACHIEVED BY 1990	COMMENTS ON PROGRESS TO DATE
Percentage of iron deficient pregnant women should be 3.5%	Iron deficiency anemia has been reduced However, no ethnic group has achieved the 3.5% goal. Low income, high parity and black pregnant females still have high prevalence of iron deficiency. (1)
Reduce prevalence of low iron stores in children 1-2 years at least 50% of levels (9%) inthe National Health and Nutrition Examination Survey 1976-1980.	Progress has been made, but iron deficiency anemia is still common. Pediatric Nutrition Surveillance systems monitoring data from 6 states showed decreases in anemia prevalence from 7.8% in 1975 to 2.9% in 1985. (2) Ethnic differences are still present among children. Low hemoglobins are greatest in blacks over 2 years, low hematocrits are greatest in Hispanics after 6 month. (1)
Less than 10% of children in the population should be under the 5th percentile of height for age on growth charts because of dietary inadequacy.	Low height for age is greater than 10% prevalence for all ethnic groups 3 months to 5 years and in all ethnic groups except Blacks from 6 to 9 years. (1) Differences in weight and fatness for age are poorly correlated with dietary intake: other health related factors such as illness prevalence may be involved, or dietary measures are poor. (3)
Children 1-14 years of age should have serum cholesterol at or below 150mg/dl (In 1971-74, for children aged 1-17 years of age, mean serum cholesterol level was 176mg/dl).	Progress has been made: mean serum cholesterol values for children aged 0-9 years are 160mg/dl; 10-14 years 156mg/dl; and 150mg/dl for ages 15-19 years. (4)
75% of women will exclusively or partially breast feed their babies at discharge from the hospital and 50% of them will continue to do so until 3-4 months of age.	Breast feeding has continued to increase within the last 8 years to 63% at hospital discharge and 37% at 4 months. (1)
States should document the inclusion of a nutrition education component in their k-to-12 curriculum. States should include the completion of at least college level course in nutrition beyond one year of biological sciences in certification requirements for elementary and secondary school teachers.	Few states to not have such provisions. It is important to keep upgrading the nutrition science-based knowledge of the nation's educators. (5)
Improve health and health habits and deaths among those aged 15 to 24 by at least 20%, to fewer than 90 per 100,000.	Some efforts have been made to reduce teenage pregnancy, sexually transmissible diseases, and mental health problems, but this goal has not been reached. (5)
Low birth weight babies (weighing less than 2,500 grams) should constitute no more than 5% of all live births.	Some progress: a reduction from 7.1% (1978) to 6.7% (1984). However, low birth weight births continue to be high in teenaged and black women. (1) Declines may have stopped in low birth weight rates.

(Continued on next page)

(TABLE 3 – Continued)

Reduce untreated gestational diabetes by early screening and management. Prevalence is presently 1-5% in this country. (6)	Prenatal screening for glucose intolerance is, and better prenatal management for all forms of diabetes is receiving more attention.
Decrease the prevalence (currently 1-2 per 1,000) of featl alcohol syndrome and also the fetal alcohol effects. (7)	Some progress has been made in identifying and treating heavy drinking and chronic alcoholism m in pregnancy, and for aftercare.
The proportion of women aware of risks associated with pregnancy and drinking should be greater than 90%. (In 1979, it was 73%.) (5)	In 1985, 87% of the women surveyed were aware of that alcohol has negative effects on pregnancy outcome. No baseline (1980) data available.

SOURCES:

1. Report of the Scientific Community's Views on Progress in Attaining the Public Health Service Objectives for Improved Nutrition in 1990. Edited by K.D. Fisher and R.B. Bennett. Maryland, Life Sciences Research Office Federation of American Societies for Experimental Biology, 1986.

2. Leads for the MMWR: Declining Anemia Prevalence Among Children Enrolled in Public Nutrition and Health Programs Selected States. JAMA 256 (16): 2165, 1985.

3. Jones DY, Weshan MC, Habicht JP Influences on child growth associated with poverty in the 1970's: an examination of HANES I and HANES II cross sectional U.S. National Surveys. Am J. Clin. Nutr. 42:714-724, 1985.

4. U.S. Department of Health and Human Services: The Lipid Research Clinics Population Studies Data Book. Volume I. Physiological and Sociodemographic Characteristics. Washington, D.S., Public Health Services, July 1980, pp 28-81.

5. U.S. Department of Health and Human Services: Health United States 1986, Washington, D.C., U.S. Government Printing Office, 1986.

6. Freinkel N Summary and Recommendations of the Second International Workshop — Conference of Gestational Diabetes Mellitius. Diabetes 34 (suppl 2):123-126, 1985.

7. Rosett HL, Weiner L: Identification and Prevention of Fetal Alcohol Syndrome. Fetal Alcohol Education Program. Boston, MA>

REFERENCES

1. U.S. Department of Health and Human Services: Chapter 17: Nutrition in Pregnancy, Infancy and Childhood, Surgeon Generals Report on Nutrition and Health, Washington, D.C., 1988.

2. Dwyer JT. Nutrition, Education and Information: In: Select Panel of Child Health, Better Health for Our Children: a national strategy, Vol 1V. Washington, D.C., U.S. Department of Health and Human Services, 1981, p 31-86.

3. Wallace HM, Gold EM, Ogelsby AC (ed). Maternal Child Health Practices. Second edition, New York, John Wiley and Sons, 1982, pp 1-861.

4. U.S. Department of Health and Human Services: Forward Plan: Maternal and Child Health, Fiscal years, 1984-1989. Rockville, MD, U.S. Government Printing Office, 1984, pp 5-6.

5. Young EA, Bingham C, Sims O, et al. Fast Foods 1986: Nutrient Analyses. Dietetic Currents 13(6): 26-36, 1986.

6. U.S. Department of Health, Education, and Welfare, Guide for Developing Nutrition Services in Community Health Programs, Rockville MD, U.S. Government Printing Office, 1978, pp 1-27.

7. Egan MC, Hallstrom BJ. Building Nutrition Services in Comprehensive Health Care. J Am Diet Assoc 61(5) 491-496, 1972.

8. Free BB. Identifying Available Resources and Planning Nutrition Services, Right to Grow. Edited by J.T. Dwyer and M.C. Egan. Boston, Frances Stern Nutrition Center, 1986, pp 72-77.

9. U.S. Department of Health, Education, Welfare: Guide for Developing Nutrition Services in Community Health Programs, Rockville, MD, U.S. Government Printing Office, 1978, pp 8-10.

10. Dwyer JT, with the assistance of Jacobson, HJ. Maternal Nutrition - Its Implications for Health Officers, Part 2 14 (4):1-6, July-August, 1974.

11. Dwyer JT (ed). The Role of MCH and WIC in the Delivery of Local Health Services Ross Roundtable on Current Issues in Public Health. Columbus, Ohio,Ross Laboratories, December 1987.

12. U.S. Department of Health and Human Services: Forward Plan: Maternal and Child Health, Fiscal years, 1984-1986. Rockville M.D.. U.S. Government Printing Office, 1984, pp 37-38.

13. U.S. Department of Health, Education and Welfare: Guide for Developing Nutrition Services in Community Health Programs (8)32-34.

14. Kaufman M (ed). Personnel in Public Health Nutrition for the 1980's. McLean, VA, Association of State and Territorial Health Officials Foundation, 1982, pp 10-11, 37.

15. Ritchey SJ, Taper J. Nutrition programs for mother and child, Maternal and Child Nutrition. New York, Harper and Row, 1983, pp 403-408.

16. Beck A. How to Find a Nutritionist: A Consumer Guide to Diet Advice. BostonGlobe Jan 6, 1988 (Food section) pp 25-26.

17. Dwyer JT. Assessment of Dietary Intake, Modern Nutrition in Health and Disease. Seventh Edition. Edited by M. E. Shils and V.R. Young. Philadelphia, Lea and Febiger, 1988, pp 887-905.

18. U.S. Department of Agriculture and U.S. Department of Health and Human Services: Dietary Guidelines for Americans. Washington, D.C., U.S. Government Printing Office,1985.

19. Dwyer JT. Diets for Children and Adolescents that Meet the Dietary Goals. Am J Dis Child, 134:1073-1080, 1980.

20 Gortmaker SL. Chronic Childhood Disorders: Prevalence and Impact on Planning Services, Now and in the Future, Right to Grow. Edited by JT Dwyer and MC Egan. Boston, Frances Stern Nutrition Center, 1986, pp 37-46.

21. Gortmaker SL. Sappenfield W, Chronic Childhood Disorders: Prevalence and Impact, Ped Clin of North America 31(1): 3-18, 1984.

22. Blackburn GL. A Look at the Facts - Home Care is a Reality, Home Care Concept. Sponsored by Travenol Laboratories, Inc. 1983, pp 1-13.

SECTION III

REPRODUCTIVE HEALTH CARE

REPRODUCTIVE HEALTH CARE IN THE UNITED STATES: CURRENT ISSUES AND CLINICAL CONTENT

19

George M. Ryan, Jr.

SUCCESS AND FAILURES IN REPRODUCTIVE HEALTH CARE TODAY

While both successes and failures have been notable in the U.S., in recent decades, related to reproductive health care, perhaps the most viable documented success has been the continued reduction in maternal mortality, perinatal mortality, and infant mortality. Maternal mortality in 1960 was 37.1 per 100,000 live births, and by 1985 this had fallen to 7.8.[1]

Infant mortality dropped from 26 per 1,000 live births in 1960 to 10.6 in 1985.[1] Perinatal mortality decreased from 28.9 per 1,000 births in 1960 to 11.6 in 1983. In spite of these successes, it should be noted that 16 countries reported lower infant-mortality rates in 1984 than did the U.S.[2] This disparity is directly related to the high rate of low birthweight in the U.S., which has remained near seven percent for the last decade, much higher than many other industrialized nations. Therefore, much of the improvement in perinatal mortality stems from the increased survival of low birthweight infants, which has produced improved neonatal death rates.[3]

The concept of neonatal intensive-care units and high-risk maternity units to serve as regional centers for the care of these mothers and infants has had an important impact upon neonatal death rates. The principles of such regional planning were outlined in 1977.[4] These guidelines for development of a regional perinatal care system stress the point that the rate of maternal-fetal and neonatal mortality could be reduced if maternity patients and their newborns at high risk were identified early, and optimal obstetric and pediatric care appropriately applied. Guidelines for referral of patients to these regional centers, and standards of services and personnel within these facilities, were outlined. The subsequent development and certification of subspecialists in maternal-fetal medicine and neonatology provided the needed medical expertise, as these centers have been established throughout the U.S.

One of the major factors in the rate of low birthweight is prenatal care.[3] At present, almost 20 percent of all pregnant women in the U.S. fail to begin prenatal care in early pregnancy, and approximately five percent receive little or no prenatal care.[5] There is no evidence of improvement in these figures over the last five years. Another disturbing statistical finding is that the perinatal mortality and infant mortality of the U.S. nonwhite population continues to greatly exceed that of the white population. In 1985, the perinatal mortality rate for white infants was 9.3, while that of nonwhite infants was 18.2 per 1,000 live births.[1] These differences clearly reflect the impact of poverty within the nonwhite population on access to reproductive health care, as well as the quality of that care. Jointly funded federal and state Medicaid programs, designed to remove fiscal barriers for the lower socioeconomic group, have undoubtedly increased access to care for many, but a complex series of barriers, including lack of education, transportation, program eligibility, and child care, still exists to explain the difference in perinatal mortality rates between racial groups.

The U.S. continues to have a high rate of unwanted pregnancy and teenage pregnancy compared to other western nations.[6] The availability of legal abortion in the U.S. has allowed the termination of approximately 45 percent of teenage pregnancies, but 55 percent go on to delivery and the cycle of poverty and early childbearing is renewed. Efforts at public education, particularly to the teenage group, have not been widely effective. Attempts to introduce sex education into school curricula have been bitterly contested by those who feel that this type of information implies consent of the adults to teenage sexual activity. The resulting politicization of the issue has stymied many of the efforts of health professionals and educators to effectively address the teenage pregnancy problem. More recently, the introduction of general health care programs into school systems, with these programs providing information as to reproductive health, has seemed to offer a new approach to the prevention of teenage pregnancy.[7]

Infection and hemorrhage are the classic causes of maternal mortality, and the dramatic reduction in maternal mortality previously cited is largely a result of improvement in the management of these two conditions. Hemorrhage control has been addressed by both refinements in the use of blood and blood products, as well as the more important development of blood-bank facilities as a standard component of hospitals providing maternity services. The control of infection has been greatly enhanced by a better understanding of the flora involved in pelvic infection, as well as continuing development of effective antibiotics. Perhaps one of the most important concepts in the last two decades has been the recognition that pelvic infections usually involve mixed bacterial flora, with anaerobic organisms a frequent and major component, and the use of multiple antibiotic regimes to provide coverage for gram positive, gram negative, and anaerobic organisms.[8] However, in spite of all of these developments, we have failed to control sexually transmitted diseases and the resulting pelvic inflammatory disease which so tragically effects the reproductive ability of young women. The sexual behavior of young people, coupled with the failure of public education to prevent transmission of these diseases, has contributed to this outcome. Today, the wide dissemination of information concerning such diseases as herpes genitalis and, more recently, acquired immune deficiency syndrome, should be expected to produce changes in the sexual behavior of young people, specifically in the reduction of the frequency of "casual sex." This change should produce a decrease in all sexually transmitted diseases.

Anesthesia for obstetrics is another area in which marked changes have occurred. Over the last 20 years, the concept of "natural childbirth" has been widely accepted and has been reflected by a decrease in the use of sedation during labor. In addition, anesthesia for labor and delivery has been enhanced by the development of epidural anesthesia and its wide usage to offer pain relief without fetal depression. Women desiring anesthesia can usually plan to be awake at the time of birth, though relatively pain-free.

Of concern is the fact that cesarean section rates have dramatically increased in the U.S. over the last two decades, from five percent in 1965, to 15 percent in 1978, and to 17.9 percent in 1981.[9] Preliminary figures for 1986 suggest a rate of 24.8 percent. Rates exceeding 20 percent have been reported in some hospitals.[10] It was readily recognized that one of the factors forcing cesarean section rates higher was the dictum "once a cesarean section, always a cesarean section,"[11] which obstetricians had followed for many years. In the last decade, we have seen increasing numbers of vaginal births after cesarean section, and have found that almost 80 percent of these patients will deliver vaginally.[12] Nevertheless, there is no immediate prospect for reduction in cesarean section rates and no hard evidence that reduction in those rates would improve perinatal outcome. While there is some small theoretical risk to the mother from cesarean section,[13] as a practical matter, it is of little significance.[10] Most cesarean sections are done for fetal indications, and these indications outweigh the risk to the mother of cesarean section. One of the factors in the increasing rate of cesarean section is the frequency of suits against physicians and hospitals following an unsatisfactory pregnancy outcome. This has tended to create an adversarial relationship between health care providers and patients, and has been termed a professional liability *crisis*. The resulting practice of defensive medicine has seen much greater usage of cesarean section and high technology with a resulting increase in the cost of maternity care. Tort reform efforts have not as yet been successful, and obstetrics remains a very high-risk specialty in terms of potential litigation.

Perhaps the most dramatic success in the clinical management of pregnancy has been the ability to assess the intrauterine status of a fetus in late pregnancy. The use of non-stress testing, stress testing, ultrasound, and amniocentesis with pulmonary maturation studies have all greatly advanced the obstetrician's ability to recognize a fetus in jeopardy and act accordingly. Today, the status of the feto-placental unit can be assessed for gestational age, fetal growth, and lung maturation in suspected cases of intrauterine growth retardation (IUGR), in patients with medical complications, such as diabetes and hypertension, and even to help determine the optimal time for elective repeat cesarean section. This is a dramatic change from the days when judgment of the fetal status represented the "art" of medicine, with little objective guidance.

Finally, no cataloging of successes and failures in reproductive health care today would be complete without mentioning data collection. While it is clear that state data collection from birth certificates has improved, in that data are now being collected as to the time of the first prenatal visit and the number of prenatal visits, as well as other data, data collection has not been standardized nationally. The ability to monitor trends in care and quality of care has been hampered by this failure. Recently, a private corporation has established the National Perinatal Information Center, which is attempting to standardize data collection on a national basis and provide data analysis for participating hospitals. It remains to be seen whether this program will attract wide enough hospital enrollment to truly offer a national data set on a valid sample of U.S births.

CONTENT OF CURRENT CLINICAL CARE IN OBSTETRICS
ANTEPARTUM CARE

Current maternity care is increasingly beginning with a pre-pregnancy visit to the physician. Many times this is because the patient is practicing contraception and seeks the advice of the physician as to cessation of contraception and how long to wait before becoming pregnant. At other times, it is the recognition by the patient that she is in a high-risk category either because of complications of previous pregnancies or because of significant medical problems. These pre-pregnancy visits give the physician a chance not only to advise the patient as to correct diet and general care during the early pregnancy but also to offer pre-pregnancy screening that would ordinarily be delayed until the first prenatal visit, well after the patient has become pregnant. This screening can allow for detection of potential problems prior to the patient becoming pregnant, and allow for a reassessment of the desirability of pregnancy (e.g., in a patient with a positive screening for Tay-Sachs disease) or to take action to avoid some risks (e.g., vaccination for rubella in a school teacher who is not immune and is planning her first pregnancy). Public and professional recognition of the benefits of such pre-pregnancy visits is just beginning.

Prenatal care should begin as soon after conception as is practical. When the patient suspects she is pregnant, she should seek medical attention, and the initial visit promptly scheduled. The purpose of the initial visit should be to establish a trusting relationship between the physician and the patient, document the medical history, perform a complete physical examination, establish the patient's risk status, counsel her as to lifestyle during the pregnancy, provide her with educational material as well as educational opportunities (i.e., childbirth education classes), and discuss the choices available to her in regard to the type of childbirth experience available. Out of this initial visit should come a plan for management during the pregnancy, as well as assessment of any known risks to an optimal pregnancy outcome. Prenatal laboratory tests at the time of the initial prenatal visit should include cervical cytology and cervical culture for gonorrhea, a clean-catch urine specimen for complete urinalysis, as well as culture and colony count for the detection of asymptomatic bacteriuria. Blood is drawn by venipuncture for a prenatal profile that includes hematocrit, white blood cell count, serologic tests for syphilis, blood type and Rh determination, antibody screen, rubella titer, and, in Black patients, a sickle cell prep. A tuberculin test should be administered, and some physicians will screen at this time for gestational diabetes by administering to the patient orally a 50-gram glucola solution and drawing blood one-hour later for determination of blood glucose. Other physicians prefer to wait until approximately 26 weeks of gestation to perform screening for gestational diabetes.

A genetic history should be sought from each patient. Factors increasing the risks for producing abnormal offspring include previous offspring with a chromosomal abnormality, particularly autosomal trisomy; chromosomal abnormality in either parent, particularly a translocation; family history of a sex-linked condition; inborn errors in metabolism; neural tube defects; and hemoglobinopathies. Tests used to evaluate these conditions include amniocentesis, fetoscopy, chorionic villus sampling, ultrasound examination, and cytogenetic assessment. Specialists in the antenatal diagnosis of genetic disorders should be consulted as appropriate.[14] All patients 35 years of age or over should be offered genetic counseling and possible amniocentesis for chromosomal studies. These patients are at increased risk of infants with Down's syndrome, and over the age of 40, such studies should be strongly encouraged. More recently, routine screening of all pregnant women for elevated maternal serum alpha fetoprotein (MSAFP) has been shown to detect 85 percent of neural tube defects, as well as some other abnormalities.[15] Genetic counseling, follow-up, and amniocentesis for patients with elevated MSAFP are an essential part of such a program. The patient may indicate she will not accept abortion if an abnormal fetus is identified, but she should still receive counseling and be encouraged to undergo amniocentesis, since once she is forewarned of an abnormal infant she may change her mind or at least be better prepared to accept the abnormal infant.

Patient education at the time of the first visit is important since the physician can reassure the patient of the normality of the pregnancy, or if there are complications or risk factors present point out these problems and indicate plans for management. The patient should be encouraged to participate in moderate, regular exercise during her pregnancy, and a total weight gain of 22 to 27 pounds is generally advisable. Instructions are given as to smoking limitation or cessation, the dangers of alcohol, the principles of a sound nutritional diet, cautions against the intake of any drugs without consulting with her physician, and danger signs and symptoms for which the patient should immediately contact the physician. At this time, the subject of childbirth education classes should be discussed, as these are available in almost every community.

The frequency of return visits in uncomplicated pregnancies is generally every four weeks for the first 28 weeks of pregnancy, every two to three weeks until 36 weeks of gestation, and weekly thereafter. Those women with risk factors or complicating diseases should be seen more frequently, as necessary, for careful monitoring of the condition. At subsequent visits, a brief interval history of events since her previous visit should be taken and the patient's weight, blood pressure, measured fundal height, fetal presentation, and fetal heart rate should be documented. Routine laboratory determinations include a urinalysis for protein, sugar, and ketone at each visit.

At the start of the third trimester, a reassessment of risk factors should be performed, screening for gestational diabetes performed, if not done previously; repeat tests done for sexually transmitted diseases, if the patient belongs to a high-risk population; and an unsensitized Rh-negative patient should have a repeat antibody test done.

During the third trimester, final discussions between the physician and patient should take place concerning plans for hospital admission, labor, and delivery. These discussions can take into account changes in the patient's risk staus or other relevant findings during the prenatal period.

LABOR AND DELIVERY

In the U.S., almost all births take place in hospitals, with out-of-hospital births constituting approximately one percent of the total.[16] It is generally conceded that the hospital provides the safest environment for the mother and baby during labor, delivery, and the postpartum period, though for low-risk uncomplicated pregnancies, free-standing Birthing Centers may offer safety nearly equal to the hospital's, in warmer, more-personal surroundings. Mention should be made of the growing popularity of family-centered care and the use of birthing rooms, both within hospitals and in free-standing centers to provide a single room for labor, delivery, and postpartum recovery, so that a woman may complete this whole process with her family support and with a minimum of interference by traditional hospital patterns of care. Labor and delivery should be an emotionally satisfying process, and the birthing room development indicates that hospitals and health care professionals are not only aware of this but are attempting to provide such an experience accompanied by the safety of the hospital setting.

Minimum services to be available include identification of high-risk mothers and fetuses, continuous electronic fetal monitoring, cesarean delivery capabilities within 30 minutes, blood and fresh-frozen plasma for transfusion, anesthesia on a 24-hour basis, radiology and ultrasound examination, neonatal resuscitation, laboratory services on a 24-hour basis, consultation and transfer agreement, nursery, and data collection and retrieval.[14] Those hospitals serving as referral centers for high-risk obstetrical patients or seriously ill newborns will provide special services, including the capabilities for fetal assessment during the latter part of pregnancy, a maternal high-risk unit, and a neonatal intensive-care unit.

The maternity high-risk unit will be utilized for the management of patients with complications, such as pregnancy induced hypertension, antepartum bleeding, premature rupture of the membranes, multiple gestation, or other conditions which may require admission prior to the onset of labor. There, these patients can be monitored and appropriate determination of the fetal status made to allow for optimal intervention by the attending physician.

All hospitals providing obstetrical services should be prepared to handle obstetric and neonatal emergencies and should have access to a neonatal intensive-care unit. If such a unit is not available within the hospital, well-planned transportation of sick neonates to the regional newborn center should be available. Ideally, maternity patients likely to deliver a markedly premature or otherwise compromised newborn should be transferred for delivery to a hospital with an intramural newborn intensive care unit. Technological capability required for the practice of obstetrics today would seem to necessitate the provision of ultrasonography and electronic fetal heart rate monitoring in all obstetrical units.

Patients admitted to the labor and delivery unit include those at term in labor, those in premature labor or with premature rupture of the membranes, and those with late complications of pregnancy, such as vaginal bleeding or pre-eclampsia, which may require delivery for treatment. For those patients in premature labor, the use of tocolytic agents, such as ritodrine hydrochloride, may prove advantageous when the fetus is healthy, gestational age is 20-34 weeks, and cervical dilatation is less than four centimeters with intact membranes. Ritodrine is a β-mimetic adrenergic agent, approved for tocolytic therapy in the U.S. The ability to delay labor with such drugs represents significant progress in the management of premature labor.

Patients admitted in labor require an initial evaluation of their status and subsequent monitoring of the progress of labor. The initial evaluation includes a recording of the maternal vital signs, the fetal heart rate, assessment of the fetal size and presentation by abdominal examination, and pelvic examination to confirm the status of the cervix and membranes, as well as the position of the presenting part. In addition, hematocrit and urinalysis are routinely performed.

During labor, surveillance requires the recording of maternal temperature at least every four hours, maternal blood pressure every hour, the fetal heart rate at least every 30 minutes, and recording of the fluid intake and output.[14] During the second stage of labor, the fetal heart rate is recorded every 15 minutes, and when the patient is ready for delivery the fetal heart rate should be checked at least every ten minutes. At any time the membranes rupture, the fetal heart should be checked immediately thereafter. If an electronic fetal monitor is used, a constant record of the fetal heart rate, as well as beat-to-beat variability and any patterns of deceleration, allow for assessment of the fetal status. Today's obstetricians do not generally require the patient to receive either an enema or a perineal "prep." Intravenous fluids may be used, depending upon risk factors present or the duration of labor. Management of pain during labor is generally accomplished using techniques discussed with the patient during antepartum care.

It is also generally accepted that the father or other support person may be with the patient during labor and delivery. Wide experience would indicate there is no increased hazard to mother, baby, or physician.

Immediately following delivery, the resuscitation of the newborn infant is the responsibility of the obstetrician. However, should the obstetrician recognize in advance the need for the neonatologist, arrangements are made to have this specialist in the room to undertake the care of the infant at birth. In the case of an emergency with the mother, another qualified person must be present to provide initial care to the newborn. If a cesarean section is planned, the obstetrician will usually notify the pediatrician, who will be present at the time of birth.

Low birthweight infants, depressed infants, or infants with other evidence of difficulty should be sent to a newborn intensive-care unit as soon as possible after initial resuscitation.

POSTPARTUM CARE

During the immediate postpartum period, the maternal blood pressure and pulse should be recorded at least every 15 minutes during the first hour, and thereafter until stable.[14] The amount of bleeding and the ability of the uterus to contract is also evaluated at frequent intervals, and any abnormality reported to the responsible physician. Following stabilization of all signs in the recovery room, the patient may be returned to her room, where the vital signs are again recorded and followed for the next several hours. The purpose of postpartum hospital care is to allow the patient a chance to stabilize and begin recovery from labor and delivery, to provide patient education for care of both the infant and the mother following their return home, and to identify any maternal or infant complications. A planned program of patient education to instruct the mother on the care and feeding of her new infant is carried out within the first 48 to 72 hours, and uncomplicated patients may be discharged at that time. During this first 72 hours, the unsensitized Rho (D)-negative patient, who has delivered an Rh-positive infant should receive Rh immune globulin.[14] Prior to discharge, all patients should be informed of scheduled visits to both the pediatrician and the obstetrician for follow-up examinations.

SUMMARY

While there have been many advances in maternal and newborn care in the U.S. in recent decades, they have mostly related to the individual care of those patients who are in the mainstream of care within the system. However, too many women in the U.S. do not enter the system because of barriers to care including fiscal problems and a lack of appropriately available and accessible services. The lack of national policy for such issues as child care, maternity leave, sex education in the public schools, and the prevention of unwanted pregnancy all contribute to deficiencies in maternity care in the U.S..

Recent changes in the attitudes of health care providers have led to a broadened participation by patients in decisions related to their own care during pregnancy. The increased marketing competition in the field has also led to rapid acceptance by providers of those changes desired by patients.

Technologic advancements, including ultrasound, antepartum assessment of the intrauterine fetal status, electronic fetal monitoring, scalp pH, increased use of the cesarean section, and the development of maternal and newborn high-risk centers, have all contributed to an improved pregnancy outcome while changing the face of maternity care today.

REFERENCES

1. National Center for Health Statistics: Advance Report of Final Mortality Statistics, 1985. Monthly Vital Statistics Report, Vol 36, Supplement 5, Aug 28, 1987.

2. Wegman ME. Annual Summary of Vital Statistics-1985. Pediatr 78:983-994, 1986.

3. Institute of Medicine, Committee to Study the Prevention of Low Birthweight: Preventing Low Birthweight, Wash DC, 1985.

4. The National Foundation—March of Dimes, Committee on Perinatal Health: Toward Improving the Outcome of Pregnancy. White Plains, NY, 1977.

5. National Center for Health Statistics: Advance Report of Final Natality Statistics. Monthly Vital Statistics Report, DHHS, Vol 36, Supplement 4 , July 17, 1987.

6. Jones EF, Forrest JD, Goldman N, et al. Teenage Pregnancy in Developed Countries; Determinants and Policy Implications. Family Planning Perspectives, 17:53-63, 1985.

7. Dryfoos J. School Based Health Clinics: A New Approach to Preventing Adolescent Pregnancy? Family Planning Perspectives, 17:70-75, 1985.

8. Ledger WJ. Infection in the Female. Lea & Febiger, Philadelphia, 1986.

9. Placek PJ, Taffel S, Moien M. Cesarean Section Delivery Rates: United States, 1981. Am J Public Health 73:861-862, 1983.

10. Frigoletto FD, Jr., Ryan KJ, Phillipe M. Maternal Mortality Rate Associated with Cesarea Section. An Appraisal. Am J Obstet Gynecol 126:969-970, 1980.

11. Cragin ER. Conservatism in Obstetrics. NY Med J 54:1, 1916.

12. Stovall TG, Shaver DC, Solomon SK, et al. Trial of Labor in Previous Cesarean Section Patients, Excluding Classical Cesarean Sections. Obstet Gynecol 70:713-717,1987.

13. Evrard JR, Gold FM. Cesarean Section and Maternal Mortality in Rhode Island. Obstet Gynecol 50:594-597, 1977.

14. American College of Obstetricians and Gynecologists: Standards for Obstetric Gynecologic Services. 6th ed, p 19, Wash DC, 1985.

15. Niebyl JR. Update on Alpha Fetoprotein. Postgrad Obstet Gynecol 6:13, 1986.

16. American College of Obstetricians and Gynecologists: Trends in Out-of Hospital Births in the United States in Manpower Planning in Obstetrics and Gynecology. Wash DC, 1985.

COMPREHENSIVE HEALTH CARE FOR WOMEN OF THE CHILDBEARING AGE

20

Charles S. Mahan

CONTENT OF "COMPREHENSIVE" CARE

Comprehensive health care for women can be defined as care that provides the most accurate, up-to-date, cost-effective diagnostic techniques to help detect common existing diseases and potential health problems. Further, it provides treatment, health education, and referral; all based on intelligent and timely interpretation of the diagnostic work-up.

For purposes of this discussion, health care for women will be divided into "pregnant" and "non-pregnant" sections, even though the majority of American women use the same health provider for both situations.

NON-PREGNANT WOMEN

It would be hoped that all American men and women would receive progressive health education starting in the preschool years. This would include comprehensive reproductive family life and sex education, and would be provided by family, schools, the media, churches and, very importantly, by health care professionals in all of the various work settings. In addition to the standard teachings, such items as breast self-examination, nutrition and reproduction, and perineal and urinary tract hygiene should be taught.[1]

If a woman has not become sexually active and has had normal, regular menses, a baseline first pelvic and breast examination would generally not become a part of the total physical examination until around age 18. In today's time, the above situation should not put a heavy burden on most college health services.

Papanicolau (Pap) smears should be started as soon as the woman, even if a young teen, is sexually active; otherwise, at age 18. The schedule of subsequent examinations is still the subject of some controversy between those who recommend "screening Paps" for asymptomatic women at intervals as close as six months to one year and the American Cancer Society (ACS) Guidelines listed in Table 1. The ACS Guidelines are gaining favor as the passage of time underscores their validity and especially as more women enter the work force and want to decrease the frequency of their health care visits. Women who perform breast self-examination and have no symptoms of ill-health need a breast examination and general history, physical examination, and laboratory work-up only at the time of their Pap smear, using the ACS Guidelines for appropriate intervals.

Women's health care professionals should be able to provide a complete spectrum of family planning teaching, drugs, and devices. Clinics or offices that do not provide a complete range of services, including pregnancy termination and outpatient sterilization, should have referral arrangements with providers of such services who are known to be of high quality. Clinics that specialize in *only* family planning services should employ health providers that can provide comprehensive examinations and care as described above. The perimenopausal woman may need special help if she develops irregular bleeding. A bleeding calendar, endometrial biopsy, and increased frequency of visits may be important while altering the family planning method accordingly. Women who have not had a sterilization procedure should continue to use family planning protection until at least one year after their last menstrual period.[2] This is an excellent time to underscore the importance of starting prenatal care in the first trimester of pregnancy.

PREGNANT WOMEN

Prenatal care *does* reduce the number of low birthweight babies and *does* improve pregnancy outcomes, although the relative importance of the various elements of prenatal care is still under debate.[3] Much recent work has been done with the goal of fine-tuning prenatal care so that it will be even more effective and better serve the individual needs of each family.[4,5] An outline of the important elements of modern prenatal care is listed in Table 2.[6]

Since low birthweight is by far our most serious problem in American pregnancy outcomes, much attention has finally been turned to this area in recent years. Preterm birth-prevention programs in France, San Francisco, North Carolina, and Florida have shown significant reductions in low birthweight using similar

TABLE 1

**SUMMARY OF AMERICAN CANCER SOCIETY RECOMMENDATIONS
FOR THE EARLY DETECTION OF CANCER IN ASYMPTOMATIC PEOPLE**

Test or Procedure	Population		
	Sex	Age	Frequency
Sigmoidoscopy	M & F	Over 50	After 2 negative exams 1 year apart, perform every 3-5 years
Stool Guaiac Slide Test	M & F	Over 50	Every year
Digital Rectal Examination	M & F	Over 40	Every year
Pap Test	F	All women who are, or who have been, sexually active, or have reached age 18, should have an annual Pap test and pelvic examination. After a woman has had three or more consecutive satisfactory normal annual examinations, the Pap test may be performed less frequently at the discretion of her physician.	
Pelvic Examination	F		
Endometrial Tissue Sample	F	At menopause, women at high risk*	At menopause
Breast Self-examination	F	20 and over	Every month
Breast Physical Examination	F	20-40 Over 40	Every 3 years Every year
Mammography	F	35-39 40-49 50 and over	Baseline Every 1-2 years Every year
Chest X-ray			Not recommended
Sputum Cytology			Not recommended
Health Counseling and Cancer Checkup**	M & F M & F	Over 20 Over 40	Every 3 years Every year

*   History of infertility, obesity, failure to ovulate, abnormal uterine bleeding, or estrogen
therapy.

**   To include examination for cancers of the thyroid, testicles, prostate, ovaries, lymph
nodes, oral region, and skin.

TABLE 2

MINIMUM STANDARD PREGNANCY HEALTH CARE VISIT CONTENT

FIRST VISIT

A. **Health Questionnaire—Filled out by patient**

Should include family-centered questions such as:
- father at labor and birth?
- breast feeding?
- rooming-in?
- early discharge?
- circumcision?
- post-partum sterilization?

B. **History**
- **Past** - include detailed reproductive history
- **Family** - include genetic
- **Review of systems** - include sexual activity and satisfaction, family relationships, drugs, smoking, alcohol, and nutrition

C. **Physical Examination**
- Complete general
- Breasts
- Abdominal
- Pelvic (include pap smear, gonorrhea culture, and measurements of bony pelvis)

D. **Laboratory Testing–First Visit**

1. **All women**
- Hemoglobin or hematocrit
- Urine test for protein, sugar, and ketones
- Bacteriuria screen
- Rubella screen (if status in doubt)
- Sickle screen (if status in doubt and if black, or of Mediterranean origin)
- Blood group and Rh
- Atypical blood antibody screen if Rh negative or if history of blood transfusion
- Serologic test for syphilis
- Blood glucose screen at 24-28 weeks

2. **As indicated by first prenatal work-up**
- Genetic amniocentesis
- Pregnancy test
- Ultrasound for dating purposes (18-22 weeks)
- HIV testing
- Hepatitis B testing
- TB skin test
- Chlamydia test
- Alpha fetoprotein

E. **General Risk Assessment and Preterm Labor Risk Screen**

F. **Referral**
- Other members of health care team
- High-risk pregnancy center
- Hospital
- Birth center
- Dental care

G. **Subsequent Visits**

1. **Low risk**
- 1st trimester, 18, 22, 28, 32, 36, 38, 40, 41, 42 weeks
- Repeat syphilis and gonorrhea tests at 32 weeks; other tests repeated as indicated

2. **Medical high risk**
- Frequent visits as determined by obstetrical specialist following woman

3. **Preterm labor high risk**
- Weekly visits to nurse or physician after 22 weeks, including cervical checks

protocols. [7,8,9,10] Some of the unique elements of this care include risk-scoring, case management, more frequent visits, stress-reduction counseling, same health provider at each visit, and extensive patient education.

The importance of risk-scoring for all pregnant women cannot be overemphasized. A *general* risk evaluation should be done after the history, physical examination, and laboratory work are completed, looking for the "classical" high-risk problems of hypertension, diabetes, etc. After that, a *separate* risk evaluation should be done specifically for assessing the chance of the occurrence of preterm labor. The most commonly used scoring system for this latter effort is the Papiernik/Creasy. [10]

Bacteriuria screens at the first prenatal visit and blood glucose screens at 24-28 weeks of pregnancy have been proven to be extremely valuable adjuncts to prenatal care and should be performed for all pregnant women. [11]

PROBLEMS IN THE DELIVERY OF COMPREHENSIVE CARE FOR WOMEN

EDUCATION AND PREPARATION OF PRACTITIONERS

The majority of residency training programs in obstetrics and gynecology stress care for the *hospitalized* patient and offer very little in the way of instruction directed at holistic health care or care of the woman in the *ambulatory* setting. This situation is slowly changing as residency review committees emphasize the fact that the average obstetrician-gynecologist spends 75 percent of his/her practice time in the office. Family practice residencies and nurse-midwife/nurse practitioner training programs place a much heavier emphasis on preparation of students to deal with the ambulatory setting. The majority of nurse and physician training programs still do not have adequate segments exposing their students to the practical aspects of public health care, including home visits, clinic or office management, and sociology and anthropology of health in diverse cultural groups, etc.

DELIVERY OF PREGNANCY AND GYNECOLOGIC CARE

Pregnancy Care Health providers of pregnancy care have been loathe to adjust their prenatal care routines to new information. It took over ten years for the majority of pregnancy care specialists in the U.S. to stop restricting weight in pregnant women after *all* of the major obstetric textbooks recommended against it. The same scenario is unfolding with low birthweight prevention, where successful techniques to deal with the problem have only been instituted primarily in public health and academic settings even though the problem cuts through all classes of society. The same problem exists with vaginal birth after cesarean section. [12] This reluctance to change old practice habits needs to be dealt with by national provider organizations, training programs, and a better informed public.

The problem of access to *early* prenatal care is a serious one throughout the U.S. and needs to be conquered by better office and practice management for private physicians and midwives, and less arcane eligibility determination systems for low-income women trying to gain access to public health or academic care providers. Constant attention needs to be paid to innovative media reminders about the importance of early prenatal care.

Pregnancy care has been less-easily accessible in many parts of the U.S., in the past few years, due to the liability insurance crisis. This has resulted in many physicians dropping obstetrics, or at least high-risk obstetrics; nurse-midwives losing their physician back-up; home-birth services run by licensed lay midwives, losing doctor back-up; hospitals closing obstetric units; and doctors refusing low-income patients because they are "more likely to sue"—a common idea that runs converse to all insurance statistical reports. Many think a "Workman's Compensation" system of insurance for babies with poor outcomes is the only way to reverse the above problems in pregnancy care access.

It has been shown that legal liability problems are decreased and patient outcomes are better if the pregnant woman can see the same care provider throughout pregnancy, and also if that care provider gives enough time for all questions to be answered. This would involve reorganizing the group practices of many physicians and midwives, but would pay big dividends in women's satisfaction with the care they receive.

A reorganization of pregnancy care into a "tiered" system of care, based on risk status of mother and fetus, makes sense and helps one think more clearly about the logical stratification of such care (Table 3). No matter how one feels about home birth, the fact is that one percent of Americans *do* give birth at home and it is our duty as health care professionals to do what we can to help them have the safest birth outcomes possible, whether this is through providing prenatal care supervision, hospital back-up, and licensing and supervision of home-birth midwives, etc. Out-of-hospital birth centers have proliferated in the U.S. in the past five years, and now number over 200, with much current interest in future expansion of such by the large national hospital chains. Care of normal pregnancies in such centers costs approximately half that of hospital birth and has been reported to be at least as safe as hospital birth.[13,14] Most birth centers in the U.S. are run by certified nurse-midwives, with obstetric back-up.

Gynecologic Care Even though Medicaid programs have been expanded recently in many states to cover more low-income pregnant women, there remains a widespread problem of difficulty in paying for any extraordinary gynecologic care needed by that same group. If any of those women need colposcopy, sterilization, pregnancy termination, diagnostic laparoscopy, breast biopsy, hysterectomy, or cancer surgery, there is frequently difficulty in receiving these needed services because there is no source of funding for them. This problem has become much more acute recently as more public hospitals have "gone private," having been acquired by major for-profit national hospital chains.

DELIVERY OF FAMILY PLANNING SERVICES

Since 1970, family planning services have been made available to most American women of all income levels. Since 1973, abortion has been available to women in all states, but only a handful of states help low-income women pay for abortions and this seems unlikely to change in the near future.

In spite of the close proximity of the various forms of family planning services to most Americans, there is a clear need in many of those services for better office or clinic management to increase efficiency and client acceptance. This would include night and weekend hours for both men and women, and the ability to choose a place for family planning help that is not limited by political boundaries. The reason for this is that research has shown that many teenagers (and some adults) prefer to travel across town or to another city for family planning services than be seen in a clinic in their own neighborhood.

TABLE 3

TIERED SYSTEMS OF PREGNANCY CARE

Risk Determination	Practitioner	Facility
Low	Lay Midwife	Home/Birth Center
	Nurse Midwife	Home/Birth Center/ Level I Hospital
	Physician (Family Practice)	Home/Birth Center/ Level I Hospital
Medium	Nurse-Midwife with Physician Co-Management Physician (Family Practice or OB/GYN)	Level II Hospital
High	Physician (OB/GYN or Maternal-Fetal OB/GYN Specialist)	Level III Hospital

Another serious weakness of many family planning providers is a willingness to accept the "status quo" and to passively await client applications to their program rather than taking an aggressive "marketing" approach to the community they serve. Targeting recruitment and public information programs to high-risk groups, such as sexually active teenagers, women who have already had poor pregnancy outcomes, and men and women with serious health programs, has a more positive effect on the general health of the public than a passive approach.[15] This has recently been seen in the efforts made to inform the gay population about methods to prevent the spread of Acquired Immune Disease Syndrome (AIDS).

The offering of free pregnancy tests has been used for years by private abortion clinics to "capture" clients for their services. This has been shown to be an excellent measure for public health clinics to use, to enroll clients into immediate family planning help or early prenatal care. To be successful, the pregnancy test results should be reported to the woman rapidly and by a health professional who can *immediately* counsel the woman and enroll her in whatever service she needs. This proactive approach will very quickly have a pay-off much greater than any that could be gained by charging $5.00 a pregnancy test, as many clinics currently do—a charge that in itself may serve as a barrier to care.

GENERAL HEALTH CARE SERVICES FOR WOMEN

The content of a general health care visit for women is listed in Table 4. Approximately 85 percent of American women have health insurance or are enrolled in HMO-type care. This leaves 15 percent of women who are poor or in minimum wage jobs with no insurance, who have to use public health clinics or sometimes hospital emergency rooms for care. This latter group may include runaway teenagers thrown into prostitution, homeless women who are mentally ill, or women who have been the victims of violence and then abandoned. Some arrangement to provide decent health care to these women would be helpful, but their problems transcend even the best health care and involve better housing, job training, education, and even perhaps a greater effort to tone down violence to women portrayed in movies and on television.

Much more can be done to promote self-care and individual responsibility through innovative educational approaches. Techniques, such as breast self-examination and skin cancer surveillance, along with preventive nutrition ideas and the effects of substance abuse, need to be constantly in the public eye, not just sporadic media blitzes.

The concept of team care has been a very successful one in modern health care. As health and medical knowledge proliferates and increases in complexity, no one practitioner can hope to be able to provide sound, timely advice and counseling to adequately cover all of the needs of most women. The team may consist of

TABLE 4

MINIMUM STANDARD GENERAL HEALTH CARE VISIT CONTENT

1. **Health Questionnaire–Filled out by patient**

2. **History**
   - Present illness (if any)
   - Past history (include detailed reproductive history)
   - Family history
   - Review of systems (includes sexual activity and satisfaction, drugs, smoking, alcohol, nutrition)

3. **Physical Examination**
   - Complete general
   - Pelvic (includes Pap Smear and STD Testing)
   - Recto-vaginal (included test for occult blood in stool if over age 40)

4. **Laboratory Testing**
   - **A. All women**
     - Hemoglobin or Hematocrit
     - Urinalysis

   - **B. If indicated by history or physician exam:**
     - serologic test for syphilis
     - chlamydia culture
     - gonorrhea culture
     - vaginitis testing
     - HIV test
     - Hepatitis B testing
     - urine culture
     - serum cholesterol, triglycerides, HDL, and LDL
     - blood glucose screen
     - electrocardiogram
     - sigmoidoscopy
     - cystoscopy
     - colposcopy
     - urodynamics
     - other

5. **Referral**
   - To other team members
   - Hospital
   - Medical Specialist

6. **Patient Education–Should give adequate time to answer all of the woman's or family's questions**

a mixture of any or all of the types of professionals listed in Table 5, depending on the specific and unique health care needs of the community being served.

WOMEN'S SATISFACTION WITH PRESENT SERVICES

Surveys performed by the American College of Obstetricians and Gynecologists find that women receiving private OB/GYN care are *highly* satisfied with the services they receive. A survey of low-and middle-income women done by the University of Florida found the majority of those women to be highly pleased with the services they received in public family planning clinics.

In spite of the results reported above, a significant minority of women, perhaps having had their awareness of the issues heightened by the Women's Movement or feminist writings, have complaints about their care. And in an era of stiff health care service competition for the paying customer, providers are paying much more attention to these complaints and are altering services accordingly.[5,16,17,18]

It is important for all providers to poll each of their clients yearly as to their satisfaction with all aspects of the services being provided. Even if the woman elects not to fill out an offered survey, she feels good that the provider cared enough to ask her opinion.

UNMET NEEDS IN WOMEN'S HEALTH CARE

Parental leave at the time of childbirth The U.S. is the only Western industrialized country that does not guarantee a working mother or father time off

---

TABLE 5

THE WOMEN'S HEALTH CARE TEAM
(Components Depend on Needs of Office or Clinic and Clientele)

Physician	Nurse-Midwife
Nurse	Lay-Midwife
Social Worker	Nutritionist
Child-Development Specialist	Psychologist (counseling)
Childbirth Education Instructor	Physical Therapist
Nurse-Practitioner (OB/GYN, Family Planning, Family, Pediatric)	Genetic Counselor

from the work place after a birth. This time is important for parent-infant attachment, strengthening the family, and for the stabilization and continuation of breast feeding.[19] Efforts are currently underway in some states and at the national level to correct this situation, but progress has been slow. In this same area, serious efforts to decrease low birthweight baby numbers in the U.S. must consider that France and other European countries have reduced their low birthweight numbers dramatically by offering elective, or in some cases mandatory, maternity leave starting at 28-32 weeks of pregnancy and continuing for an extended period after birth. Income during the time off is provided by either insurance or social security.[20,21]

The 15 percent of women using emergency rooms for problems need a "health care home." Some states are starting to provide this by using federal Primary Care Centers and county or city health departments to help reduce dependency on emergency rooms for ambulatory care visits.

Health education, especially emphasizing prevention, is a serious unmet need in many parts of the country. School-based clinics and innovative media programs have been established in many areas, as well as ongoing efforts to educate school children as to good health practices starting in day-care facilities.

Other common unmet needs are safe, well-run day-care facilities; child-care areas in offices and clinics; adequate numbers of shelters with medical back-up for women and children who are victims of violence; a broader array of family planning choices; the provision of family-centered care in public clinics; more women physicians in OB/GYN and Family Practice specialties; and more nurse-midwives and nurse practitioners due to the current shortage.

Progress has been, and is being, made, but there are still many long miles to go in our quest for comprehensive health care with a high standard of excellence that is available to all American women.

REFERENCES

1. Boston Women's Health Book Collective: The new our bodies, ourselves. New York, Simon and Schuster, 1984, pp 489-491, 507.

2. Hatcher RA, Guest F, Stewart F, et al. Contraceptive technology 1984-1985. New York, Irvington Publishers, Inc., 1984, pp 31-32.

3. Committee to Study the Prevention of Low Birthweight: Preventing Low Birthweight. Washington DC, National Academy Press, 1985.

4. Mahan CS, McKay S. Let's reform our antenatal care methods. Cont Obstet Gynecol 23:147, 1984.

5. Enkin M, Chalmers I (ed). Effectiveness and satisfaction in antenatal care. Philadelphia, J.B. Lippincott Co, 1982, pp 266-286.

6. Department of Health and Rehabilitative Services, State of Florida: Maternal and Child Health Services Manual 150-13. Tallahassee, Fl, 1987.

7. Papiernik K, Bouyer J, Dreyfus J, et al. Prevention of preterm births: a perinatal study in Haguenau, France. Pediatrics 76:154, 1985.

8. Herron MA, Katz M, Creasy RK. Evaluation of a preterm birth prevention program: preliminary report. Obstet Gynecol 59:452, 1982.

9. Mies PJ, Ernest JM, Moore ML. Regional program for prevention of premature birth in northwestern North Carolina. Am J Obstet Gynecol 157:551, 1987.

10. Mahan CS. New strategies for preventing an old problem: low birthweight. J Florida MA 70:722, 1983.

11. Whalley PJ. Bacteriuria of pregnancy. Am J Obstet Gynecol 97:723, 1967.

12. Taffel SM, Placek PJ, Liss T. Trends in the United States cesarean section rate and reasons for the 1980-85 rise. Am J Public Health 77:955, 1987.

13. McLead D. Birth centers deliver lower maternity costs. Business Insurance, October 25, 1982, p 1.

14. Scupholme A, McLeod AGW, Robertson EG: A birth center affiliated with the tertiary care center: Comparison of outcome. Obstet Gynecol 67:598, 1986.

15. Perkin GW. Assessment of reproductive risk in nonpregnant women. Am J Obstet Gynecol 101:709, 1968.

16. Jolly C, Held B, Caraway AF, et al. Research in the delivery of female health care: The recipients' reaction. Am J Obstet Gynecol 110:291, 1971.

17. Connell EB. Meeting the ambulatory health care needs of women. Ambulatory Care in Obstetrics and Gynecology. Edited by GM Ryan. New York, Grune and Stratton, Inc., 1980, pp 31-37.

18. Rusley RL. In the practice-building game, nice guys finish first. Medical Economics. April 27, 1981, p 171.

19. Young D. ICEA Resolution on parental leave after childbirth. International Childbirth Education Association. Minneapolis, MN, 1987.

20. Chamberlain G. Effect of working during pregnancy. Obstet Gynecol 65:747, 1985.

21. Miller CA. Maternal Health and Infant Survival. Washington DC National Center for Clinical Infant Programs, 1987, pp 27-28.

PREVENTING LOW BIRTHWEIGHT

21

Sarah S. Brown

INTRODUCTION

Low birthweight babies—those born too soon, too small, or both—have long been a source of deep concern to theMCH profession. Among such experts is a solid appreciation of the increased risks of both mortality and morbidity that accompany low birthweight. Two-thirds of deaths in the first four weeks of life are of infants weighing 2,500 g or less; and, of these, half are deaths of very-low birthweight newborns, 1500 g or less. Low birthweight babies are almost 40 times more likely to die in the neonatal period than are heavier newborns, and infants of very-low birthweight are 200 times more likely to die. Even when all other factors known to affect neonatal deaths are accounted for, low birthweight remains the major determinant.

Those who survive face increased risks of various childhood illnesses and developmental problems. Although the impact of low birthweight on morbidity is less well-established than is its contribution to mortality, the association between low birthweight and neurodevelopmental problems, such as cerebral palsy, is well-documented. Low birthweight infants are more likely than others to be susceptible to lower respiratory tract infections, learning disorders, behavior problems, and complications of the neonatal care interventions themselves. Such infants and children account for more hospital visits than do those who were of normal birthweight.[1] And, of course, the human and financial costs can be staggering.

As the 1980s draw to a close, there is clear evidence that ever-increasing numbers of non-expert citizens are coming to appreciate the burdens associated with prematurity and fetal growth retardation, the twin contributors to low birthweight. Much of the concern is embedded in the larger context of infant mortality, but it is real nonetheless, and heartening. In this chapter, a few aspects of this "growing audience" are discussed, the relationship of infant mortality and low birthweight is outlined, the risk factors are catalogued, and possible approaches to reducing low birthweight are described.

THE RELATIONSHIP OF INFANT MORTALITY AND LOW BIRTHWEIGHT

On July 1, 1987, the National Commission to Prevent Infant Mortality became formally constituted. The 15-member group was established by the 99th Congress to "develop a national strategy for reducing infant mortality in the United States." As this chapter is being drafted, the commission is holding hearings to learn from both national and international experts about approaches to improving infant survival, and is working with numerous private and public organizations to mobilize action on numerous perinatal issues.

Because congressional actions of this nature—impaneling expert groups with high visibility and lofty mandates—is usually a response to broad political movements or changing opinions in the country, it is helpful to consider the commission's antecedents. What lies at the base of this recent, top-level expression of concern about infant mortality?

An important ancestor of the group is unmistakably the Surgeon General. In 1980, that office (then occupied by Dr. Julius Richmond) issued the publication *Promoting Health/Preventing Disease: Objectives for the Nation.*[2] Numerous experts and a long and publicly open process generated this document, which included 226 objectives (19 concerning pregnancy and infant health), many of which stated numerical goals.

These national objectives have been cited repeatedly since their publication, in countless texts, articles, reports, funding applications, and media segments, and have clearly met one of their goals: to serve as guideposts for measuring progress or lack thereof. In those health areas where positive change since 1980 has been significant, leaders have taken great pride in announcing that the 1990 goals have already been met, or soon will be. However, in areas where progress has been slow, the 1990 goals have made it relatively easy to pinpoint failure or, at least, lack of progress and, to a certain extent, have increased the pressure on responsible officials to redouble their efforts to solve troubling problems.

Infant mortality, unfortunately, is one of those areas where progress seems too slow. In its *Midcourse Review of the 1990 Objectives*, the Public Health Service states quite simply that based on progress to date, achievement of the 1990 goal of no more than nine deaths per 1,000 births is "questionable."[3] This cautious assessment reflects the fact that although the infant mortality rate in the U.S. has declined steadily since the mid-1960s, its rate of decline has slowed (Table 1), a discouraging development that advocacy groups such as the Children's Defense Fund have brought to clear public prominence.[4]

Concern about the infant mortality level and the nation's probable failure to meet the 1990 goals is heightened by international comparisons. It is widely acknowledged that the U.S. ranks behind 17 other industrialized nations in infant mortality rates (Table 2). With regard to number-one ranked Japan, the National Commission noted that, in 1955, Japan ranked 17th in infant mortality. In 1985, Japan ranked first, with the lowest recorded infant mortality rate in the world. The U.S., by contrast, has dropped from 6th, in rank, in 1955, to 18 in 1985. Clearly, the Congress accurately identified a troubling—and internationally embarrassing—health problem in creating its National Commission.

In some states, cities, and smaller areas, of course, the rates are significantly higher than the U.S. national average—the 1985 infant mortality rate for the District of Columbia, for example, was 20.8—and cities such as Detroit and Hartford actually reported increasing rates in the early 1980s. In response to distressing infant-mortality data, over half the states, and countless cities and communities have organized infant mortality reduction initiatives, ranging from sophisticated statewide efforts, such as California's Obstetrical Access project, to grass roots "outreach" and public awareness programs, such as the District of Columbia's campaign,

TABLE 1

INFANT MORTALITY RATE - UNITED STATES - ALL RACES

1985	10.6	1974	16.7
1984	10.8	1973	17.7
1983	11.2	1972	18.5
1982	11.5	1971	19.1
1981	11.9	1970	20.0
1980	12.6	1969	20.9
1979	13.1	1968	21.8
1978	13.8	1967	22.4
1977	14.1	1966	23.7
1976	15.2	1965	24.7
1975	16.1	1955	26.4

SOURCE: National Center for Health Statistics, Vital Statistics of the United States

"Beautiful Babies Right from the Start." Although no comprehensive list exists detailing the hundreds of initiatives, knowledgeable sources report a major outpouring of community concern, creativity, and even money.

One very interesting aspect of these numerous initiatives—national, state, local—is their tacit appreciation of the intimate relationship between infant mortality and low birthweight. A common scenario is that a city, for example, notes with concern its high rate of infant mortality, compared to national estimates, and such targets as the 1990 goals. It then establishes a Blue Ribbon Commission to determine the underlying causes of the area's high rates of infant mortality and to make recommendations for remedial action. With the assistance of vital statistics experts, it is gradually understood that over the first half of this century, infant mortality declined from about 100 to about 30 deaths per 1,000 live births. Most of this decline has been attributed to decreases in the rate of post-neonatal mortality (deaths from 28 days to the first birthday), brought about largely by environmental changes, especially a reduction in infectious diseases, and by better nutrition. An improved birthweight distribution probably did not make a significant contribution to decreases in post-neonatal deaths. By 1950, neonatal mortality accounted for about two-thirds of all infant deaths, and it became clear that further substantial decreases in infant mortality rates would require reducing the proportion of infants who are born underweight or increasing the survival rates of vulnerable babies. For a variety of reasons, the latter approach has been emphasized— primarily through hospital-based management of high-risk pregnancies and neonatal intensive care. It is generally agreed that improvements in the survival of tiny, often ill newborns has been largely responsible for the 55 percent reduction in infant mortality rates

TABLE 2

INTERNATIONAL COMPARISON OF INFANT MORTALITY

Country	Rate	Country	Rate
Japan	6.0	Singapore	8.8
Sweden	6.0	Hong Kong	9.0
Finland	6.5	Australia	9.2
Switzerland	7.5	Belgium	9.4
Denmark	7.7	FRG	9.6
France	8.2	UK	9.6
The Netherlands	8.3	Spain	9.7
Norway	8.3	GDR	10.0
Canada	8.5	U.S.	10.6

SOURCE: National Center for Health Statistics, provisional 1984 data except for (1) U.S., which is 1985 data, and (2) Hong Kong, which is from UNICEF.

between 1965 and 1985, to 10.6 deaths per 1,000 live births. Such a belief is consistent with the fact that although birthweight-specific neonatal mortality rates have fallen dramatically in recent years, the proportion of infants born underweight has declined only modestly—from 7.6 percent of all babies born in 1971 to about 6.8 percent currently.[5] The decline has been concentrated mostly among infants of moderately low birthweight delivered at full term. There has been almost no change, and perhaps even a slight increase, in the proportion of infants whose birthweights are very low, currently a little more than one percent of all live-borns.[6]

In short, a substantial proportion of recent (since 1965) declines in infant mortality is due to the increased survival of low birthweight infants rather than to an improved birthweight distribution. In fact, birthweight-survival rates in the U.S. may be the best in the world.

The slowed rate of decline in infant mortality documented in the mid-1980s may reflect the decrease in federal support for selected perinatal programs seen in the early 1980s and also the fact that the technology of neonatal care has not altered dramatically in the last few years. For example, it has been suggested that no recent development in neonatology has had the same impact as the widespread introduction of artificially assisted ventilation in the early 1960s. Whatever the cause of the slowed decline in infant mortality, accelerating the rate of decrease, or perhaps even sustaining its current sluggish decline, will require action on one or both of the following fronts: some dramatic new progress in neonatology, such that even tinier, sicker babies can be helped to survive and/or some lowering of the low birthweight rate.

Relying primarily on neonatal intensive care as the principal means of reducing infant mortality is a troubling strategy, for at least two reasons. First is the concern about poor quality of life for infants born less than 1500 g who survive. Up to now, the increased survival of low birthweight infants has not been associated with an increase in the proportion of infants born with handicaps. Concerns remain, however, about the effect of increased survival of the very smallest infants—especially those weighing less than 1000 g. For example, in a recent study of 57 infants <1500 g, close to half (46 percent) were classified as having severe morbidity, and 42 percent required one or more readmissions to the hospital within the first month of life, compared with an expected percentage of about 14.[7] The U.S. Congress' Office of Technology Assessment (OTA) recently concluded that "neonatal intensive care has contributed to improved long-term developmental outcomes for premature infants. The great decline in mortality among all subgroups of very low birthweight infants over the last ten years, however, means there are now larger absolute numbers of both seriously handicapped and normal survivors. For every 100 very low birthweight infants treated in today's NICUs (neonatal intensive care units), about 27 will die before hospital discharge, 16 will be seriously or moderately disabled, and 57 will be normal children, though some will develop mild learning disabilities."[8]

Reluctance to rely on the salvage efforts of neonatal care to reduce infant mortality also is cost-based. The OTA has noted that neonatal intensive care for very-low birthweight infants ranks among the most costly of all hospital admissions. "A primary predictor of cost is birthweight; costs increase as birthweight falls. The average cost for a very-low birthweight survivor is from $31,000 to $71,000. The tiniest infants who survive, those with birthweights under 750 grams, have the longest average hospital stay, about 98 days, and the highest costs, averaging $62,000 to $150,000. Hospitals report increasing numbers of these tiniest babies in their NICUs. (About 8,500 infants weighing less than 750 grams are born each year in the U.S.)"[8]

The choice of strategy, of course, is not "either-or." The miracle and promise of neonatal intensive care will continue to be a cornerstone of perinatal medicine. But what are the prospects for pursuing the other strategy—preventing low birthweight in the first place? Cannot a similar investment and intensity of effort be brought to the goal of producing bigger, healthier babies in the first place?

RISK FACTORS FOR LOW BIRTHWEIGHT

It is usually easier to design preventive interventions if underlying cause is known. Unfortunately, the basic mechanisms of both preterm labor and fetal growth retardation are not well understood. Although a range of clues and hypotheses can be outlined, the fact is that clinicians caring for women in whom such conditions are or may be present must rely more on art than science in understanding etiology or planning treatment. In the absence of adequate information about the basic causes of low birthweight, a large body of information has developed about "risk factors," or factors whose presence in an individual woman indicates an increased chance of bearing a low birthweight infant. These factors are listed in Table 3. They include demographic characteristics, medical risks that can be identified before pregnancy, several that can only be identified during pregnancy, behavioral and environmental factors, risks associated with health care (such as inadequate prenatal care), and a separate group of factors whose relationship to low birthweight is more tenuous, such as stress, uterine irritability, and inadequate plasma volume expansion.[9]

Grouping the risk factors, as noted on Table 3, helps one to identify those that can be detected before pregnancy and reinforces the concept that interventions can begin before the prenatal period. Smoking is perhaps the best example of this perspective. The grouping also emphasizes the importance of behavioral and environmental risks and the need for interventions that go beyond medical care. The demographic measures can help to define target populations. The cluster of health care factors highlights the fact that not all risks for low birthweight derive from characteristics of women themselves. And, finally, the category of evolving concepts of risk suggests some important research areas.

TABLE 3

PRINCIPAL RISK FACTORS FOR LOW BIRTHWEIGHT

1. **Demographic Risks**
   A. Age (less than 17; over 34)
   B. Race (black)
   C. Low socioeconomic status
   D. Unmarried
   E. Low level of education

2. **Medical Risks Predating Pregnancy**
   A. Parity (0 or more than 4)
   B. Low weight for height
   C. Genitourinary anomalies/surgery
   D. Selected diseases such as diabetes, chronic hypertension
   E. Nonimmune status for selected infections such as rubella
   F. Poor obstetric history including previous low birthweight infant, multiple spontaneous abortions
   G. Maternal genetic factors (such as low maternal weight at own birth)

3. **Medical Risks in Current Pregnancy**
   A. Multiple pregnancy
   B. Poor weight gain
   C. Short interpregnancy interval
   D. Hypotension
   E. Hypertension/preeclampsia/toxemia
   F. Selected infections such as symptomatic bacteriuria, rubella, and cytomegalovirus
   G. 1st or 2nd trimester bleeding
   H. Placental problems such as placenta previa, abruptio placentae
   I. Hyperemesis
   J. Oligohydramnios/polyhydramnios
   K. Anemia/abnormal hemoglobin
   L. Isoimunization
   M. Fetal anomalies
   N. Incompetent cervix
   O. Spontaneous premature rupture of membranes

4. **Behavioral and Environmental Risks**
   A. Smoking
   B. Poor nutritional status
   C. Alcohol and other substance abuse
   D. DES exposure and other toxic exposures, including occupational hazards
   E. High altitude

5. **Health Care Risks**
   A. Absent or inadequate prenatal care
   B. Iatrogenic prematurity

6. **Evolving Concepts of Risk**
   A. Stress (physical and psychosocial)
   B. Uterine irritability
   C. Events triggering uterine contractions
   D. Cervical changes detected before onset of labor
   E. Selected infections such as mycoplasma and Chlamydia trachomatis
   F. Inadequate plasma volume expansion
   G. Progesterone deficiency

SOURCE: Committee to Study the Prevention of Low Birthweight: Preventing Low Birthweight. Institute of Medicine. National Academy Press. Washington, D.C., 1985.

Although a variety of factors are clearly and consistently linked to low birthweight, there are important limits to neat, easily comprehensible listings, such as Table 3. It is known, for example, that the magnitude of risk posed by each factor for an individual or for a group cannot always be calculated easily, that the risks for low birthweight are widely distributed throughout the population, and that a substantial number of low birthweight deliveries will continue to occur outside of groups currently defined as high risk. Some additional aspects of selected risk factors merit comments.

Black newborns are more than twice as likely to weigh less than 2,500 grams as white infants. The race-specific low birthweight rates among live births in the U.S. in 1984 were 12.4 percent for Blacks and 5.6 percent for whites. The reasons for the higher risk among Blacks are not clear and recent research in this area has produced conflicting results.[10,11] It has been speculated that maternal age may account for part of the difference—twice as many Black births are to teenagers— but when Black and white mothers of the same age are compared, Blacks are at higher risk of low birthweight in every age group. Similarly, Black mothers, as a group, have less education than white mothers, but when Blacks and whites are matched by level of education, Blacks still have a higher risk of low birthweight. Other factors that have been studied, but fail to account for the white-Black differential, include delay in initiating prenatal care, smoking status, height and weight distributions of the mother, and obstetric history.

The conclusion to be drawn from the complicated data on race, low birthweight, and race-specific birthweight mortality rates is that the reasons for the risk differentials between white and Black newborns are not well understood. The cumulative effects over time, of Black poverty and lower social status, and the interaction of such factors with biological processes, undoubtedly have played a role in these racial differences; other factors remain to be defined. Research should be pursued to improve our understanding of these important issues.

Obstetric history has emerged as a potent predictor of future poor outcomes. In particular, the history of a woman's previous pregnancies is of prime importance in the prediction of a subsequent low birthweight infant. A detailed study of the weights and gestational ages of all births in Norway from 1967 through 1973 showed that a premature first birth is the best predictor of a premature second birth, and that growth retardation in a first pregnancy is the most powerful predictor of growth retardation in a second pregnancy.[12] Previous fetal and neonatal deaths also are strongly associated with preterm low birthweight, and the risk increases as the number of poor fetal outcomes increases. Nutritional status and smoking are two additional risk factors to be underscored. Numerous studies point to the common conclusion that good nutrition has a positive influence on birthweight, but the extent of the effect is unclear. The magnitude of nutritional effects on low birthweight is not easily assessed because nutritional status is difficult to isolate from other socio-economic characteristics and because of the complicated relationship between pre-pregnant weight and weight gain during pregnancy. A reasonable conclusion is that poor nutritional status before pregnancy and inadequate nutrition during pregnancy have a negative impact on fetal weight gain, thereby increasing the risk of IUGR.

One recent study explored the relationship between a mother's weight gain during pregnancy and the occurrence of low birthweight by analyzing data from the 1980 National Natality and Fetal Mortality Surveys. The investigators found that many groups of women known to have an increased risk of delivering a low birth-weight infant also were more likely to have inadequate weight gains. For example, they found that Black mothers were twice as likely as white mothers to gain less than 16 pounds during pregnancy. In addition, mothers 35 years of age or older, and teenage girls, were less likely to gain at least 16 pounds as were unmarried women, poorly educated women, and women of lower socio-economic status. A further analysis of numerous risk factors among white mothers only indicated that, except for period of gestation, weight gain has the strongest impact on birthweight.[13]

And finally, smoking is one of the most important and preventable determinants of low birthweight in the U.S. A recent survey of the literature on smoking and birthweight indicates that smoking during pregnancy is associated with a reduction in birthweight ranging from 150 to 250 grams.[14] This relationship has persisted for at least 20 years, despite reported reductions in the average tar and nicotine yields of cigarettes on the market. The reasons for the detrimental effects of cigarette smoking are not fully understood, but the fact than an estimated 20 to 30 percent of pregnant women in the U.S. smoke underscores the importance of this risk factor.[15]

APPROACHES TO PREVENTION

Faced with the data on trends in infant mortality and low birthweight, and the voluminous literature on risk factors, the Institute of Medicine published *Preventing Low Birthweight,* in 1985, which included recommendations for action in both the private and public sector to reduce the incidence of low birthweight.[9] A key conclusion of the authoring committee was that enough is known about low birthweight to do more than we are currently doing to prevent it and, further, that preventive efforts are likely to prove less costly, both socially and economically, than additional investment in intensive neonatal services. The committee noted that reducing poverty and improving education could probably do much to decrease low birthweight, given the strong associations among birthweight, socio-economic status and education, but even absent such basic improvements some promising steps can be taken in the interim.

The five major activities advocated by the committee were:

1. Reduce the risks associated with low birthweight before pregnancy by means of risk identification and counseling; enlarge the content of

general health education related to reproduction; expand and improve the provision of family planning services.

2. Increase the availability of early and regular high-quality prenatal care; systematically remove major barriers that women encounter in obtaining prenatal services.

3. Strengthen and expand the content of prenatal services; make them more flexible to meet individual needs; emphasize certain components of care for particular high-risk women.

4. Mount an extensive and sustained public information campaign to convey a few well-chosen messages aimed at preventing low birthweight.

5. Conduct a multifaceted research program into the causes of, and interventions to reduce, low birthweight; involve scientists from numerous disciplines, including physiologists, epidemiologists, social and behavior scientists, and health services researchers and evaluators in such a program.

The balance of this chapter comments further on goals 1, 2, and 3.

PREGNANCY INTERVENTIONS

Because many risks associated with low birthweight can be identified before conception (Table 3, categories 1, 2, and 4), numerous opportunities exist before pregnancy to reduce the incidence of the problem. Yet, these are often overlooked in favor of interventions during pregnancy. Among the risk factors that can be addressed before pregnancy are various maternal chronic illnesses, smoking, poor nutrition, alcohol use, inadequate weight for height, susceptibility to rubella and other infectious agents, very young or old age, a very short interval since the last birth, and high parity. For some of these factors, such as nutritional status, reducing the risk before conception may offer more protection against having a low birthweight infant than doing so after pregnancy has been established. Accordingly, some experts have suggested that more attention be given to health assessment of women before they become pregnant, to identification of risk factors and, where possible, to interventions for reducing them.

A major limitation of this approach is that those most in need of pre-pregnancy counseling and services—particularly, the very poor and the very young—are the least likely to be in a service system that offers such assistance. This fact lends importance to the provision of such help in many different kinds of settings.

Family planning is also a key element of pre-pregnancy interventions to reduce low birthweight. Several studies have shown that the reduction in infant mortality over the past 20 years has been due in part to more effective family planning.[16] There is also some evidence that family planning services have contributed to the more modest decline in the incidence of low birthweight, presumably by preventing pregnancies among high-risk groups, including low income women and teenagers, and by helping women to space their pregnancies at longer intervals. Evidence from the 1980 National Natality Survey supports the belief that women who plan for and welcome their pregnancies are more likely than those who do not to obtain prenatal services early in pregnancy, which, in turn, increases the chances of a successful pregnancy outcome. Accordingly, the Institute of Medicine committee argued forcefully in its report that family planning services be an integral part of overall strategies to reduce the incidence of low birthweight. Title X of the Public Health Service Act—the major source of federal funds for family planning services—should be regarded as an important part of public efforts to prevent low birthweight because it specifically aimed at low-income and adolescent women who are at especially high risk of having low birthweight babies.

ACCESS TO PRENATAL CARE

A second approach to reducing low birthweight rests on drawing more pregnant women into prenatal care. Though seemingly a straightforward proposition, it is unfortunately the fact that, in 1985, approximately one-fourth of all infants in the U.S. were born to women who failed to begin prenatal care early in pregnancy. More than five percent of women received little or no care at all. For certain groups, the rates were even worse. Of infants born to Black teenagers, only 47 percent were to teens who began care in the first trimester and 14 percent were to teens who had little or no care at all. Moreover, recent trends in the use of prenatal care are not improving for all groups. In 1985, for the sixth consecutive year, there was no progress in reducing the percentage of infants born to women who received late or no prenatal care. For Blacks, the size of this group actually appears to be increasing. In 1980, 8.8 percent of Black infants were born to mothers having had little or no prenatal care; by 1985, this number had grown to 10.3 percent.[4]

These disturbing recent trends are important challenges to public policy and to the health care system, for several reasons. First, the consensus is broad and deep that prenatal care represents an effective intervention that is strongly and clearly associated with improved pregnancy outcomes. Declines in rates of low birthweight, maternal mortality, and infant mortality have been repeatedly linked to full participation in high-quality prenatal care offering a wide variety of services and social supports, well-connected to hospital-based services, such as intrapartal and neonatal care. Moreover, the evidence suggests that prenatal care is especially important for those women at highest risk because of their social condition, their health status, or both. Because of difficulties in evaluation methodology and because randomized clinical trials are precluded on ethical grounds, incontrovertible scientific proof of the degree of prenatal care's effectiveness is not available.

Nevertheless, exhaustive reviews of the literature, and recent analyses, continue to underscore the value of this basic health service.[9]

The importance of prenatal care is also underscored by evidence of its cost-effectiveness, particularly for low-income women who obtain relatively inadequate prenatal care and who are at increased obstetrical risk. For example, in 1985, the Institute of Medicine calculated that each additional dollar spent on providing more adequate prenatal care to a cohort of low income, poorly educated women could reduce total expenditures by $3.38 for direct medical care of their low birthweight infants during the first year of life. Such savings would occur if increasing the amount of prenatal care obtained by these women decreased their rate of low birthweight from the current level of about 12 percent to the Surgeon General's 1990 goal of nine percent.[9] Other investigators have computed different cost saving ratios for prenatal care, but virtually all analyses find evidence of cost-effectiveness.[17]

As noted earlier, rates of infant mortality are notably lower in many other countries than in the U.S. It is also apparent that rates of low birthweight are better in several other European countries (Table 4), a difference due in part to the better participation in prenatal care evident in these countries. As elaborated most recently by Miller, it is apparent that many countries approach the provision of care to pregnant women as a form of social investment. In these settings, prenatal care, like health care generally, is offered with few barriers or preconditions in place. Such services are seen as part of a broad social strategy to protect and support childbearing and to produce healthy future generations.[18]

TABLE 4

LOW BIRTHWEIGHT RATE – 1982-83

Belgium	5
Denmark	6*
France	5
FRG	5
Ireland	4
Netherlands	4
Norway	4
Spain	NA
Switzerland	5
United Kingdom	7
U.S.A.	7

SOURCE: UNICEF, The State of the World's Children, 1987, Oxford Press.

* According to other sources, the rate of low birthweight for Denmark is 3% (World Health Organization, 7th Annual Report on World Health Situation, 1986, Geneva).

Our limited progress in extending prenatal care appears to be only part of the larger problem of poor access to health services for low income and minority populations, in general. In the face of an increasingly competitive, profit-oriented medical care system, this nation has failed to find adequate ways to finance health care services for the poor. Unfortunately, in 1988, socio-economic status remains a major influence on both health status and use of medical services. Moreover, there is some evidence that access to health care may be deteriorating for the nation's poor, minorities, and the uninsured. For example, Freeman, et. al. found, in 1986, that, "poor and black Americans have experienced a reversal of the gains in access to physician care made over the previous two decades."[19]

As for risk factors for low birthweight, a list of barriers to prenatal care can be developed (Table 5). Although the relative salience of each factor probably varies enormously among individual women, there is ample evidence to suggest that financial barriers (particularly absence of private insurance) and an undervaluing of prenatal care contribute substantially to poor participation in this basic health service. A number of surveys have recently been completed in which women who have obtained inadequate prenatal care are asked to characterize the obstacles to care they may have encountered. Typical of such surveys is that published by the General Accounting Office (GAO). In 1987, the GAO interviewed 1,157 women in eight states to determine the timing and number of their prenatal visits and the barriers they perceived as preventing them from obtaining care earlier or more often. Cited barriers varied according to such factors as age, race, and size of community, with about half of the women listing multiple barriers. However, three barriers predominated in virtually every demographic group of women—lack of money to pay for care, lack of transportation to the provider of care, and unawareness of pregnancy. The importance of these and other barriers differed, however, by community.[20]

In response to the poor use of prenatal care by some women, states, and communities have over the years developed numerous programs to draw more women into prenatal care early in pregnancy and to sustain their participation. At least five program types can be identified:

1. Reducing the financial obstacles to care experienced by poor women through provision of insurance or other sources of payment;

2. Reducing these same financial barriers through increasing the basic capacity of the prenatal care system used by low-income women, which includes health department clinics, hospital outpatient departments, community health centers, and similar settings;

3. Revising institutional practices to make services more genuinely available and acceptable to potential users;

4. Conducting active case-finding through a wide variety of methods, including hotlines, community canvassing via "outreach workers," or

TABLE 5

BARRIERS TO USE OF PRENATAL CARE

1. Sociol-Demographic Correlates

Poverty
Inner city or rural resident
Minority
Under 18
Higher parity
Recent immigrant (?)
Non-English speaking
Unmarried
Less than high school education
Medicaid eligible
No private health insurance

2. Prenatal Care System Barriers

Coverage limits in private health insurance policies
Poorly "advertised" Medicaid program
Complicated and demeaning process to secure Medicaid
Inadequate/absent maternity resources for low-income women and other at-risk groups (long wait for appointment; few or no providers taking uninsured or Medicaid women, etc.)
Inadequate transportation services and/or long travel time to service sites
Poor child care supports
Inadequate coordination among such services as pregnancy testing, WIC, and prenatal care services
Requirements for "up front" payments

Limited information on where precisely to get care – phone numbers and addresses
Clinic hours rarely on evenings and weekends
Long waits to see physician
Language incompatibility

Poor communication between clients and providers, exacerbated by little continuity in providers and brief interactions with providers
Negative clinic attributes, including rude clerks and other personnel, uncomfortable surroundings, complicated registration procedures, etc.

3. Barriers Based in Beliefs, Knowledge and Attitudes

Pregnancy unplanned and/or viewed negatively
Ambivalence
Prenatal care not valued or understood
Fear of doctors, hospitals and/or procedures
Fear of parental discovery
Fear of deportation
Lifestyles likely to be criticized by providers (drug abuse, smoking, eating disorders)
Inadequate social supports and personal resources
Excessive stress
Denial/apathy
Concealment

other paraprofessional personnel, cross-agency referrals, and the provision of incentives; and

5. Providing social supports to encourage continuation in prenatal care and, more generally, to increase the probability of healthy pregnancies and a smooth transition into parenthood.

At present, a study committee within the Institute of Medicine is assessing the relative value of these different strategies for drawing women into prenatal early in pregnancy and sustaining their participation.

Improving access to prenatal care will likely require action at two levels. First, the consensus seems to be growing that the nation's patchwork, non-systematic approach to providing prenatal care will continue to leave some women out.[21] The overly complicated Medicaid program; the limited capacity of local health departments, hospital outpatient departments, and other systems used by low-income women; inadequate numbers of maternity care providers for some groups of women and in some areas, due to malpractice issues and changes in obstetric practice; an often dehumanizing public health care system—these barriers in the aggregate form a maze in which even the most socially organized woman may become lost. Accordingly, it is increasingly common for various groups to call for a major overhaul of the health care system for pregnant women and young children, such that services during pregnancy and infancy become, in effect, an entitlement.

The second set of needed action is characterized by work for incremental improvements in the maternity care system. While the consensus grows that major restructuring is needed, numerous groups continue to advocate smaller changes at the margin, particularly for expansions in the Medicaid program. Whether such incrementalism will ease the major access problem in the U.S. at present is questionable, perhaps unlikely.

CONTENT OF CARE

Returning to the Institute of Medicine's list of five promising approaches, the content-of-care topic deserves emphasis, even if only briefly. While it is true that drawing more women into prenatal care is a key element in preventing low birthweight, the actual content of those prenatal visits deserves careful scrutiny. Many of the risk factors for low birthweight could be reduced by prenatal care, if it is broadly defined to include such actions as help in smoking cessation, detailed attention to nutrition, perhaps the detection of the early signs of preterm labor, prompt linkage to other needed services (AFDC, housing assistance, etc.), and counseling about various psychosocial issues. Unfortunately, it is probably true that not all women receive prenatal care that includes such enrichments. Indeed, the precise definition of prenatal care is not clear. In most contexts, the term *prenatal care* describes an inexact constellation of individual procedures and interactions between a pregnant woman and a health care provider. To some, the term suggests a minimum set of medical procedures offered by a health care provider on a well-defined schedule, while to others prenatal care means these services plus a broad array of medical, educational, social, and nutritional services provided in a flexible fashion dictated by the needs of the individual patient. Many groups have called for additional research necessary to specify the content of this form of health care and the value of each of its components for different groups of women. Clearly a final resolution of the question of what is useful within the "black box" termed prenatal care, whether defined narrowly or broadly, must await further understanding of the physiology of pregnancy, of threats to maternal and fetal health during pregnancy, and of the specific antenatal interventions needed to minimize these threats.

Progress in this direction is promised by the work of the Public Health Service's Expert Panel on the Content of Prenatal Care. Among other activities, this committee has proposed a set of outcome variables by which the effectiveness of various aspects of prenatal care can be judged. The list is particularly valuable for its breadth. It suggests that the worth of prenatal care services should not rest solely on its effect on either infant mortality or birthweight—a focus which has dominated recent discussions of prenatal care—but should instead consider a much broader array of measures, including, for example, maternal and fetal mortality, the developmental progress of preterm infants, family functioning, intendedness of future pregnancies, child abuse and neglect, and maternal stress.

COMMENT AND CONCLUSION

Infant mortality and its major underlying contributor, low birthweight, have recently attracted attention in the broader population, as evidenced by the formation of the National Commission on Infant Mortality and by numerous state and local initiatives. Interestingly, the majority of these programs have highlighted access to prenatal care as the principal means of attacking infant mortality and low birthweight. The focus on prenatal care is useful, given the evidence that prenatal care improves birth outcome. It is unfortunate, however, that some of the additional approaches to reducing low birthweight that the Institute of Medicine and other expert groups have advocated have not "caught on" as dramatically. Increased investment in family planning services and education, for example, could likely make a major contribution to improved infant well-being, as could detailed attention to the content of prenatal care, particularly for low-income women who often have multiple risk factors and who typically obtain prenatal services in clinics that are understaffed, rushed, and not financed adequately enough to provide a rich array of services. And stronger public education about reproductive health—planning for pregnancy, avoiding drugs, alcohol and tobacco while pregnant, seeking out prenatal care—could probably help considerably. Unfortunately, most public education in this field consists of brief media flurries that have no long-term follow-up, are inadequately financed, and are not packaged creatively. Finally, the research imperative in this field is pressing and exists at many levels, all the way from the need for increased research on the etiology of low birthweight to such applied research as learning how best to conduct case-finding for prenatal care in both rural and inner-city communities. Challenging though it may be, preventing low birthweight probably will require work in all of these disparate domains. There is, unfortunately, no single magic bullet, no simple solution that glows in the dark.

REFERENCES

1. McCormick MC. The Contribution of Low Birthweight to Infant Mortality and Childhood Morbidity. New England Journal of Medicine 312: 82-90, 1985.

2. U.S. Department of Health and Human Services: Promoting Health/Preventing Disease: Objectives for the Nation. U.S. Government Printing Office. Washington, D.C., 1980.

3. Office of Disease Prevention and Health Promotion, Public Health Service, Department of Health and Human Services: The 1990 Health Objectives for the Nation: A Midcourse Review. U.S. Government Printing Office, Washington, D.C., November 1986, p. 36..

4. Hughes D, Johnson K, Rosenbaum S, Simons J and Butler E: The Health of America's Children: Maternal and Child Health Data Book Children's Defense Fund, Washington, D.C., 1987.

5. National Commission to Prevent Infant Mortality. Infant Mortality: Care for Our Children, Care for Our Future. January, 1988, p. 13.

6. Brown SS. Can Low Birthweight Be Prevented: Family Planning Perspectives, 17(3):112, May/June, 1985.

7. Skeoch C, Rosenberg K, Turner T, Skeoch H, and McIlwaine G. Very Low Birthweight Survivors: Illness and Readmission to Hospital in the First 15 Months of Life, British Medical Journal 295:579-580. Sept 5, 1987.

8. U.S. Congress, Office of Technology Assessment. Neonatal Intensive Care for Low Birthweight Infants: Costs and Effectiveness (Health Technology Case Study 38), OTA-HCS-38. Washington, D.C.: U.S. Congress, Office of Technology Assessment, December, 1987, p. 5.

9. Institute of Medicine: Preventing Low Birthweight. National Academy Press, Washington, D.C., 1985.

10. Kleirman J, and Kessel S. Racial Differences in Low Birthweight: Trends and Risk Factors. New England Journal of Medicine 317:749-753, Sept 17, 1987.

11. Lieberman E, Ryan K, Monson R, Schoenbaum S. Risk Factors Accounting for Racial Differences in the Rate of Premature Birth. New England Journal of Medicine 317:743-748, Sept 17, 1987.

12. Bakketeig LS, Hoffman HJ, and Harley EE. The tendency to repeat gestational age and birthweight in successive births. Am J Obstet Gynecol 135:1086-1103, 1979.

13. Taffel SM, and Keppel KG. Implications of mother's weight gain on the outcome of pregnancy. Paper presented at the American Statistical Assoc. meeting. Philadelphia, PA, Aug 13-16, 1984.

14. Stein Z and Kline J. Smoking, Alcohol and Reproduction. <u>Am J Pub Health</u> 73:1154-1156, 1983.

15. Office on Smoking and Health: <u>The Health Consequences of Smoking for Women: A Report of the Surgeon General.</u> Public Health Service. U.S. Government Printing Office, Washington, D.C., 1980.

16. Grossman M and Jacobowitz S. Variations in Infant Mortality Rates Among Counties of the United States; The Roles of Public Policies and Programs. <u>Demography.</u> 18:695-713, 1981.

17. Corman H and Grossman M. Determinants of Neonatal Mortality Rates in the U.S.: A Reduced Form Model. <u>J. Health Econ 4(3)</u>, Sept, 1985.

18. Miller CA: <u>Maternal Health and Infant Survival</u> National Center for Clinical Infant Programs, Washington, D.C., July, 1987.

19. Freeman H, Blendon R, Aiken L, Sudman S, Mullinex C, and Corey C: Americans Report on Their Access to Health Care. <u>Health Affairs</u> p. 6, Spring 1987.

20. General Accounting Office: <u>Prenatal Care: Medicaid Recipients and Uninsured Women Obtain Insufficient Care.</u> GAO/HRD 87-137. U.S. Government Printing Office, Washington, D.C., 1987.

21. The Alan Guttmacher Institute: <u>Blessed Events and the Bottom Line: Financing Maternity Care in the United States</u>, New York, 1987.

METHODS OF FERTILITY CONTROL

22

Robert A. Hatcher, Felicia Jane Guest,
Felicia Hance Stewart, Gary K. Stewart,
James Trussell, Sylvia Cerel Bowen, and
Willard Cates, Jr.

INTRODUCTION

The focus of attention in this chapter is on several important subjects in the vast field of fertility control:

- The most important contraceptive methods used in the U.S.
- The effectiveness or lack of effectiveness of these methods
- Management issues in the delivery of contraceptive services
- Condoms and the prevention of human immunodeficiency virus infection

HEALTH BENEFITS OF FAMILY PLANNING

The ability to determine when or even whether to have children is an extraordinarily important human right that benefits not only the individual woman, who is able to control her fertility, but also others—the husband, the couple, the family, and the community. The ways in which family planning improves family health are outlined in Deborah Maine's monograph, *Family Planning: Its Impact on the Health of Women and Children*,[2] and in the following mnemonic that spells out, *Family Health*:

FOOD and other key resources are available in greater amounts for all of the family, when children are spaced and when total family size is small.

325

ANEMIA, particularly iron-deficiency anemia, is diminished in women and children.

MATERNAL MORTALITY rates fall.

INFERTILITY may be prevented by family planning programs, both by prompt treatment of pelvic inflammatory disease and by the protective effect, against pelvic inflammatory disease of condoms, foams, diaphragms with a spermicide, and oral contraceptives.

LOW BIRTHWEIGHT deliveries, a major cause of mental retardation, are less likely to occur.

YOUNG children and infants are less likely to die of infectious diseases.

HAPPIER SEXUAL RELATIONSHIPS can develop as the fear of unplanned and unwanted pregnancy diminishes.

EDUCATIONAL OPPORTUNITIES may increase for mothers, fathers, and children.

ABORTIONS performed are more often legal and safe.

LACTATION can continue for a longer period of time when babies are not born very close together; in some environments, this may provide better emotional, as well as nutritional health.

TEENAGE PREGNANCY rates are decreased.

HEALTH SCREENING TESTS, such as breast exams, blood-pressure readings, hematocrits, weights, Pap smears, and pelvic examinations, are done while providing family planning services.

COMBINED ORAL CONTRACEPTIVES

As of 1984, oral contraceptive (OCs) were being used by 55-56 million women throughout the world.[3] Pills have been used by more than 150 million women worldwide, 50 million of them in the U.S.[4] Currently, approximately ten million women in the U.S. use the pill. Use in developed nations has stabilized since 1977 at around 20 million. In developing nations other than China, the number of women using oral contraceptive pills increased from 14 to 18 million in the four-year span from 1977 through 1980.

Effectiveness

The lowest expected first-year reported failure rate is 0.1 percent. It is important to realize that pregnancies can occasionally occur even though the patient has taken all of her pills on schedule. The Royal College of General Practitioners' study reported a failure rate, over time, of 0.34 pregnancies per 100 woman-years.[5] A typical first-year failure rate is three percent. A typical first-year failure rate for users less than 22-years old is 4.7 percent.[6]

Choosing a Combined Oral Contraceptive

Today's combined oral contraceptives contain far less estrogen or progestin than the combined and sequential pills first available in 1960. For example, Ovcon-35 exposes a woman to 0.4 mg of norethindrone or 1/25th of the norethindrone, as did the early pill, Ortho Novum 10, which exposed a woman to 10 mg of the same progestin daily. Similarly, Loestrin 1/20 provides a woman with 20 mcg of ethinyl estradiol, which is one-fifth of the amount of ethinyl estradiol that was in the sequential pill, Oracon (now discontinued).

Triphasic Oral Contraceptives

Triphasil was introduced in Europe in 1979 and in the U.S. in 1985. Ortho-Novum 7/7/7 and Tri-Norinyl were introduced in 1984. Advantages of triphasic OCs include:

1. *Less progestin* than one of their already-available, low-dose, combined pills. Ortho-Novum 7/7/7 provides 15.75 mg of norethindrone per cycle, which is 25 percent less than the 21 mg of norethindrone in Ortho-Novum 1/35. Tri-Norinyl provides 15.0 mg of norethindrone, or about 29 percent less than the 21 mg in Norinyl 1/35. Modicon and Brevicon, with 0.5 mg of norethindrone, both provide less progestin than either Ortho-Novum 7/7/7 or Tri-Norinyl. Triphasil provides 1.925 mg of the more powerful progestin levonorgestrel, which is about 39 percent less than the amount of levonorgestrel in Nordette.

2. *Fewer metabolic effects* related to the progestin in their pill. Fewer effects on lipids, blood pressure, and carbohydrate metabolism.

3. *They are new and different.* In some instances, the new approach employed with these triphasic pills probably does lead to increased patient and/or physician acceptance.

CLINICAL MANAGEMENT ISSUES

Some Practical Considerations

1. AIDS, which causes several thousand deaths a year, is far more likely to kill sexually active women and men than are OCs, to which several hundred deaths appear to be attributable annually. AIDS must be kept in mind as clinicians provide OCs. Pills do not protect against the virus that causes AIDS. Women who want to use OCs but who will have several sexual partners in the course of their reproductive years should be strongly encouraged to use condoms as well as birth-control pills.

2. Women initiating OC use should be re-evaluated during the first three to six months. After a woman has used the pill for three to six months, is having no problems, and wants to continue the pill, seven packets (a

six-month supply) may be provided. *After a woman has used pills for one year (cumulative year of pill use), a full-year's supply of pills may be provided in an effort to decrease pill discontinuation rates.*

3. It is important to find out for patients where they can fill their prescriptions most inexpensively. In drug stores, the price of pills in mid-1985 ranged from $9.00 to $19.95 per cycle. In the summer of 1987, the average price paid for one cycle of OCs in six Atlanta pharmacies was $12.73. For the same OCs, a woman could pay $8.99 to $12.00 per cycle at one pharmacy while, at another, the range was from $12.99 to $20.49. In subsidized clinics, pills are sold to women for $1.00 to $11.00 per cycle.

4. Each provider must decide what medical history should be taken each time a woman returns for a pill refill. Clear and concise self-administered questions can protect the pill user from continuing to use pills when she has developed medical problems or is experiencing one of the pill danger signs.

EARLY PILL DANGER SIGNS

CAUTION

A – Abdominal pain (severe)
C – Chest pain (severe), cough, shortness of breath
H – Headache (severe), dizziness, weakness, numbness
E – Eye problems (vision loss or blurring), speech problems
S – Severe leg pain (calf or thigh)

The woman should see her clinician if she has any of these problems, or if she develops depression, yellow jaundice, or a breast lump.

5. A sample informed-consent form for pill users is presented in Figure 1.

6. Weight, blood pressure, Pap smear, and pelvic examination should be done at the time of the initial examination and at each annual exam. In women at high risk of cardiovascular disease, a lipid profile and two-hour postprandial glucose determinations should be performed prior to initiating OCs, and annually thereafter. Baseline mammography is recommended for women once between the ages of 35 and 40, and every other year in the 40s.

7. The pill danger signs should be conveyed to women *at each visit.* Women should also receive the patient package insert for the pill they are using. Some clinicians provide patients with additional instructions that explain OCs in language that is clearer than the package inserts.

FIGURE 1
ORAL CONTRACEPTIVE CONSENT FORM
Grady Memorial Hospital
Atlanta, Georgia
Revised May 1985

I hereby acknowledge that I am voluntarily receiving birth control Pills. Pills are the method of family planning which I have chosen from the methods that have been explained to me. The advantages and disadvantages of the other methods of contraception have been explained to me.

BENEFITS: I am aware that oral contraceptives are *not* guaranteed to be 100% effective. It is my understanding that combined birth control Pills can be close to 99% effective if I take them consistently and correctly. It is my understanding that progestin-only Pills (Mini-Pills) are slightly less effective even if taken consistently. I have been told that in addition to their benefits as a method of birth control, some women experience the following benefits from using birth control Pills:

- Decreased menstrual cramps
- Decreased menstrual bleeding
- More regular menstrual bleeding
- Decreased pain at the time of ovulation
- Less risk of acute gonococcal pelvic inflammatory disease
- Improvement in acne
- Less risk of developing ovarian and/or endometrial cancer
- Less risk of developing benign breast tumors and/or ovarian cysts

RISKS: I have been told to watch out for the following Pill Danger Signals and to return to the clinic or make contact with my clinician at once if I develop one of these problems. These could be warnings of serious or even life-threatening illness.

EARLY PILL DANGER SIGNS

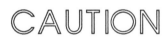

A • Abdominal pain (severe)
C • Chest pain (severe) • cough • shortness of breath
H • Headache (severe) • dizziness • weakness • numbness
E • Eye problems (vision loss or blurring) • speech problems
S • Severe leg pain (calf or thigh)

See your clinician if you have any of these problems,
or if you develop depression, yellow jaundice or a breast lump.

I am aware that while using oral contraceptives, I could experience the following side effects, many of which can be temporary:

Major Problems	*Minor Problems*
• Blood clots of the legs or the lungs	• Nausea
• Strokes or heart attacks	• Spotting between periods
• Gallbladder disease	• Less menstrual bleeding
• One type of liver tumor	• Breast tenderness
• Death	• Weight gain
	• Headache
	• Depression
	• High blood pressure
	• Darkening of the skin on my face
	• Worsening of acne
	• Infections in the vagina

I have been informed that a majority of the serious complications in Pill users occur in women over 30 who are heavy smokers (15 or more cigarettes a day).

Stopping Pills: I have been told that I may stop using the Pills *at any time.* I have been told I should use another means of birth control until I have had three regular periods before attempting to become pregnant. I have also been informed that if my periods were very irregular, very heavy, and/or very painful before taking Pills, they may return to this pattern when I stop taking birth control Pills.

Instructions for the use of birth control Pills have been given to me and I have been given a patient package insert for my specific type of Pill

Questions: I have been given the opportunity to ask questions about all forms of birth control and about the Pill in particular. My questions have been answered to my satisfaction.

8. Consider inviting patients to obtain pills by mail. A patient may be offered the opportunity to send in a stamped, self-addressed envelope and a completed pill-resupply form. If the pill-resupply form indicates a possible problem, the patient is contacted, and, depending on the problem, a clinic visit may be necessary. *Many women who really need the pills will discontinue them because they cannot get back to a public clinic to pick up new supplies.*

NONCONTRACEPTIVE BENEFITS OF PILLS

Relief of Cyclic Problems

In the Royal College of General Practitioners' study, combined oral contraceptive users frequently experienced relief of unwanted symptoms of their menstrual cycles.[7] The pill minimizes menstrual cramps, decreases the number of days of bleeding and the amount of blood loss, produces more regular menstrual periods, decreases the incidence of functional ovarian cysts, and eliminates mittelschmerz (pain at the time of ovulation). Also, iron-deficiency anemia is decreased in pill users. Other women notice that their premenstrual tension, anxiety, or depression may be diminished (or increased) while taking oral contraceptives.

Extensive evidence exists showing that the pill exerts a protective effect against pelvic inflammatory disease (PID), a major cause of female infertility worldwide.[8,9] Pill users are *less* likely to develop more severe forms of PID than nonusers of contraceptives. Why might combined birth control pills decrease a woman's risk of developing acute PID? Considerable evidence suggests that the pill protects against both ovarian and endometrial cancer.[8,10,11,12,13,14] A recent multicenter study, conducted by the Centers for Disease Control (CDC), in Atlanta, investigated the association between oral contraceptive use and a woman's risk of developing endometrial and ovarian cancer.[15,16,17] When compared with never-users, users of combined oral contraceptives were found to be at half the risk of developing endometrial and ovarian cancer.[18] In both cases, the protective effect was conferred after at least 12 months of use. The protective effect against endometrial and ovarian cancer appears to persist for a number of years after pills have been discontinued.

PROGESTIN-ONLY PILLS (MINI-PILLS)

Mini-Pills have been marketed in the U.S. since January 1973. They contain the same progestins available in combined oral contraceptives but in smaller doses. Three products are available in the United States:

- Ovrette: 0.075 mg norgestrel (28-day pack)
- Micronor: 0.35 mg norethindrone (28-day pack)
- Nor-Q.D.: 0.35 mg norethindrone (42-day pack)

Ovrette provides 25 percent of the progestin dose found in Lo/Ovral and about half the progestin dose in Triphasil. Nor-Q.D. and Micronor provide 35 percent of the progestin dose found in Norinyl 1+35 and Ortho-Novum 1/35, about half the progestin dose in Tri-Norinyl and Ortho-Novum 7/7/7, and just slightly less than the lowest norethindrone-containing combined pill, Ovcon-35 (which provides 0.4 mg of norethindrone per pill).

The absence of estrogen and the low dose of progestin are responsible for both the advantages and disadvantages of Mini-Pills, as compared with the more commonly used combined oral contraceptives. Women who experience unacceptable estrogen-related side effects with pills may be able to use Mini-Pills successfully. At least theoretically, certain significant medical risks may be lower with Mini-Pills than with combined pills. Some serious adverse effects of the pill are definitely related to estrogen, and progestin dose is also a significant determinant of risk. Research to document enhanced safety, however, is lacking.

On the other hand, low progestin dose and the absence of estrogen are associated with less predictable menstrual patterns and, for some users, unacceptable, irregular, bleeding problems. Abnormal bleeding is particularly troublesome among older women.

Reported failure rates for various kinds of Mini-Pills (including some products not available in the U.S.) range from 0.9 to 9.6 pregnancies per 100 woman-years. The range for U.S. products reported is somewhat narrower, 0.5 to 2.5. Manufacturers of Micronor and Nor-Q.D. cite a slightly higher failure rate (3.7) for first-time pill users, probably reflecting less consistent use,[19] and on this basis they caution that failure rates may be higher during the initial six months of Mini-Pill use. "Fresh" Mini-Pill users in this study, however, were compared with women who changed from combined oral contraceptives to Mini-Pills. This choice for a comparison group involves significant bias because the resumption of fertility is known to be delayed for women who discontinue combined pills; therefore, their failure rates with any subsequent method are predictably lower than rates for women who have not used pills. Investigators who conducted a British study that included similar progestin-only pills did not find that effectiveness changed with duration of Mini-Pill use.[20] Younger women (aged 25 to 29) in this study, however, experienced a slightly higher failure rate (3.1) than did older women aged 35-39 (1.0), or aged 40+ (0.3).

INTRAUTERINE DEVICES

Despite the discontinuation of production and distribution of all intrauterine devices (IUDs) in the U.S.—except for the Progestasert system and the Copper-T 380A—the IUD remains a medically sound and excellent contraceptive method for many women. When the Copper-T 380A became available in early 1988, one of the best IUDs ever distributed was available for U.S. women. In 1987, the U.S.

Agency for International Development made the decision to provide only the Copper-T 380A to nations receiving contraceptive aides.

Women wearing IUDs are at increased risk for developing the serious sequelae of sexually transmitted diseases, i.e., pelvic inflammatory disease (PID), infertility, and ectopic pregnancy. The IUD affords no protection against the virus that causes AIDS. If a woman or her partner has other sexual contacts, she should be strongly discouraged from using an IUD. Likewise, if she has a history of having had PID or an ectopic pregnancy, she should be strongly discouraged from using an IUD.

The Progestasert-T, which has been marketed since 1976, comes in separate sterile packages and has a wide inserter barrel diameter at the end nearest the non-movable plastic phalange. The inserter narrows down so that the end that must go through the internal cervical os is a good bit narrower than the distal position. The Progestasert-T must be inserted by the plunging technique. This IUD must be replaced every 12 months. Longer-acting progestin IUDs may eventually be marketed in this country.

THE DIAPHRAGM, CONTRACEPTIVE SPONGE, AND CERVICAL CAP

How Effective are These Methods?

In choosing among birth control options, the patient needs to know just how effective each method is likely to be for her. In the case of vaginal barrier/spermicide methods, this is a simple, very important question that does not have a simple answer. The range of failure rates reported for these methods is so wide that choosing one published rate would be dishonest, while quoting the whole range is of little help to the patient's decision.

Numerous factors, including the following, which will be discussed subsequently, can potentially influence the effectiveness found for any birth control method in a research study:

1. Inherent fertility of the user (couple).
2. Frequency of intercourse.
3. Ability of the user to master proper use.
4. Risk-taking attitudes and habits of the user.
5. Motivation of the user regarding pregnancy prevention.
6. Clinical and educational measures to ensure that each user learns proper use.
7. Clinical skills in providing a method or in fitting a device optimally, and in identifying those women who cannot be fit or should not rely on the method.

8. Technical attributes of the method that facilitate or interfere with proper use.

9. Inherent effectiveness of the method being studied.

For some birth control methods, factors 8 and 9, above, are so excellent that extremely low-failure rates are found in all studies, and the range of reported failure rates is narrow. Surgical sterilization, injectable progestins, and progestin implants are good examples. For other methods, such as the IUD and oral contraceptives, inherent effectiveness is high, but because other factors do play a role, a slightly wider range of failure rates in research is to be expected.

For vaginal barrier/spermicide methods, the very-wide range of documented failure rates suggests that factors 1 through 7, above, are extremely important. Understanding these factors is key in interpreting the meaning of research results and in helping patients predict (guess) how successful these methods will be.

In the past, attention has focused on the role of correct and consistent method use (factors 3, 4 and 5, above) and the clinician's role in providing excellent education. This approach carries an implied (and sometimes stated) hypothesis that any conscientious user can achieve excellent success: that the difference between low-failure rates and typical-failure rates is accounted for entirely by misuse or risk-taking. Research does not support this hypothesis. Misuse is an important factor, but it accounts for only about half the failures in most studies. Moreover, it is implausible that women (couples) in three major U.S. studies,[21,22,23] who all received excellent education and intensive follow-up, would have differed so drastically in how they used the method that misuse could account for the disparate effectiveness observed (Table 1).

The importance of factor 1, above, inherent fertility of the couple, is intuitively obvious, but probably impossible to measure because many components contribute to this factor. In a research population, the prevalence of pelvic inflammatory disease, for example, might affect results of a study. Age is also a component,

TABLE 1

DIAPHRAGM: DISPARATE FAILURE RATES IN SIMILAR STUDIES

Study	N	Pregnancies per 100 women during first 12 months of use
Lane, 1976	2,168	2.1
Edelman, 1984	721	12.5
Bernstein, 1987	572	16.7

with reduced fertility anticipated for women who are at either age-extreme in the reproductive-age range. Investigators have documented significant differences in failure rates relative to age for several contraceptive methods. [24, 25, 26] (Table 2)

To what extent these observed differences reflect inherent fertility, however, is uncertain because age is also an important determinant of factor 2, above, *frequency of intercourse*. Few researchers have reported results that were analyzed for intercourse frequency, but a multicenter study comparing diaphragm and sponge use provides some evidence of its importance (Table 3). [24]

Comparing vaginal barrier/spermicide methods with each other is also problematic. Results of independent studies cannot be directly compared because study populations differ in obviously significant ways that result in the wide range of disparate rates. The identity and relative importance of such factors is unknown, so it's not possible to make statistical adjustments to compensate for the impact of such factors. Two studies, with randomized assignment of the methods being

TABLE 2
AGE AND CONTRACEPTIVE FAILURE

Study Group	N	Pregnancy Rate
Vessey, 1982 a/, b/		
Condom use		
Women aged 25-34		6.0
Women aged 35 or more		2.9
Diaphragm use		
Women aged 25-34		5.5
Women aged 35 or more		2.8
Vessey, 1985 c/, d/		
Progestin-only Pill use		
Women aged 25-29	117 b/	3.1
Women aged 30-34	492	2.0
Women aged 35-39	996	1.0
Women aged 40 or more	1,257	0.3
McIntyre, 1986 e/		
Diaphragm use		
Women aged 25 or more	339	17.6
Women aged 26 or more	378	9.2

a/   24 months or less duration of use; all estimates based on 250 or more woman-years of use.
b/   Woman-years of use.
c/   Pearl Index; pregnancies per 100 woman-years of exposure.
d/   Life-table first-year failure rate.
e/   36 months or less duration of use.

compared, however, have been undertaken (Table 4).[21,24] What conclusions can be drawn from vaginal barrier/spermicide efficacy studies?

- A woman who is at high risk for pregnancy—has a steady, accessible partner, is in the peak reproductive age range (20 to 30 or 35), and has

TABLE 3

INTERCOURSE FREQUENCY AND CONTRACEPTIVE FAILURE

Study Group	N	Pregnancies Per 100 Women During First 12 Months of Use
(McIntyre, 1986)		
Nulliparous Diaphragm Users		
Intercourse < 4 times/week	399	9.9
Intercourse ≥ 4 times/week	161	20.7
Nulliparous Sponge Users		
Intercourse < 4 times/week	358	12.7
Intercourse ≥ 4 times/week	161	16.6
Parous Diaphragm Users		
Intercourse < 4 times/week	118	10.8
Intercourse ≥ 4 times/week	39	21.2
Parous Sponge Users		
Intercourse < 4 times/week	138	27.3
Intercourse ≥ 4 times/week	46	31.1

TABLE 4

COMPARISON OF METHODS

Study	Pregnancies Per 100 Women During First 12 Months of Use	
Bernstein, 1987	Cap Users (581 a/)	Diaphragm Users (572)
Overall	17.4	16.7
McIntyre, 1986	Sponge Users (723)	Diaphragm Users (717)
Nulliparous	13.9	12.8
Parous	28.3	13.4
Overall	17.4	12.9

a/ ( ) indicates N for study group.

intercourse frequently—four times weekly—should not expect highly effective contraceptive protection with any of these methods, unless she uses them perfectly. Even then, failure rates are likely to be at least three-five percent during the first year.

- A woman whose risk of pregnancy is low because of intermittent sexual exposure, age less than 16 or 17 or over 35 to 40, and infrequent intercourse, can reasonably expect a fairly low failure rate with conscientious use of a diaphragm or cap and, if she is nulliparous, with use of sponges as well.

- Recommending an alternative method of birth control or concomitant use of condoms, with a vaginal barrier/spermicide method, for any woman who would find pregnancy devastating, or for any woman who has already experienced a contraceptive failure, is reasonable. Alternatively, concomitant use of condoms for one week each cycle, beginning four to five days before ovulation is anticipated, may improve efficacy with less inconvenience.

- For nulliparous women, the diaphragm, cervical cap, and sponge probably all provide similar contraceptive efficacy.

- For parous women, the efficacy of the sponge is significantly lower than that of the diaphragm or cervical cap.

- Although excellent patient education and conscientious use are important for success with vaginal barrier/spermicide methods, factors such as socio-economic status and young age are not valid reasons for clinicians to discourage patients from using the diaphragm.[27] Investigators have documented low failure rates for nulliparous women and for teenagers.[17] Despite the fact that many women have significant concerns about effectiveness, vaginal barrier/spermicide methods have many advantages and may be an entirely reasonable contraceptive choice. In overall safety, these methods, backed up by abortion in case of failure, are second only to consistent use of condoms. For many women, relying on their partners to use condoms is not a realistic (feasible) option, so the fact that vaginal barrier/spermicide methods do not necessitate partner involvement in the decision or implementation may prove particularly important. For women who need contraception only intermittently, these methods are also attractive. This contraceptive choice is available for immediate protection whenever it is needed, no matter how long the interval between uses. No doubt many pregnancies have been prevented (uncounted in research) because a woman had an available vaginal barrier/spermicide product obtained months or years before.

VAGINAL CONTRACEPTIVE SPONGE

Natural sea sponges have been used since antiquity, for contraception. In 1983, the FDA approved the first vaginal contraceptive sponge for use in the U.S. This product, the Today Vaginal Contraceptive Sponge, is a small, pillow-shaped polyurethane sponge that contains 1 gram on nonoxynol-9 spermicide.

First-year failure rates reported for sponge use range from 17 to 24.5 pregnancies per 100 women who initiate use of the method. These rates, however, may not fairly represent sponge effectiveness for nulliparous women and may overestimate effectiveness for parous users. Analyzing data from the Edelman study, McIntyre found that parous sponge users were twice as likely as nulliparous users to become pregnant (failure rates of 28 versus 13).

Data on sponge continuation are limited. In the diaphragm/sponge study, continuation rates for both methods were similar. Fifty-four percent of sponge users and 57 percent of diaphragm users continued their method for 12 months or more.[9]

VAGINAL SPERMICIDES

Because of their safety and simplicity, spermicides, barrier contraceptives, and combinations of these approaches have received extensive attention.[28,29] Most spermicidal preparations consist of two components: an inert base (usually foam, cream, or jelly), which is a medium used to hold the spermicidal agent in the vagina against the cervix, and a spermicidal chemical (usually nonoxynol-9 or a second spermicide called octoxinol-9) which kills the sperm.

Vaginal spermicides are relatively ineffective at preventing accidental pregnancy, when used (or misused) by the typical woman. The first-year failure rate among typical users is about 21 percent. According to the National Survey of Family Growth (NSFG), women using vaginal spermicides experienced a failure rate of 14.9 percent in 1973, 17.5 percent in 1976, and 17.9 percent in 1982.[30] Studies suggest that using spermicides at point of conception or during pregnancy may result in a higher risk of birth defects for the infant born to the spermicide user.[22,31,32,33,34]

The majority of those who have written on this subject conclude that there is not a significant association between the use of spermicides and teratogenic effects on the fetus. However, this remains a controversial issue. The authors of *Contraceptive Technology* suggest that, during possible pregnancies, a conservative approach to spermicide use be taken until more conclusive results are reported. Other side effects include:

- Rare allergic reactions may occur in either the male or female.
- Couples having oral-genital sex may note that spermicides have a very unpleasant taste.
- Suppositories fail to melt or foam in the vagina.

FILM

The FDA has officially approved VCF, a vaginal contraceptive film made in England that is marketed over-the-counter in the U.S. It is marketed in Europe as C-film, where it has been used for the past ten years. The paper-thin, 2" x 2" films are available in packages of 12. Apotheca, Inc., the importer, suggests a retail price of $6.98. The VCF film contains 72 mg of the spermicide nonoxynol-9. It is recommended that the film should be inserted on the tip of a finger (either partner can insert the film) into the vagina no less than five minutes before intercourse; it remains effective for two hours after it has dissolved. Its small size and convenience is a clear advantage. The VCF film is probably comparable in effectiveness to other over-the-counter spermicidal contraceptives.

THE CONDOM

In 1986, New York City's health commissioner declared, to ringing applause: "The day of the condom has returned."[35]

With the exception of coitus interruptus, condoms are the only easily-reversible method of birth control for men. Today, condoms are the second most-widely used reversible contraceptive in the U.S. after the pill. Contrary to lingering myths, condoms are a safe and effective method of birth control.

Condoms are rubber or processed collagenous tissue ("skin") sheaths that fit over the erect penis and act as a barrier to the transmission of semen into the vagina. About one percent of condoms are made of skin from the intestinal caecum of lambs.

In late 1982, the first spermicidal condom became available in the U.S. Ramses Extra has 0.5 grams of the spermicide nonoxynol-9 on the inner and the outer surfaces of the condom. Sperm ejaculated into spermicidal condoms are quickly inactivated. In one study, the percentage of motile sperm in spermicidal condoms was 10.3 percent at 30 seconds, 4.3 percent at 60 seconds, and 1.5 percent at 120 seconds after ejaculation. In regular condoms, the percentage of motile sperm was 55.9 percent at 30 seconds, 52.3 percent at 60 seconds, and 50.2 percent at 120 seconds.[36] Clearly, the spermicidal condom is highly effective at killing sperm within the condom. The effectiveness of the spermicides on the outside of the condom, should the condom break, has not been evaluated. The spermicidal condom has become very popular in the United Kingdom over the past several years.

In a 1987 Population Reports review,[37] Gallen suggests that, worldwide, at least one-third of couples (138.8 million) use a method that requires active male participation: condoms (46 million), vasectomy (41 million), periodic abstinence (17 million), or withdrawal (35 million). Although married U.S. men are second to those in the United Kingdom in their use of vasectomy as a contraceptive at ten percent of all married couples, condoms are used less extensively in the U.S. than in a number of other nations. Gallen reports that condoms are used by 43 percent of married couples in their reproductive years in Japan and by 32 percent in Finland, 25 percent in Denmark, 17 percent in the United Kingdom, ten percent in the U.S. and by 15 percent of married couples in developed countries as a whole. However, condoms are used by only three percent of married couples in developing countries as a whole, by one percent in Guatemala, Egypt, Mexico, and China and by virtually zero percent of married couples in Benin, Cameroon, Kenya, Nepal, Sudan, and Zaire.

In one study of the heterosexual transmission of the virus that causes AIDS, 79 percent of couples using condoms experienced condom breakage at least once in the 18-month study period. Another eight percent experienced leakage at least once. The heterosexual partners of HIV-positive individuals were least likely to seroconvert if abstinence was employed (zero percent or zero of 12). Of the 18 couples using condoms consistently, three (17 percent) seroconverted to become HIV-positive over 18 months. If condoms were not used, or used erratically, as was the case in 17 couples, where one person was infected with HIV, then 82 percent (14 of 17) became HIV-positive during the study period. Consistent condom use thus helped decrease, from 82 percent to 17 percent, but did not eliminate the risk of HIV transmission.[38]

In an attempt to determine the risk of condom breakage in another group of individuals, attendees at reproductive health and family planning conferences were asked several questions about their prior condom use, condom breakage, and pregnancies specifically attributed by the respondent to a condom that broke. During the first half of 1987, a total of 320 individuals were asked if they had ever in their lifetime used condoms. The 282 (88.1 percent) who had used condoms experienced breakage of the condom 244 times. The overall risk of condom breakage was one broken condom per 161 acts of intercourse. In the three states where respondents were asked if the condom break had led to an unplanned pregnancy, there were nine pregnancies that were directly attributed to condom breakage, or one pregnancy per 4,005 acts of intercourse protected by condoms. Condom breakage did not always lead to pregnancy; one pregnancy resulted for every 26 times a condom broke.[39] (Table 5)

If couples have intercourse 100 times a year on the average (two times a week) and the anticipated rate of condom breakage is one broken condom per 161 acts of intercourse, this survey suggests that just under two-thirds of couples using condoms for one year might anticipate a condom breakage to occur.

NATURAL MEMBRANE CONDOMS VERSUS LATEX CONDOMS

Natural membrane condoms, often called "skin" condoms or "naturalskin" condoms, are actually made from the caecum of lamb intestine. Most are produced in Australia. The hepatitis B virus (HBV), which is approximately 42nm (nanometers) in diameter, has been demonstrated to pass through natural membrane condoms.[40] The same investigator found that larger viruses, such as the retrovirus causing AIDS (HIV) (100-150nm), cytomegalovirus (CMV) (150-200nm), and herpes simplex virus (HSV) (150-200nm) did not pass through natural membrane condoms.[40] At a conference convened in early 1987 to discuss the use of condoms in the prevention of sexually transmitted diseases, a number of participants expressed the opinion that they could "see no reason why anyone would recommend natural skin condoms for the prevention of disease."

At Grady Memorial Hospital in Atlanta, Georgia, condoms were offered to 165 women during the summer of 1986. Women were encouraged to pass these condoms on to family and friends as well as use these condoms themselves; 73.3 percent of women took up to 50 condoms (an average of 27 per person). Within two weeks, when they were contacted by phone, they had given condoms to boyfriends, to be given to someone else (8.4 percent); to male friends (9.9 percent); to female friends (13.0 percent); to brothers (15.8 percent); to sisters (4.8 percent); or to other individuals (18.0 percent). Another 30.2 percent of condoms had not been distrib-

TABLE 5

CONDOM BREAKAGE AND UNPLANNED PREGNANCIES
EXPERIENCED BY 282 INDIVIDUALS* FOLLOWING USAGE
OF CONDOMS AT THE TIME OF 39,383 ACTS
OF SEXUAL INTERCOURSE, FOUR U.S. CITIES, 1987

	#Individuals		Total Times Condoms Utilized	# Times Condom Broke	# Pregnancies** Experienced Attributed To a Condom Break	Condom Breaks Acts of Intercourse
	Ever Used Condoms	Never Used Condoms				
Ohio	37	8	9,063	19	0	1:477
South Dakota	25	6	3,336	13	unk	1:257
Pennsylvania	134	8	15,453	140	6	1:115
Minnesota	86	6	11,531	72	3	1:160
TOTAL	282 (88.1%)	38 (11.9%) never used a condom	39,383	244	9	1:161

* Individuals working in family planning, reproductive health, gynecology, and obstetrics surveyed in the first half of 1987; information collected at family planning conferences.

** In 3 of the locations, women were asked how many pregnancies they had experienced which were attributed to a broken condom. Women using condoms 36,047 times experienced 231 condom breaks of which 9 led to pregnancy or approximately 1 pregnancy for each 4,005 acts of sexual intercourse protected by condoms and 1 pregnancy for each 26 condom breakages.

uted and were available for future distribution or for future use. A 1987 project, called CONDOM SENSE, at this hospital family planning program, provided 500,000 condoms to women and men in the clinic for redistribution in their communities. The number of individuals served by the condom distribution program and the number of woman-years of birth control provided, at a cost just under ten percent of the program's current operating budget, approximately doubles the total service provided by this large program.

MARCH, or Men Acting Responsibly for Contraception and Health, is a remarkable public awareness/service program in Philadelphia, Pennsylvania. The centerpiece of MARCH is a series of citywide posters. One poster used extensively in the public transportation system is a transit card that lists "5 Good Reasons to Use a Condom: Herpes, Gonorrhea, Syphilis, Chlamydia and 'Honey, I'm pregnant!" This poster may be adapted to local use, and AIDS may be added to the list.

CHARTING MENSTRUAL CYCLES
AND FERTILITY AWARENESS METHODS

Some patients who use charting skills for birth control choose to abstain from all sexual activity on fertile days; others engage in non-coital sexual activities; still others use a diaphragm, condom, or other form of birth control. *Each patient should be offered a full range of options so that the patient and partner can make the best decision for themselves.*

Charting is only moderately effective for preventing pregnancy when couples have unprotected intercourse both before and after ovulation; it can be quite a bit more effective when unprotected intercourse is limited to postovulatory days only. Among typical users, approximately 20 percent fail during the first year of use. A sizable but unknown portion of the failures is attributable to improper use of the method. Experts at the World Health Organization suspect that sexual risk-taking during fertile days accounts for more accidental pregnancy than does inability to interpret chart records accurately.[41]

POSTCOITAL CONTRACEPTION

As long as condoms break, inclination and opportunity unexpectedly converge, men rape women, diaphragms and cervical caps are dislodged, people are so ambivalent about sex that they need to feel "swept away," IUDs are expelled, and pills are lost or forgotten, we will need morning-after birth control. Our birth-control technology is imperfect, and human behavior is imperfect. Family planners who don't offer postcoital contraception shortchange their patients. In 1981, the International Planned Parenthood Federation addressed this issue, endorsing the use of postcoital contraceptives: "There is still no ideal contraceptive to fit every circumstance. For women exposed to a single unexpected and unprotected act of sexual intercourse, postcoital contraception can be used to avoid an unwanted pregnancy.[42]

Several studies have indicated that postcoital pills that contain 50 mcg of ethinyl estradiol and .5 mg of dl-norgestrel (marketed in the U.S.as Ovral) compare favorably with another older morning-after regimen, diethylstilbestrol (DES). The Ovral regimen has a low failure rate similar to the DES regimen but causes fewer adverse side effects. When used as morning-after pills, two Ovral tablets are taken within 72 hours (preferably within 12-24 hours) of coitus, and two more tablets are taken 12 hours later. The total dosage is therefore 2.0 mg of norgestrel and 200 mg of ethinyl estradiol. In multicenter clinical trials in Canada, Yuzpe tested this approach on 1,300 women. The failure rate in the first trial was 0.16 percent[43] and in the second was 1.6 percent.[44,45] The second figure appears to be more accurate, since similar results have been reported by others. Shilling reported no failures after treating 115 university students with the regimen, in California.[46]

ABORTION

Before 1970, legal abortion was generally unavailable in the U.S. Beginning in that year, several large states on the east and west coasts passed legislation that allowed abortion under many circumstances. During the next three years, New York and California accounted for the bulk of the legal abortions performed domestically.

The decision-making process regarding abortion begins when the patient first suspects she is pregnant. Women need to be aware of both the timing of their menstrual cycle and also the symptoms of pregnancy. Any delay in confirming pregnancy increases the risks whether a woman chooses to terminate her pregnancy or to continue it.

RU 486 and prostaglandins, for use in early pregnancy are being researched but, despite success overseas, none appears near the marketing stage in the U.S.[47] RU486 is a progesterone antagonist that has been investigated both as an early abortifacient and as a mid-cycle contraceptive.[48,49] When administered orally within ten days of the expected onset of the missed menstrual period, RU 486 produced a complete abortion in 85 percent of women. Prolonged uterine bleeding occurred in nearly one in five women with a successful abortion, but neither blood transfusions nor curettage was required.

STERILIZATION

With the removal of many legal and cultural barriers, and the development of acceptable, low-risk sterilization techniques for men and women, permanent contraception has become increasingly important in family planning in the U.S. For the past decade and a half, an estimated 1,150,000 sterilization procedures have been performed annually in the U.S. (Figure 2) By 1982, sterilization had become the most prevalent method of contraception among married women in the U.S.[50] The total number of sterilized adults in the U.S., in 1983, was estimated to be more than 16.5 million,[51] whereas the worldwide estimate of people who have undergone sterilizations is about 100 million.

In no other phase of family planning is it more important that the patient's decision be based on clear, complete information than when the patient is considering sterilization. Candidates must be told repeatedly that, at present, our sterilization procedures for both men and women are to be considered irreversible. Couples wishing to maintain the option of having children in the future should be

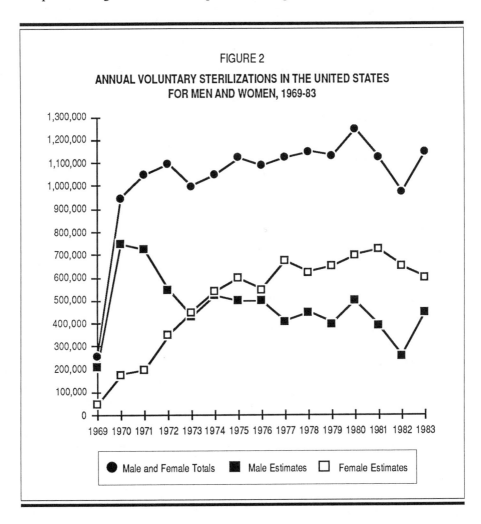

FIGURE 2

ANNUAL VOLUNTARY STERILIZATIONS IN THE UNITED STATES
FOR MEN AND WOMEN, 1969-83

encouraged to use other approaches to birth control. Significant numbers of sterilization procedures are performed on women under the age of 25. Informed consent is particularly important in these younger women and men.

Our modern methods of birth control provide couples with extensive options. If provided thoughtfully and used correctly and consistently, they can effectively minimize unplanned and unwanted pregnancies.

REFERENCES

1. Hatcher RA, Guest F, Stewart F, Stewart GK, Toussell J, Bowen SC, Cates W. Contraceptive Technology 1988-1989. Atlanta, Georgia, Printed Matter Inc and Irvington Publishers, New York.

2. Maine D: Family planning: its impact on the health of women and children (monograph). New York, The Center for Population and Family Health, College of Physicians and Surgeons, Columbia University, 1981.

3. Liskin L, Rutledge AH. After Contraception. Popul Rep J(28):697-731,1984.

4. American College of Obstetricians and Gynecologists: Oral contraceptives. ACOG Technical Bulletin No. 106, July, 1987.

5. Royal College of General Practitioners: Oral contraceptives and health: report of Royal College of General Practitioners. New York, Pitman Publishing Corporation, 1974.

6. Ory HW, Forrest JD, Lincoln R. Making choices: evaluating the health risks and benefits of birth control methods. New York, The Alan Guttmacher Institute, 1983.

7. Gallup Organization Inc: Attitudes toward contraception. Princeton, NJ, March 1985:4.

8. Ory HW. The noncontraceptive health benefits from oral contraceptive use. Fam Plann Perspect 14:182-184, 1982.

9. Senanayake PL, Kramer D. Contraception and the etiology of pelvic inflammatory disease: new perspectives. Am J Obstet Gynecol 138(7)852, 1980.

10. Casagrande JT, Pike MC, Ross RK, Louie EW, Roy S, Hendersen BE. Incessant ovulation and ovarian cancer. Lancet 2:170, 1979.

11. Kaufman DW, Shapiro S, Slone D, et al. Decreased risk of endometrial cancer among oral contraceptive users. N Engl J Med 303:1045, 1980.

12. Kowal D. OCs do not raise breast, endometrium ovary cancer risks. Contraceptive Technol Update 3:69, 1982.

13. Rosenberg L, Shapiro S, Slone D, et al. Epithelial ovarian cancer and combination oral contraceptives. JAMA 247:3210-3212, 1982.

14. Weiss NS, Sayvetz TA. Incidence of endometrial cancer in relation to the use of oral contraceptives. N Engl J Med 302:551, 1980.

15. Centers for Disease Control, Center for Health Promotion and Education, Division of Reproductive Health: Oral contraceptive use and the risk of endometrial cancer. JAMA 249:1600-1604, 1983.

16. Centers for Disease Control, Center for Health Promotion and Education, Division of Reproductive Health: Oral contraceptive use and the risk of ovarian cancer. JAMA 249:1596-1599, 1983.

17. Dicker RC, Webster LA, Layde PM, Wingo PA, Ory HW. Oral contraceptive use and the risk of ovarian cancer. Presentation at EIS Conference, 1982. DHHS, Centers for Disease Control, Atlanta, Georgia.

18. Rubin GK, Peterson HB. Oral contraceptive use and cancer. Contraceptive Technol Update January, 1985.

19. Physicians' desk reference. 41st edition. Oradell, New Jersey, Medical Economics Co, 1987.

20. Vessey MP, Lawless M, Yeates D, McPherson K. Progestin-only oral contraception: findings in a large prospective study with special reference to effectiveness. Br J Fam Plann 10:117-121, 1985.

21. Bernstein GS. Personal communication. July, 1987.

22. Edelman DA, McIntyre SL, Harper J. A comparative trial of the Today contraceptive sponge and diaphragm. Am J Obstet Gynecol 150:869-876, 1984.

23. Lane M, Arceo R, Sobrero AK. Successful use of the diaphragm and jelly by a young population: report of a clinical study. Fam Plann Perspect 8:81-86, 1976.

24. McIntyre SL, Higgins JE. Parity and use-effectiveness with the contraceptive sponge. Am J Obstet Gynecol 155:796-801, 1986.

25. Vessey M, Wiggins P. Use-effectiveness of the diaphragm in a selected family planning clinic population in the United Kingdom. Contraception 9:15-21, 1974.

26. Vessey MP, Lawless M, Yeates D. Efficacy of different contraceptive methods. Lancet 1:841-842, 1982.

27. Oliva G, Cobbie J. A reappraisal of the use and effectiveness of the diaphragm: an appropriate modern contraceptive. Adv Plann Parenthood 14:27-32, 1979.

28. Anonymous: Vaginal spermicides. The Medical Letter 5:13-16, 1986.

29. Fihn SD, Latham RH, Roberts P, et al. Association between diaphragm use and urinary tract infection. JAMA 254:240-245, 1985.

30. Grady WR, Hayward MD, Yagi J. Contraceptive failure in the United States: estimates from the 1982 National Survey of Growth. Fam Plann Perspec 18:200-209, 1986.

31. Austin H, Louv WC, Alexander J. A case-control study of spermicides and gonorrhea. JAMA 251:282-284, 1984.

32. Bernstein GS, Kilzer LH, Coulson AH, et al. Studies of cervical caps: I. vaginal lesions associated with use of the Vimule cap. Contraception 5:443-446, 1983.

33. Bracken MB. Spermicidal contraceptives and poor reproductive outcomes: The epidemiologic evidence against an association. Am J Obstet Gynecol 151:552-556, 1985.

34. Faich G, Pearson K, Fleming D, et al. Toxic shock syndrome and the vaginal contraceptive sponge. JAMA 255:216-218, 1986.

35. Leinster C. The rubber barons. Fortune, November 10-118, 1986.

36. Dale E. A laboratory investigation of the anti-spermatozoal action of condoms treated with a spermicidal preparation. 1982 paper available through Schmid Products Company.

37. Gallen ME, Liskin L, Kak N. Men—new focus in family planning. Popul Rep J(33), 1987.

38. Fischl M. Heterosexual AIDS transmission. Proceedings of conference: condoms in prevention of sexually transmitted diseases, Atlanta, Georgia, February 20, 1987.

39. Hatcher RA. Condom breakage. In press, 1987.

40. Minuk G. Passage of viral particles through natural membrane condoms. Proceedings of conference: condoms in prevention of sexually transmitted diseases, Atlanta, Georgia, February 20, 1987.

41. World Health Organization. Special programme of research, development and research training in human reproduction: seventh annual report. Geneva: World Health Organization, November, 1978.

42. Johnson JH. Contraception—the morning after. Perspectives Nov/Dec 16:226-27, 1984.

43. Yuzpe AA, Lancee WJ:. Ethinyl estradiol and dl norgestrel as a post-coital contracepton. Fertil Steril 9:932-936, 1977.

44. Yuzpe AA. Post-coital contraception. Int J Gynaecol Obstet 16:497-501, 1979.

45. Yuzpe A, Smith P, Rademaker A. A multi-center clinical investigation employing ethinyl estradiol combined with DL norgestrel as a postcoital contraceptive agent. Fertil Steril 37 508-513, 1982.

46. Schilling LH. An alternative to the use of high-dose estrogens for post-coital contraception. JACHA 247-249, 1979.

47. Population Information Program. Prostaglandins. Popul Rep 1976:G(7).

48. Couzinet B, LeStrat N, Ulmann A, Boulieu EE, Schaison G. Termination of early pregnancy by the progesterone antagonist RU 486 (Mifepristone). N Engl J Med 315:1665-1670, 1986.

49. Nieman L, Choate TM, Chrousos GP. The progesterone antagonist RU 486: a potential new contraceptive agent. N Engl J Med 316:187-191, 1987.

50. Bachrach CA, Mosher WD. Use of contraception in the United States, 1982 NCHS Advance data. National Center for Health Statistics No. 102, Dec. 4, 1984.

51. Association for Voluntary Surgical Contraception: Vasectomy deaths in the United States. Personal communication, July 1987.

SEXUALLY TRANSMITTED DISEASES

23

David A. Grimes

INTRODUCTION

In the U.S., women and their children bear the brunt of sexually transmitted disease (STD), other than the acquired immunodeficiency syndrome (AIDS). For too many years, the prototype "STD patient" has been a young single male with urethral discharge. This focus is misleading. Aside from AIDS, most deaths and serious morbidity related to STDs occur in women and children.

This chapter will briefly outline the scope of STDs as an MCH problem, estimate the medical and economic consequences of several key infections, emphasize the role of primary prevention, and review educational efforts concerning STDs.

SCOPE OF THE PROBLEM

The most serious and deadly consequences of STDs disproportionately affect women and infants. Each year, pelvic inflammatory disease (PID) kills over 150 women in the U.S.[1], contributes to at least 30,000 ectopic pregnancies (and hence 30,000 fetal deaths), and involuntarily sterilizes 100,000 to 500,000 women. PID remains the single most-frequent cause of death from STDs, far surpassing deaths from syphilis; and PID persists as the single most-frequent preventable cause of infertility in the U.S. In 1984, over 1.7 million visits to private physicians were made for infertility services.[2] In addition, STDs and their sequelae cause adverse pregnancy outcomes (such as prematurity, infant pneumonia and conjunctivitis, mental retardation, and neoplasia).

The victims of STDs tend to be young; most of the estimated 14 million cases each year in the U.S. (Table 1) occur among adolescents and young adults. Sixty-five percent of these infections occur among persons younger than 25 years of age, and 2.5 million of these are teenagers. [2] STDs and unplanned pregnancy are the twin scourges of adolescent sexual activity.

STDs have also been linked with cancer. Among these cancers are carcinomas of the anus, cervix, vulva, penis, and liver. Both epidemiologic and virologic evidence points to these cancers as sexually transmitted. Human papilloma virus types 16, 18, 31, 33, and 35 are linked with cancers of the male and female genital tract, [3] and hepatitis B virus with cancer of the liver. In the U.S. alone, nearly 7,000 women die each year of cervical cancer.[1]

GONORRHEA

Gonorrhea remains the most-frequently reported communicable disease in the U.S. In FY 1986, 392,984 cases (321 per 100,000 women) were reported among women, a 1.3 percent increase over 1985. [2] Rates of gonorrhea in the U.S. peaked in the mid-1970s and have generally been declining since then.

In FY 1986, grant funds were directed toward targeted screening programs for gonorrhea in women. These federally supported programs obtained cultures from 7.4 million women, of whom 4.1 percent were found to be infected. Of those

---

TABLE 1

**ESTIMATED ANNUAL NUMBERS OF CASES OF SELECTED
SEXUALLY TRANSMITTED DISEASES, UNITED STATES**

DISEASE	ESTIMATED NUMBERS (Millions)
Chlamydial infection	4
Trichomoniasis	3
Gonorrhea	1.8
Urethritis (non-gonococcal, non-chlamydial)	1.2
Mucopurulent cervicitis (non-gonococcal, non-chlamydial)	1.0
Human papillomavirus infection	1.0
Herpes simplex virus infection	0.2 - 0.5
Hepatitis B	0.2
Syphilis	0.09

SOURCE: Reference 2

infected, 95 percent were found and treated. On a nationwide basis, gonorrhea control programs are estimated to have prevented over 160,000 new cases in that year.

CHLAMYDIA TRACHOMATIS

Chlamydia trachomatis is the most frequent bacterial STD pathogen in the U.S. Since these infections are not reportable, the incidence can only be estimated (about 4 million cases per year)[.2] *C. trachomatis* is an important cause of mucopurulent cervicitis, which can lead to PID in non-pregnant women and to maternal and neonatal infections associated with pregnancy. Approximately seven to 12 percent of pregnant women in the U.S. are infected with *C. trachomatis*, with the rates being highest among unwed teenagers in urban areas. An estimated 40 percent of PID in the U.S. is caused by *C. trachomatis*.

Vertical transmission of *C. trachomatis* has a number of adverse consequences for infants. Each year, about 155,000 newborns are exposed to *C. trachomatis* during birth. Inclusion conjunctivitis and pneumonia are caused by *C. trachomatis*, and exposed infants have a slightly increased risk of otitis media and bronchiolitis.

SYPHILIS

Syphilis remains the third most common reportable disease in the U.S. In FY year 1986, 26,678 cases of primary and secondary syphilis were reported among both sexes, a decrease of 2.0 percent from 1985. The rate of primary and secondary syphilis among women increased by 4.6 percent, from 6.6 per 10,000 in 1985 to 6.9 in 1986. Since 1969, the number of cases of primary and secondary syphilis in women have fluctuated between 6,000 and 9,000 per year. However, in the first months of 1987, a number of states reported a dramatic increase in cases of syphilis among heterosexuals, which raises concerns about the adverse impact on rates of congenital syphilis. [4]

Recent trends in congenital syphilis are even more worrisome. Since 1983, the number of such cases has increased each year, from 210 in FY 1983 to 391 in 1986. [2] Most of these cases came from four states: California, Florida, New York, and Texas. A number of explanations account for the recrudescence of this old problem. Nearly half of the mothers involved received no prenatal care. Among those who did receive prenatal care, about two-thirds did not have their syphilis diagnosed because of clinical errors. The other one-third received a recommended antibiotic which failed to prevent fetal disease. Over half of these treatment failures occurred in the third trimester of pregnancy. Nearly a quarter of these treatment failures were related to use of erythromycin or other alternative antibiotics in women who reported an allergy to penicillin. [2,5]

HUMAN PAPILLOMA VIRUS INFECTIONS

Human papilloma virus (HPV) may be the most common viral STD in the U.S. Since genital warts are not a reportable condition, the incidence can only be estimated, as is the case with *C. trachomatis* infections. However, about five percent of all STD clinic visits are for warts, and the number of office visits to physicians because of genital warts increased over 500 percent, from 180,000 cases in 1966 to 1,148,600 in 1984. [2]

An alternative means of estimating the prevalence of HPV infection in women is the Pap smear. Authorities now believe that about 90 percent of what has been termed "dysplasia" of the cervix is due to HPV infection. About two percent of all smears taken are suggestive of HPV infection. In several investigations, the prevalence of HPV infection has ranged from five to ten percent of women seen in family planning or student health clinics, and 25 to 30 percent of women in STD clinics. [6]

Genital HPV infections are highly contagious, stubborn to treat, and often recurrent. Part of the last problem stems from poor evaluation and treatment of male sex partners, the majority of whom have obvious or subclinical penile infections. Infants can acquire HPV infection during birth, and laryngeal papillomatosis is an uncommon but potentially serious sequelae.

HERPES SIMPLEX VIRUS

Genital herpes simplex virus (HSV) infection is another extremely common, yet unreportable, viral STD. An estimated 200,000 to 500,000 cases occur annually, and, since infection is life-long, as many as 40 million persons may harbor the virus in the U.S. Office consultations for genital herpes increased 14-fold, from 31,000 in 1966 to nearly 451,000 in 1984.

The neonatal consequences of vertical transmission can be severe. As many as three of every 10,000 newborns are infected during birth.[2] Without treatment, half of these will die, and half of the survivors will suffer from serious neurologic handicaps. Vital statistics data indicate that the number of neonatal deaths due to herpes infection nearly quadrupled between 1968 and 1978.[6] Control efforts are hampered by the fact that most genital HSV infections are transmitted by persons unaware that they are infected and by the lack of a rapid and accurate test for infection.

OTHER STDs

Other STDs, less well-documented, carry substantial risks for women and children. Two genital mycoplasmas (*Ureaplasma urealyticum* and *Mycoplasma hominis*) have been linked with low birth weight and postpartum fever, respectively. Over a million office visits each year are related to *Trichomonas vaginalis* vaginitis. Hepatitis B virus (HBV) is now recognized as an important STD pathogen among heterosexual women. [7] Congenital cytomegalovirus infection is thought to occur in about 55,000 babies per year, or about 1.5 percent of all births. Of these, about 8,200 will be retarded, deaf, or visually impaired. Each year, group B streptococcus probably causes clinical illness in 12,000 infants younger than three months and nearly 5,000 infant deaths. Chancroid, caused by Haemophilus ducreyi, is appearing in community outbreaks on both coasts of the U.S. [2]

PRIMARY PREVENTION

Preventive medicine has three tiers. Primary prevention avoids the occurrence of illness. Secondary prevention minimizes morbidity once illness is present. Tertiary prevention reduces late sequelae of disease. For decades, the thrust of STD control in the U.S. has been at the secondary level. With the advent of a range of viral STDs, primary prevention has assumed greater importance.

Use of barrier contraceptives provides powerful (but not complete) protection against STDs. In clinical studies, condoms have been found to protect against gonorrhea, non-gonococcal urethritis, urethral mycoplasma infection, and PID. Use of a diaphragm with spermicide reduces the risk of gonorrhea and PID, and two studies have indicated protection against cervical neoplasia, as well. [8] Spermicides kill or inactivate sperm and a number of STD pathogens, as well. Clinical studies have shown protection against gonorrhea, chlamydial cervicitis, and PID. [8]

Development of vaccines against STD organisms has been slow and frustrating. Only one STD (hepatitis B) is preventable by vaccination at present, and immunization should be encouraged for persons at risk, such as those with multiple sex partners. Although hepatitis B vaccine is safe and effective, it is expensive and requires three injections over a six-month period.

Practical advice for preventing infection with an STD includes the following: [8]

1. Limit the number of sexual partners.
2. Avoid sexual encounters with anonymous persons or those with multiple sex partners.
3. Avoid sexual contact with infected persons or those undergoing treatment for STD.
4. Inspect the genitals of potential sex partners for lesions or discharge; ask them if they have STD.
5. Use barriers and spermicides as disease prophylactics, regardless of the need for contraception.
6. While infected with an STD, refrain from sexual activity until treatment has been completed and symptoms have subsided.

GOVERNMENT RESPONSIBILITIES IN STD CONTROL

Three levels of government cooperate in a coordinated effort to control STDs. At the federal level, the Centers for Disease Control [2] is charged with responsibility for developing and implementing nationwide control strategies. The agency also conducts epidemiologic studies of STDs, ranging from outbreak investigations to studies of the association between HPV and genital cancers. The National Institutes of Health funds both basic research and applied clinical studies.

States have primary responsibility for the control of communicable diseases, and these include the STDs. States are also the focus for disease reporting and evlauation of control programs. The federal government funds STD control activities in states and some large cities through program project grants; these numbered 63 in 1987. [6]

Local health departments have the responsibility for providing direct patient care, counseling, and partner-contact tracing. Using epidemiologic indices, the three levels of government work together to orchestrate the national control effort.

COSTS AND BENEFITS

Expenditure of money for STD prevention and control is money well-spent. As has been shown for both syphilis and gonorrhea, expenditures are inversely related to rates of disease. [2] The disheartening news, however, is that funding of STD control programs has not kept pace with the expanding array of STDs and the challenge they pose. After taking into account the effect of inflation, the peak year for federal funding of STD control was 1947. In that year the equivalent of over 127 million dollars was spent on control of syphilis alone. By 1986, this figure had declined to 45 million dollars, which was spread across the broad spectrum of STDs, including AIDS. [6] Over half of these grant operations monies (27 million dollars) were designated for gonorrhea control, followed by syphilis (eight million dollars), and chlamydia (six million dollars). [2]

The yield on these investments is large. Control of gonorrhea provides a good example. In 1986, prevention of uncomplicated gonorrhea saved at least 28.7 million dollars, and prevention of PID and its sequelae another 53.1 million dollars. Thus, for these crude estimates related to only one disease, nearly 82 million dollars in federal funds were saved, yielding a 3:1 return on the investment. [2]

Traditional STD educational methods, often sober depictions of the ravages of gonorrhea and syphilis, have been largely abandoned. These strategies, which carried pejorative messages, not only were largely ineffective but also may have had a paradoxical effect. They may have delayed seeking care among infected persons because of the stigma associated with "venereal disease."

More enlightened approaches seem to be working better. These emphasize the benefits of primary prevention and responsible decision-making about sexual behavior. Messages stressing discrimination in the choice of sex partners and practices rather than total abstinence (an unacceptable notion for many) may be helpful. For example, among unmarried persons who perceive themselves at risk of contracting genital herpes in the U.S., over half report having changed their sexual behavior to reduce their risk. [9] Among hepatitis B carriers who had been advised of the potential for sexual transmission, the number of reported sex partners decreased after receiving this counseling. [8] The changes in rates of syphilis and gonorrhea observed in recent years among gay men in the U.S. stem largely from behavioral changes prompted by fear of AIDS.

Health education strategies extend beyond primary prevention. By encouraging prompt treatment, compliance with therapy, and follow-up evaluation, counseling can minimize the morbidity caused by STDs. For example, use of videotapes to promote these behaviors has been encouraging, in early experience. [10] These teaching aids can complement the verbal instructions given during counseling of STD patients.

STD education in public schools has been deficient for many years—both in scope and thrust. For decades, school-based teaching had a myopic preoccupation with gonorrhea and syphilis. Generations of Americans have grown up with knowledge of only two STDs. Moreover, when STD material has been delivered in health science rather than sex-education texts, the thrust has not been toward prevention. [11] To remedy this, pilot materials for teachers and students in grades six through 12, based on a self-instructional format and with an emphasis on primary prevention, have been developed.

Telecommunications play an important role as well. Public awareness of both AIDS and genital herpes is due primarily to the news media. Indeed, a 1982 survey found that two-thirds of Americans had heard of herpes only since 1980. [9] Public awareness clearly lags behind public infection. Since teenagers spend an average of 23 hours per week listening to radio or watching television, they comprise a critical target population for STD prevention messages. [6] At present, network television portrays a distorted and dangerous view of sexuality: desirable men and women hop from bed to bed without consequence. Realistic portrayals of sexual activity, public service announcements about STD, and advertisements for condoms have, until recently, been shunned as being "offensive."

Telephone "hot lines" are an important source of information and referrals for treatment. In the U.S., hot lines exist for both AIDS and general STD information and referrals. In 1986, more than 60,000 calls were placed to the STD hot line, and half of these callers received referrals to health care providers. [6] These hot lines are a unique national resource.

PROFESSIONAL EDUCATION

The training of health care providers in the diagnosis and treatment of STDs has not kept pace with the growing problem. To address this deficiency, the U.S. Public Health Service has used four approaches. [12] The first was the establishment of ten STD Prevention/Training Centers in prominent institutions across the country. These Centers provide intensive training and clinical experience to mid-career clinicians who have direct patient care responsibilities. The second was the development of an innovative STD curriculum for six medical schools. Preliminary evaluations indicate that in these six schools, an average of ten hours is now devoted to STD topics, while nearly half of the U.S. medical schools offer no formal instruction in STD at all. Generations of physicians have been graduated who may be more knowledgeable about glycogen storage diseases than about gonorrhea. The third approach was the funding of a growing number of STD Research Training Centers to foster research careers in STD. Finally, the U.S. Public Health Service has sponsored the development of an instructional package for clinicians who see STD patients infrequently. [12]

CONCLUSION

STDs comprise one of the most important threats to the health of women and infants in the U.S. The growing number of viral STDs has reemphasized the importance of primary rather than secondary prevention of illness. Changes in sexual behavior and use of barrier contraception with spermicides can play an important role in primary prevention of STD. As AIDS diverts both money and effort from the more traditional STDs such as syphilis, the consequences may be grim. That cases of congenital syphilis are increasing in the U.S. is a national tragedy.

Health care workers in MCH must help to reestablish priorities for federal expenditures. For example, in recent years, the U.S. has spent huge amounts of money subsidizing a moribund passenger train system. What benefits would have accrued had the same amount of money been spent on STD control for American women and children?

REFERENCES

1. Grimes DA. Deaths due to sexually transmitted diseases. The forgotten component of reproductive mortality. JAMA 255:1727, 1986.

2. Centers for Disease Control: Division of sexually transmitted diseases and STD laboratory program, annual report, fiscal year 1986. Atlanta, Centers for Disease Control, 1987.

3. Grubb GS. Human papillomavirus and cervical neoplasia. Int J Epidemiol 15:1, 1986.

4. Centers for Disease Control: Increases in primary and secondary syphilis—United States. MMWR 36:393, 1987.

5. Mascola L, Pelosi R, Blount JH, et al. Congenital syphilis. Why is it still occurring? JAMA 252: 1719, 1984.

6. Cates W Jr. Epidemiology and control of sexually transmitted disease: strategic evolution. Infect Dis Clin N Am 1:1, 1987.

7. Alter M, Ahtone J, Weisfuse I, et al. Hepatitis B virus transmission between heterosexuals. JAMA 256: 1307, 1986.

8. Stone KM, Grimes DA, Magder LS. Personal protection against sexually transmitted disease. Am J Obstet Gynecol 155: 180, 1986.

9. Aral SO, Cates W Jr, Jenkins WC. Genital herpes: does knowledge lead to action? Am J Public Health 75: 69, 1985.

10. Solomon MZ, DeJong W. Recent sexually transmitted disease prevention efforts and their implications for AIDS health education. Health Ed Q 13: 301, 1986.

11. Kroger F, Yarber WL. STD content in school health textbooks: an evaluation using the worth assessment procedure. J School Health 54:41, 1984.

12. Centers for Disease Control: Progress toward achieving the national 1990 objectives for sexually transmitted diseases. MMWR 36: 173, 1987.

ACQUIRED IMMUNODEFICIENCY SYNDROME

24

Margaret J. Oxtoby and James W. Curran

INTRODUCTION

In 1981, the first few cases of *Pneumocystis carinii* pneumonia and Kaposi's sarcoma in previously healthy young men were reported from a few metropolitan areas in the U.S. [1,2] These were the first of numerous unusual infections and cancers to be described in persons afflicted with this new disease, later named, *acquired immunodeficiency syndrome* (AIDS). Only 6 1/2 years later, over 50,000 persons with AIDS have been reported in the U.S. alone, and over 130 countries worldwide are reporting cases of this new and highly fatal disease.[3] Although homosexual men were the first cases described, women, children, and heterosexual men clearly constitute an important part of the epidemic.

Much had been learned about the disease's clinical spectrum and the risk factors for transmission even before the causative agent was discovered in 1983. Cases of AIDS were documented in homosexual men, intravenous drug abusers, persons with hemophilia who had received clotting factor concentrates, and persons who had received transfusions from donors who later developed AIDS. Cases were also documented in heterosexual partners of persons at risk for AIDS and in infants born to mothers who had AIDS or who were in high-risk groups for AIDS. Thus the three routes of transmission could be clearly delineated: sexual transmission, bloodborne transmission, and transmission from women to their fetus or infant.

One aspect of this new disease was immediately apparent—the severe immune suppression that developed in previously well persons and left them susceptible to a variety of unusual infections and malignancies. One particular cell type, the T-helper lymphocyte, is specifically depleted in AIDS patients; because these cells coordinate the body's response to pathogens, their loss leads to a breakdown of the entire immune system and an inability to combat pathogens unable to cause disease in the normal host.

ETIOLOGY

Two aspects of AIDS—the spectrum of illness in affected persons, ranging from mild swelling of lymph nodes to life-threatening infections and malignancies, and the apparent patterns of transmission—pointed to an infectious agent as the cause. This was most likely a virus infecting lymphocytes and manifesting a long latent period between infection and disease. This agent, a retrovirus now called *human immunodeficiency virus* (HIV), was discovered in 1983 and proved to be the cause of AIDS in 1984.[4,5,6] A test to detect HIV antibody permitted detection of virus in blood of infected persons. This test allowed the screening of blood and plasma donations, helped to define more fully the spectrum of HIV infection and risk factors for transmission, and allowed diagnosis of HIV infection. Studies have documented presence of HIV in a stored sample from Zaire, from 1959;[7] by the time the first case of the disease later known as AIDS was reported in 1981, many people in widely separated countries had already become silently infected with HIV.[8,9]

HIV is a retrovirus with an enzyme called reverse transcriptase that allows it to convert its ribonucleic acid (RNA) genetic material into deoxyribonucleic acid (DNA). The viral DNA copy of the RNA is then inserted into the host cell DNA. In 1986, a second closely related retrovirus, HIV-2, was discovered in persons from West Africa. HIV-2 has been isolated from persons with AIDS and from asymptomatic persons, but the entire epidemiologic and clinical spectrum has not yet been elucidated.[10]

EPIDEMIOLOGY OF AIDS

After the first cases were reported in 1981, national surveillance was established. The surveillance definition of AIDS is based on clinical and laboratory criteria; it includes persons with a reliably diagnosed disease indicative of underlying cellular immunodeficiency, who lack any other known cause of immunosuppression. The AIDS case definition was revised in 1987,[11] based on new knowledge about the clinical spectrum of HIV infection, to include a broader range of indicator diseases, as well as certain HIV-related signs, such as HIV encephalopathy (progressive neurologic impairment caused by HIV invasion of the central nervous system) and wasting syndrome (marked by weight loss, chronic diarrhea, and fever).

As of the end of 1987, over 50,000 AIDS cases had been reported in the U.S., with each year bringing substantially more cases than the previous year (Figure 1). Ninety-one percent of U.S. cases have been in men, of whom 70 percent are homosexual or bisexual without a history of IV-drug abuse, 15 percent are present or past IV-drug abusers, and eight percent are homosexual/bisexual and IV-drug abusers. Of the 3500 women reported with AIDS, 50 percent have a history of intravenous drug abuse, while 30 percent have had a sexual partner at risk for AIDS, often an intravenous drug abuser (Table 1).[12] Of the 730 children (diagnosed under 13 years of age), 77 percent acquired the disease perinatally from their mothers, 13 percent were transfusion-associated, five percent are hemophiliacs who have received clotting factor, and risks for the remaining five percent are undetermined or under investigation.[13] Risk factors for mothers of children with perinatally acquired

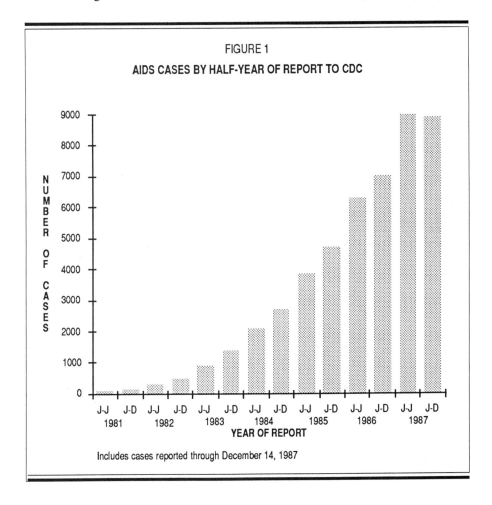

FIGURE 1

AIDS CASES BY HALF-YEAR OF REPORT TO CDC

Includes cases reported through December 14, 1987

AIDS parallel those for women with AIDS (Table 2). Nearly all persons with transfusion- or hemophilia-associated AIDS received their blood or blood products before universal donor screening and heat treatment of clotting factor concentrates.

TABLE 1

ADULTS WITH AIDS, BY SEX AND TRANSMISSION CATEGORY
1981-1987*

	Number (Percent) of Cases	
Risk Factor	Men	Women
Homosexual/bisexual male	31,120 (70%)	—
Intravenous drug abuser	6,436 (15%)	1,755 (50%)
Homosexual male and IV drug abuser	3,604 (8%)	—
Transfusion recipient	709 (2%)	380 (11%)
Hemophilia/coagulation disorder	460 (1%)	19 (1%)
Heterosexual contact	241 (1%)	845 (24%)
Born in country with predominant heterosexual transmission	645 (1%)	189 (5%)
Undetermined	1,133 (3%)	309 (9%)
TOTAL	44,348 (100 %)	3,497 (100 %)

*   Cases reported to CDC as of December 14, 1987.

TABLE 2

RISK FACTORS ASSOCIATED WITH PEDIATRIC AIDS CASES*

Risk Factor	Number, Percent of Cases	
Congenital/Perinatal Infection	560	(77%)
Mother's Risk Factor:		
IV drug abuser	312	
Partner of IV drug user	100	
Haitian born**	71	
Partner of man with other or unknown risk	37	
Received transfusion	13	
Infected, risk unknown	27	
Recipient of Blood (before 1985)	96	(13%)
Hemophilia	39	(5%)
No identified Risk	35	(5%)
TOTAL:	730	(100%)

*   Total includes children younger than 13 years of age at diagnosis and reported as of December 14, 1987.
**   Country where heterosexual transmission plays a major role.

AIDS has been reported from every state, but has had the most impact in certain metropolitan centers. In particular, 70 percent of women and children with AIDS reside in primarily urban areas of New York, New Jersey, and Florida; however, the proportion reported from other areas is steadily increasing. Similarly, the burden of disease falls disproportionately on minority communities; the cumulative incidence rates of AIDS for Black and Hispanic adults are three times that for white adults. The disparity is greatest in women and children; 55 percent of cases occur in Black children and 23 percent in Hispanic children, giving cumulative incidence rates 15 and nine times, respectively, than for white children.[14,15]

PREVALENCE OF HIV INFECTION

Since the time between HIV infection and development of AIDS varies from several months to several years, it is necessary to monitor HIV infection rates to determine present patterns of transmission and occurrence. Prevalence of infection varies widely. Seroprevalence rates for IV-drug abusers in the U.S. range from five percent in cities on the West Coast to 65 percent in New York.[16] Antibody seroprevalence for steady heterosexual partners of infected persons has been between ten percent and 60 percent. In the U.S. and Europe, most HIV-seropositive prostitutes have been IV-drug abusers; however, the pattern is different in cities in Central Africa, where drug use is rare yet a high proportion of prostitutes have been infected through heterosexual contact.[9] Rates of infection in childbearing women have been studied; data from Massachusetts, in 1987, suggested an overall seroprevalence of 2 per 1000,[17] while in New York City the rate was shown to be 1.6 per 100 among women presenting for delivery during the same period.[18,19] In a few African cities, seroprevalence rates are even higher, with over five percent of young adults infected with the virus.[20,21]

TRANSMISSION OF HIV

Studies incorporating HIV antibody testing have further added to our knowledge about virus transmission.[22] Studies have documented that sexual intercourse can result in transmission of HIV to either partner.[23,24] Among homosexual men, risk of infection increased with the number of sexual partners and the frequency with which they are the receptive partner in anal intercourse. The virus can be transmitted through penile-vaginal intercourse. Coexisting infections, such as those producing genital ulcers, or sexual practices that result in mucosal tears, may increase the likelihood of HIV transmission. Infectiousness may vary over the course of the infection, with more immunosuppressed persons being more efficient transmitters.

Receipt of blood from an HIV-infected donor is the most efficient route of transmission. Over 90 percent of persons receiving blood or blood products from a seropositive donor will become infected. Sharing contaminated needles or syringes by IV-drug abusers is also an efficient means of transmission.

Transmission from an infected mother to her infant can occur during pregnancy through transplacental passage, at the time of delivery by contact with infective blood, or, rarely, postpartum through breastfeeding. Overall, it is estimated that transmission occurs in 30-50 percent of pregnancies of infected women. More advanced disease in the mother, or delivery of a previously affected child, may be associated with an increased likelihood of transmission. Further studies are needed to determine the precise timing of infection and which infants acquire HIV by each route, so that means of preventing transmission from mother to infant can be developed. Systematic studies of HIV antibody in households and other settings have further strengthened the evidence for lack of transmission through casual contact. Studies of health-care workers and laboratory workers with intensive occupational exposure have documented a very low risk of infection, although a few cases of infection apparently acquired through needlesticks or direct exposure to blood have occurred. Risk of infection after a needlestick with contaminated blood is less than one percent. Routine use of blood and body fluid precautions for all patients will minimize the risk of occupational exposure.[25]

CLINICAL ASPECTS

The antibody test has furthered understanding of the natural history of HIV infection. An acute transient viral syndrome, similar to mononucleosis, occurs in some individuals a few weeks after HIV infection. Most infected adults do not develop AIDS for several years. Once infected, a person probably remains infected and potentially infectious for the remainder of his/her life, and remains at risk for developing the more severe manifestations known as AIDS. Studies suggest that the proportion of persons developing AIDS five years after becoming infected is ten-30 percent and that most infected persons develop some symptoms by then.[26-28] AIDS cases continue to occur among persons transfused with infected blood before antibody screening of donations (instituted in the U.S. in early 1985). Children may develop symptoms more rapidly after infection; among AIDS patients who acquired the infection perinatally from their mothers, the median age at diagnosis is nine months (Figure 2). However, as the epidemic continues, there will likely be more and more children and adults with long incubation periods.

Classification systems have been developed for both adults [29] and children[30] to provide a framework for evaluating patients with the protean clinical symptoms of HIV infection. Some persons are asymptomatic; others manifest only a persistent generalized lymphadenopathy. Certain constitutional findings, including weight loss, chronic unexplained diarrhea, and persistent fever are frequent harbingers of severe HIV disease; persistent and severe oral candida infections (thrush) and recurrent bacterial infections (particularly in children) also occur. As the immune deficiency worsens, opportunistic infections—fungal, parasitic, bacterial and viral—occur; cancers, such as Kaposi's sarcoma and lymphoma, also develop. A progressive encephalopathy, probably caused by HIV invasion of the brain, can also occur. In children, neurologic findings include loss of developmental milestones, acquired microcephaly, and progressive symmetrical motor deficits.

Children rarely present with malignancies; rather, they often show the constitutional signs, suffer frequently from infections including common bacterial infections, and often have a characteristic chronic pulmonary condition, lymphoid interstitial pneumonitis.[31,32] Children under one year of age more frequently present with failure to thrive or with a wasting syndrome, and have opportunistic infections, such as *Pneumocystis carinii* pneumonia; older children often present with a more insidious course, with lymphadenopathy and chronic pneumonitis. Prognosis for both adults and children with symptomatic HIV infection is poor. After diagnosis with AIDS, patients survive a median of one year, and few survive more than three years after diagnosis.

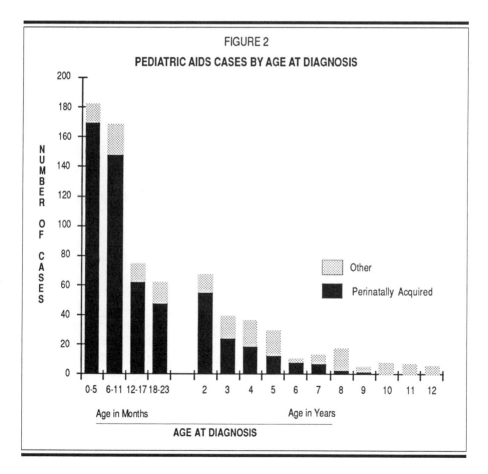

FIGURE 2
PEDIATRIC AIDS CASES BY AGE AT DIAGNOSIS

LABORATORY ASSESSMENT

Evaluation of the clinical status of infection can be aided by immunologic and other laboratory studies. Persons with severe symptomatic HIV infection characteristically have depletion of their CD4 cells (helper lymphocytes), and this is sometimes reflected in a inverted CD4/CD8 ratio. Children with HIV-related disease show altered antibody function sometimes long before displaying inverted T-cell ratios; they often have increased levels of immunoglobulins, although antibody-mediated immunity may be relatively poor. A few children, especially those with advance wasting syndrome or opportunistic infections, conversely, are severely hypogammaglobulinemic. Chronic anemia and thrombocytopenia are also commonly seen.

The principal method to detect HIV infection is the HIV-antibody ELISA test, followed by a confirmatory test. The ELISA is a reliable, easily performed and widely available assay; positive ELISAs require confirmation by a more specific antibody test (usually a Western blot immunoprofile or an immunoflourescence assay). The antibody test is highly sensitive and specific, although it is occasionally falsely negative early or late in infection. However, its diagnostic usefulness is limited in infants born to infected mothers. The mother's immunoglobulin G crosses the placenta regardless of virus transmission and is reflected as positive HIV antibody in the baby's blood. Maternal antibody is usually lost between three and nine months of age but can persist until 15 months of age. [29] Other tests, including viral isolation, antigen tests, and IgM tests have also been used, but each has limitations. It is likely that a combination of these tests, together with careful clinical followup for frequent infections or growth or development problems will prove necessary in following children born to HIV-infected mothers.

THERAPY

Clinical management of persons with HIV-related disease is challenging because of the complexity and severity of HIV-related illnesses. General supportive measures, such as maintaining good nutrition, should be combined with aggressive diagnosis and treatment of secondary infections. Several agents directed against HIV, or meant to boost the immune system, are under study. Azidothymidine, a reverse transcriptase inhibitor, has demonstrated promising short-term benefit, although it has some serious side-effects, including suppression of blood-forming cells; [33,34] this drug is licensed for adults and is being studied in children.

Vaccination against the usual childhood diseases is recommended for HIV-infected persons. [35,36] However, if their immune system is already affected they will not respond optimally to these vaccines. Limited studies have revealed no major adverse reactions after immunization of HIV-infected persons. Diphtheria, pertussis, and tetanus immunizations, as well as other inactivated vaccines, such as

Haemophilus influenzae β should be given routinely. Effective inactivated vaccines, where they exist, are preferred to live vaccines because of the potential for vaccine-related disease in immunosuppressed persons; thus, inactivated polio vaccine is preferred over polio vaccine for children possibly infected with HIV or for children in areas where there is risk of exposure to the natural diseases, since the risk of complications due to the natural disease is much lighter than the risk due to rare vaccine-associated complications.

Passive protection can also be helpful, including specific immunoglobulin prophylaxis after exposure to viruses such as varicella or measles. In some symptomatic HIV-infected children, periodic immunoglobulin infusions have been used by some clinicians to decrease susceptibility to bacterial and viral infections, but the efficacy of this intervention has not been rigorously evaluated. [37]

For an asymptomatic HIV-infected person, there is no reason to restrict usual daily contacts at work or in school. However, persons with advanced disease may benefit from more limited exposure, for their own protection. While some caution must be stated about the attendance of HIV-infected infants in daycare settings, because of the theoretical possibility of transmission to other young children through exchange of body fluids, there is no need to restrict older children if they are toilet trained, do not exhibit certain behaviors such as biting, and have no uncovered, oozing lesions.[38-40]

Optimal care of HIV-infected persons involves attention to their emotional well-being and social-service needs. IV-drug abusers, for instance, are often without community support or family structure, so housing needs and other not-strictly medical concerns need to be addressed.[41] Underlying social problems, such as drug abuse and prostitution, must also be addressed.

IMPACT OF THE AIDS EPIDEMIC

Since its appearance, HIV has proven itself a formidable public health challenge. By 1985, it was one of the leading causes of death among young men in the U.S., with particularly severe effects among homosexual men, and was rapidly sweeping through IV-drug-using communities, with further spread to sex partners and offspring of these drug users. The chronic nature of the disease and the complexity of treatment necessitate careful medical care, including sometimes lengthy inpatient care. In several metropolitan areas, over ten percent of hospital beds are needed for persons suffering complications of HIV infection. The social, medical, and economic burdens of this new disease are even more striking in certain developing countries, where HIV has already begun to add substantially to infectious disease morbidity and mortality among young adults and children.

As severe as the epidemic has been, trends in HIV seroprevalence and in the incidence of AIDS cases, together with the virus' long incubation period, suggest a continued increase in the number of cases over the coming years. In 1986, the Public Health Service projected that 270,000 cases of AIDS would be diagnosed by the end of 1991, with 54,000 deaths in that year alone. These projected cases will occur mainly in persons already infected by 1987.[42]

Public health policy must be carefully and wisely developed. HIV infection can be devastating, not only physically and emotionally but also socially because of potential effects on a person's ability to attend school, to work, or to otherwise function in society. Antibody testing must be combined with counseling and continued support to be effective. Unfounded fears of transmission through casual contact can hinder prevention efforts by adding to the emotionally charged atmosphere surrounding this disease.

It is highly encouraging that within a few years of its appearance, the etiology of AIDS and the clinical spectrum and routes of HIV transmission have been clearly delineated. Search for better treatments and for an effective vaccine are clearly of high priority. However, effective education about AIDS can help lead to a decreased rate of new infections and to more humane treatment of persons already infected. [43]

PREVENTION

Prevention of new HIV infections can best be accomplished by preventing transmission through each of the three major routes (Table 3). Sexual transmission can be prevented through abstinence or through mutually monogamous relationships between uninfected partners. Proper and consistent use of condoms markedly decreases transmission of various sexually transmitted infections. While most condom failures result from failure to use them properly, breakage also occurs. Spermicides have been shown to inactivate HIV and other viruses in the laboratory and may provide additional protection when used with condoms.

In most industrialized and some developing countries, universal antibody screening of blood donors has been instituted. This public health measure, in concert with deferral of donors with increased risk of HIV exposure and heat treatment of clotting-factor concentrates, has drastically reduced the risk of transfusion-associated HIV infection. The current challenge is to establish such programs in all countries and continue to monitor their effectiveness.

In the U.S. and Europe, IV-drug abuse accounts for a major proportion of all HIV infection. Effective HIV prevention programs must seek to decrease the number of persons newly adopting illicit drug habits. Interim measures must also focus on providing effective treatment programs for current IV-drug abusers and on providing education about clean needles and syringes for those unable to stop their drug habit.

Transmission to children can best be prevented by preventing infection in young women. Testing and counselling of high-risk women should be *routine* in all health-care settings.[44,45] Highest priority must be given to providing optimal inexpensive (or free) family planning services for HIV-infected or high-risk women. For a woman already infected with HIV, pregnancy carries a very grave risk to the child, and pregnancy may harm the mother's own health. The mother has to also consider that if she becomes ill or dies she will not be able to care for her child. In all developed countries where safe and effective breast-milk substitutes are available, HIV-infected mothers should avoid breastfeeding to prevent possible transmission to an uninfected child.[46] However, in many developing areas of the world, breastfeeding will continue to be the preferred method of feeding even for the HIV-infected mother, because the immunological, nutritional, psychological, and child-spacing advantages of breastfeeding outweigh the small incremental risk to her infant of becoming infected through breastfeeding.

Health-care workers need to routinely follow blood and body fluid precautions for all patients to avoid acquiring not only HIV but other, more contagious bloodborne infections, such as hepatitis B virus.[23] In health care settings, and in

---

TABLE 3
MEASURES TO PREVENT HIV TRANSMISSION

─ **MEASURES TO PREVENT SEXUAL TRANSMISSION** ───────────────
    Abstinence, mutual monogamy between uninfected partners
    Limit number of sex partners
    Avoid sexual contact with high risk partners
    Use condoms if sexually active with possibly infected partner
    Avoid anal intercourse with possibly infected partner

─ **MEASURES TO PREVENT BLOODBORN TRANSMISSION** ───────────
    Do not use intravenous drugs
    Do not share or reuse needles or drug works
    High risk persons should not donate blood, semen, milk or organs
    Blood banks should screen blood of donors of r HIV antibody
    Health care workers should use universal blood and body fluid precautions
    Heat treat clotting factor to inactivate virus

─ **MEASURES TO PREVENT TRANSMISSION FROM MOTHER TO INFANT** ──────
    Health care providers must provide effective contraceptive options to high-risk communities
    Women should defer childbearing, if infected
    HIV-infected women should avoid breast-feeding, in settings where safe and effective
      substitutes are available

─ **GENERAL EDUCATION MEASURES** ───────────────────────
    Educate children, adolescents and young adults about AIDS and means of spread
    Offer HIV antibody test routinely in appropriate settings
    Provide accurate and supportive counseling

other settings where needles or other sharp objects are used for tatooing, other scarifications, or for injections, reuse of needles must be avoided.

Education must include both broad-based prevention messages and more individual counseling.[44] The HIV-antibody test should be routinely offered in a variety of medical settings. Counseling must ensure understanding about HIV infection and how to avoid transmission. Confidentiality of test results must be assured. HIV-infected persons must be protected from unwarranted discrimination.

As a society, AIDS requires that we plan ahead in providing preventive, treatment, and social services, while continuing to emphasize research on this disease. The worldwide extent of the infection necessitates collaboration between nations and compassion among people within them, in all aspects of response to this epidemic.

REFERENCES

1. Pneumocystis pneumonia: Los Angeles. MMWR 1981;30:250-2.

2. Kaposi's sarcoma and Pneumocystis pneumonia among homosexual men: New York City and California. MMWR 1981, 30:305-8.

3. Communication, World Health Organization Special Programme on AIDS, 1987.

4. Barre-Sinoussi F, Chermann JC, Rey F, et al. Isolation of a T-lymphotropic retrovirus from a patient at risk for acquired immune deficiency syndrome (AIDS). Science 1983, 220:868-71.

5. Gallo RC, Salahuddin SZ, Popovic M, et al. Frequent detection and isolation of cytopathic retroviruses (HTLV-III) from patients with AIDS and at risk for AIDS. Science 1984; 224:500-3.

6. Levy JA, Hoffman AD, Kramer SM, Landis JA, Shimabukuro JM, Oschiro LS. Isolation of lymphocytopathic retroviruses from San Francisco patients with AIDS. Science 1984;225:840-2.

7. Nahmias AJ, Weiss J, Yao X, et al. Evidence for human infection with an HTLV III/LAV-like virus in Central Africa, 1959. Lancet 1986; 1:1279.

8. Jaffe HW, Darrow WW, Echenberg DF, et al. The acquired immunodeficiency syndrome in a cohort of homosexual men: a six-year follow-up study. Ann Intern Med 1985:103:210-214.

9. Quinn TC, Mann JM, Curran JW, Piot P. AIDS in Africa: An epidemiologic paradigm. Science 1986:234:955-963.

10. AIDS due to HIV-2 infection: New Jersey. MMWR January 29, 1988, 33-35.

11. Revision of the CDC surveillance case definition for acquired immunodeficiency syndrome: MMWR 1987; 36 (suppl no. 1S):3S-15S.

12. Guinan ME, Hardy A. Epidemiology of AIDS in women in the United States. JAMA 1987; 257:2039-2042.

13. Rogers MF, Thomas PA, Startcher ET, Noa MC, Bush TJ, Jaffe HW. Acquired immunodeficiency syndrome in children: report of the Centers for Disease Control National Surveillance, 1982-1985. Pediatrics 1987; 79:1008-1014.

14. Acquired immunodeficiency syndrome (AIDS) among blacks and hispanics: United States. MMWR 1986; 35:656-666.

15. Rogers MF, William WW. AIDS in blacks and hispanics: implications for prevention. Issues in Science and Technology, 1987;3:89-94.

16. Human immunodeficiency virus in the United States: MMWR 1987; 36:801-804 and supplement, 36:S-6.

17. Medical News and Perspectives: HIV antibody prevalence data derived from study of Massachusetts infants. JAMA 1987; 258:171-172.

18. Landesman S, Minkoff H, Holman S, McCalla S, Sijin O. Serosurvey of HIV infection in parturients: implications for HIV testing programs of pregnant women. JAMA 1987; 258:2701-2703.

19. Data from the New York Department of Health, January 1988.

20. Mann JM, Bila K, Colebunders RL, et al. Natural history of HIV in Zaire. Lancet, 1986; 2:707-709.

21. Nzila N, Ryder RW, Behets F, et al. Perinatal HIV transmission in two African hospitals In: III International Conference on AIDS Abstracts volume, Washington, D.C.,1987;158.

22. Friedland GH, Klein RS. Transmission of the human immunodeficiency virus. N Engl J Med 1987, 317:1125-1135.

23. Peterman TA, Curran JW. Sexual transmission of human immunodeficiency virus. JAMA 1986; 256:2222-6.

24. Padian NS. Heterosexual transmission of acquired immunodeficiency syndrome: international perspectives and national projections. Rev Infect Dis 1987; 9:947-960.

25. Recommendations for prevention of HIV transmission in health-care settings. MMWR 1987; 36(suppl 2S):3S-18S.

26. Eyster ME, Gail MH, Ballard JO, Al-Mondhiry H, Goedert JJ. Natural history of human immunodeficiency virus infections in hemophiliacs: effects of T-cell subsets, platelet counts, and age. Ann Intern Med 1987; 107:1-6.

27. Goedert JJ, Biggar RJ, Melbye M, et al. Effect of T4 count and cofactors on the incidence of AIDS in homosexual men infected with human immunodeficiency virus, JAMA 1987; 257:331-334.

28. Hessel NA, Rutherford GW, O'Ma lley PM, Doll LS, Darrow WW, Jaffe HW. The natural history of human immunodeficiency virus infection in a cohort of homosexual and bisexual men: a 7-year prospective study. In: III International Conference on Acquired Immunodeficiency Syndrome, Washington, DC, 1987:1.

29. Classification system for human T-lymphotropic virus type III/lymphadenopathy-associated virus infections: MMWR 1986; 35:334-339.

30. Classification system for human immunodeficiency virus (HIV) infection in children under 13 years of age: MMWR 1987; 36:225-236.

31. Parks WP, Scott GB. A overrview of pediatric AIDS: approaches to diagnosis and outcome assessment. In: AIDS: Modern Concepts and Therapeutic Challenges. New York, Marcel Dekker, Inc, 1987:98-121.

32. Rubinstein A. Pediatric AIDS . Current Probl Pediatr, 1986; 26:362-409.

33. Fischl MA, Richman DD, Grieco MH, et al. The efficacy of 3'azido-3'-deoxythymidine (azidothymidine) in the treatment of patients with AIDS and AIDS-related complex: a double-blind placebo-controlled trial. N Engl J Med 1987; 317:185-191.

34. Richman DD, Fischl MA, Grieco MH, et al. The toxicity of azidothymidine (AZT) in the treatment of patients with AIDS and AIDS-related complex: a double-blind placebo-controlled trial. N Engl J Med 1987; 317:192-197.

35. von Reyn CF, Clements CJ, Mann JM. Human immunodefiency virus infection and routine childhood immunization. Lancet 1987; 2:669-672.

36. Immunization of children infected with human T-lymphotropic virus, type III/lymphadenopathy-associated virus: MMWR 1986:35:595-606.

37. Ochs HD. Intravenous immunoglobulin in the treatment and prevention of acute infections in pediatric acquired immunodeficiency syndrome. Pediatr Infect Dis J, 1986; 6:509-511.

38. Education and foster care of children infected with human T-lymphotropic virus type III/lymphadenopathy-associated virus: MMWR 1985; 34:517-521.

39. American Academy of Pediatrics: Health guidelines for the attendance in daycare and foster care settings of children infected with human immunodeficiency virus. Pediatrics 1987; 79:466-469.

40. American Academy of Pediatrics.: School attendance of children and adolescents with human T-lymphotropic virus/lymphadenopathy-associated virus infection. Pediatrics 1986; 77:430-432.

41. Report of the Surgeon General's workshop on children with HIV infection and their families: Washington, D.C.: U.S. Department of Health and Human Services, 1987.

42. Morgan WM, Curran JW. Acquired immunodeficiency syndrome: current and future trends. Public Health Rep 1986; 101:459-466.

43. Surgeon General's report on acquired immune deficiency syndrome: Washington, D.C.: U.S. Department of Health and Human Services, 1986.

44. Public Health Service guidelines for counseling and antibody testing to prevent HIV infection and AIDS: MMWR 1987; 36:509-515.

45. Minkoff HL. Care of pregnant women infected with human immunodeficiency virus. JAMA 1987; 258:2714-2717.

46. Recommendations for assisting in the prevention of perinatal transmission of human T-lymphotropic virus type III/lymphadenopathy-associated virus and acquired immunodeficiency syndrome: MMWR 1985; 34:721-6, 731-2.

SURVEILLANCE FOR GENETIC DISORDERS AND CONGENITAL ANOMALIES*

25

Joe Leigh Simpson

Impressive genetic advances have been made in only a few decades. The first human chromosomal abnormality was delineated in 1958, and prenatal diagnosis of genetic disorders first achieved in 1968. Increasing public and professional awareness of genetic issues further dictates attention by the MCH specialist to clinical genetics. Concurrently, public and professional awareness has increased because the relative burden of major birth defects (two to three percent of all deliveries) has increased, as deaths due to infectious causes decrease. MCH delivery systems must therefore adapt to genetic advances.

In this chapter, we shall discuss selected aspects of clinical genetics. Initially, we shall discuss the routine genetic history. Next, we shall delineate those disorders amenable to genetic screening, along with the principles underlying initiation of screening programs. Finally, we shall survey the most common indications for prenatal diagnosis of genetic disorders. Further details are published in other articles by the author.[1]

I. THE ROUTINE GENETIC HISTORY

For all pregnancies, it is standard practice to determine whether a couple, or anyone in their families, has a disorder that might prove heritable. One should

---

* There are a large number of tables and figures in this chapter. They are placed at the end of the text in order to facilitate the ease of reading. Also, footnotes for the figures appear at the end of the references.

inquire about the health status of first-degree relatives (sibs, parents, offspring), second-degree relatives (uncles, aunts, nephews, nieces, and grandparents), and third-degree relatives (first cousins). Record abnormal reproductive outcomes, such as repetitive spontaneous abortions, stillborns, and anomalous liveborn infants. Couples having such histories should undergo chromosomal studies[2] and other evaluations.[3] The subsequent counsel may be sufficiently complex to warrant referral to a geneticist, or it may prove sufficiently facile for the informed clinician to handle. If a birth defect is detected in a second- or third-degree relative, only rarely will the likelihood of that anomaly occurring be substantively increased in the pregnancy in question. For example, identification of a second- or third-degree relative with an autosomal recessive trait will ordinarily place the couple at little increased risk for an affected offspring, the exception occurring if the patient and her husband are consanguineous. Nonetheless, one should inquire about the status of relatives as distant as first cousins (of the fetus) because identification of certain disorders in distant relatives may be the only clue that the couple may be at increased risk for autosomal dominant disorders characterized by decreased penetrance, or for X-linked recessive disorders.

If a polygenic/multifactorial trait (Table 1) is identified in a first-degree relative of the fetus, the likelihood of recurrence is usually two-five percent. If such a trait is identified in second- or third-degree relatives, likelihood of recurrence is increased only slightly over that of the general population, a possible exception existing for neural tube defects. Empiric risk for specific polygenic/multifactorial traits are provided elsewhere by the author,[4] as are discussions of principles of Mendelian traits.

In addition to identifying relatives with genetic disorders, one should record drug exposure by the woman and her partner. Identify not merely those agents currently received but also noxious agents to which exposure occurred prior to pregnancy. The latter could be mutagenic. Again, deleterious agents are identified elsewhere.[5] Table 2 lists unequivocal teratogens.

Parental ages should also be recorded. Indeed, the most common indication for prenatal diagnosis is advanced maternal age (Table 3). Advanced maternal age warrants discussion irrespective of a patient's difficulties in achieving pregnancy, and irrespective of a physician's personal convictions regarding pregnancy termination. Offspring of fathers in the fifth and sixth decade are at increased risk for new dominant mutations. Unfortunately, the latter are not amenable to prenatal diagnosis.

Finally, ethnic origin should be recorded. This will be relevant to the genetic screening issues discussed in the next aspect. Ashkenazi Jews are at increased risk for offspring with Tay-Sachs disease and, hence, should be screened to determine heterozygote status (frequency 1/27). In the U.S., Jewish individuals are often uncertain whether they are of Ashkenazic or Sephardic descent; thus, we offer screening and to all Jewish couples, including couples in which only one partner is Jewish. Increasing availability of prenatal diagnostic techniques also makes advisable routine heterozygote screening for β-thalassemia in Italians and Greeks, sickle cell anemia in Blacks, and a-thalassemia in Southeast Asians and Philippinos.[1,6] When heterozygote testing becomes feasible for cystic fibrosis, Caucasians should surely be screened for this condition.

Some obstetricians consider it useful to obtain genetic information through use of questionnaires or checklists, often constructed to require action only to positive responses. Table 4 reproduces a form recommended by the American College of Obstetricians and Gynecologists (ACOG).[6] Use of a similar form by the author revealed that 21.4 percent of couples in a prenatal clinic showed at least one positive response, with 7.8 percent of the original sample requiring formal genetic counseling[7] (Figure 1). Advanced maternal age was the most common indication.

II. PRINCIPLES AND PREREQUISITES OF GENETIC SCREENING

Genetic screening implies monitoring a population to identify individuals having genotypes that are associated with a detectable disease or may lead to that disease in their offspring. Several aspects of genetic screening deserve emphasis.

One principle is that genetic screening should be voluntary unless specifically mandated by law.[8] Legal requirements usually dictate neonatal screening for phenylketonuria (PKU) and hypothyroidism, but not for other disorders. Of course, voluntary screening does not mean that a physician must remain neutral or even fail to express his/her opinion. However, a given test should not be performed without a patient's knowledge. The reason is that a patient may not wish to be faced with the dilemma of deciding among options raised by the screening process.

Second, in genetic screening one does not expect to detect all affected individuals in a given population. For example, in neonatal screening for phenylketonuria PKU, one fails to detect 16 percent of affected infants if screening is performed on the first day of life, three percent if performed on the second day, and 0.3 percent if performed on the third day.[9] (Coincidentally, these figures should give pause to those advocating same-day discharge for a newly delivered mother and infant.) A further example is that only 80-90 percent of NTD cases are detected in maternal serum alpha-fetoprotein (MSAFP) screening (discussed in third aspect).

Third, establishing technical feasibility for screening does not alone suffice to justify screening. Indeed, many genetic disorders could be subjected to screening. For example, all chromosomal abnormalities could be detected during the neonatal period, and almost all disorders of amino-acid metabolism are amenable to screening. On the other hand, screening is actually recommended only for those disorders that fulfill prerequisites essential for initiating screening programs. Four generally accepted prerequisites[8] (Table 5) are elaborated upon below.

A. CAPACITY TO ALTER CLINICAL MANAGEMENT

Although screening to achieve research objectives (e.g., determining the incidence of a disorder) is sometimes appropriate, widespread testing is ordinarily performed only if an abnormal finding would alter clinical management. Thus, *neonates* are screened for those metabolic disorders that are amenable to treatment (e.g., PKU and hypothyroidism), but not for those disorders that are untreatable (e.g., Lesch-Nyhan syndrome). Neonatal screening for sickle cell anemia has recently been recommended, but only after it became clear that prophylactic antibiotics might prevent life-threatening infections. Relatively common disorders that are not treatable, and therefore for which *neonates* should not be subjected to screening, include chromosomal abnormalities, Tay-Sachs disease, Duchenne muscular dystrophy, and probably cystic fibrosis.

If neonatal screening is undesirable for a given disorder, it may still be reasonable to screen *adults* to determine whether they are at increased risk for offspring with the same disorder. Identification of individuals heterozygous for an autosomal recessive disorder could alter reproductive choices and thus clinical management. The object is to identify mating between two individuals heterozygous for the same mutant allel. Screening adults to determine heterozygote status is, however, ordinarily applicable only if prenatal diagnosis is possible. Common Mendelian disorders thus amenable to heterozygote determination include Tay-Sachs disease, β-thalassemia, ∂-thalassemia, and sickle cell anemia (ACOG, 1987).[1,6] Ideally, screening should be performed prior to pregnancy; however, if the patient is already pregnant, screening should be completed as early in gestation as possible in order to allow maximum reproductive options.

B. COST-EFFECTIVENESS

Ability to identify a heterozygote, or even to detect an affected neonate with a treatable disorder, still does not necessarily dictate that screening be undertaken. For only a few disorders does the cost of screening justify the monetary and emotional savings of detecting the rare affected case. Indeed, technology now exists to screen scores of Mendelian disorders. Yet only hypothyroidism, PKU, and perhaps sickle cell anemia currently fulfill criteria of cost-effectiveness in neonatal screening. Screening for other treatable disorders is arguable, although some states mandate screening for galactosemia, maple-syrup-urine disease, and adenosine deaminase deficiency. Chromosomal analysis and alpha feto-protein (AFP) assays are routinely performed whenever amniotic fluid is obtained at amniocentesis, but testing for other detectable disorders (e.g., rare metabolic traits) is not pursued. In the future we can anticipate that virtually all common Mendelian disorders will be detectable in utero.[10] However, for only a few disorders will neonatal screening, heterozygote detection, or prenatal testing be recommended for the general population.

C. RELIABLE MEANS OF ASSESSMENT

The requisite assay must have a high predictive value. Although a general axiom of laboratory medicine, this statement is especially applicable for genetic diseases. Because genetic disorders are individually rare, even low false-negative rates could result in a given abnormal value being more likely to represent a false-positive than a true-positive value.

D. CAPACITY TO HANDLE PROBLEMS

Fulfilling all the above prerequisites still does not mean that screening for a particular disorder should be initiated. A final requirement is the ability to handle difficulties that inevitably arise in screening programs. Sometimes the inability to handle these problems obviates initiation of a screening program that would otherwise be attractive.

It should be specifically anticipated that unexpected problems will arise. After screening programs for PKU were initiated, it became clear that elevated neonatal phenylalanine was often not the result of PKU, but rather the result of other conditions that required no dietary treatment. Ability to separate false-positive from true PKU proved crucial.

In screening normal populations to detect heterozygotes (sickle cell disease, Tay-Sachs disease, ∂-thalassemia, β-thalassemia), one must assure that individuals identified as heterozygotes do not become stigmatized or do not develop erroneous impressions that their own health is threatened.

E. SPECIFIC INDICATIONS FOR PRENATAL GENETIC SCREENING

Prenatal genetic screening is obviously undertaken to facilitate prenatal diagnosis. Table 6 summarizes disorders warranting screening, details of which are provided in the fourth aspect.

III. INDICATIONS FOR
PRENATAL CYTOGENETIC STUDIES

All chromosomal disorders are detectable in utero. It is not appropriate, however, to perform amniocentesis or chorionic villus sampling (CVS) in every pregnancy, because for many couples the risks of these invasive procedures outweigh diagnostic benefits. Elsewhere, these risks are reviewed in detail.[1] Briefly, procedure-related loss rates are 0.5 percent for amniocentesis and no more than one-two percent for CVS. These losses are in addition to background rates of perhaps three percent in the first trimester[11] and one percent at 16 weeks[1,3]. Given these risks, let us then assess the propriety of prenatal cytogenetic studies for specific indications.

A. ADVANCED MATERNAL AGE

The most common indication for antenatal cytogenetic studies is advanced maternal age. The overall incidence of trisomy 21 is 1 per 800 liveborn births in the U.S., but the frequency increases with age (Table 3). Above age 30, the rate increases exponentially. Thus, the likelihood of a 35-year-old mother being delivered of a child with trisomy 21 is 1 in 385; at age 39, the likelihood is 1 in 137; and at age 45, the likelihood is 1 in 30.[12] Trisomy 21 is not the only chromosomal abnormality that increases with maternal age. Trisomy 13, trisomy 18, 47,XXX, and 47,XXY also increase.[13] No biologic explanation has been found for the relationship between aneuploidy and advanced maternal age.

On the basis of these data, it is now standard medical practice to offer prenatal chromosomal diagnosis to all women who, at their expected delivery date (Estimated Date of Confinement, E.D.C.), will be 35 years or older.[6] The choice of age 35 is largely arbitrary, however, chosen at a time when the risk figures were available only for five-year intervals (i.e., 30-34 years, 35-39 years, 40-44 years, etc.). Thus, flexibility is appropriate when answering inquiries from women younger than 35 years.

The risk figures shown in Table 3 are applicable only for liveborns. The prevalence of abnormalities in antenatal studies at 16 to 18 weeks gestation is about 30 percent higher.[13,14] The prevalence of aneuploidy in CVS studies (nine to 11 weeks) appears comparable or slightly higher than that found at amniocentesis.[15] The discrepancy between frequencies of chromosomal abnormalities in liveborn infants and in fetuses is presumably due to the disproportionate likelihood that chromosomally abnormal fetuses will abort spontaneously between prenatal sampling (nine to 16 weeks) and term (40 weeks). In fact, five percent of stillborn infants show chromosomal abnormalities.[16,17] That is, some therapeutically aborted fetuses would have aborted spontaneously had not iatrogenic intervention occurred.

Low maternal serum alpha-fetoprotein (MSAFP) is associated with increased risk of aneuploidy. A logical deduction is that normal or slightly elevated MSAFP [1.0-2.4 multiple of the median (MOM)] should *decrease* the risk of aneuploidy for older women. Although some British workers recommend against amniocentesis in older women (35-37 years) having such MSAFP values, U.S. workers do not appear to agree because of the potential legal hazards.[18]

B. PREVIOUS CHILD WITH CHROMOSOMAL ABNORMALITY

After the occurrence of a child, or probably also an abortus with trisomy 21, the likelihood that subsequent progeny will also have autosomal trisomy is traditionally considered increased, even if parental chromosomal complements are normal. Although the risk is perhaps not so great as once believed, parental anxiety alone dictates that antenatal chromosomal studies should be discussed for couples having a trisomy 21 child. Risks of perhaps one percent are considered appropriate for counseling.

Recurrence risk data following the birth of a liveborn infant trisomic for chromosome other than No. 21 are limited. However, the risk seems to be increased (perhaps one percent) for recurrence of either the same or for a different chromosomal abnormality. Thus, antenatal studies should be offered to such couples.

C. PARENTAL CHROMOSOMAL REARRANGEMENTS

Another indication for prenatal cytogenetic studies is the presence of a parental chromosomal abnormality. A balanced translocation is the usual indication, but inversions and other chromosomal abnormalities also occur.

A simple way to appreciate the clinical significance of translocations is to recall Robertsonian translocations, the most common type of translocation in humans. These translocations involve centromeric fusion of acrocentric chromosomes (Nos. 13, 14, 15, 21, or 22). Centric fusion involving two acrocentrics results in a single chromosome that has the information ordinarily carried by two separate chromosomes (Figure 2); thus, the chromosome number is reduced from 46 to 45. If there exists not only the translocation chromosome but 45 additional chromosomes, an imbalance (triplication) exists.

If a child has Down syndrome as result of a Robertsonian translocation [e.g., 46,XX,-14,+(14q;21q)], the rearrangement will prove to have originated *de novo* in 50 to 75 percent of cases. That is, the translocation will be present in neither parent, having arisen in oocyte or sperm. The likelihood of Down syndrome recurring in progeny of parents whose offspring have a *de novo* translocation is no greater than that for any other woman of similar age.

On the other hand, one parent may have a *balanced* Robertsonian translocation. If so, that parent will have only 45 chromosomes, with only one separate No. 21 [e.g., 45,XX,-14,-21,+(14q;21q)]. If this circumstance exists, the risk to offspring is much higher. The theoretical risk that a parent carrying a t(14q;21q) chromosome will have a child with Down syndrome is 33 percent (Figure 2); however, empiric risks are much lower. The likelihood is no more than two percent if the father carries translocation, and ten to 15 percent if the mother carries the translocation.[19,20] For other Robertsonian translocations, risks are usually lower. In t(13q;14q), the risk for unbalanced liveborns (namely trisomy 13) is one percent or less.[19,20] This low risk probably reflects the lethality of unbalanced products. Finally, homologous translocations [e.g., 45,XX,-13,-13,+t(13q;13q)] carry prohibitive (100 percent abnormal outcome) risks; the only possible outcomes are abortions or liveborns with anomalies.

Reciprocal translocations differ from Robertsonian translocations in that the former involve an exchange of chromosome material between two or more chromosomes. Acrocentric chromosomes are usually not involved. Unbalanced products show duplication for some chromosomal regions and, concomitantly, deficiencies for others. Empiric data for specific translocations are rarely available, but some generalizations can be made by pooling data derived from different translocations. Again, theoretical risks for abnormal (unbalanced) offspring are far greater than empiric risks. Risks approximate 11 percent for offspring of female heterozygotes and 11 percent for offspring of male heterozygotes.[20]

Another chromosomal rearrangement is an inversion, either pericentric or paracentric. Clinical significance and management following detection of an inversion are similar to that discussed for a translocation. However, inversions are far less common.

IV. COMMON INDICATIONS FOR PRENATAL DIAGNOSIS OF MENDELIAN DISORDERS

Originally possible only for certain inborn errors of metabolism, increasing numbers of Mendelian disorders have become detectable *in utero*. Moreover, techniques for diagnosis are changing. Antenatal diagnosis of hemoglobinopathies and hemophilia initially required fetal blood, obtainable only by fetoscopy; more recently, DNA analysis suffices, allowing diagnosis with any nucleated cell (chorionic villi, amniotic fluid cells). The changing status and increasing complexity required to diagnose Mendelian traits dictate close liason between MCH teams and geneticists.

A. INBORN ERRORS OF METABOLISM

Antenatal diagnosis is possible for approximately 100 inborn errors of metabolism.[21] Most are transmitted in autosomal recessive fashion, although a few are transmitted in X-linked recessive or autosomal dominant fashion. Couples will usually be identified to be at risk for an affected child because they previously had such a child. Most metabolic disorders are so rare that it is unreasonable to expect physicians who are not geneticists to remain current concerning prenatal diagnosis. On the other hand, screening programs can readily identify heterozygotes prior to the birth of a child with an autosomal recessive disorder. This situation now exists for Tay-Sachs disease, ∂-thalassemia, β-thalassemia and sickle cell anemia.

Several general principles should be kept in mind:

First, the basis for offering an invasive prenatal diagnotic test should always be verified. Otherwise, an inappropriate test may be performed. Unfortunately, confirmation is not always easy. If the affected child is no longer alive, verification may be difficult or even impossible.

Second, detection of a metabolic error usually will require that the enzyme be expressed in amniotic fluid cells or chorionic villi. This requirement is fulfilled by most, but unfortunately not by all, metabolic disorders, a prominent exception being PKU. It is for this reason that PKU must be sought not by enzymatic but by molecular techniques (see below).

Third, metabolic disorders detectable in amniotic fluid have also proved detectable in chorionic villi, although enzyme activity levels may differ between the two tissues.[22] Occasionally, one can arrive at a diagnosis on the basis of a product in amniotic fluid, the most prominent example being 17a-hydroxyprogesterone for detection of adrenal 21-hydroxylase deficiency.

Fourth, biochemical analyses require more planning than is necessary for cytogenetic studies. Often fluid or cultured cells must be transported to a referral laboratory, no single lab being capable of performing all analyses.

B. MENDELIAN DISORDERS CHARACTERIZED BY DISTINCTIVE CHROMOSOMAL FEATURES

Several autosomal recessive disorders are characterized by chromosomal breakage, in vivo and in vitro. Individuals with these abnormalities show growth retardation, various somatic anomalies and increased propensity for neoplasia. Bloom syndrome, ataxia teleangiectasia, and Fanconi anemia are examples. In those disorders in which the precise molecular defect is not known, distinctive cytogenetic features still permit antenatal diagnosis.

The "fragile X" syndrome is an X-linked disorder characterized by mental retardation, prognathism, and macroorchidism. The syndrome accounts for a significant proportion of familial X-linked mental retardation. However, the condition is not well understood. Some males carrying the mutant are affected and heterozygous females may sometimes be retarded. The gene responsible for the fragile X syndrome is linked or identical to a "fragile site," a staining gap on the long arm of the X chromosome (Xq27).

C. GENODERMATOSIS AND OTHER DISORDERS DETECTABLE ONLY BY TISSUE SAMPLING (BLOOD, SKIN, LIVER)

If a gene causing a given disorder is expressed in neither amniotic fluid nor chorionic villi, analysis of such tissues will provide no information concerning presence or absence of the disorder. However, the gene might still be expressed in other tissues—blood alone, skin alone, or liver alone. Such tissues can be obtained through fetoscopic or other ultrasound-directed sampling. Unfortunately, the likelihood of abortion following these invasive procedures is at least one to three percent over the background loss rate thus, (the total absolute loss rate is perhaps five-six percent).[25] Despite these high risks, the severity of some disorders may justify tissue sampling if no other diagnostic method is available.

Initial experience in blood sampling was obtained in the diagnosis of hemo-globinopathies. In sickle cell anemia, β-thalassemia, ∂-thalassemia, and a few other hematologic disorders, the derangement is limited to a single tissue, erythrocyte. Prior to the availability of molecular techniques (see *D*, below), antenatal diagnosis of hemoglobinopathies required fetal blood obtained by fetoscopy. In some countries fetoscopic blood sampling is still used for the diagnosis of β-thalassemia. Disorders once diagnosable only by analysis of fetal sera, namely hemophilia A, are also now detectable through molecular techniques. Again, the clinical significance of molecular diagnosis is that such tests can utilize amniotic fluid cells or chorionic villi. Fetal blood is not required. However, some parents have uninformative restriction fragment length polymorphisms (RFLP), thus necessitating analysis of fetal blood. In such cases, needle aspiration under concurrent high-quality ultra-sound guidance can allow blood to be obtained with less trauma than previously possible.

Obtaining fetal liver was originally necessary for detection of urea cycle defects, such as ornithine transcarbamylase (OTC) deficiency.[26] Molecular tech-niques now allow detection of OTC deficiency, replacing liver biopsy in most cases.

Sampling fetal skin allowed diagnosis of dermatologic abnormalities, such as epidermolysis bullosa and congenital ichthyosis (harlequin ichthyosis). Auto-somal dominant and X-linked recessive forms of each condition exist, but it is usually the autosomal recessive forms that warrant antenatal diagnosis. The meta-bolic basis of these disorders is unknown, and the gene locations are often not known; thus, antenatal detection is currently possible through histologic and elec-tron-microscope analysis of fetal skin biopsies. Our group utilizes ultrasound-directed biopsy without introducing a fetoscope for direct visualization.

D. DIAGNOSIS DETECTABLE BY MOLECULAR TECHNIQUES

Prenatal diagnosis by molecular techniques has several advantages. The most obvious advantage is that all cells contain the same DNA. Thus, any available nucleated cells (villi, amniotic fluid) would allow prenatal diagnosis by DNA analysis. That is, the gene sought need not be expressed in villi or amniotic fluid, unlike the situation when a gene product (protein) is being analyzed. Thus, one need not obtain fetal blood to detect hemoglobinopathies; villi or amniotic fluid will suffice.

1. General Principle of DNA Analysis Within the past decade, several important analytic techniques have been developed. Pivotal was the discovery of restriction endonucleases, bacterial enzymes that recognize specific nucleotide se-quences and cut DNA at those sequences. For example, the restriction enzyme Pvu II recognizes the following sequences of nucleotides: cytosine, adenine, guanine, cytosine, thymine, guanine (CAGCTG). Pvu II will cut DNA wherever the se-quence CAGCTG exists, and at no other site (Figure 3). Many different restriction enzymes are known, each recognizing a specific and often unique sequence of base pairs.

Restriction enzymes permit DNA to be divided into fragments whose lengths are reproducible from experiment to experiment. Analysis of the DNA fragments is accomplished using a labeled single-stranded gene probe.

2. Diagnosis When the Molecular Basis is Known For disorders characterized by absence of DNA, one can determine whether a probe able to recognize (hybridize to) a normal sequence of DNA will recognize the DNA from an individual of unknown genotype. Failure of hybridization indicates that the individual lacks the DNA sequence in question; thus, the disorder must be present. This approach can be used for all forms of ∂-thalassemia, for 50 percent of Duchenne muscular dystrophy, for a few forms of hemophilia, and for a few forms of β-thalassemia.

If the nucleotide sequence responsible for a point mutation is known, another approach becomes applicable. In sickle cell anemia, the triplet (codon) designating the sixth amino acid has undergone a change from the nucleotide adenine to thymine. As result, codon No. 6 now signifies valine rather than glutamic acid, leading to an abnormal protein, B^S. There exist restriction enzymes capable of recognizing the normal DNA sequence at codon 6. Such enzymes would not, however, recognize the mutant sequence because it would differ from the normal. Altering the normal sequence thus results in loss of a restriction site for certain enzymes. The pattern of DNA fragments will thus differ in B^A and B^S for such enzymes. Use of a B-globin probe can readily demonstrate differences in sickle cell anemia and in some forms of β-thalassemia. Most cases of β-thalassemia require the study of restriction fragment length polymorphisms (RFLPs).

A variant of the direct approach involves construction of probes that hybridize only to a specific sequence of nucleotides. Oligonucleotide synthetic probes are designed to hybridize, if and only if, the (complementary) DNA of the individual to be tested contains every single nucleotide in its correct sequence. If even one nucleotide is absent or altered (i.e., as result of a point mutation as in sickle cell anemia), the oligonucleotide probe will fail to hybridize.

3. Diagnosis When Molecular Basis is Not Known The direct approaches described above are applicable only when the precise molecular basis of a disorder is known. This criterion is presently fulfilled by only a few diseases. However, prenatal diagnosis may still be possible by taking advantage of the ostensibly innocuous differences in DNA that exist among different individuals in the general population. These differences, termed, *restriction fragment length polymorphism* (RFLPs), allow linkage analysis to be applied for prenatal diagnosis.

All individuals contain repetitive DNA sequences, DNA not coding for protein and thus lacking ostensible functional significance. As an example, a noncoding sequence of 500 to 1000 base pairs may be present (inserted) in some but not other individuals. These ostensibly innocuous DNA differences can be recognized through the analytic techniques already described. Loss of a given restriction site through alteration or loss of DNA might result in a relatively longer fragment than otherwise existing, whereas addition of a new restriction site might result in a shorter fragment. These DNA differences, which occur normally among individuals, are termed, *restriction fragment length polymorphisms* (RFLPs). (A polymorphism is defined as existence of more than one allele at a given locus, the minority allele being relatively frequent i.e., present in at least one percent of the population). An example of a blood group polymorphism involves the ABO locus with alleles A, B and O.

The inheritance of RFLPs can be traced in a given family, the differing patterns being inherited as co-dominant alleles. Suppose a given RFLP lies close to or preferably within the mutant gene of interest. The principles of linkage analysis can then be used to deduce presence or absence of the mutant gene. That is, one can test for the presence or absence of a "marker," in this case the RFLP. The status of the mutant is inferred indirectly by the status of the marker, even though the two are functionally quite independent. (Figure 5)

There are limitations in RFLP analysis. Although the nature of the mutant gene need not be known, its distance from the RFLP must be known because the likelihood of recombination is inversely related to accuracy of diagnosis. To understand this limitation, let us recall meiosis during meiosis I, recombination can occur between homologous chromosomes. Genes are linked to one another if, after meiosis I, they remain together more often than expected by chance. That is, genes are linked if they segregate to the same gamete more often than segregating to complementary gametes. Distance between loci can be determined by calculating the frequency with which genes on the same chromosome become interchanged (recombine) during meiosis I. If genes at different loci remain on the same parental chromosome with a frequency of 90 percent, they are said to be ten centimorgans (cM) apart. If genes remain together with a frequency of only 50 percent, one cannot distinguish loose linkage from absence of linkage (i.e., presence of genes on different chromosomes). However, recombination can occur even between closely linked loci; thus, prenatal diagnosis based on linkage analysis is never 100 percent accurate. Using RFLPs or other polymorphic markers on both sides of the mutant can, however, allow recombination to be recognized.

Another limitation of RFLP analysis for prenatal diagnosis is the possibility that an informative RFLP may not exist in a given family. Unaffected individuals should be distinguishable unequivocally from affected individuals. If all family members show the same DNA fragment pattern, that particular RFLP is useless because affected and unaffected individuals show identical patterns. Other RFLPs must then be sought. A further problem arises if DNA of the proband is unavailable (e.g., deceased), in which case the cis-trans relationship between the mutant gene and a given RFLP pattern cannot be deduced.

Despite these caveats, RFLP analysis permits prenatal diagnosis of many disorders not heretofore detectable. Furthermore, linkage analysis is becoming increasingly useful because potentially limitless number of RFLPs exist. Furthermore, their identification is becoming easier, as a more complete map of the human genome is developed.

Using RFLPs, prenatal diagnosis should eventually be possible for all common Mendelian disorders. Autosomal dominant and X-linked recessive traits prove especially easy to diagnose. Still the extent of linkage remains to be established for some probes, and the percentage of families in whom a given RFLP will be informative will vary. Nonetheless, Huntington chorea, Duchenne muscular dystrophy, hemophilia A and B, phenylketonuria, cystic fibrosis, β-thalassemia, and adult-onset polycystic kidney disease are already among the detectable disorders. Details about diagnosis of these disorders is discussed elsewhere.[1].

V. PRENATAL DIAGNOSIS AND GENETIC SCREENING FOR POLYGENIC/MULTIFACTORIAL DISORDERS

A. NEURAL TUBE DEFECTS, AND ALPHA-FETO PROTEIN

Failure of neural tube closure during embryogenesis leads to anencephaly, spina bifida (myelomeningocele or meningocele), and other less common midline defects, such as encephalocele. Anencephaly is not compatible with long-term survival. Spina bifida is compatible, albeit frequently leading to hemiparesis, urinary incontinence, and sometimes hydrocephalus.

Anencephaly and spina bifida represent different manifestations of the same pathogenic process; thus, couples who have had a child with any type of neural tube defect (NTD) incur approximately one percent risk for subsequent offspring having spina bifida and one percent for anencephaly.[27]. This holds true irrespective of the type of NTD present in the index case (proband). Second-degree relatives (nieces, nephews, grandchildren) and third-degree relatives (first cousins) are less likely to be affected. However, the risk of NTD in first cousins of affected individuals seems to be increased over that of the general population, more than for most polygenic/multifactorial traits. A woman whose sister had a child with NTD carries a 0.5 to 1.0 percent risk for NTD offspring.[27]

1. Amniotic Fluid Alpha-Feto Protein Analysis Antenatal diagnosis of NTD can theoretically be accomplished by either high-quality ultrasound or assay of amniotic fluid alpha feto-protein (AFP). Ultrasonography by experienced physicians should readily exclude anencephaly, and spina bifida can be detected by serial views of the vertebral column and third ventricle. Unfortunately, few centers can state their own sensitivity or specificity, essential components of genetic testing and counseling. Unless such figures are available in a given center, analysis of amniotic fluid AFP (AF-AFP) levels should be considered the standard method for detecting NTD. Through AF-AFP analysis, a diagnosis of NTD is possible in all except the five percent of spina bifida cases in which skin covers the lesion. Meticulous ultrasonographic study may or may not detect such lesions. Irrespective, we recommend both amniocentesis and ultrasound in couples having at least a two percent risk of NTD.

Amniotic fluid AFP may be spuriously elevated if the amniotic fluid is contaminated with fetal blood. However, this pitfall can be eliminated if amniotic fluid acetylcholinesterase (AChE) is assayed simultaneously. (Acetycholinesterase is normally not detectable in amniotic fluid.) Presence of AChE verifies that elevated AFP is due to NTD or other fetal defect. If fetal hemoglobin is present but AChE is absent, the elevated AFP can be deduced to be due to either presence of fetal blood or to an anomaly other than NTD.

Elevated AFP is also associated with other polygenic/multifactorial anomalies (e.g., omphalocele, cystic hygroma) and with certain Mendelian traits (e.g., congenital nephrosis). In these disorders, AChE may or may not be elevated. Ultrasonographic studies should therefore be undertaken to corroborate an abnormal AFP result and to determine the nature of any defect present. On the other hand, failure to detect an anomaly by ultrasound does not indicate that elevated amniotic fluid AFP was spurious. A subtle anomaly may still exist. If amniotic fluid AFP is elevated and ACE is present, we would consider the fetus to be abnormal irrespective of ultrasound findings.

2. Maternal Serum Alpha Feto Protein (MSAFP) Screening Relatively few (five percent) NTDs occur in families having a previously affected offspring. Thus, a method other than family history is needed to identify couples in the general population who are at risk for NTD. Maternal serum AFP elevations serve this purpose, identifying couples at sufficient risk to justify amniocentesis.

Maternal serum alpha feto-protein (MSAFP) is elevated typically greater than 2.5 multiples of the median (MOM), in 80 to 90 percent of pregnancies in which the fetus has a NTD. However, considerable overlap exists between MSAFP in normal pregnancies and MSAFP in pregnancies characterized by a fetus with NTD. Thus, protocols for determining the explanation for a single elevated MSAFP value NTD are needed. Specifically, elevated MSAFP occurs for the following reasons: (1) under-estimation of gestational age, inasmuch as MSAFP increases as gestation progresses (Figure 6); (2) multiple gestation, 60 percent of twins and almost all triplets showing an elevated value; (3) threatened abortion, presumably due to fetal blood extravasting into the maternal circulation; (4) Rh disease and other conditions associated with fetal edema; (5) anomalies other than NTD generally characterized by edema or skin defects; and (6) fetal demise.

Maximum accuracy of MSAFP screening requires that the initial assay be performed at 15 to 18 weeks gestation. Corrections for maternal weight are necessary, using various algorithms (Table 7). Some groups also correct for race. At the University of Tennessee, Memphis, we pursue weight-adjusted MSAFP values of 2.5 MOM or greater in the general population. We follow-up values of 2.0 MOM in women with insulin-dependent diabetes mellitus. Conversely, in twin gestations, MSAFP is considered abnormal only if 4.5 MOM or greater. If MSAFP lies between 2.50 and 2.99 MOM, and if gestational age is 18 weeks or less, we perform a second MSAFP sample one week after the initial sample. If the second value is also elevated, ultrasound is necessary in order to exclude erroneous gestational age, multiple gestations, or fetal demise. After a single elevated value, many centers go directly to ultrasound. Indeed, at the University of Tennessee, Memphis, we do not obtain a second sample if the initial MSAFP is greater than 3.0 MOM or obtained after 18 weeks gestation. Irrespective, amniocentesis for amniotic fluid AFP and AChE is necessary if no explanation for elevated MSAFP is evident at ultrasound.

MSAFP programs identify about 90 percent of anencephaly and 80 percent of spina bifida, albeit at the cost of one-two percent of all pregnant women undergoing amniocentesis. Of approximately 15 women having a single elevated serum AFP, only one will prove to have a fetus with NTD. If gestational age assessment is vigorously pursued before MSAFP sampling, the number of women undergoing amniocentesis is lower.[28]

Observations of great potential importance to MCH are studies showing that women with MSAFP elevations whose fetuses do *not* have a NTD may be at increased risk for other obstetric complications: intrauterine growth retardation (IUGR), fetal demise, and placental abruption. The predictive value of this association is being investigated. Conversely, we have alluded previously to the relationship of MSAFP to autosomal trisomy. We correctly follow-up weight-adjusted MSAFP less than 0.4 MOM.

3. Legal Status of MSAFP Screening MSAFP programs are increasingly being initiated in the U.S.[29] Again, screening should always be voluntary, with patients informed about the benefits and risks of testing. Since the 1983 U. S. Food and Drug Administration (FDA) approval of test kits for serum AFP reagents, it is becoming prudent for obstetricians to inform their patients of the availability of MSAFP screening. Indeed, we believe that MSAFP screening will soon be considered standard. Before initiating a screening program, however, one must ensure the availability of laboratory, ultrasound, and counseling.[29] All this will be necessary to reassure women initially having one or more elevated MSAFP values but later having normal tests.

B. DISORDERS DETECTABLE ONLY BY ULTRASOUND

Defects inherited in polygenic/multifactorial fashion usually carry recurrence risks of one to five percent for first-degree relatives (sibs, offspring, parent).

Traits inherited in polygenic/multifactorial fashion include most of the common anatomic defects limited either to one organ system or to a single embryologically related system (Table 1). Because the number of genes responsible for these defects is unknown, diagnosis by enzyme assays or even linkage analysis cannot seriously be proposed at the present time.

The only remaining method of assessment is visualization of fetal anatomy. Of course, fetal visualization is also useful for certain Mendelian disorders, e.g., autosomal recessive polycystic kidney disease, X-linked recessive aqueductal stenosis (hydrocephaly), and various skeletal dysplasias.

Ultrasonography, fetoscopy, and roentgenography have, in the past, all been employed for fetal visualization; however, ultrasound is now the primary modality for visualization. The typical couple at risk previously had a child with the anomaly in question, thus incurring a one to five percent risk for another affected child. In order to alter clinical management, defects should be detectable by 20 to 24 weeks gestation. This is sufficiently early for the alternative reproductive options of termination, fetal surgery, or preterm delivery followed by neonatal surgery. (Percutaneous uterine blood sampling or transabdominal chorionic villus sampling to exclude chromosomal abnormalities would be appropriate prior to either of the latter two options.)

Some conditions—hydrocephaly, NTDs, omphalocele, renal, and bladder anomalies—are more readily detectable than others. Detection of certain cardiac anomalies is more difficult, often requiring echographic studies. Gastrointestinal obstructions, such as duodenal atresia, are often difficult to detect prior to the third trimester. In many centers, diagnosis of fetal sex is offered with some success. However, chromosomal analysis should still be used if fetal sexing is truly important, as in X-linked recessive traits. Similarly, certain infants with Down syndrome can be detected on the basis of nuchal pads and shortened femur [30]; however, chromosomal analysis by amniocentesis should not be eschewed in favor of ultrasound in women having a traditional indication for cytogenetic studies (third aspect). Finally, it seems hazardous to render a diagnosis on the basis of assessing fetal motion, as might be attempted in arthrogryoposis with multiple flexion contractures.

As mentioned previously, antenatal ultrasonography for anomaly detection should be performed only by highly experienced physicians. Brief examinations by primary providers should not be used to derive information regarding presence or absence of anomalies. In fact, clinics or physicians scanning obstetrical patients for fetal viability, presence or absence of twins, and placental location should explicitly inform their patients that no attempt at anomaly assessment is being made.

Information on a given unit's sensitivity and specificity ideally should be communicated to patients. Unfortunately, determining the predictive value of ultrasonography for anomaly detection is difficult. Even the definitions of "correct" and "incorrect" diagnosis are uniform. How should one classify cases in which the anomaly was not evident on second-trimester examinations, but did become evident in the third trimester? Does this represent a diagnostic error, or merely reflect the natural developmental process? In addition, outcome data will be altered by choice of equipment, befitting an evolving technology. A 1982-1985 study by our group revealed the predictive values of a normal and abnormal ultrasound finding for anomaly detection to be 90 percent and 99 percent, respectively.[31] A similar study conducted in 1988 may or may not show similar results.

TABLE 1
POLYGENIC/MULTIFACTORIAL TRAITS

Neural tube defects
(anencephaly, spina bifida, encephalocele)

Hydrocephaly (excepting some cases
of acqueductal stenosis and some
cases of Dandy-Walker syndrome)

Cleft lip, with or without cleft palate

Cleft lip (alone)

Cardiac defects (most types)

Diaphragmatic hernia

Omphalocele

Renal agenesis

Ureteral anomalies

Hypospadias

Posterior urethral values

Uterine (mullerian fusion) defects

Hip dislocation

Limb reduction defects

Talipes equinovarus (clubfoot)

TABLE 2
PROVEN HUMAN TERATOGENS

Chemotherapeutic agents
Folic acid antagonists (methotrexate, aminopterin)
Antimetabolites (5-fluorouracil)
Alkylating agents (busulfan)

Antibiotics
Tetracycline (after 20 weeks)
Amnioglycosides and streptomycin
(VIII nerve damage)

Anticonvulsants
Hydantoins
Valproic acid
Trimethadione

Coumarin

Lithium

Thalidomide

Androgens and selected progestins
(Virilization of females fetuses at high dose)
Danazol
Methyltetosteone
Norethindrone

Vitamin A cogeners and excess vitamin A
Isoretinoin
Etretinate

Alcohol (High and probably moderate doses)

Polychorinated biphenyls

Methyl mercury

TABLE 3
CHROMOSOMAL ABNORMALITIES IN LIVEBORNS*

Maternal Age	Risk for Down Syndrome	Total Risk for Chromosomal Abnormalities**
20	1/1667	1/526
21	1/1667	1/526
22	1/1429	1/500
23	1/1429	1/500
24	1/1250	1/476
25	1/1250	1/476
26	1/1176	1/476
27	1/111	1/455
28	1/1053	1/435
29	1/1000	1/417
30	1/952	1/385
31	1/952	1/385
32	1/769	1/322
33	1/602	1/286
34	1/485	1/238
35	1/378	1/192
36	1/289	1/156
37	1/224	1/127
38	1/173	1/102
39	1/136	1/83
40	1/106	1/66
41	1/82	1/53
42	1/63	1/42
43	1/49	1/33
44	1/38	1/26
45	1/30	1/21
46	1/23	1/16
47	1/18	1/13
48	1/14	1/10
49	1/11	1/8

*   Because sample size for some intervals is relatively small, 95% confidence limits are sometimes relatively large. Nonetheless, these figures are suit able for genetic counseling.

**   47,XXX excluded for ages 20-32 (data not available) Modified from the following sources: Hook EB, Cross PK, JAMA 249:2034, 1983; Hook EB: Obstet Gynecol 58:282, 1981.

TABLE 4

QUESTIONNAIRE FOR IDENTIFYING COUPLES
HAVING INCREASED RISK FOR OFFSPRING WITH GENETIC DISORDERS

From American College of Obstetricians and Gynecologists Technical Bulletin
Number 108, September,1987; Antenatal Diagnosis of Genetic Disorders, ACOG, Washington, D.C.

SAMPLE PRENATAL GENETIC SCREEN*

Name_____ Patient # _____ Date_____

1. Will you be 35 years or older when the baby is due?   Yes __ No __
2. Have you, the baby's father or anyone in either of your families ever had any of
   the following disorders?
   . Down syndrome (mongolism)   Yes __ No __
   . Other chromosomal abnormality   Yes __ No __
   . Neural tube defect, i.e., spina bifida (meningomyelocele oropen spine),
     anencephaly   Yes __ No __
   . Hemophilia   Yes __ No __
   . Muscular dystrophy   Yes __ No __
   . Cystic fibrosis   Yes __ No __
   If yes, indicate the relationship of the affected person to you or to the
   baby's father:_____
3. Do you or the baby's father have a birth defect?   Yes __ No __
   If yes, who has the defect and what is it?_____
4. In any previous marriages, have you or the baby's father had a child, born
   dead or alive, with a birth defect not listed in question 2 above?   Yes __ No __
5. Do you or the baby's father have any close relatives with mental retardation?   Yes __ No __
   If yes, indicate the relationship of the affected person to you or to the
   baby's father:_____
   Indicate the cause, if known: _____
6. Do you, the baby's father, or a close relative in either of your families have a birth defect,
   any familial disorder, or a chromosomal abnormality not listed above?   Yes __ No __
   If yes, indicate the condition and the relationship of the affected person to you or to the
   baby'sfather: _____
7. In any previous marriages, have you or the baby's father had a stillborn child or three or more
   first-trimester spontaneous pregnancy losses?   Yes __ No __
   Have either of you had a chromosomal study?   Yes __ No __
8. If you or the baby's father are of Jewish ancestry, have either or you been
   screened for Tay-Sachs disease?   Yes __ No __
   If yes, indicate who and the results: _____
9. If you or the baby's father are Black, have either of you been screened for
   sickle cell trait?   Yes __ No __
   If yes, indicate who and the results: _____
10. If you or the baby's father are Italian, Greek or Mediterranean background,
    have either of you been tested for β-thalassemia?   Yes __ No __
    If yes, indicate who and the results: _____
11. If you or the baby's father are of Philippine or Southeast Asian ancestry, have
    either of you been tested for ∂-thalassemia?   Yes __ No __
    If yes, indicate who and the results:_____
12. Excluding iron and vitamins, have you taken any medications or recreational
    drugs since being pregnant or since your last menstrual period? (include non-
    prescription drugs)   Yes __ No __
    If yes, give name of medication and time taken during pregnancy: _____

Any replying "YES" to question should be offered appropriate counseling. If the patient declines
further counseling or testing, this should be noted in the chart. Given that genetics is a field in
a state of flux, alterations or updates to this form will be required periodically.

TABLE 5

PREREQUISITES FOR GENETIC SCREENING

▸ Capacity to alter clinical management of affected individuals
▸ Ability to identify matings of two heterozygotes, provided reproductive options are possible
▸ Cost Effective
▸ Reliable Methods of Assessment of Genetic Status
  • Reproducible Assay
▸ Capacity to Handle Ancillary Problems
  • Variants not requiring action
  • Potential stigmitization of heterozygotes

TABLE 6

PRENATAL GENETIC SCREENING

Ethnic Group	Disorder	Initial Screening Test(noninvasive)	Definitive Tests Screening Test
Ashkenazi Jews	Tay-Sachs Disease	Decreased serum hexosamidase-A	Chorionic villus sampling (CVS) or amniocentesis for assay of hexosamidase-A
Black	Sickle cell anemia	Presence of sickle cell hemoglobin, confirmatory hemoglobin electrophoresis	CVS or amniocenetesis for determination genotype (direct molecular studies)
Greeks, Italians Mediterrean	β-thalassemia	Mean corpuscular volume (MCV) <80%, followed by hemoglobin electrophoresis	CVS or amniocentesis for determination genotype (direct molecular studies or indirect RFLP snalysis)
Southeast Asians (Vietnamese, Laotian Cambodian): Phillipinos	∂-thalassemia	MCV <80%, followed by hemoglobin electorphoresis	CVS or amniocentesis for determination genetic (direct molecular studies)
All ethnic groups: Maternal age over 35 years (EDC)	All numerical chromosomal abnormalities	CVS or amniocentesis for cytogenetic analysis	
All ethnic groups:	Elevated MSAFP (maternal serum alpha-fetoprotein)	Amiocentesis for assays of amniotic fluid (AFP) and acetylcholinesterase, if no explanation found for elevated MSAFP	

TABLE 7

RELATIONSHIP OF MATERNAL WEIGHT TO MSAFP (MOM)
ILLUSTRATIVE STUDIED AT THE UNIVERSITY OF TENNESSEE, MEMPHIS
WEIGHT IS DETERMINED AT THE TIME MSAFP SAMPLE IS DRAWN.

Patient Weight (lbs)	MSAFP ng/ml	Unadjusted MOM	Adjusted MOM
91*	115.8	3.01	2.56
119	82.6	2.58	2.44
206	15.8	0.41	0.59
285**	75.1	1.96	5.35

*   Amniotic fluid alpha-fetoprotein within normal range; normal infant subsequently delivered.
** Fetus with spina bifida

FIGURE 1

OUTCOME OF ONE GENETIC QUESTIONNAIRE,
DISTRIBUTED BY THE AUTHOR [7] IN AN EARLIER STUDY

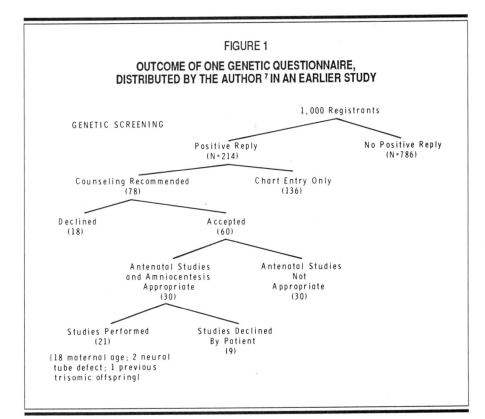

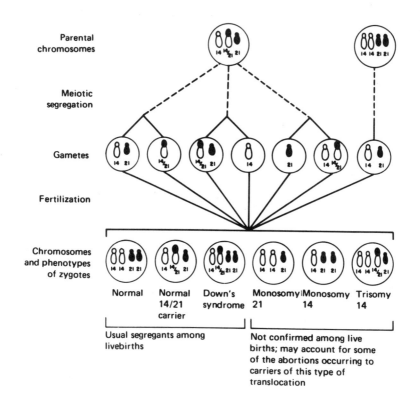

FIGURE 2

POSSIBLE GAMETES AND PROGENY OF A PHENOTYPICALLY
NORMAL INDIVIDUAL HETEROZYGOUS FOR A ROBERTSONION
TRANSLOCATION BETWEEN CHROMOSOMES 14 AND 21

Three of the six possible gametes are incompatible with life. The likelihood
that an individual with such a translocation would have a child with Down syndrome
is theoretically 33%. However, the empirical risk is considerably less.

Gerbie A, Simpson JL. Antenatal detection of genetic disorders. Postgrad Med J 59 (6): 129,
1976

FIGURE 3

THE MANNER IN WHICH A RESTRICTION ENDONUCLEASE CUTS DNAAT A SPECIFIC NUCLEOTIDE SEQUENCE.

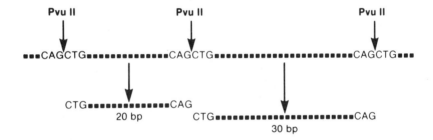

Pvu II recognizes sequence CAGCTG, and only that sequence. DNA is separated into fragments of different lengths on the basis of distances between restriction enzyme recognition sites. The greater the distance between sites, the longer the length of intervening DNA. Shorter DNA fragments (eg. 20 base pairs, bp) show greater mobility and migrate farther in an agarose gel.

Gerbie A, Simpson JL (eds). Obstetrics: Normal and Problem Pregnancies. New York, Churchill-Livingstone, 1986.

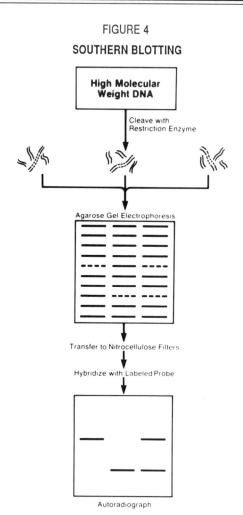

FIGURE 4

SOUTHERN BLOTTING

DNA is cleaved with restriction enzymes, and then separated by size by using agarose gel electrophoresis. The gel is laid onto a piece of nitrocellulose filter paper, and buffer allowed to flow through the gel onto the filter paper. DNA fragments also migrate out of the gel and bind to the filter paper. A replica of the gel's and DNA fragment pattern is thus made on the paper, which can then be hybridized with a suitable radioactively labeled probe.

Gabbe SG, Niebyl JR, Simpson JL (eds). Obstetrics: Normal and Problem Pregnancies. Churchill Livingstone, New York, 1986.

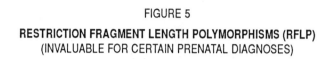

FIGURE 5

RESTRICTION FRAGMENT LENGTH POLYMORPHISMS (RFLP)
(INVALUABLE FOR CERTAIN PRENATAL DIAGNOSES)

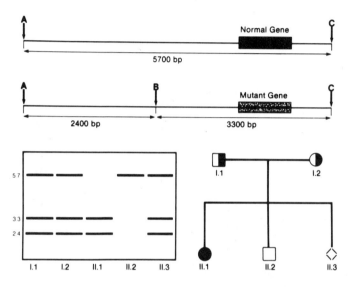

Suppose a mutant gene is linked to another gene (B) that governs whether or not a restriction site (B) is present. If the repetitive segment is present, DNA is cut by a certain restriction enzyme (arrow) to produce 3,300- and 2,400-bp fragments long. If the segment is not present, the total fragment is 5,700-bp long. The different lengths can function as markers to allow genotypes to be deduced.

Suppose two individuals (I.1 and I.2) have an affected child, demonstrating that each is an obligate heterozygote. Suppose further that a probe is available and characterized by ability to hybridize to the region from A to C. The probe can thus potentially identify three fragments (2,400-bp, 3,300-bp, 5,700-bp). If the affected child shows only the 2,400- and 3,300 bp fragments, it can be deduced that the mutant allele is in association, i.e., on the same chromosome, as the gene conferring restriction site B and thus producing both 2,400- and 3,300-bp fragments. The normal allele must then in each patient be in association with the allele not conferring restriction site B; thus it is designated by the 5,700-bp fragment. Genotypes can thus be predicted from DNA analysis of chorionic villi or amniotic fluid cells. Fetus II.3 can be assumed to be heterozygous because all three fragments are present.

Gabbe SG, Niebyl JR, Simpson JL (eds). Obstetrics: Normal and Problem Pregnancies. Churchill Livingstone, New York, 1986.

FIGURE 6

MEDIAN MATERNAL SERUM α-FETOPROTEIN (MSAFP) THROUGHOUT GESTATION

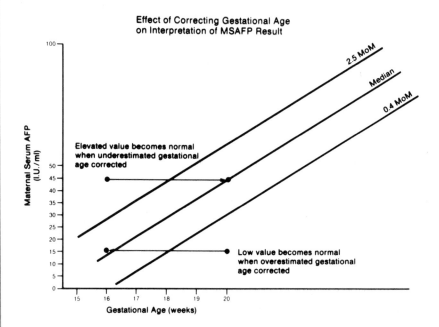

Increasing values with increasing gestational age require accurate dating to interpret low or high MSAFP.

Gerbie A, Simpson JL (eds). Obstetrics: Normal and Problem Pregnancies. Churchill-Livingstone, New York, 1986.

REFERENCES

1. Simpson JL, Elias S. Prenatal Diagnosis : Maternal-Fetal Medicine, 2nd Edition. Edited by Creasy TN, Resnik R. W.B.Saunders Philadelphia. In Press, 1988.

2. Simpson JL, Elias S, Martin AO. Parental chromosomal rearrangements associated with repetitive spontaneous abortions. Fertil Steril 36:584, 1981.

3. Carson SA, Simpson JL. Spontaneous Abortion (In) Fetal Assessment: Physiological, Clinical and Medico-Legal Principles, (R. Eden, F. Boehm, eds), New York, Appleton-Century-Croft, In Press.

4. Simpson JL, Golbus MS, Martin AO, et al. Genetics in Obstetrics and Gynecology. Grune and Stratton, New York, 1982.

5. Sever JL, Brent RL. Teratogen Update. Environmentally Induced Birth Defects Risks. New York, Liss, 1986.

6. American College Obstetricians and Gynecologists: Technical Bulletin Number 108, September 1987: Antenatal Diagnosis of Genetic Disorders. ACOG, Washington, 1987.

7. Simpson JL, Elias S, Gatlin M, et al. Genetic counselling and genetic services in obstetrics and gynecology. Am J Obstet Gynecol 140:70, 1981.

8. National Academy of Sciences, Genetic Screening: Programs, Principles and Research, Washington, DC, National Academy of Sciences, 1975.

9. Andrews LB. State laws and regulations governing newborn screening. Chicago, American Bar Association, 1986.

10. Simpson JL. Predictions for the foreseeable future. Cont Ob/Gyn , In Press, 1988.

11. Simpson JL, Mills JL, Holmes LB, et al. Low fetal loss rates after ultrasound-proved viability in pregnancy. JAMA 258:2555, 1987.

12. Hook EB. Rates of chromosome abnormalities at different maternal ages. Obstet Gynecol 58:282, 1981.

13. Hook EB, Cross PK, Schreinemachers DM. Chromosomal abnormality rates at amniocentesis and in liveborn infants. JAMA 249:2034, 1983.

14. Hook EB. Chromosome abnormalities and spontaneous fetal death following amniocentesis: Further data and association with maternal age. Am J Hum Genet 35:110, 1983.

15. Hook EB, Cross PK, Jackson LG, et al. Rates of 47,+21 and other cytogenetic abnormalities diagnosed in 1st trimester chorionic villus samples (CVS): Comparison with rates from 2nd trimester amniocentesis. Am J Hum Genet 41:A276, 1987.

16. Kuleshov NP. Chromosomal anomalies in infants dying during the perinatal period and premature newborn. Hum Genet 31:151, 1976.

17. Simpson JL, Bombard AT. Chromosomal abnormalities in spontaneous abortions: Frequency, pathology and genetic counselling. Spontaneous Abortion. Edited by Edmonds K, Bennet MJ. Blackwell Scientific Publications, London, pp. 51, 1987.

18. DiMaio MS, Baumgarten A, Greenstein RM, et al. Screening for fetal Down's syndrome in pregnancy by measuring maternal serum alpha-fetoprotein levels. N Engl J Med 317:342, 1987.

19. Daniel A, Boue' A, Gallano P. Prospective risk in reciprocal translocation heterozygotes in amniocentesis as determined by potential chromosome imbalance sizes. Data of European Collaborative Prenatal Diagnosis Centres. Pren Diagn 6:315, 1986.

20. Boue A, Gallano PA. Collaborative study of segregation of inherited chromosome structural rearrangements in 1356 prenatal diagnoses. Pren Diagn (special issue) 4:45, 1984.

21. Nyhan WL, Sakati NO. Diagnostic recognition of genetic disease. Lea & Febiger, Philadelphia, 1987.

22. Poenaru L. First trimester prenatal diagnosis of metabolic diseases: A survey in countries from the European community. Prenat Diagn 7:333, 1987.

23. Shapiro LR, Wilmot PL, Murphy PD, et al. Multiple approaches to the prenatal diagnosis of the fragile X syndrome: Amniotic fluid chorionic villi, fetal blood and molecular methods. Am J Hum Genet 41:A285, 1987.

24. Oberle I, Mandel JL, Boue J, et al. Polymorphic DNA markers in prenatal diagnosis of fragile X syndrome. Lancet 1:871, 1985.

25. Elias S. Easterly N. Prenatal diagnosis of hereditary skin disorders. Clin Obstet Gynecol 24:1069, 1981.

26. Rodeck CH, Patrick AD, Pembry ME, et al: Fetal liver biopsy for prenatal diagnosis of ornithine carbamyltransferase deficiency. Lancet 2:297, 1982.

27. Milunsky A. The prenatal diagnosis of neural tube and other congenital defects. (In) Genetic Disorders and the Fetus, 2nd Edition, Plenum Press, New York, 1986, pp. 453-519.

28. Simpson JL, Baum LD, Marder, et al. Maternal serum alpha-fetoprotein (MSAFP) screening: Low and high values for detection of genetic abnormalities. Am J Obstet Gynecol 155:593, 1986.

29. Simpson JL, Nadler HL. Maternal serum alpha feto protein screening in 1987. Obstet Gynecol 69: 134, 1987.

30. Benacereff BR, Gelman R, Frigolitto FD. Sonographic identification of second trimester fetuses with Downs syndrome. N Engl J Med 317:1371, 1987.

31. Sabbagha RE, Sheikh Z, Tamura RK, et al. Predictive value, sensitivity, and specificity of ultrasonic targeted imaging for fetal anomalies in gravid women at high risk for birth defects. Am J Obstet Gynecol 152:822, 1985.

FOOTNOTES FOR FIGURES

Figure 1.   Outcome of one genetic questionnaire, distributed by the author[7] in an earlier study.

Figure 2.   Diagram of possible gametes and progeny of a phenotypically normal individual heterozygous for a Robertsonion translocation between chromosomes 14 and 21. Three of the six possible gametes are incompatible with life. The likelihood that an individual with such a translocation would have a child with Down syndrome is theoretically 33 percent. However, the empirical risk is considerably less. (Gerbie A, Simpson JL: Antenatal detection of genetic disorders. Postgrad Med J 59(6):129, 1976).

Figure 3.   Diagram illustrating the manner in which a restriction endonuclease cuts DNA at a specific nucleotide sequence. Pvu II recognizes sequence CAGCTG, and only that sequence. DNA is separated into fragments of different lengths on the basis of distances between restriction enzyme recognition sites. The greater the distance between sites, the longer the length of intervening DNA. Shorter DNA fragments (eg 20 base pairs, bp) show greater mobility and migrate farther in an agarose gel. From Gabbe SC, Niebyl JF, Simpson JL [eds]: Obstetrics: Normal and Problem Pregnancies. New York, Churchill-Livingstone, 1986.

Figure 4. Diagram illustrating Southern blotting. DNA is cleaved with restriction enzymes, and then separated by size by using agarose gel electrophoresis. The gel is laid onto a piece of nitrocellulose filter paper, and buffer allowed to flow through the gel onto the filter paper. DNA fragments also migrate out of the gel and bind to the filter paper. A replica of the gel's and DNA fragment pattern is thus made on the paper, which can then be hybridized with a suitable radioactively labeled probe. From Gabbe SC, Niebyl JF, Simpson JL [eds]: Obstetrics: Normal and Problem Pregnancies. New York, Churchill-Livingstone, 1986.

Figure 5. Restriction fragment length polymorphisms (RFLP), invaluable for certain prenatal diagnoses. Suppose a mutant gene is linked to another gene (B) that governs whether or not a restriction site (B) is present. If the repetitive segment is present, DNA is cut by a certain restriction enzyme (arrow) to produce 3,300 and 2,400-bp fragments long. If the segment is not present, the total fragment is 5,700 bp long. The different lengths can function as markers to allow genotypes to be deduced. Suppose two individuals (I.1 and I.2) have an affected child, demonstrating that each is an obligate heterozygote. Suppose further that a probe is available and characterized by ability to hybridize to the region from A to C. The probe can thus potentially identify three fragments (2,400 bp, 3,300 bp, 5,700 bp). If the affected child shows only the 2,400- and 3,300 bp fragments, it can be deduced that the mutant allele is in association, i.e., on the same chromosome, as the gene conferring restriction site B and thus producing both 2,400- and 3,300-bp fragments. The normal allele must then in each patient be in association with the allele not conferring restriction site B; thus it is designated by the 5,700-bp fragment. Genotypes can thus be predicted from DNA analysis of chorionic villi or amniotic fluid cells. Fetus II.3 can be assumed to be heterozygous because all three fragments are present. Gabbe SG, Niebyl JR, Simpson JL (eds). Obstetrics: Normal and Problem Pregnancies. Churchill Livingstone, New York, 1986.

Figure 6. Median maternal serum a-fetoprotein (MSAFP) throughout gestation. Increasing values with increasing gestational age require accurate dating to interpret low or high MSAFP. From Gabbe SG, Niebyl JR, Simpson JL (eds). Obstetrics: Normal and Problem Pregnancies. Churchill Livingstone, New York, 1986.

SPECIFIC FEDERAL PROGRAMS FOR IMPROVING REPRODUCTIVE HEALTH CARE: WHAT HAVE WE LEARNED? 26

Donald McNellis

INTRODUCTION

An important element in the development of publicly funded health services in the U.S. is the provision of prenatal, perinatal, and infant care to high-risk women of low-economic status and their children. Since 1963, the Maternity and Infant Care Program (MICP) has exemplified the commitment of both federal and state governments to improve MCH and reduce mortality and morbidity. A special administrative initiative, the Improved Pregnancy Outcome Program (IPOP), was begun by the federal Bureau of Maternal and Child Health, in 1976, to enable selected states with relatively high infant mortality to strengthen the planning and evaluation aspects of state MCH programs, while enhancing the utilization and effectiveness of perinatal regionalization for all mothers and infants in those states.

What were the essential features of these programs? What did they accomplish? What is their legacy, both in terms of the content of current programs, as well as implications for future programs?

LEGISLATIVE BACKGROUND OF MICP

The MICP originated in 1963, when the U.S. Children's Bureau moved from the Social Security Administration to the U.S. Department of Health, Education, and Welfare. The enabling legislation for the MICP's states their purpose: "To help reduce the incidence of mental retardation caused by complications associated with childbearing." [1] Expectant mothers who were at high risk for medical or other reasons, and who were not receiving appropriate care, were the intended beneficiaries of the MICP.

Prior to 1963, there had been substantial progress afforded by Title V of the Social Security Act. This Act established the basis for a cooperative federal-state MCH program, and the resulting improvements included professional standards, maternity clinics, direct payment for services, nutrition counseling, and home visits by public health nurses.

In 1974, the MICP was well enough established in most states that an administrative change was promulgated through regulations. The MICP, along with other elements of the "program of projects" (including Children and Youth, Neonatal Intensive Care, Family Planning, and Dental Health Projects), was subsequently to be a requirement for State Title V programs rather than a discretionary grant program of the federal MCH office, as had previously been the case. This modification translated into greater flexibility and control by states of federal MCH formula funds supplied to them under Title V. The Omnibus Reconciliation Act of 1981 is the most recent legislative event affecting the MICP. This Act expanded the states' control over the content and funding allocation for MICP and similar programs, while weakening the federal role in promoting the quality and effectiveness of health services for expectant mothers and their infants.

MICP CONTENT

The original MICP projects were located in areas with concentrations of low-income families. Thus, most, but not all, projects were located in cities. Projects offered preventive, diagnostic, and hospital services to women and infants in their service areas, as well as procedures to assure follow-up and continuity of care. An important assumption of MICP was that multidisciplinary staffing was required to provide the comprehensive services typically needed by the targeted populations. Patients received services from physicians, nurses, health educators, nutritionists, psychologists, medical social workers, and other professionals.

State-to-state variability in the content of services provided directly by the MICP has been the rule. Thus, while most state programs offered comprehensive prenatal care, some projects have provided intrapartum services, and others merely assured that they were available, and strove to maximize access to hospital services. Most projects appeared to provide postpartum follow-up maternal services, as well as infant care. Family planning services were usually provided to postpartum patients, or appropriate referral arranged.

MICP EVALUATION

It has been pointed out that relatively few of the State MICP projects have been systematically evaluated.[2] Many evaluations used before-and-after designs, and suggested some decrease in the perinatal or infant mortality rate, or some increase in the proportion of women receiving early or adequate care. However, Peoples and Siegel have suggested that these designs may have used control populations with characteristics different from the intervention population.[2] The evaluation of the Cleveland MICP project by Sokol, et al, employed close matching, with both groups receiving intrapartum and neonatal care in the same care system. Thus, the effect of MICP prenatal care could be tested in a more sophisticated way.[3] The MICP patients were found to have experienced a 60 percent lower perinatal mortality rate, although the analytic techniques did not include multivariate adjustments for specific differences between the comparison group.[2]

A recent evaluation of the MICP project in North Carolina examined its effect on the use of prenatal care and on the prevalence of low birthweight. Initial analysis of vital statistics data indicated minimal MICP effectiveness. However, a weighted least squares statistical procedure suggested a differential effect of the MICP according to maternal risk status. That is, the highest-risk mothers and infants benefitted the most. While this effect tends to support the targeting of the MICP in general, the authors explore alternative explanations for the observation. Such deliberations have important implications for the targeting and delivery of maternity and infant services in an era of budgetary constraint.

CURRENT STATUS OF MICP

In 1985, Wallace et al carried out a survey of MCH divisions of in all state health departments. [4] Its purposes were to assess the viability of MICP projects, to profile the services provided by the projects, to learn the reasons for changes in projects, and to determine the unmet needs for health services for mothers and infants. The survey was clearly occasioned by concern about the budgetary impact of the Omnibus Reconcilation Act of 1981 and the implementation of the MCH Block Grant program.

Of all MCH projects ever present in the responding states, two-thirds were still operational in 1985. The vast majority of discontinued projects went out of existence since 1980, with the modal year of termination being 1982.

A major finding was that most of the continuing projects still offered an essential set of maternal preventive and follow-up services, including prenatal and postpartum care, family planning, health education, nutrition, social services, and counseling. Ancillary services, such as outreach and parenting classes, were still provided by some projects, but were most likely to have been discontinued. Some services, such as transportation and nurse-midwifery, had never been provided by most of the projects.

The infant-care services provided by the projects appeared to have been curtailed more severely, with an absence of certain important services, such as well-child care, immunization, and developmental assessment in nearly half of the projects.

Wallace views the maintenace of comprehensive services within the MICP as evidence that state MCH divisions find the MICP approach to be effective in providing critical services to the high-risk and low-income population. In fact, the majority of MCH divisions indicated that MICP concepts, particularly the multidisciplinary "team" approach to antepartum and postpartum care, had been extended to other areas of the states. Finally, the majority of states reporting terminations of MICP projects cited federal funding as the primary reason. Thus, it is probable that maintenance of MICP projects has required innovative use of available state and federal funding.

Finally, the Wallace survey revealed that MCH divisions in the states still perceive significant needs for maternal, perinatal, and infant services, particularly regarding universal availability and accessibility of appropriate services, planning of services, and adolescent pregnancy care.

NATURE OF THE IMPROVED PREGNANCY OUTCOME PROGRAM (IPOP)

In the mid-1970s, the federal MCH Bureau developed IPOP as a special initiative in response to national concerns about infant mortality and morbidity rates. Specifically, the relative international standing of the U.S., the slow rates of decline nationally, and the marked discrepancies in rates between states, regions, and racial and social-economic groups, were interpreted as evidence of need of improved health services for mothers and infants.

States were selected for IPOP participation from a rank-order list based on infant mortality in 1973 and 1974, several components of infant mortality, plus the adolescent and total birth rates for 1975. Grants of up to $400,000 per year, for five consecutive years, were made to each of 34 states, including Puerto Rico and the District of Columbia, in three successive groups, as follows: FY 1977: 13 worst-ranking states; FY 1978: next 11 states; FY 1979: next 10 states. State participation was contingent on approval of an IPOP plan, which was to be an amendment to the state's MCH plan. The IPOP plan was required to promote the implementation of regionalized perinatal care, especially the preventive and follow-up aspects, but was permitted wide flexibility to allow responsiveness to local and state needs and ongoing initiatives. Whatever the IPOP activities designed by a state, it was required also to create an evaluation plan, and an evaluation manual was provided by the national MCH office, which presented evaluation methodology and a prototype plan. [5]

CONTEXTUAL BACKGROUND OF IPOP

In the late 1970s, there was a sudden increase in diagnostic capabilities and clinical management techniques available to neonatologists and, to a lesser extent, to obstetricians. When these enhanced approaches were applied by appropriately trained personnel in perinatal centers, it was becoming clear that pregnancy outcomes, especially for neonates, could be dramatically improved.[6] The organizational challenge of how to provide the best care appropriate to maternal or infant risk was addressed by a consortium of professional societies and the National Foundation/March of Dimes. The product of this collaboration was the document, *Toward Improving the Outcome of Pregnancy*, which propounded a regionalized system of tiered perinatal care, linked by outreach, transport, educational, and other necessary elements.[7] Almost concurrently, the Johnson Foundation funded a set of demonstration programs to determine the effectiveness of regional perinatal care. Important elements in a regional system included careful planning, screening, and referral to high-risk pregnancies and newborns, transportation and communication systems, designation of hospital for level of perinatal care provided, setting of standards for each level of care, and provider and public education. IPOP sought to promulgate such elements by mobilizing public health resources within states with excessive infant mortality.

SPECIFIC IPOP ACTIVITIES

One extensive survey, in 1983, found that the predominant activity of many state IPOP projects was strengthening the perinatal management system.[8] Hiring professional program staff at the state and regional levels to administer perinatal programs was a critical step. Improving the collection and analysis of perinatal data was a frequent activity, which then enabled better needs-based planning and tracking of services. Also, linkage of various perinatal services, through better transportation and communication systems, figured prominently in the management activities. Related activities commonly undertaken included advocacy groups, monitoring quality of care, and promoting favorable state legislation and funding.

In general, however, demonstration service delivery projects and consumer education programs were not extensively emphasized.[8]

EVALUATION OF IPOP

Each yearly group of IPO states experienced a statistically significant decline in infant mortality, both since 1976 and over their respective funding periods. Moreover, each IPOP group showed a rate of decline in infant mortality rate through 1982 that was statistically different from the non-funded groups of states.[8] Thus, a likely inference is that the rapid expansion of state-wide perinatal organization and related activities was causally related to the observed improvements in infant mortality.

An opinion survey conducted by Wallace et al, in 1984, indicated that state MCH directors felt that their IPOP projects had met specific needs, particularly in prenatal care and postpartum follow-up, and in patterns of care and referral of patients.[9] Their general impression was that IPOP had considerable impact. Moreover, the analysis referred to earlier found that MCH directors believed that the general guidelines and relatively unrestricted funding of IPOP had enabled them to pull together various pre-existing resources in their states into effective perinatal systems.[8]

Finally, it is important to note that the Wallace survey found that over 80 percent of the IPOP states had managed to perpetuate IPOP activities substantially after IPOP funding expiration by incorporating them into other programs.[9] This development may be viewed administratively as a positive de facto evaluation of the effectiveness of the program. However, given the relatively strong emphasis on project evaluation by the IPOP, it is somewhat disappointing that so few evaluation reports have been published. Possibly the evaluation task seemed formidable because IPOP may have been seen as the "glue" that held many diverse parts of the perinatal care system together.

IMPLICATIONS OF MICP AND IPOP FOR THE FUTURE

There is strong, although not incontrovertible, evidence that maternal, perinatal, and infant health status can be improved significantly by both an intensive, targeted project offering comprehensive services (MICP), as well as by a broad, coordinated management effort to make existing services more efficient and effective (IPOP). It is unclear whether these programmatic examples are always the best and least-costly approaches to specific problems.

However, whatever success has been achieved by these programs, a pattern of initial central (federal) leadership, followed by state and local modification and eventual permanent adoption of MCH service innovations, seems generally acceptable, especially in states with below-average perinatal outcomes and with inadequate resources for planning, monitoring, and evaluating services programs. It may certainly be true that more fortunate states may be capable of improving MCH services without federal leadership and support.

Although specific MCH program innovations will vary over time according to changing needs, it is reasonable to assert that all programs will succeed to the greatest extent possible only when MCH programs are adequately staffed with competent health professionals and administrators. While this may seem obvious, the IPOP was able to fulfill certain staffing needs and this may have been one of the most important factors in improving perinatal outcomes in the participating states. To burden already fully committed staff with new programs does a disservice to staff and to both new and existing programs.

Given the alacrity with which state MCH divisions assimilated the planning and evaluating mandates of IPOP, it would appear that there is an increasing readiness to apply these activities more widely in administration. However, the paucity of published evaluations suggests that evaluation efforts are not involving appropriate faculty from schools of public health and other resources. Such publications could lead to faster and wider application of effective program innovations. Perhaps continuing education programs for MCH personnel could promote closer collaboration between these potential partners.

REFERENCES

1. Pearse WH. The maternity and infant care program. Obstet Gynecol 35-247, 1970.

2. Peoples MD and Siegel E. Measuring the impact of programs for mothers and infants on prenatal care and low birth weight: The value of refined analysis. Med Care 21(6)-586, 1983.

3. Sokol RJ, Woolf RB, Rosen MG, et al. Impact of a maternity and infant care project. Obstet Gynecol 56(2)-150, 1980.

4. Wallace HM, Green G, Peter W, et al. Follow-up study of maternal and infant care projects. Manuscript submitted.

5. Geomet, Inc: Improved Pregnancy Outcomes Evaluation Manual. Final Report Number HF-601. Gaithersburg, Maryland, 1977.

6. Budetti PP and McManus P. Assessing the effectiveness of neonatal and intensive care. Med Care 20(10)-1027, 1982.

7. Committee on Perinatal Health: Toward Improving the Outcome of Pregnancy. White Plains, New York. National Foundation/March of Dimes, 1976.

8. Goldenberg RL and Koski J. The improved pregnancy outcome project: An analysis of the impact of a Federal program on infant mortality. Birmingham, Alabama, University of Alabama 1984.

9. Wallace HM, Green G, Peter W, et al. Results and sequelae of improved pregnancy outcome projects. Submitted manuscript.

SECTION IV

CHILD HEALTH CARE

INFANT MORTALITY

27

Helen M. Wallace

The infant mortality rate is the most sensitive index of the status of economic and social development of any country. It is related to the socio-economic status of the family; to the educational status of the parents, and especially of the mother; the marital status of the pregnant woman; the age of the pregnant woman; and the health status of the pregnant woman, particularly to her previous reproductive history. It is related to the interpregnancy interval of the mother, and also the availability, accessibility, and utilization of medical and health care for the mother. It is related to the nutritional status of the pregnant woman, particularly because of the effects on birthweight of the infant. There are differences in infant mortality by ethnic group.

INTERNATIONAL RANKING IN INFANT MORTALITY

Prior to 1981, Sweden had led the world with the lowest reported infant mortality rate for several decades. Since 1980, Finland, Japan, and Sweden have shared this number-one ranking on a somewhat rotating basis. In 1981 and 1982, Finland had the lowest reported infant mortality rate (6.5 and 6.0 per 1,000 live births, respectively). In 1983, Finland and Japan shared the lowest reported infant mortality rate (6.2 per 1,000 live births). In 1984, Japan had the lowest reported infant mortality rate (6.0 per 1,000 live births). In 1984, the U.S. had an infant mortality rate of 10.7 per 1,000 live births, and ranked eighteenth (Tables 1 and 2).

411

TIME OF INFANT DEATHS

In 1985, the infant mortality rate of 10.6 per 1,000 live births in the U.S. was subdivided into:

Neonatal (within the first 27 days after birth) rate of 7.0 per 1,000 live births

Postneonatal (from the 28th day of life to the first birthday) rate of 3.7 per 1,000 live births (Table 3).

TABLE 1

BIRTH RATE & INFANT MORTALITY RATE – FOR 25 COUNTRIES WITH POPULATION GREATER THAN 2,500,000, 1984 AND 1985

Country	Birth Rate	Infant Mortality Rate 1985	Infant Mortality Rate 1984	% Births To Women Under 20	
Japan	12.5		6.0	1.2	
Sweden	11.8	6.7	6.4	3.8	
Finland	13.3		6.5	4.3	
Switzerland	11.5		7.1	3.2	
Denmark	10.6		7.7	4.2	
France	14.1	8.4	8.0	4.3	(1981)
Canada	14.9		8.1	7.8	(1982)
Norway	12.1		8.3	6.3	
Netherlands	12.1	7.9	8.4	2.7	
Hong Kong	14.4		8.8	3.0	(1982)
Singapore	16.6	9.3	8.8	3.2	
Australia	15.0		9.2	6.9	
German Fed. Rep.	9.6		9.6	4.4	
United Kingdom	12.9		9.6	8.6	
German Dem. Rep.	13.7	9.6	10.0	13.4	
Ireland	18.2		10.1	4.4	
Belgium	11.5	9.4	10.7	5.9	(1981)
U.S.A.	15.5	10.6	10.7	13.7	
Austria	11.5	11.0	11.5	10.4	
New Zealand	16.0	10.8	11.6	9.5	
Italy	10.1	10.9	11.6	6.9	(1980)
Spain	12.5		12.3	6.9	(1979)
Israel	23.7	12.3	12.8	5.1	
Greece	12.8	14.0	14.1	12.2	(1982)
Czechoslovakia	14.5		15.3	11.8	(1982)

Definitions:
Infant Mortality Rate: Number of deaths per 1,000 live births.
Birth Rate: Number of live births per 1,000 population.

SOURCE: Wegman, M.E. Annual Summary of Vital Statistics, 1985. Pediatrics 78:983-994, December 1986.

INFANT MORTALITY BY ETHNIC GROUP

In the U.S., in 1985, the infant mortality rate for whites was 9.3, and for Blacks was 18.2 per 1,000 live births.

INFANT, NEONATAL, POSTNEONATAL
MORTALITY RATES IN THE U.S.—1985

	Total Infant	Neonatal	Postneonatal
Total	**10.6**	**7.0**	**3.7**
Whites	9.3	6.1	3.2
Blacks	18.2	12.1	6.1

Infant, neonatal, and postneonatal mortality rates in the U.S., in 1985, among Blacks, were twice that among whites. (Figure 1) The infant mortality rate in whites, in 1985, in the U.S. (9.3), is 50 percent higher than that for Finland, Japan, and Sweden.

TABLE 2

**INFANT MORTALITY RATE IN COUNTRIES WITH THE LOWEST
IMR AND IN THE UNITED STATES**

Year	Sweden	Finland	Japan	USA	Switzerland	Denmark	Norway
1980	6.9	7.6	7.5	12.5	9.1	8.4	8.1
1981	6.9	6.5	7.1	11.7	7.6	7.9	7.5
1982	6.8	6.0	6.6	11.2	7.7	8.2	8.1
1983	7.0	6.2	6.2	11.2	7.6	7.7	7.8
1984	6.4	6.5	6.0	10.7	7.1	7.7	8.5
1985	6.7	6.7	5.5	10.6			
1986	5.9	5.9		10.4			

SOURCES: Wegman, M.E. Annual Summary of Vital Statistics.
For 1985 - Pediatrics 78:983-994, December 1986
For 1984 - Pediatrics 76:861-871, December 1985
For 1983 - Pediatrics 74:981-990, December 1984
For 1982 - Pediatrics 72:755-764, December 1983
For 1981 - Pediatrics 70:835-843, December 1982
For 1980 - Pediatrics 68:755-762, December 1981

TABLE 3

INFANT, NEONATAL, AND POSTNEONATAL MORTALITY RATES BY RACE AND SEX:
UNITED STATES, 1940, 1950, 1960, AND 1975-85 RATES ARE INFANT (UNDER 1 YEAR), NEONATAL
(UNDER 28 DAYS), AND POSTNEONATAL (28 DAYS - 11 MONTHS) DEATHS PER 100,000 LIVE BIRTHS IN SPECIFIED GROUP

| | All Races | | | White | | | All Other | | | | | |
| | | | | | | | Total | | | Black | | |
	Both Sexes	Male	Female	Both Sexes	Male	Female	Both Sexes	Male	Female	Both Sexes	Male	Female
INFANT MORTALITY RATE												
1985	10.6	11.9	9.3	9.3	10.6	8.0	15.8	17.2	14.4	18.2	19.9	16.5
1984	10.8	11.9	9.6	9.4	10.5	8.3	16.1	17.3	14.8	18.4	19.8	16.9
1983	11.2	12.3	10.0	9.7	10.8	8.6	16.8	19.3	15.2	19.2	21.1	17.2
1982	11.5	12.8	10.2	10.1	11.2	8.9	17.3	18.9	15.5	19.8	21.5	17.7
1981	11.9	13.1	10.7	10.5	11.7	9.2	17.8	19.2	16.3	20.0	21.7	18.3
1980	12.6	13.9	11.2	11.0	12.3	9.6	19.1	20.7	17.5	21.4	23.3	19.4
1979	13.1	14.5	11.6	11.4	12.8	9.9	19.8	21.5	18.1	21.8	23.7	19.8
1978	13.8	15.3	12.2	12.0	13.4	10.6	21.1	23.1	18.9	23.1	15.4	20.8
1977	14.1	15.3	12.4	12.3	13.9	10.7	21.7	23.7	19.8	23.6	25.9	21.3
1976	15.2	16.8	13.6	13.3	14.8	11.7	23.5	25.5	21.4	25.5	21.3	23.2
1975	16.1	17.9	14.2	14.2	15.9	12.3	24.2	26.2	22.2	26.2	28.3	24.0
1970	20.0	22.4	17.5	17.8	20.0	15.4	30.9	34.2	27.5	32.6	36.2	29.0
1960	26.0	29.3	22.6	22.9	26.0	19.6	43.2	47.9	38.5	44.3	49.1	39.4
1950	29.2	32.9	25.5	26.8	30.2	23.1	44.5	48.9	39.9	43.9	48.3	39.4
1940	47.0	52.5	41.3	43.2	48.3	37.8	73.9	82.2	65.2	72.9	81.1	64.6
NEONATAL MORTALITY RATE												
1985	7.0	7.9	6.1	6.1	6.9	5.3	10.3	11.3	9.4	12.1	13.2	10.9
1984	7.0	7.7	6.3	6.2	5.3	5.5	10.2	11.0	9.5	11.8	12.1	10.9
1983	7.3	8.0	6.5	6.4	7.1	5.7	10.9	11.7	9.7	12.4	13.5	11.2

(Continued on next page)

(TABLE 3 – Continued)

Year												
1982	7.7	8.0	6.5	6.8	7.5	6.0	11.3	12.4	10.3	13.1	14.3	11.8
1981	8.0	8.8	7.2	7.1	7.3	6.3	11.8	12.8	10.9	13.4	14.6	12.3
1980	8.5	9.3	7.6	7.5	8.3	6.6	12.5	13.5	11.5	14.1	15.3	12.9
1979	8.9	9.8	7.9	7.9	8.8	6.9	12.9	13.9	11.9	14.3	15.5	13.1
1978	9.5	10.5	8.4	8.4	9.3	7.4	14.0	15.5	12.4	15.5	17.2	13.7
1977	9.9	11.0	8.7	8.7	9.8	7.6	14.7	16.0	13.3	16.1	17.6	14.5
1976	10.9	12.0	9.7	9.7	10.7	8.5	16.3	17.7	14.9	17.9	19.5	16.3
1975	11.6	12.9	10.2	10.4	11.7	9.0	16.8	18.2	15.3	13.3	19.8	16.3
1970	15.1	17.0	13.1	13.8	15.5	11.9	21.4	23.9	18.9	22.8	25.4	20.1
1960	18.7	21.2	16.1	17.2	19.7	14.7	26.9	30.0	28.6	27.8	31.1	24.5
1950	20.5	23.3	17.5	19.4	22.2	16.4	27.5	30.8	24.2	27.8	31.1	24.4
1940	28.8	32.6	24.7	27.2	30.9	23.3	39.7	44.9	34.5	39.9	44.8	34.9

POSTNEONATAL MORTALITY RATE

Year												
1985	3.7	4.2	3.2	3.2	3.7	2.7	5.5	6.0	5.0	6.1	6.7	5.6
1984	3.8	4.2	3.3	3.3	3.7	2.8	5.8	6.3	5.3	6.5	7.1	5.9
1983	3.9	4.3	3.4	3.3	3.7	2.9	6.0	6.6	5.4	6.8	7.4	6.1
1982	3.8	4.3	3.3	3.3	3.7	2.8	5.9	6.5	5.3	6.6	7.3	5.9
1981	3.9	4.3	3.5	3.4	3.8	3.0	6.0	6.5	5.4	6.6	7.1	6.0
1980	4.1	4.6	3.6	3.5	4.0	3.0	6.6	7.2	6.0	7.3	7.3	6.6
1979	4.2	4.7	3.7	3.5	4.0	3.0	6.9	7.6	6.1	7.5	8.2	6.7
1978	4.3	4.7	3.9	3.6	4.0	3.2	7.0	7.6	6.5	7.6	8.2	7.0
1977	4.2	4.8	3.7	3.6	4.1	3.1	7.0	7.7	6.3	7.6	8.3	6.8
1976	4.3	4.8	3.8	3.6	4.1	3.2	7.2	7.8	6.3	7.6	8.4	6.9
1975	4.5	4.9	4.0	3.8	4.2	3.3	7.5	8.0	6.9	7.9	6.5	7.2
1970	4.9	5.4	4.4	4.0	4.4	3.5	9.5	10.3	8.6	9.9	10.3	8.9
1960	7.3	8.1	6.5	5.7	6.3	4.9	15.4	17.8	14.8	16.5	18.0	14.9
1950	8.7	9.4	8.0	7.4	8.0	6.7	16.9	19.1	15.7	16.1	17.2	15.0
1940	18.3	19.9	15.6	16.0	17.5	14.5	24.1	37.3	38.7	33.0	35.4	29.7

SOURCE: National Center for Health Statistics, Advance Report of Final Mortality Statistics, 1985. Mortality Vital Statistics Report, Vol. 36, No. 5 Supplement. August 28, 1987. 47 pages.

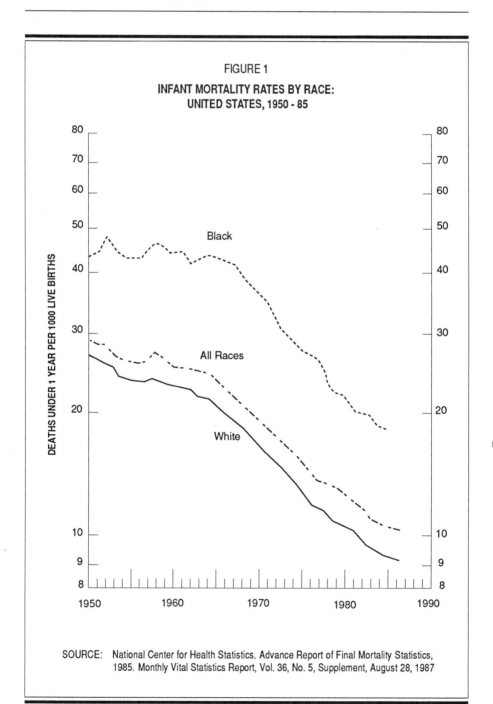

FIGURE 1

INFANT MORTALITY RATES BY RACE:
UNITED STATES, 1950 - 85

SOURCE: National Center for Health Statistics. Advance Report of Final Mortality Statistics, 1985. Monthly Vital Statistics Report, Vol. 36, No. 5, Supplement, August 28, 1987

Native American [1]

The infant mortality rate of 11.0 in Native Americans for 1981-1983 was slightly lower than that for the U.S. as a whole in 1982 (11.5 per 1,000 live births). The neonatal mortality rate for 1981-1983 was lower for Native Americans (5.0) than for the 1982 U.S. as a whole (7.7 per 1,000 live births). However, the postneonatal mortality rate in Native Americans for 1981-1983 (6.1) was substantially higher than for the 1982 U.S. as a whole (3.8 per 1,000 live births). The mortality rates for special causes of death for all Indian Health Service Areas, for 1981-1983, show that the rates for sudden infant death syndrome, birth trauma/asphyxia, pneumonia, injuries, and diarrhea are higher than for the U.S. as a whole. For this reason, the American Academy of Pediatrics is launching a three-year project with the Indian Health Service, specifically aimed at postneonatal deaths in three Indian Health Service Areas.

TRENDS IN INFANT MORTALITY IN THE U.S.[2]

INFANT MORTALITY

In 1985, there were 40,030 deaths of infants under one year of age. The infant mortality rate of 10.6 infant deaths per 1,000 live births was the lowest final rate ever recorded for the U.S., and it compares with a rate for the previous year of 10.8. Among white infants, the rate was 9.3, essentially the same as the rate of 9.4 in 1984; the rate for Black infants in 1985 was 18.2 compared with a rate of 18.4 in 1984. For all infants and for infants of both major ethnic groups considered separately, the change in infant mortality rates between 1984 and 1985 was not statistically significant (Table 3).

The absolute difference in infant mortality rates between Black and white infants has been narrowing; in 1960, the difference in rates was 21.4 deaths per 1,000 live births, compared with 8.9 in 1985. However, because the infant mortality rate for both whites and Blacks has been decreasing by the same average annual percent (3.5) between 1960 and 1985, the Black infant mortality rate in 1985 was 1.95 times the white rate, approximately the same ratio as in 1960 (1.93). The downward trend in infant mortality has slowed for both whites and Blacks—since the late 1970s for white infants, and since 1981 for Black infants (Table 3).

The infant mortality rate for 1986 was 10.4 per 1,000 live births, two percent lower than the rate of 10.6 for 1985.

NEONATAL MORTALITY

Between 1984 and 1985, the neonatal mortality rate remained the same, 7.0 deaths in infants under 28 days per 1,000 live births. By ethnic group, the rate for whites was 6.1 per 1,000 live births, and for Blacks 12.1. For both groups, differences in neonatal mortality rates between 1984 and 1985 were not statistically significant. Neonatal mortality rates have declined since 1960 for both ethnic groups, but the rate for whites has declined relatively faster than that for Blacks—an average annual decrease of four percent per year for white infants compared with 3.3 percent for Black infants (Table 3).

For 1986, the estimated mortality rate for infants under 28 days was 6.7 deaths per 1,000 live births. Between 1985 and 1986, the change in mortality was not statistically significant.

POSTNEONATAL MORTALITY

The postneonatal mortality rate—deaths to infants 28 days to 11 months per 1,000 live births—for 1985 was 3.7, three percent lower than in 1984. For whites, the postneonatal mortality rate in 1985 was 3.2 compared with 3.3 in 1984, a change that was not statistically significant. For Black infants, the rate for 1985 (6.1) declined from 6.5 in 1984 and 6.8 in 1983. In contrast to the trend for neonatal mortality, between 1960 and 1985, the postneonatal rate decreased relatively faster for the Black population than for the white population; an average annual decline of 3.9 percent per year for Black infants compared with 2.3 percent for white infants (Table 3).

For 1986, the estimated postneonatal mortality rate was 3.7 per 1,000 live births. Between 1985 and 1986, the change in postneonatal mortality rate was not statistically significant. The downward trends in infant, neonatal, and postneonatal mortality rates have slowed recently for both whites and Blacks.

Infant Mortality by Sex

Infant mortality is higher for males than for females, for the total population, and for whites and Blacks. The difference between males and females is greater for whites (24.5 percent) than for Blacks (17.1 percent) (Table 3).

Infant Mortality by Cause of Death

Major reported causes of death, as reported on death certificates, are congenital anomalies, sudden infant death syndrome, respiratory distress syndrome, disorders relating to short gestation and unspecified low birthweight, intrauterine hypoxia and birth asphyxia, and "other conditions originating in the perinatal period" (Table 4).

Infant Mortality in the States

The U.S. infant mortality rate, in 1985, ranged from a low of 8.2 in Rhode Island to a high of 20.8 in the District of Columbia. In 1985, no state had an infant mortality rate as low as Sweden (Table 5).

TABLE 4

INFANT MORTALITY RATES BY AGE AND FOR 10 SELECTED CAUSES OF DEATH: UNITED STATES, 1983-86*

Age and Cause of death (Ninth Revision, International Classification of Diseases, 1975)		1986 (prov.)	1985 (prov.)	1984 (prov.) a/	1984 (final)	1983 (final)
Total, under 1 year		1,039.2	1,057.0	1,068.8	1078.7	1,116.5
Under 28 days		669.5	692.6	691.8	700.2	728.4
28 days - 11 months		369.7	364.1	377.0	378.5	388.0
Certain gastrointestinal diseases	008-009, 535, 555-558	5.9	4.8	7.6	7.2	7.4
Pneumonia and influenza	480-487	18.0	17.9	17.2	18.7	21.1
Congenital anomalies	740-759	218.9	236.7	230.0	233.0	240.0
Disorders relating to short gestation and unspecified low birth weight	765	87.9	83.3	94.1	88.9	91.6
Birth trauma	767	8.6	7.5	9.0	10.2	12.2
Intrauterine hypoxia and birth asphyxia	768	24.2	28.4	26.4	31.9	
Respiratory distress syndrome	769	94.4	100.7	104.8	96.9	101.2
Other conditions originating in the prenatal period	760-764, 766, 770-779	266.2	264.5	275.0	281.2	288.5
Sudden infant death syndrome	798.0	130.4	129.6	132.9	142.9	145.8
All other causes	Residual	184.7	183.9	171.5	167.8	175.8

SOURCE: National Center for Health Statistics. Annual Summary of Births, Marriages, Divorces, and Deaths: United States, 1986. Monthly Vital Statistics Report, Vol. 35, No. 13. August 24, 1987.

* Provisional data for 1984-86 based on a 10% sample of deaths. Rates per 100,000 live births. For information on standard errors of the estimates and further discussion, see Technical Notes.

TABLE 5

TOTAL DEATHS AND DEATH RATES, AND INFANT AND NEONATAL DEATHS AND MORTALITY RATES FOR THE UNITED STATES, EACH DIVISION, AND STATE, AND BY RACE AND SEX FOR THE UNITED STATES: 1986

Race, Sex, and Area	Total deaths Number	Rate a/	Infant deaths (under 1 year) Number	Rate b/	Neonatal deaths (under 28 days) Number	Rate b/
United States	2,086,440	873.9	40,030	10.6	26,179	70
Male	1,097,758	945.0	22,958	11.9	14.948	7.8
Female	988,682	806.6	17,072	9.3	11,231	6.1
White	1,819,054	897.1	27,864	9.3	18,231	6.1
Male	950,455	960.0	16,218	10.6	10,536	6.9
Female	868,599	837.1	11,646	8.0	7,697	5.3
All Other	267,386	743.3	12,166	15.8	7,946	10.3
Male	147,303	858.6	6,740	17.2	4,412	11.3
Female	120,083	638.1	5,426	14.4	3,534	9.4
Black	244,207	845.7	11,063	18.2	7,340	12.1
Male	13,610	976.8	6,127	19.9	4,075	13.2
Female	110,597	727.7	4,936	16.5	3,265	10.9
New England	117,975	932.1	1,654	9.2	1,207	6.7
Maine	11,420	979.4	154	9.1	110	6.5
New Hampshire	9,483	849.1	144	9.3	98	6.3
Vermont	4,662	871,4	68	8.5	43	5.4
Massachusetts	55,593	955.4	743	9.1	535	6.5
Rhode Island	9,647	997.6	107	8.2	78	6.0
Connecticut	28,170	888.4	438	10.0	343	7.8
Middle Atlantic	367,099	987.6	5,676	10.8	3,903	7.4
New York	172,117	969.9	2,791	10.8	1,912	7.4
New Jersey	71,128	940.7	1,119	10.6	764	7.2
Pennsylvania	123,954	1,043.9	1,766	11.0	1,227	7.6
East North Central	369,629	887.5	6,912	10.9	4,612	7.3
Ohio	98,941	920.6	1,660	10.3	1,082	6.0
Indiana	48,195	876.3	883	10.9	604	7.5
Illinois	102,279	886.5	2,123	11.7	1,441	8.0
Michigan	78,722	866.2	1,572	11.4	1,070	7.8
Wisconsin	41,492	868.8	674	9.1	415	5.6
West North Central	162,194	923,9	2,609	9.5	1,633	5.9
Minnesota	34,801	830.2	594	8.8	366	45.4
Iowa	27,834	966.1	391	9.5	243	5.9
Missouri	50,368	1,000.4	789	10.2	500	6.5
North Dakota	5,628	821.6	100	8.5	63	5.4
South Dakota	6,603	932.6	120	9.9	65	5.4
Nebraska	14,903	928.5	246	9.6	159	6.2
Kansas	22,057	900.3	369	9.3	237	6.0

(Continued on next page)

(TABLE 5 – Continued)

Race, Sex, and Area	Total deaths Number	Rate a/	Infant deaths (under 1 year) Number	Rate b/	Neonatal deaths (under 28 days) Number	Rate b/
South Atlantic	363,649	904.3	7,261	12.1	4,938	8.2
Delaware	5,475	880.2	142	14.8	102	10.6
Maryland	36,620	833.6	808	11.9	556	8.2
District of Columbia	5,981	1,120.5	205	20.8	157	15.9
Virginia	45,277	794.1	989	11.5	695	8.1
West Virginia	19,444	1,003.8	259	10.7	177	17.3
North Carolina	52,988	846.3	1,051	11.8	695	7.8
South Carolina	27,099	812.6	738	14.2	519	10.0
Georgia	48,657	814.3	1,222	12.7	829	8.6
Florida	121,108	1,065.6	1,847	11.3	1,208	7.4
East South Central	140,385	927.7	2,701	12.1	1,762	7.9
Kentucky	34,865	935.0	594	11.2	396	7.5
Tennessee	43,226	906.8	759	11.4	503	7.5
Alabama	37,603	934.9	752	12.6	496	8.3
Mississippi	24,691	944.6	596	13.7	367	8.4
West South Central	209,284	788.6	4,968	10.4	3,144	6.6
Arkansas	24,137	1,022.8	409	11.6	249	7.1
Louisiana	37,029	825.4	968	11.9	629	7.7
Oklahoma	29,782	900.8	577	10.9	363	6.8
Texas	118,336	722.2	3,014	9.8	1,903	6.2
Mountain	88,021	687.8	2,317	9.6	1,344	5.7
Montana	6,724	815.0	139	10.3	68	5.0
	7,115	708.7	183	10.4	111	6.3
			114	12.2	60	6.4
New Mexico	9,763	672.8	295	10.6	174	6.3
Arizona	24,619	771.5	577	9.7	352	5.9
Utah	9,049	550.1	360	9,6	204	5.4
Nevada	7,236	772.3	130	8.5	73	4.8
Pacific	268,204	765.7	5,932	9.7	3,636	5.9
Washington	34,504	792.8	752	10.7	435	6.2
Oregon	22,896	889.7	389	9.9	209	5.3
California	201,911	766.0	4,490	9.5	2,820	6.0
Alaska	2,068	396.2	139	10.8	65	5.1
Hawaii	5,825	554.2	162	8.6	107	5.8

SOURCE: National Center For Health Statistics, Advance Report of Final Mortality Statistics, 1985. Monthly Vital Statistics Report, Vol. 36 No. 5, Supplement. August 28, 1987
a/ Per 100,000 population in each race-sex group and area.
b/ Per 1,000 live births in each race-sex group and area.

The Role of Sudden Infant Death Syndrome in Infant Mortality

In 1985, out of a total of 40,030 infant deaths, 5,315 (13.3 percent) were attributed to sudden infant death syndrome (SIDS). The rate of SIDS for all races in 1985 was 141.3 per 100,000 live births; for whites it was 125.6 and for Blacks it was 223.1 per 1,000 live births [2,A] (Table 4).

LOW BIRTHWEIGHT

In 1984, 6.7 percent of newborn infants in the U.S. were low birthweight (2500 grams or less), and slightly more than one percent were very-low birthweight (1500 grams or less). The incidence of low birthweight in the U.S. is shown in Table 6. For the total population, the incidence of low birthweight has declined slowly. The incidence is over twice as high in Blacks as in whites; it is also higher in Native Americans and Hispanics than whites (Table 6).

In 1984, the incidence of low birthweight in the U.S. was 6.7 percent compared with 4.1 percent in Sweden. In 1983, the incidence in the U.S. was 6.8 percent compared with 4.0 percent in Finland.

The Significance of Low Birthweight [3]

Low birthweight is an indicator of inadequate fetal growth, resulting from premature birth (duration of pregnancy less than 37 weeks from the last menstrual period), poor weight gain for a given duration of gestation (intrauterine growth retardation), or both. Two-thirds of deaths in the neonatal period occur among infants born at 2500 grams or less. The risk of mortality increases with decreasing birth weight; the risk of neonatal death is 200 times greater for the very-low birthweight infant than for the normal birthweight infant. Low birthweight infants are five times more likely than normal birthweight infants to die later in the first year, and account for 20 percent of postneonatal deaths. The higher neonatal mortality rates for babies born of non-white mothers, adolescent mothers, and mothers with less than a high school education are largely explained by higher proportions of low birthweight infants in these groups. Furthermore, the association between low birthweight and neurodevelopmental problems, such as cerebral palsy and seizure disorders, has been well documented. Low birthweight infants are three times as likely as normal birthweight infants to have neurodevelopmental handicaps; the risk increases with decreasing birthweight.

The first step in prevention of low birthweight at present is early risk assessment. The Institute of Medicine group [3] has concluded that the majority of 13 risk classification systems examined in the U.S. correctly identify as high-risk about 65 percent or more of those pregnancies with eventual adverse outcomes. Essential steps include pre-pregnancy risk identification and reduction; enlarging the content of health education; making family planning information, education, services, and supplies easily available for all women of childbearing age; making prenatal education and care of high quality available and accessible for all women of the child-bearing age, and ensuring access to care for all, including transportation, child care, and outreach; improving the content of prenatal care; risk-scoring for all pregnant women early in pregnancy and providing special care for those of high risk; and provision of an extensive public information program (Table 7).

The obstetrical (OB) access program in California is an example of a successful Medicaid pilot project.[4] It operated in 13 California counties from July 1979 through June 1982. The goals were to improve access to care in under-served areas and improve pregnancy outcomes by providing enhanced prenatal care, including psychosocial, health education, and nutrition services. OB access mothers had a low birthweight rate of 4.7 percent, compared with 7.0 percent for a matched control group, suggesting a 33 percent reduction in low birthweight.

PRENATAL CARE

Table 8 provides data on the status of prenatal care in the U.S. For 1984, 76.5 percent of pregnant women delivering a live baby began prenatal care in the first trimester of pregnancy; 1.7 percent had no prenatal care. Over the five years (1980-1984), there has been essentially no improvement in the picture of entry to prenatal care in the U.S. (Table 8).

The Institute of Medicine report[3] concludes its review of the value of prenatal care by stating that the overwhelming evidence is that prenatal care reduces low birthweight.

TABLE 6
INCIDENCE OF LOW BIRTH WEIGHT - USA
(2500 GRAMS OR LESS)

Year	Total	White	Black	Native American	Hispanic
1960	7.7	6.8			
1965	8.3	7.2			
1970	7.9	6.8	13.9	8.0	
1975	7.4	6.3	13.1	6.6	
1976	7.3	6.1	13.0	6.9	
1977	7.1	5.9	12.8	6.6	
1978	7.1	5.9	12.9	6.7	6.7
1979	6.9	5.8	12.6	6.4	6.1
1980	6.8	5.7	12.5	6.5	6.1
1981	6.8	5.7	12.5	6.3	6.1
1982	6.8	5.6	12.4	6.2	6.2
1983	6.8	5.7	12.6	6.4	6.3
1984	6.7	5.6	12.4	6.2	6.2
1985	6.8	5.6	12.4	5.9	6.2

TABLE 7

SUMMARY OF PRINCIPAL RISK FACTORS
FOR LOW BIRTH WEIGHT

1. **Demographic Risks**
   A. Age less than 17; over 34
   B. Race (black)
   C. Low socioeconomic status
   D. Unmarried
   E. Low level of education

2. **Medical Risks Predating Pregnancy**
   A. Parity (0 or more than 4)
   B. Low weight for height
   C. Genitourinary anomalies/surgery
   D. Selected diseases such as diabetes, chronic hypertension
   E. Nonimmune status for selected infections such as rubella
   F. Poor obstetric history including previous low birthweight infant, multiple spontaneous abortions
   G. Maternal genetic factors (such as low maternal weight at own birth)

3. **Medical Risks in Current Pregnancy**
   A. Multiple pregnancy
   B. Poor weight gain
   C. Short interpregnancy interval
   D. Hypotension
   E. Hypertension/preeclampsia/toxemia
   F. Selected infections such as symptomatic bacteriuria, rubella, and cytomegalovirus
   G. 1st or 2nd trimester bleeding
   H. Placental problems such as placenta previa, abruptio placentae
   I. Hyperemesis
   J. Oligohydramnios/polyhydramnios
   K. Anemia/abnormal hemoglobin
   L. isoimmunization
   M. Fetal anomalies
   N. Incompetent cervix
   O. Spontaneous premature rupture of membranes

4. **Behavioral and Environmental Risks**
   A. Smoking
   B. Poor nutritional status
   C. Alcohol and other substance abuse
   D. DES exposure and other toxic exposures, including occupational hazards
   E. High altitude

5. **Health Care Risks**
   A. Absent or inadequate prenatal care
   B. Iatrogenic prematurity

6. **Evolving Concepts of Risk**
   A. Stress, physical and psychosocial
   B. Uterine irritability
   C. Events triggering uterine contractions
   D. Cervical changes detected before onset of labor
   E. Selected infections such as mycoplasma and Chlamydia trachomatis
   F. Inadequate plasma volume expansion
   G. Progesterone deficiency

SOURCE: Institute of Medicine. Preventing Low Birthweight. Summary. 1985. Washington D.C. Page 7.

INTERPREGNANCY INTERVAL

Interpregnancy interval is a factor in influencing low birthweight. Spratley and Taffel [5] reported that 19.2 percent of the 1977 births occurring within one year of a previous live birth were of low birthweight, about three to 4-1/2 times the proportion observed for longer interbirth intervals. The percent of infants of low birthweight was lowest when the interval between live births was between two and four years. The opportunity for the role of family planning in reducing infant mortality is clear.

STEPS NEEDED TO REDUCE INFANT MORTALITY

In order for the U.S. to achieve significant further reduction in its infant mortality rate, top priority needs to be given this problem in our national agenda, over a substantial period of time. The national agenda needs to be comprehensive in scope, including:

1. Maternity benefits for all pregnant women.

2. Parental leave, or at least maternity leave, for employed parents.

3. Protection of women of the childbearing age on the job, and re-assignment from hazardous job assignments.

4. Family planning education, services, and supplies for all women and couples of the childbearing age who wish to use them.

5. Preconceptional care for young women and couples prior to pregnancy.

TABLE 8

**ENTRY TO PRENATAL CARE: UNITED STATES,
SELECTED YEARS, 1970-1984**

Month of Pregnancy Entered Prenatal Care	Percentages of Live Births by Year					
	1970	1980	1981	1982	1983	1984
1-3 months	68.0	76.3	76.3	76.1	76.2	76.5
4-6 months	24.1	18.6	18.5	18.5	18.2	17.9
7-9 months	6.2	3.8	3.8	3.9	3.9	3.9
No Care	1.7	1.3	1.4	1.5	1.6	1.7

6. Primary health care for all women of the childbearing age, screening for high risk, and special care of those of high risk, prior to and during pregnancy.

7. Extension of the WIC Program to all pregnant and lactating women.

8. Extension of regionalized perinatal care, with more emphasis of transfer of the mother, and fetus in utero.

9. Special follow-up of all high risk women *after delivery* to assist them in achieving optimal health prior to the next pregnancy.

10. Offering of interdisciplinary team reviews for maternity, perinatal, and infancy community programs in all states, large counties, and cities, in an effort to strengthen organized community efforts.

11. Support and organization of intensive efforts to study individual infant and perinatal deaths on a community basis, to utilize the information gained to improve community efforts and services, and for educational purposes of the health professions.

12. Extension of family life education to all pupils and to all parents.

13. Extension of efforts to decrease smoking and the use of alcohol and drugs during pregnancy.

REFERENCES

1. AAP Joins Indian Health Service in Postneonatal Mortality Study. American Academy of Pediatrics Newsletter June 1987.

2. National Center for Health Statistics:
    A. Advance Report of Final Mortality Statistics, 1985. Monthly Vital Statistics Report, Vol. 36, No. 5 Supplement. August 28, 1987. 47 pages.
    B. Annual Summary of Births, Marriages, Divorces, and Death: United States 1986.Monthly Vital Statistics Report, Vol. 35, No. 13, August 24, 1987. 27 Pages.

3. Committee to Study the Prevention of Low Birthweight, Institute of Medicine. Preventing Low Birth Weight.
    A. Full Report. Washington, D.C. 1985.
    B. Summary. Washington, D.C. 1985.

4. Lennie, JA; Klun, JR; and Hausner, T. Low-birth-weight reduced by the obstetrical access project. Health Care Financing Review 8:83-86, Spring 1987.

5. National Center for Health Statistics. Interval Between Births: United States, 1970-1977. Prepared by E. Spratley and S. Taffel. Vital and Health Statistics, Series 21, No. 39. DHHS No. (PHS) 81-1917. Public Health Service, Washington, D.C. U.S. Government Printing Office, August 1981.

THE HEALTH STATUS OF PRESCHOOL AND SCHOOL-AGE CHILDREN

28

Mary Grace Kovar and Deborah Dawson

INTRODUCTION

The purpose of this chapter is to present a brief overview of the health of children in the U.S., using indicators ranging from parental evaluation to illness, disability, and death. Use of medical services, such as doctor visits and hospitalizations, also are indicators of health. The focus of the chapter is on national data, with differences by sex and by race.

Mortality data are from the vital statistics system.[1] The age groups used in describing child mortality are ages one-four and five-14. Unless otherwise noted, all other data are from the National Health Interview Surveys of 1985 and 1986.[2,3] Preschool children are defined as those of ages 0-four years, and school-age children are defined as those of ages five-11. Many of the data have not been published before; references are given only for published data.

MORTALITY

If mortality is used as a health indicator, there have been substantial improvements in the health of children over the past few decades. The decline in infant mortality, discussed in another chapter, has been dramatic. Declines in mortality for other age groups of children, while less spectacular, have been impressive as well. In 1950, the death rates for children ages one-four and five-14 were 139.4 and 60.1, respectively. By 1985, these rates had decreased to 51.1 and 27.9, and the provisional estimates for 1986 are 50.8 and 26.4. While most of this decline occurred prior to 1980, child mortality has continued to decrease in the 1980s (Table 1). For children ages one-four, the death rate decreased by 21 percent between 1980 and 1986; for children ages five-14, there was a 14 percent reduction in mortality.

Although improvements in mortality have been greater for Black than for white children, Black children are still at greater risk of death than white children at each age. The racial differential is greatest for infants and decreases with advancing age of child. The death rate for Black children is 75 percent higher than the rate for white children at ages one-four, and 51 percent higher at ages five-14.

Death rates are higher for boys than girls throughout childhood. The gender difference is larger among older than younger children. The rate for boys is 24 percent higher at ages one-four. At ages five-14, it is 55 percent higher. Boys' excess mortality reflects their higher rates of accidental injuries, homicides, and suicides. Despite the general decline in child mortality, death rates for these three causes have increased since the 1950s for boys and girls of both races.[4]

HEALTH STATUS

Injuries

Each time a child is involved in an accident or non-accidental violence that causes an injury resulting in medical attention or at least one day of restricted activity, it is considered an episode of injury. Thus, a child may have more than one episode of injury in a year, and a single episode may result in more than one injury. In the mid-1980s, there were 28.6 episodes of injury per 100 children ages 0-four and 31.6 for children ages five-11 (Table 2).

For episodes of injury where the site of the accident was reported, 85 percent of the episodes for children ages 0-four occurred at home. Four percent occurred at school, five percent on the street (e.g., traffic accidents), and six percent took place in other locations, such as recreational facilities, stores, etc. For older children, those ages five-11, about half (50 percent) of the episodes of injury occurred at home. Accidents or non-accidental violence taking place on the street accounted for 13 percent of all episodes, and those occurring at school or other places made up 18 percent each of the total.

Boys are more likely than girls to be injured, except among Black children ages five-11, for whom there is no differential by sex. The rates are higher for white children than for Black children, especially among school-age children. At ages five-11, there are more than twice as many episodes of injury reported per 100 white children as per 100 Black children. This differential is surprising, especially in view of the fact that deaths from accidental or non-accidental injury are more common among Black than white children. If there is no strong racial differential in reporting, the proportion of injuries resulting in death (such injuries are excluded from

TABLE 1

NUMBER OF DEATHS PER 100,000 POPULATION, BY AGE, RACE, AND SEX, FOR CHILDREN UNDER 15 YEARS OF AGE: UNITED STATES, 1980, 1985, AND 1986*

| | All Races | | | White | | | All Other | | | | | |
| | | | | | | | Total | | | Black | | |
	Both Sexes	Male	Female	Both Sexes	Male	Female	Both Sexes	Male	Female	Both Sexes	Male	Female
				Deaths per 100,000 population								
Ages 0-1 Years:												
1980	1288.3	1428.5	1141.7	1099.9	1230.3	962.5	2148.5	2350.2	1944.1	2356.6	2586.7	2123.7
1985	1055.2	1178.0	927.1	930.0	1046.7	806.8	1600.0	1762.0	1435.2	1817.1	2000.0	1643.9
1986*	1036.7	1156.7	911.5	877.3	989.7	758.2	1723.0	1884.8	1557.5	1952.1	2140.4	1759.9
Ages 1-4 Years												
1980	63.9	72.6	54.7	57.9	66.1	49.3	91.4	103.0	79.5	97.6	110.5	84.4
1985	51.1	56.7	45.1	46.1	52.6	39.1	72.6	74.6	70.5	79.3	80.0	78.5
1986*	50.8	56.1	45.2	45.7	51.0	40.2	72.0	77.6	66.3	80.2	84.0	76.2
Ages 5-14												
1980	30.6	36.7	24.2	29.1	35.0	22.9	37.4	44.9	29.8	39.0	47.4	30.5
1985	27.9	33.3	22.2	26.1	31.6	20.3	35.5	40.5	30.4	37.3	43.2	31.3
1986*	26.4	32.0	20.6	24.5	29.9	18.8	34.6	40.7	28.3	36.9	44.2	29.3

SOURCE: National Center for Health Statistics, Monthly Vital Statistics Report, Vol 35, No. 13, August 24, 1987

* Provisional data

TABLE 2

NUMBER OF EPISODES OF INJURY PER 100 CHILDREN AND PERCENT DISTRIBUTION OF EPISODES OF INJURY BY LOCATION, BY AGE, RACE, AND SEX: UNITED STATES, 1985/86

	All Races			White			All Other — Total			All Other — Black		
	Both Sexes	Male	Female	Both Sexes	Male	Female	Both Sexes	Male	Female	Both Sexes	Male	Female
Episodes Of Injury Per 100 Children												
Ages 0-4 Years	26.9	27.7	26.0	27.5	28.5	26.4	24.2	24.1	24.2	24.9	29.2	20.4
Ages 5-11 Years	31.0	32.2	29.8	34.8	36.0	33.6	14.3	15.3	13.3	16.5	16.9	16.1
Percent Distribution Of Episodes Of Injury												
Ages 0-4 Years												
At Home	61.8	69.0	53.5	59.3	67.9	49.5	73.6	75.0	72.3	79.3	75.0	85.7
On The Street	2.8	5.3	0.0	2.8	5.3	0.0	2.4	4.9	0.0	2.9	4.9	0.0
In School	3.6	2.3	5.0	4.3	2.7	6.1	0.0	0.0	0.0	0.0	0.0	0.0
Other	4.4	6.1	2.5	5.2	7.2	3.0	0.0	0.0	0.0	0.0	0.0	0.0
Unknown	27.6	17.3	39.1	28.3	16.8	41.5	23.9	20.1	27.7	17.8	20.1	14.3
Ages 5-11 Years												
At Home	44.4	51.1	36.8	46.0	51.9	39.3	27.8	42.9	9.6	24.5	37.9	9.6
On The Street	11.8	8.0	16.1	11.4	7.0	16.3	16.1	18.3	13.4	16.8	20.0	13.4
In School	16.4	15.3	17.6	15.3	15.4	15.1	28.1	14.2	44.8	29.4	15.5	44.8
Other	16.4	17.1	15.6	16.9	17.2	16.5	12.0	16.4	6.7	12.5	17.8	6.7
Unknown	11.0	8.4	13.9	10.5	8.4	12.9	16.0	8.1	25.5	16.7	8.8	25.5

SOURCE: National Health Interview Survey, 1985 and 1986

NOTE: Includes only those episodes of injury that resulted in medical attention or at least one day of restricted activity.

Table 2) must be greater for Black than white children. However, the episodes of injury included in Table 2 are only those that resulted in medical attention or restriction of activity, and there may be a racial differential in whether injuries result in medical treatment or in restriction of a child's usual activity.

Limitation of Activity Due to Chronic Conditions

Very few children are limited in the activities usual for their age (Table 3). Two percent of all children ages 0-four have some form of long-term activity limitation due to a chronic condition. At ages five-11, the proportion of children limited in activity rises to six percent. The higher rate of limitation among school-age children may reflect the fact that their normal activities are more physically and mentally demanding than those of preschool children, or it may be due to the fact that older children have had more time in which to contract the types of chronic illness or impairment generally associated with limitation of activity.

Black children are more likely to be limited in activity than white children, especially at preschool ages. In general, boys are more likely than girls to have some form of activity limitation. Black children ages 0-four are the exception to this rule, with the two sexes equally likely to be limited.

TABLE 3

**PERCENT OF CHILDREN WITH LIMITATION OF ACTIVITY
DUE TO CHRONIC CONDITIONS, BY AGE, RACE, AND SEX:
UNITED STATES, 1985/86**

Race and Sex	Age	
	0-4 Years	5-11 Years
All races	2.3	5.9
Male	2.6	7.1
Female	2.0	4.6
White	2.1	5.7
Male	2.4	6.9
Female	1.7	4.5
Nonwhite:		
Total	3.2	6.5
Male	3.3	7.9
Female	3.1	5.0
Black	3.4	6.7
Male	3.4	8.2
Female	3.4	5.1

SOURCE: National Health Interview Survey, 1985 and 1986

Perceived Health Status

The majority of children are classified by a household respondent as being in excellent health relative to other children the same age. The distribution by perceived health status is almost identical for preschool and school-age children. There is little difference by sex of child, but there is a racial differential. As shown in Table 4, the proportion of Black children judged to be in excellent health is 12 percentage points lower than the proportion of white children for both preschool and school-age children. Black children in both age groups are almost twice as likely as white children to be reported in fair or poor health.

To a large extent, the racial differential is a function of differences in socioeconomic status. Black children are far more likely than white children to live in poverty,[5,6] and low income is positively associated with the probability that a child will be in poor health. Other data from the National Health Interview Survey show that the proportion of children who are perceived as being in excellent health increases with family income.[7] After adjusting for poverty status, the racial differential in perceived child health status is greatly reduced.

Bed Days

While limitation of activity entails long-term disability resulting from a chronic condition, a child's activities also may be restricted on a temporary basis. A bed day—a day during which a child spends at least half of the day in bed—is one measure of such temporary restriction. Children can be expected to have a few bed days each year; however, an excessive number of bed days may be indicative of overall poor health.

As shown in Table 5, children have an average of four to five bed days per child per year. Thirteen percent of all children spend seven or more days in bed per year. At ages 0-four, boys have more bed days, on average, than girls; at ages five-11, the opposite is true.

USE OF MEDICAL CARE

Hospitalization

Hospitalization is relatively rare among children. Only six percent of children ages 0-four and three percent of those ages five-11 were reported to have had one or more short stay hospital episodes in the preceding year. The average annual numbers of hospital episodes and hospital days per 100 preschool children were 7.5 and 50.2, respectively. For children who were hospitalized at least once, this is an annual average of 1.3 hospital episodes and 8.5 hospital days per child. Thus, the average length of stay was approximately seven days. The average numbers of hospital episodes and hospital days, and the average length of hospital stay, were all less for school-age than for preschool children. Children ages five-11 with at least one hospitalization in the preceding 12 months had an average of 1.1 hospital episodes and 4.2 hospital days per year, for an average length of stay of about four days.

TABLE 4

PERCENT DISTRIBUTION OF CHILDREN BY ASSESSED* HEALTH STATUS, BY AGE, RACE, AND SEX: UNITED STATES, 1985/86

| | All Races | | | White | | | All Other | | | | | |
| | | | | | | | Total | | | Black | | |
	Both Sexes	Male	Female	Both Sexes	Male	Female	Both Sexes	Male	Female	Both Sexes	Male	Female
Ages 0-4 Years:												
Excellent	54.2	53.7	54.8	56.5	55.6	57.6	44.1	45.2	42.9	42.3	43.7	40.9
Very Good	26.2	26.0	26.4	26.6	27.0	26.2	24.2	21.5	26.9	24.9	22.0	27.8
Good	17.1	17.7	16.4	14.8	15.4	14.2	27.1	28.1	26.1	28.1	29.2	27.0
Fair or Poor	2.5	2.7	2.4	2.1	2.1	2.0	4.6	5.2	4.0	4.7	5.1	4.4
Ages 5-11 Years:												
Excellent	52.6	53.6	51.5	54.7	56.3	53.1	42.9	41.7	44.2	41.3	40.4	42.2
Very Good	27.0	26.0	28.0	27.3	26.3	28.5	25.4	24.9	26.0	25.6	24.5	26.7
Good	18.1	17.8	18.4	16.0	15.2	16.7	27.3	28.9	25.7	28.6	30.8	26.3
Fair or Poor	2.4	2.7	2.2	2.0	2.2	1.7	4.4	4.5	4.2	4.5	4.4	4.7

SOURCE: National Health Interview Survey, 1985 and 1986
    * Assessed by household respondent

TABLE 5

AVERAGE ANNUAL NUMBER OF BED DAYS PER CHILD AND PERCENT OF CHILDREN WITH 7 OR MORE BED DAYS IN PRECEDING YEAR, BY AGE, RACE, AND SEX: UNITED STATES, 1985/86

	All Races			White			All Other Total			Black		
	Both Sexes	Male	Female	Both Sexes	Male	Female	Both Sexes	Male	Female	Both Sexes	Male	Female
Average Annual Number Of Bed Days Per Child:												
Ages 0-4 Years	4.7	4.9	4.4	4.5	4.7	4.4	5.3	5.9	4.7	5.5	5.8	5.2
Ages 5-11 Years	3.9	3.4	4.5	4.1	3.5	4.7	3.3	2.7	4.0	3.5	2.8	4.3
Percent Of Children With 7+ Bed Days:												
Ages 0-4 Years	12.7	12.9	12.5	12.5	12.6	12.4	13.7	14.6	12.6	13.6	14.3	13.2
Ages 5-11 Years	12.7	12.3	13.1	12.5	13.0	14.0	9.0	9.2	9.0	9.1	9.3	8.7

SOURCE: National Health Interview Survey, 1985 and 1986

One reason school-age children have fewer hospital days is that data on preschool children include hospitalization associated with complications of birth. In the case of infants who are born prematurely or with birth defects requiring immediate treatment, post-delivery hospital stays are protracted, adding to the average number of hospital days and average duration of hospitalization for the 0-four year age group. Data from the National Hospital Discharge Survey show that the average length of hospital stay was between two and three days longer for children under age one than for those of ages one-four or five-14.[8]

A higher proportion of boys than of girls have had at least one short stay hospital episode in the preceding year. Among children who have been hospitalized, the average number of hospitalizations is almost identical for the two sexes, but girls have more hospital days than boys at ages 0-four. As a result, the average duration of hospital stay is greater for girls than boys of preschool age. For children ages five-11, the average annual number of hospital days per hospitalized child and the average duration of hospital stay are similar for boys and girls.

At ages 0-four, the proportion of Black children who have been hospitalized in the preceding year is higher than the proportion of white children, while the opposite is true at ages five-11. Among children who have been hospitalized at least once, the average number of hospital episodes is similar for children of both races, but the average number of hospital days is higher for Black than for white children in this age group (Table 6).

Ambulatory Physician Contacts

Unlike hospitalization, which almost always indicates a health problem, contact with a physician outside a hospital does not necessarily mean that there is a problem. Much of the care of children, especially very young children, is preventive. In 1982, 96 percent of all children under 16 years of age had had a routine physical exam, 79 percent in the preceding year. Sixty-two percent of children ages three-16 had had an eye exam in the preceding year.[9] While a large number of physician contacts is likely to be a sign of poor health, too few contacts can mean that a child is not obtaining the recommended screening and preventive care.

Ninety percent of all preschool children had at least one contact with a physician or someone working under a physician's supervision during the year, as did 75 percent of school-age children. Boys and girls were equally likely to have had a physician contact. The proportion of children with at least one contact was slightly higher for white than for Black children.

Preschool children had an average of 6.5 physician contacts per-child per-year. This average, which includes visits for routine immunizations, is considerably higher than that for school-age children: 3.4 contacts per-child per-year. The average number of physician contacts is slightly larger for boys than girls at ages 0-four and ages five-11. Among preschool children, Black children had an average

TABLE 7

PHYSICIAN CONTACTS BY AGE, RACE, AND SEX: UNITED STATES, 1985/86

| | All Races | | | White | | | All Other | | | | | |
| | | | | | | | Total | | | Black | | |
	Both Sexes	Male	Female	Both Sexes	Male	Female	Both Sexes	Male	Female	Both Sexes	Male	Female
Percent Of Children With 1+ Physician Contacts in Preceding Year:												
Ages 0-4 Years	90.3	90.2	90.5	91.1	90.7	91.5	87.0	87.7	86.2	86.5	87.1	85.8
Ages 5-11 Years	75.0	74.6	75.3	76.3	75.9	76.8	69.1	69.2	69.1	69.1	69.1	69.2
Average Annual Number Of Physician Contacts Per Child:												
Ages 0-4 Years	6.5	6.6	6.3	6.9	7.0	6.7	4.6	4.8	4.5	4.5	4.8	4.2
Ages 5-11 Years	3.4	3.5	3.3	3.7	3.8	3.6	2.2	2.4	2.0	2.2	2.2	2.2

SOURCE: National Health Interview Survey, 1985 and 1986

of 4.5 contacts per child, compared to 6.9 for white children. The racial differential is smaller for school-age children.

Most of the ambulatory care of children and youth is received in physicians' offices. About 56 percent of the physician contacts for children under age 18 are in a doctor's office.[10] Fourteen percent are in a hospital, and these visits are fairly evenly divided between outpatient clinics and emergency rooms. Telephone contacts account for 18 percent of the total, and other places for the remaining 12 percent (Table 7).

SUMMARY

Most children living in households in the U.S. appear to be physically healthy. Very few of those who survive infancy die, and few of the children living in the community are reported as spending a week or more in bed during the year or being limited by a chronic condition.

One indicator of children's health has worsened in the past decade. The proportion of school-age children limited in activity by a chronic condition has increased, from four percent in 1975/76 to six percent in 1985/86. Among preschool children, however, there has been no change.

The increase in limitation among school-age children is difficult to explain. If it were due to improved survival of high-risk newborns, one would expect an increase in the proportion of preschool children who are limited. If it were due to greater parental awareness, or better diagnosis via improved access to medical care, one would expect it to be observed for children of all ages. The fact that an increase occurred only among school-age children suggests that other factors are responsible. Improved school-based testing or teachers' awareness could be factors. More children in programs designed to bring disabled children into public school systems and out of institutions may be contributing, as well.

Racial differences are observed for several health indicators, including mortality, disability, and hospitalization. Since white children have more acute conditions than Black children at all ages under 18,[2,3] it is surprising that Black preschool children have the greater number of bed days. One possibility is that the acute conditions are more severe for Black than white children at the youngest ages. increased severity could be a long-term consequence of excess low birthweight among Black infants. It also could be a consequence of delays in receiving medical care.

TABLE 6

SHORT-STAY HOSPITAL EPISODES, BY AGE, RACE, AND SEX: UNITED STATES, 1985/86

| | All Races | | | White | | | All Other | | | | | |
| | | | | | | | Total | | | Black | | |
	Both Sexes	Male	Female	Both Sexes	Male	Female	Both Sexes	Male	Female	Both Sexes	Male	Female
Percent Of Children With 1+ Short-Stay Hospital Episodes In Preceding Year:												
Ages 0-4 Years	5.8	6.5	5.1	5.7	6.4	4.9	6.3	7.0	5.7	6.2	7.7	7.0
Ages 5-11 Years	2.8	3.0	2.6	3.0	3.1	2.8	2.2	2.6	1.7	2.3	2.7	1.8
Average Annual Number Of Short-Stay Hospital Episodes Per 100 Children:												
Ages 0-4 Years	7.5	8.7	6.2	7.3	8.5	6.0	8.5	9.7	7.3	8.7	9.6	7.7
Ages 5-11 Years	3.1	3.4	2.9	3.2	3.3	3.0	2.9	3.6	2.2	3.0	3.5	2.5
Average Annual Number Of Short-Stay Hospital Episode Days Per 100 Children:												
Ages 0-4 Years	50.2	52.3	48.0	45.3	48.4	42.0	71.5	69.7	73.4	73.4	71.6	75.3
Ages 5-11 Years	12.3	13.2	11.2	11.9	12.8	11.1	13.8	15.2	12.4	15.3	15.9	14.6

SOURCE: National Health Interview Survey, 1985 and 1986

REFERENCES

1. National Center for Health Statistics: Annual summary of births, marriages, divorces, and deaths, United States, 1986. Monthly Vital Statistics Report . Vol. 35, No. 13. DHHS Pub. No (PHS) 87-1120. Public Health Service, Hyattsville, MD, 1987.

2. National Center for Health Statistics, Moss AJ and Parsons, VL: Current estimates from the National Health Interview Survey, United States, 1985. Vital and Health Statistics. Series 10, No. 160. DHHS Pub. No. (PHS) 86-1588. Public Health Service. Washington. U.S. Government Printing Office, 1986.

3. National Center for Health Statistics, Dawson, DA and Adams, PF: Current estimates from the National Health Interview Survey, United States, 1986. Vital and Health Statistics. Series 10, No. 164. DHHS Pub. No. (PHS) 87-1592. Public Health Service. Washington. U.S. Government Printing Office, 1987.

4. National Center for Health Statistics: Health, United States, 1986. DHHS Pub. No. (PHS) 87-1232. Public Health Service. Washington. U.S. Government Printing Office, 1986.

5. U. S. Bureau of the Census: Economic Characteristics of Households in the United States: Fourth Quarter 1984. Current Population Reports, Series P-70, No. 6. Washington. U.S. Government Printing Office, 1986.

6. U.S. Bureau of the Census: Characteristics of the Population Below the Poverty Level. Current Population Reports, Series P-60, No. 147. Washington. U.S. Government Printing Office, 1985.

7. Kovar, M.G.: Health status of U.S. children and use of medical care. Public Health Reports 97:3-15, 1982.

8. Kozak, LJ, Norton C, McManus M and McCarthy E: Hospital use patterns for children in the United States, 1983 and 1984. Pediatrics 80(4):481-490, 1987.

9. U.S. National Center for Health Statistics, Bloom B: Use of selected preventive care procedures, United States, 1982. Vital and Health Statistics. Series 10, No. 157. DHHS Pub. No. 86-1585. Public Health Service. Washington. U.S. Government Printing Office, 1986.

10. U.S. National Center for Health Statistics, Ries P: Physician contacts by sociodemographic and health characteristics, United States, 1982-83. Vital and Health Statistics. Series 10, No. 161. DHHS Pub. No. (PHS) 87-1589. Public Health Service. Washington. U.S. Government Printing Office, 1987.

DAY CARE OF CHILDREN

29

Patricia T. Schloesser

As the century draws to a close, a social revolution is taking place, with day care replacing home care as a cultural institution for the rearing of young children. In increasing numbers, infants and preschool children are spending their days away from their own homes or relative care as their mothers enter the job market. In 1985, 20 million, or 62 percent, of women with children under 18 were employed.[1] The most dramatic rise in employment is among mothers of preschool children, with more than 52 percent in the labor force, affecting over nine million children under six years of age in 1984.[2] If present trends continue, the Children's Defense Fund projects that, by 1995, 34.4 million school-age children and 14.6 million preschool children will have mothers in the work force.

Mothers have joined the work force for a variety of personal and economic reasons. For most women, the primary reason is financial necessity. Only one job in five in the U.S. today will support a family of four at an acceptable standard of living. Although community day care arrangements have expanded, they have not kept pace with the needs of increasing numbers of single or two-parent working families. Relative care is also in decline, as other family members are also employed outside the home. The cost of paying a child care provider to come to the family home is prohibitive for many parents. Qualified persons willing to accept such employment, however, are on the increase as a result of a thriving nationwide "Nanny" training and placement program.

In 1958, 57 percent of young children whose mothers worked full time were cared for in their own homes, decreasing to 29 percent by 1977. The Bureau of the Census reported, in 1982, that 42.3 percent of children whose mothers worked were cared for by non-relatives. The care by site was in the child's own home, 13 percent; in a family day care home, 52 percent; and in a day care center, 35 percent.[3]

The types of child care arrangements available to working parents can be divided almost equally between care within the family or a relative's home and care in a community facility.[4] "Family care" may include care by parents with staggered working hours, a parent working in the home, relative care in the child's home or relative's home, and an employed child care provider who comes to the family home. Other family plans include care of younger children by an older sibling during part of the day, or self-care by the child (particularly those of school age), referred to as a "latchkey" arrangement. (Approximately five million children, six to 13 years of age, provide self-care before and after school.) Care in a community setting consists of purchased care from a facility, either regulated or non-regulated, which is operated by persons not related to the child. These arrangements also take several forms:

- Family day care homes for six or fewer children in a home setting.

- Group day care homes for seven to 12 children, with usually two adult care givers.

- Day care centers for 13 or more children on a part or full-day basis, including preschools, Head Start programs, school-age programs, infant/toddler care and care for children with special needs.

Most of the group day care homes are located in family homes. The setting for the centers may be a free-standing building designed specifically for day care or a church, school facility, or worksite such as a hospital. Of all types of community care, the family day care home, whether licensed, registered or unregulated, is the most common arrangement. Family day care homes tend to offer less permanent arrangements for children than day care centers, due to high turnover, and they may be unrecognized or in some states excluded from public regulation. All states regulate centers, although coverage varies, as some exclude certain categories, such as church operated facilities.

A HISTORICAL PERSPECTIVE

Group care of infants and young children outside of the family home originated in nurseries associated with orphanages for the poor. The Hospital of the Innocents, in Florence, established during the Middle Ages is perhaps one of the best known. A Della Robbia terra-cotta portrayal of a foundling at this early orphanage is the insignia of the American Academy of Pediatrics. In the U.S., the first recorded "day nursery" was opened in 1828 in Boston. The day nurseries established under charitable auspices in New York City, in the 1850s, were regulated by the sanitary code of the city health department, and came under the supervision of the Bureau of Child Hygiene when it was established in 1908.[5] In Kansas, the current child care licensing act, enacted in 1919, specifically included day nurseries. This category was cited as needing special protection in recognition that infants in orphanages were cared for in day nurseries during the day and were dying of infections and of "marasmus."[6]

Group education of preschool children began in the early nineteenth century with its future course set by Friedrich Froebel, a German educator, who named his school a *kindergarten*, or a "children's garden." In 1828, he wrote: "I shall not call this an infant school, because I do not intend children to be schooled, but to be allowed under the gentlest treatment to develop freely." These first kindergartens served children primarily from underprivileged homes, with an effort to provide good experiences for children as early as three years of age. Froebel reasoned that young children learned by doing things and their play could be organized to teach as well as to amuse. Modern preschools, Head Start, and kindergarten programs all incorporate much of this philosophy.

Early in the twentieth century, nursery schools became a popular supplement to home care for middle-class families for socialization and preschool educational purposes. It was not until the depression era of the 1930s that publicly run full-time day care centers for working families emerged. World War II gave further impetus to full-time day care programs. Federal funds were provided by the Lanham Act to provide day care for women joining the labor force to assist in the war effort. These centers were located at or near factories, hospitals, or community service agencies. Although the Lanham Act was repealed after the war, the need for child day care remained as an ever increasing number of women continued in the work force. During the 1950s, private day care arrangements in family homes and centers emerged to replace these earlier publicly operated facilities.

National policy considerations regarding working women and their need for day care surfaced at the Midcentury White House Conference on Children and Youth, in 1950. Among the recommendations was the call "that appropriate public bodies establish minimum standards for licensing or authorization with respect to plant, program, and staff, for all child care and preschool groups." By the 1960 White House Conference on Children and Youth, the recommendations took on greater substance and urgency—"that governmental assistance and support be given to the establishment and/or expansion of day care services for children of working mothers.[11]

The expansion of federal support in the 1960s and 1970s included the Head Start Program for disadvantaged preschool children, retraining programs for women entering the work force, a child care food program, a child care tax credit, employer tax incentives, and governmental funding of day care services for poor families. In

1971, a coalition of labor and social service agencies was credited with the passage by Congress of a wide-ranging, two billion dollar child care bill. It was vetoed by President Richard Nixon, who cited its high cost and "family weakening implications." Associated with increased federal funding of day care services for the poor, through the Title XX Program, were the Federal Interagency Day Care Regulations (FIDCR).[8] Although the federal standards served as a model for some states to upgrade day care requirements, they were never fully implemented, as many states did not comply. They were repealed in 1981, when federal responsibilities were transferred to states and the Social Service Block Grant replaced Title XX as a source of funding day care for the poor.

In the absence of federal standards and in an effort to upgrade day care programs, guidelines have been issued through the years by a number of private agencies, i.e., the Child Welfare League of America, American Academy of Pediatrics (AAP), American Public Health Association (APHA), and National Association for the Education of Young Children. [9,10,11,12]

CURRENT POLICY CONSIDERATIONS

Recent surveys point to an insufficient supply of quality, affordable day care for working families. As demand exceeds supply, day care facilities have less motivation to provide appropriate staff-child ratios, particularly for infants and toddlers, or to limit the number or group size of children in care. There is a high turnover of day care staff due to low wages, with potential harm for children because of ever-changing relationships. In January 1988, the Child Welfare League of America's biennial survey reported that adults who care for children earn only $12,800/year, less on the average than janitors, cleaners and garbage collectors. To assure quality and a stable nurturing environment, the child care staff must receive increased compensation and recognition. There is also a growing recognition that increased financial support of day care for families on public assistance will be necessary if they are to become self-sufficient.

The average cost of day care for a child is $3,000 a year, far beyond the reach of families below the poverty level (one-fifth of men heading two-parent families and two-thirds of women heading single-parent families). The major source of federal funding for child care assistance is from the Title XX Social Service Block grants to states which, when adjusted for inflation, in 1987, is worth only half of its 1977 level.[13] During this same period, preschool children living in poverty increased from 3.4 million to 4.9 million. Eighteen states have allocated state funds for day care, to increase the number of poor children served, yet 22 states provided care for fewer children in 1987 than they did in 1981.[13]

Contributions are being made by the private sector, with churches being the greatest resource. Child care assistance by employers is a relatively new phenomenon. An estimated 3,000 of the six million employers provide some type of employee benefit, such as on-site centers, vouchers for purchase-of-care in the community resource and referral services, and salary reduction plans. Hospitals are the primary employer providing on-site child care, largely as a means to recruit and retain hospital staff. Community-sponsored centers, supported in part by voluntary contributions, have also increased in numbers. These combined efforts, at the current level, cannot assure a sufficient quantity and quality of affordable day care for the nation's families.

In response to the urgent need for a national policy in support of day care, a coalition of over 90 organizations composed of religious groups, labor unions, and child care and health advocates established an Alliance for Better Child Care (ABC). Their recent lobbying resulted in the introduction by Congress of the "Act for Better Child Care Services of 1987."[14] The bill would authorize $2.5 billion a year, through 1993, to establish federal child care standards, help low- and marginal-income families pay for care, increase salaries for child care workers, and expand day care services across the country. Seventy-five percent of the funds would subsidize day care for families whose incomes are not more than 115 percent above a state's median income. Other funds would assist states in starting child care services through grants or loans, train child care providers, develop resource and referral services, and assure the monitoring and enforcement of standards. National standards of quality with particular reference to health and safety would be established. This act would benefit working families of all economic means by developing additional resources and upgrading the quality of existing day care programs.

DAY CARE RISKS

Beginning in 1983, the national news media increasingly focused on risks associated with day care, primarily infectious disease outbreaks and growing reports of physical and sexual abuse of children. Epidemiological studies by the Centers for Disease Control (CDC) and state and local public health authorities reported situations where infectious disease (hepatitis, giardiasis, salmonellosis, and meningitis) were being spread to the community from day care centers.[15, 16,17] The source was usually traced to overcrowded day care centers, especially those caring for infants and toddlers in diapers, which also had questionable hygiene practices and too few adults caring for the children.

At the National Conference on Infectious Diseases in Day Care, held in Minneapolis in 1984, the major recommendations were for improved environmental and staffing standards, basic hygiene measures, emphasizing handwashing, prevention, and management of infectious diseases, and training of child care providers.[18] During the same year, the APHA adopted a resolution urging the expansion of disease prevention and health promotion activities in day care programs for children.[19] This resolution was sent to the nation's governors and to the state health and social agencies, with an inquiry about state day care initiatives. Most states responded, describing new activities such as upgrading licensing standards, appointing inter-agency task forces, immunization surveillance, provision of Hemophilus Influen-zae Type b vaccine, provider education programs, abuse and injury prevention programs, and before and after school programs.[20]

The sensational news coverage of sexual abuse occurring in day care cen-ters in California, Minnesota, and New York City led to public concern and the enactment by Congress of Public Law 98-473, in 1984. This legislation made available federal funds to states for training programs in the prevention of child abuse in day care settings, and required states to establish procedures for checking employment and criminal record history for operators and employees of child care facilities. The law required the U.S. Department of Health and Human Services (DHHS) to provide guidance to states by distributing a Model Child Care Standards Act for state consideration. These standards addressed training, development, super-vision and evaluation of staff, staff qualifications, staff-child ratios, probation period for new staff, employment history checks for staff, and parental access to facilities.[21]

Risks from fire, unsafe playground equipment, poisons, drowning, safety hazards in the facility, and sudden infant death syndrome are all highly publicized whenever they occur in a day care setting, even though the incidence is less than in the family's own home. Risks requiring special attention to reduce potential harm to children in day care can be classified by four broad categories: physical plant, health, program, and care, as follows: [22]

Risks in Day Care Facilities

Physical Plant	**Program**
Fire	Staff/Child Ratio
Play Equipment	Activities/Equipment
Safety	Over-Enrollment
Transportation	Qualifications
Sanitation	
Building	
Environment	
Health	**Care**
Health Practices	Discipline
Staff Assessments	Neglect
Child Assessments	Physical Abuse
Immunizations	Sexual Abuse
Nutrition	
Injuries	
Emergency Procedures	

Kansas Department of Health and Environment, 1984.

Most of these risks can be lessened by accepted regulatory procedures. Others will require upgrading the training and skills of child care providers, improved involvement by parents, and increased economic support by society.

UPGRADING HEALTH AND SAFETY
OF DAY CARE FOR CHILDREN

Federal public health agencies, the CDC, and the DHHS are becoming increasingly involved with day care issues, and are targeting their funds to address problem areas. CDC has issued educational packets for national distribution to state licensing agencies, *What To Do To Stop Disease in Child Day Care Centers*, as a follow-up preventive effort to their investigations of disease outbreaks in day care facilities. Projects concerning health and safety issues in day care, such as injuries, child abuse, sudden infant death syndrome, Pediatric AIDS, and Hemophilus Influenzae Type b are being initiated. The health component of Head Start has been transferred to improve the integration of day care with MCH programs from the DHHS branch of Administration for Children, Youth and Families to the new Bureau of Maternal and Child Health and Resource Development. Beginning in 1985, three projects were funded to develop guidance publications for health professionals, providers, and parents. These projects consisted of grants to the American Academy of Pediatrics for the publication of *Health in Day Care: A Manual for Health Professionals*, to the Kansas Department of Health and Environment for the publication of *Health of Children in Day Care–Public Health Profiles*, and to Georgetown University for selected training materials for providers and parents.[23,24,25] Additionally, SPRANS grants (Special Projects of Regional and National Significance) have been awarded to Massachusetts to improve the health of children in family day care, to Connecticut for upgrading health and safety for infant and toddler care in centers, and to the APHA and AAP to develop national performance standards for health and safety in day care.

States administer a system of public regulation of out-of-home child care in the form of licensing of day care centers, including preschools, and licensing or registration of family day care homes. An effective regulatory system can reduce risks for children in day care and assure that the care they receive will be nurturing, educational, and meet their developmental needs. Through licensing standards, an acceptable quality is set which will permit a facility to operate legally. At present there is no national definition of acceptable standards, so that each state has set its own minimal standards, with considerable variation in quality. These variations are influenced both by public understanding of the needs of young children and economic factors which often conflict. The staff/child ratio is a good illustration of both factors. The younger the child, the smaller the group size should be, which means increased costs for additional staff. In the case of infants, the National Association of Education of Young Children (NAEYC) recommends one adult to three infants, yet only three states meet this standard,[26] with some states allowing seven infants to one adult. The extent of regulatory coverage also differs between states, with some states exempting programs such as church-operated programs, part-day programs, or by number or age of children in care, as in small family day care homes or programs for school-age children. A well-designed regulatory system will encompass all non-relative out-of-home care. For programs operated by public schools, standards at least equivalent to those of the licensing agency should be maintained.

The administrative responsibility for regulating day care has been assigned by state statutes primarily to the social welfare agency, as an extension of a basic child welfare concern for the protection of children in 24-hour care. However, there are seven states—Arizona, Connecticut, Kansas, Maryland, Mississippi, New Hampshire, and New Mexico, and several cities and counties where the licensing authority is assigned to the public health agency. In the other states, public health agencies participate primarily through sanitation inspections, immunization surveillance, epidemiological investigations, and with the formulation of health and safety standards.

In recent years, many public health agencies have become involved in innovative day care activities which promote the health of children in day care. Some examples include a multidisciplinary consultative and educational team service of the Minneapolis Health Department, the Infectious Disease and Injury Prevention Programs of Seattle/King County Health Department, an interagency Maternal and Child Health Council with day care a priority in Marin County, California, and programs relating to Hemophilus Influenzae Type b and diagnostic services for the handicapped of Dallas, Texas.[26]

PUBLIC HEALTH DAY CARE ISSUES

Often preschoolers are seen by health care providers only during illness. The day care setting offers new opportunities for extending preventive health services to "well" children. Through day care programs, public health professionals can also have access to other family members who may benefit from preventive health services. Since children in day care are a "captive group," as is the school population, the public health experience with school health programs (environment, health services, and health education) is easily transferable to the preschool population.

ENVIRONMENT CONCERNS

The basic environmental inspections of day care facilities by local health department sanitarians and by local fire officials have received the most attention from the public health community. These inspections are generally limited to centers which provide care to less than half of the nation's children in out-of-home care. The sanitation areas addressed are food protection, safety and health, staff education concerning emergencies and hygiene, facility construction, and disease reporting. According to the APHA's *Model Standards: A Guide for Community Preventive Health Services*, a sanitation program should ensure that "every child in child care facilities will be protected from health and safety hazards."[27] In recent years, the safety of playground equipment and education about car restraints have received renewed attention.[28,29]

DISEASE PREVENTION AND CONTROL

Almost all local health departments have been called on for advice and control measures when outbreaks of childhood or diarrheal diseases occur in day care centers. Reporting, investigations, surveillance, and preventive measures have intensified as an increasing number of infants and toddlers are placed in out-of-home group care. Day care providers frequently seek out local and state public health agencies and the CDC for assistance about hygiene, control measures, and educational programs for day care providers.

Disease prevention and control is an area for which health departments are often the only community resource for day care providers. The Seattle-King County Department of Public Health does not have regulatory or licensing jurisdiction over child care. However, due to the need of child care providers for guidance of dealing with accident prevention, communicable disease, and illness management on a daily basis, the county health department has increased its resources to provide expertise and technical assistance regarding illness and its prevention in day care centers. A day care handbook focusing on illness prevention and management was developed by the health department's nurse epidemiologist and distributed to licensed day care sites.[30]

IMMUNIZATIONS

An immunization schedule is an integral component of state regulatory programs. Many state health departments have developed interagency agreements with the regulatory agency to determine the percentage of children in regulated day care programs who have completed the total immunization series. The results have been favorable. More than 95 percent of the preschool children in day care are fully immunized in Kansas, as compared with 80 percent to 85 percent of preschoolers who are not in day care. Connecticut and Maryland also report that 95 percent of children in regulated facilities are completely immunized.[30]

NUTRITION

A child care setting provides opportunities to improve the nutritional status of the child and can serve as a model for education parents. Children in full-day care, nine-ten hours a day, often receive two meals a day in out-of-home care; thus the meals need to be nutritious and well-balanced. The posting of a daily menu at the center provides a guide for parents and aids in planning the appropriate remaining meals at home. The child care food program of the U.S. Department of Agriculture has become an important resource in upgrading the nutrition of children in day care. As public health agencies have increased their nutritionist staffing, primarily through the WIC Program, nutrition consultation has also become available to day care facilities through public health departments.

Nutritional assessment evaluations and training of all newly licensed facilities in Mississippi was implemented by the public health agency, following a 1985 nutritional evaluation of licensed day care centers which found that newly licensed facilities were often not aware, or did not adhere, to nutritional care standards.[30]

PROMOTION OF CHILD HEALTH

Health supervision, screening, and early identification of problems may be the area of public health expertise that has received the least attention. State licensing regulations for day care require an initial health assessment for admission; however, the degree of compliance, follow-up of problems, and continuing well-child supervision are often not documented or carried out. The Head Start Program is probably the best model of a comprehensive service that assures child health supervision according to the schedule of the AAP.

In the early 1980s, the MCH agency in Massachusetts reassessed its role of serving the general population of preschool children. Renewed emphasis was placed on the child health and development of over 125,000 preschool children receiving child care within an identifiable and organized day care system. A preschool health program was established to address the health concerns of day care providers, primarily communicable diseases. Development of a comprehensive health guide for day care providers, statewide training conferences and workshops, and participation in state level/interagency policy-development and standard-setting task forces were initial activities of the Massachusetts Public Health Department's Preschool Health Program. A number of other public health agencies, such as those in Seattle and Minneapolis, have developed health manuals as guidance for day care providers and parents. Screening for vision and hearing is another service offered to day care programs, as reported by agencies in Illinois, Nebraska, and Baltimore.[30]

A day care program, where health checkups, screenings, and immunizations are provided, is a valuable asset for working parents reluctant to take time off to keep appointments for well-child care. The day care center also provides a good setting for discussions between health professionals, parents, and day care staff members of child health needs, nutrition, discipline, growth and development, and injury prevention.

EMERGING ISSUES AND BEGINNING SOLUTIONS

The next generation of adults will be affected profoundly by how we address the child care challenge in this country. Affordable quality care must be available for children of working parents to assure the growth of healthy, secure children. Legislators, governors, business and community leaders, child care providers, and families are banding together to establish child care policies and standards at the national, state and local levels. Public health officials are actively involved in these discussions.

Individuals concerned with the needs of children and families should take an active role in supporting policies allowing more liberal parental leave for sick child care. Care for the sick children, by their primary caretaker, appears to be optimum from the child's viewpoint by providing for the emotional, developmental, and cognitive needs of the child.[31] However, working parents may not be able to take leave, given the lack of a national leave policy in this country, and alternatives need to be developed. A number of services have been established to care for mildly ill children. Traditional child care centers usually exclude ailing children, thus working parents often have to face difficult choices between employment responsibilities and care of their sick child. Thus, sick child care services, ranging from in-home care by paraprofessionals or nurses in specialized hospital-based settings attached to pediatric units, have been developed to address the needs of working parents with mildly ill children. Employers are increasingly contracting for sick child care services for their employees or subsidizing their employee's sick child care expenses and cost-savings measures. Parents who stay home to mind sick children cost their employers in sick time, overtime, and temporary replacement expenses. A number of policy issues need to be addressed, as day care and illness are researched and child care services for mildly ill children are established. Local health departments will become increasingly involved in licensing standards, infection control training, staff-child ratios, and health and safety requirements.[32]

Another area which states are currently addressing is services for economically disadvantaged children. The National Conference of State Legislatures issued a recent report on alternatives states use to finance child care and early childhood education programs, which outlined states' efforts to meet the needs of academically and socially at-risk children.[33] Findings from a growing body of research demonstrate that early childhood education is effective with children from economically disadvantaged families in improving school performance, reducing drop out and teen pregnancy rates, decreasing delinquency and arrest rates, decreasing welfare dependency, and increasing the likelihood of employment in young adulthood.[34]

Coordination of child care and early childhood education policies will benefit families and children by providing a coordinated approach to both child care and early education needs. The Head Start Program is an excellent model of comprehensive developmental services for low-income preschool children which provides educational, social, and health services with a strong emphasis on parental involvement. The Report of Select Panel for the Promotion of Child Health (1980) recommended the Head Start model as a vehicle for improving the health care of children. The health component of Head Start arranges for, or provides, a broad array of preventive, diagnostic, treatment, and rehabilitative services for enrolled children.[35]

Another early education issue is how to address child care for special needs (handicapped) children. During the preschool years, the development of social interaction skills is particularly important for special needs children and a child care program is an ideal setting for this development. Both age-appropriate and special-needs children can benefit from mainstreaming experiences. States will need to take action to integrate their PL 99-457 preschool responsibilities with their child care policies.

Increasing attention needs to be given to the proper care of infants in child care. Obviously, the younger the child the greater is the need for individualized care and continuity of relationships. The debate must center on the best placement for meeting an infant's developmental needs. Child development specialists differ as to when parents should return to work after the birth of a child and whether care in the family home, a family day care home, or a day care center can best meet their needs.

Another growing issue is the provision of subsidized child care to enable women with families to leave public assistance rolls. Poor women and their children are often caught in a vicious cycle of poverty and dependence. Subsidized quality child care can enable families to break the cycle of welfare dependency and insure economic self-sufficiency.

Attainment of a children's potentials depends on the understanding, insight and skill of those who guide them—their parents or others, as well as their own capacities. The environment provides the key to the child's realization of a maximum degree of health, education and happiness.[36] The child care challenge in this country is growing and public health will play a critical role in determining the course of that challenge.

REFERENCES

1.   U.S. Department of Labor, Women's Bureau, Facts on Women Workers Fact Sheet No. 86-1, March 1985.

2.   Hayghelt. Working Mothers Reach a Record Number in 1984, Research Summaries in Monthly Labor Review, Office of Employment and Unemployment Statistics, U.S. Bureau of Labor Statistics, Washington, D.C., December 1984, pp 31-34.

3. Bureau of the Census, 1982.

4. Morgan G. Child Care Options for Working Parents, in Sharp MC, Henderson FW (eds): Daycare, Report of the Sixteenth Ross Roundtable on Critical Approaches to Common Pediatric Problems. Columbus, Ohio: Ross Laboratories, 1985, pp. 4-9.

5. Goldsmith C. Child Day Care, A Public Health Responsibility. Am Jour of Public Health, 1959, 49:1069-1073.

6. Tenth Biennial Report and Bulletins, 1920, Kansas Board of Health.

7. White House Conference on Children and Youth, Recommendations by Forum II 1950, and Recommendations by Forum II, III, 1960.

8. Federal Interagency Day Care Requirements, Washington, D.C., Government Printing Office, 1968 (Revised 1980, as DHHS Day Care Report).

9. Child Welfare League of America: Standards for Day Care Services, New York, 1984.

10. Health in Day Care: A Manual for Health Professionals, American Academy of Pediatrics, Elk Grove, Illinois, 1987.

11. Dittman L. (with the Committee on Day Care, Maternal and Child Health Section, American Public Health Associates) Children in Day Care with Focus on Health, Children's Bureau, DHEW, Washington, D.C., 1967.

12. National Association for the Education of Young Children, Accreditation Criteria and Procedures, 1985.

13. State Child Care Fact Book 1987, Children's Defense Fund, Washington, D.C.

14. Act for Better Child Care Services of 1987, 100th Congress, 1st Session, S. 1885.

15. Hadler SC, Erben JJ, Francis PO, et al. Risk factors for Hepatitis A in Day Care Centers, Jour of Infectious Diseases 145:255-261, 1982.

16. Goodman RA. Infectious Diseases and Child Day Care. Pediatrics 74:134-139, 1984.

17. Pickering LK. The Day Care Center Diarrhea Dilemma. Am Jour of Pub Health 76:623-624, 1986.

18. Osterholm MT, Klein JO, Aronson SS, and Pickering LK. Infectious Diseases in Child Care: Management and Prevention. Minneapolis, MN, June 21-23, 1984. Reviews of Infectious Diseases, Vol 8, No 4, July-Aug, 1986.

19. American Public Health Association: Health Risks and Infectious Diseases Associated with Child Day Care: Resolution 8402. Am Jour of Pub Health 75:295-296, 1985.

20. Schloesser PT. Children in Day Care: A Public Health Challenge, Public Health Currents, Vol 26, No 5, 1986. Ross Laboratories, Columbus, Ohio.

21. Model Child Care Standards Act: Guidance to States to Prevent Child Abuse in Day Care Facilities, Jan, 1985.

22. Schloesser PT, Cameron EL, Class NS. Kansas Public Health Intervention to Reduce Risks for Children in Day Care. Paper presented at Am Public Health Assoc, 1984.

23. Health in Day Care: A Manual for Health Professionals, Am Academy of Pediatrics, Elk Grove Village, Illinois, 1987.

24. Schloesser PT, et al. Health of Children in Day Care: Public Health Profiles, Kansas Dept of Health and Environment, 1987.

25. Health in Day Care—A Manual for Day Care Providers, Georgetown University Child Development Center, Washington, D.C., December, 1986.

26. State Child Care Fact Book 1987, Children's Defense Fund, Washington, D.C.

27. Model Standards: A Guide for Community Preventive Health Services, ed 2. Washington, D.C.: Am Public Health Association, 1985.

28. Aronson SS. Injuries in Child Care. Young Children 38:19-20, 1983.

29. Chang A, Dillman AS, Lenard E, English P. Teaching Car Passenger Safety to Preschool Children. Pediatrics 76:425-428, 1985.

30. Schloesser PT, et al. Health of Children in Day Care. Public Health Profiles, Kansas Dept of Health and Environment, 1987.

31. Stern G. Day Care for Sick Children. Pediatrics, Vol 79, No. 3, March 1987, p. 446.

32. Haskins R, Kotch J. Day Care and Illness: Evidence, Costs, and Public Policy. Pediatrics, June 1986, Vol 77, No 6, Part 2 Supplement.

33. National Conference State Legislators: State Fiscal Policies for Child Care and Early Childhood Education. Gnezda, T: State Legislative Report, Vol 12, No. 7, Denver, CO, Oct 1987.

34. 1) Consortium for Longitudinal Studies, Lasting Effects After Preschool, Final Report. Washington, D.C.: U.S Govt Printing Office, 1978.

   2) Consortium for Longitudinal Studies, Persistence of Preschool Effects: Status, Stress and Coping Skills, Final Report. Washington D.C.: U.S. Govt Printing office, 1980.

35. U.S. Department of Health and Human Services, Better Health for Our Children: A National Strategy, Report of the Select Panel for the Promotion of Child Health. Vol 1, Major Findings and Recommendations, 1981, p. 253.

36. Dittman L. (with the Committee on Day Care, Maternal and Child Health Section, Am Pub Health Associates): Children in Day Care with Focus on Health. Children's Bureau, DHEW, Washington, D.C., 1967.

‖ HEAD
‖ START 30

Phyllis E. Stubbs

The Head Start program was first funded under Title V of the Economic Opportunity Act of 1964, 42 U.S.C. 2921, et seq. Twenty-three years later, the program continues to deliver a comprehensive child development program to preschool-aged children from low-income families.

The Head Start program is currently authorized under Title I of the Human Services Reauthorizations Act of 1986, P.L. 99-425.[1] This legislation authorized a funding level of up to $1,198 million for Fiscal Year (FY) 1987. This funding level represents an increase of $90,327 million over the final FY 1986 appropriation. Section 639 of this funding legislation authorizes spending through FY 1990, when the authorized appropriation level will be $1,405 million.

The program is administered by the Head Start Bureau, which is located in the Administration for Children, Youth and Families, Office of Human Development Services, U.S. Department of Health and Human Services. Head Start programs are funded through grants from the Administration for Children, Youth and Families' Regional Offices, and the Native American Migrant Program Branches. These grants are awarded to a variety of local public agencies, private non-profit organizations and public school systems.

The first Head Start programs offered preschool children from disadvantaged families an eight-week summer experience built around four program components. Today, the Head Start program operates as a full-year program serving

451,732 children and their families from urban, rural, suburban, Native American, and migrant farm worker communities. This represents approximately 17 percent of the Nation's low-income preschool children who are eligible for program enrollment.[2]

Head Start programs serve a multi-racial/multi-ethnic group of children and families. Of the children served: 40 percent are Black; 32 percent white; 21 percent Hispanic; four percent American Indian; and three percent Asian.[2]

All Head Start programs must offer four major components: education, social services, parent involvement, and health. With the goal of meeting each child's individual needs, the program offers a wide variety of learning experiences aimed at fostering intellectual, social, and emotional growth. Head Start also aims to meet the ethnic and cultural characteristics of the communities served. For example, when programs have a majority of children who are bilingual, the program must also have at least one teacher, or teacher's aide, fluent in the native language of the enrolled children.

Head Start program learning experiences engage the children in indoor and outdoor play, introduce them to the concept of words and numbers, encourage the expression of feelings, and the development of self-confidence and social competency.

The major objectives of Head Start social services component include:[3]

- outreach and recruitment of eligible children;
- support and assistance to families in improving the quality of family life; and
- make parents aware of community services and resources and facilitate their use.

Social Services program staff work to assist families in assessing their needs. Based on the family needs assessment, services are awarded that build on the individual strengths of families as they attempt to meet their own needs.

Head Start's parent-involvement component operates on the premise that in order for gains to be made by the Head Start child, these gains must not only be understood by the family but also supported by both the child's family and community. Head Start encourages involvement of the child's parent in every aspect of the child development center and its operation. Head Start parents are an important part of child development activities, health services, program planning, and operating activities, such as serving on policy councils where decisions are made about the program and its administration. With the Head Start belief that parents are the most important influence on a child's development, parent involvement has become a major influence in every part of the Head Start program.

The health component is designed to provide a comprehensive approach to the delivery of medical, dental, nutrition, and mental health services. The major objectives of the component include:

> arranging or providing a broad range of health maintenance or prevention, diagnostic treatment and rehabilitative services; and linking the Head Start child and family to an ongoing source of health care that will be available to the family after the child has left the Head Start program.[3]

Medical services received by all Head Start children include a complete examination; growth assessment; vision and hearing screening; anemia screening; development assessment; immunizations; and identification of handicapping conditions. Dental examination, treatment for problems found on examination, and dental health education are the major dental services offered by the program. Head Start's nutrition program provides nutritious meals for enrolled children and nutrition education for children, staff, and parents.

Head Start's mental health services work with other program components to encourage the emotional and social development of enrolled children. A mental health professional must be available to every Head Start program to provide mental health training to staff and parents; and to make them aware of the need for early attention to the special problems of children.

Health education for children, parents, and staff is a major part of all Head Start health programs. A variety of educational approaches have traditionally been used by Head Start staff to prepare children for what many of them will experience as their first visits to physician and dental offices. More recently, delivery of health education has focused on the integration of health information into the ongoing classroom activities.

Working with the American Dental Association, Head Start developed an integrated Dental Health Education curriculum[4] for preschool children, in 1984. In addition to classroom dental health-education modules, the curriculum also includes materials for the child to take home in order to inform parents of dental health-education principles learned by their children, and instruct parents on activities they can carry out in the home in order to reinforce the dental health-education practices their children have learned in Head Start.

In 1985, a Head Start grant to Montclair State College supported the development of an integrated nutrition education curriculum[5] that has been well-received by the field. Both the dental and nutrition health-education curriculum represented a major departure from the Head Start health component's traditional approach to the delivery of health materials for program staff. Where earlier health materials focused on supporting the Head Start health-program health-coordinators in their charge to administer the health component, the new health education curriculum has been developed for use by classroom teachers.

Program Information Report [6] show that Head Start's efforts in facilitating the delivery of health care services to preschool children from low-income families has been successful. For program year 1985-1986, 97 percent of the children served by the program 90 days and longer completed all medical screenings, and treatment services were provided to 97 percent of the children needing further services. In the dental area, 95 percent of the children enrolled at least 90 days completed required dental examinations. Dental treatment services were provided to 96 percent of the children needing these services. For immunization services, 96 percent of the children either completed or were up-to-date in required immunizations.

THE HEAD START PROGRAM
FOR CHILDREN WITH HANDICAPS

Head Start is the largest provider in this country of services for preschool children with handicapping conditions, in a mainstream setting. Head Start has successfully carried out a 1972 congressional mandate requiring that at least ten percent of its national enrollment consist of handicapped children. Head Start is now applying that mandate on a state-by-state basis and requiring that special education and related services be provided to meet the needs of enrolled handicapped children.[7] In FY 1986, Head Start served 69,990 children who were certified by professionals as handicapped. This constitutes 12.5 percent of the total enrollment.

Head Start is mandated to serve preschool children who have a broad range of handicaps. Diagnostic categories for Head Start handicap services are shown in Table 1. In program year 1985, the speech impairment diagnostic category repre-

---

TABLE 1

HEAD START HANDICAP DIAGNOSTIC CRITERIA

MENTALLY RETARDED

HARD OF HEARING

DEAF

SPEECH IMPAIRED

VISUALLY HANDICAPPED

SERIOUSLY EMOTIONALLY DISTURBED

ORTHOPEDICALLY IMPAIRED

HEALTH IMPAIRMENTS

SPECIFIC LEARNING DISABILITY

---

sented 61.9 percent of the handicapped children served in Head Start, and health impairment diagnostic category represented 11.1 percent. The remaining percentage distribution of diagnostic categories for all handicapped children served that year are shown in Figure 1.

Head Start also serves a significant proportion of children with severe or multiple handicaps. Such children present additional challenges to Head Start staff in the planning and provision of individual services. Program requirements call for individualized plans for special education, treatment, and related services for all handicapped children served by Head Start. These plans must be based on the child's specific handicapping conditions, as well as the unique needs arising from those conditions.

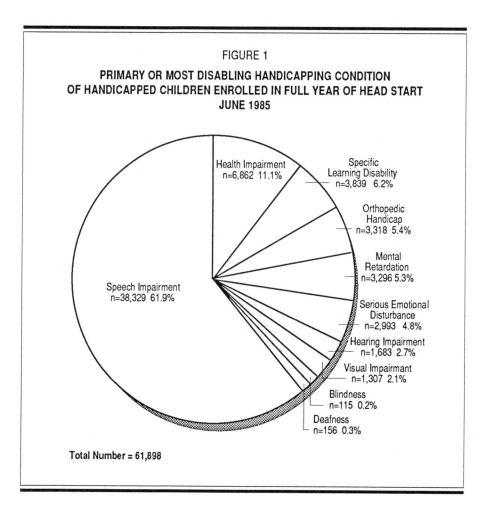

FIGURE 1

PRIMARY OR MOST DISABLING HANDICAPPING CONDITION OF HANDICAPPED CHILDREN ENROLLED IN FULL YEAR OF HEAD START JUNE 1985

Health Impairment
n=6,862 11.1%

Specific
Learning Disability
n=3,839 6.2%

Orthopedic
Handicap
n=3,318 5.4%

Mental
Retardation
n=3,296 5.3%

Serious Emotional
Disturbance
n=2,993 4.8%

Hearing Impairment
n=1,683 2.7%

Visual Impairmant
n=1,307 2.1%

Blindness
n=115 0.2%

Deafness
n=156 0.3%

Speech Impairment
n=38,329 61.9%

Total Number = 61,898

TRAINING AND TECHNICAL
ASSISTANCE FOR HEAD START HEALTH SERVICES

A very important part of the Head Start program's philosophy has always been to support upward mobility of Head Start families. One of the ways this is encouraged is through the involvement of Head Start parents, first as volunteers, classroom, and component aides, and ultimately as coordinators for the program's four components. This is also true in the health area. Whereas, a large number of Head Start health coordinators will have health backgrounds, a large number of Head Start health coordinators may have first come to the Head Start program as parents, later to become health aides and eventually function as health, nutrition, and mental health coordinators.

In attempting to support this type of upward mobility by Head Start parents and staff members, the Head Start program has had to make a major commitment to the establishment of strong training/technical assistance (T/TA) networks in each of the four component areas.

Head Start health services has a long history of T/TA support. The first national health T/TA network was with the U.S. Public Health Service (PHS) division of Dentistry, in support of T/TA and monitoring of Head Start grantees in the dental services area. This network is currently in its 22nd year of ongoing Intra-Agency Agreements between the Head Start Bureau and the Public Health Service.

In the late 1960s, through 1975, the American Academy of Pediatrics served as the major medical T/TA provider to Head Start programs. From 1976-1982, Westinghouse Health Systems served as T/TA provider for the medical, nutrition and mental health disciplines. From 1982-1986, the national medical, nutrition, and mental health T/TA network was discontinued, and T/TA support to Head Start grantees was attempted through a variety of different methods, including statewide and regional networks. Although some excellent models of state and regional T/TA networks were developed over this five-year period, it eventually became obvious that T/TA for Head Start medical, nutrition and mental health services was being attempted on a seriously unequal level of effort throughout the country. If a national level of excellence in Head Start health program performance was to be accomplished, a more uniform system of T/TA would have to be established.

In January 1987, an Intra-Agency Agreement was signed between the Office of Human Development Services, Administration for Children, Youth and Families, Head Start Bureau, and PHS, Health Resources and Services Administration, Bureau of Maternal and Child Health and Resources Development. The purpose of the agreement was to develop and implement a T/TA support system for Head Start health services in the medical, nutrition and mental health areas. The agreement was modified the following year to include training, technical assistance, and program monitoring of the Head Start dental services. With the signing of this modified agreement, the PHS now has responsibility for T/TA support to all four disciplines making up Head Start's health services component.

Internally, within the Head Start Bureau and the PHS, major shifts of existing Head Start Bureau health services staff and identification of new PHS staff members of Head Start occurred shortly after the signing of the new Intra-Agency Agreement. The Directory of Head Start Health Services Branch was reassigned to the PHS Bureau of Maternal and Child Health and Resources Development to direct the newly created Early Childhood Health Branch within the Division of Maternal, Child and Infant Health.

Within the ten PHS Regional Offices, public health nurses and nutritionists have been designated regional Head Start health services consultants. Their first charge was to develop the regional Head Start health services T/TA network by identifying, recruiting, and training state and local nurses and nutritionists to be T/TA consultants to Head Start grantees. The regional PHS public health nurses and nutritionists, along with the established network of regional PHS dental Head Start consultants, now function as regional PHS Head Start T/TA consultation teams.

As of September 1987, over 500 nutrition and nursing consultants have been brought on board as state and local PHS Head Start Health Consultants. These consultants will be providing training and on-site technical assistance to Head Start grantees all over the country. With time, it is hoped that this consultant network will prove to be a critical factor in the forging of a stronger link between Head Start and public health programs. Public health staff involvement in the Head Start programs can be most helpful when directed towards assisting Head Start grantees to provide the preventive health services and health education programs mandated by the Head Start program's health services performance standards. It is hoped that state and local health departments that do not currently have linkages with the Head Start programs in their service areas will be able to join Head Start in providing a comprehensive health services program to preschool children from low-income families.

REFERENCES

1. Human Services Reauthorization Act of 1986: Title I - The Head Start Program,Sec. 635. Head Start Act. P.L. 99-425.

2. Administration for Children, Youth and Families: Project Head Start Statistical Fact Sheet. Office of Human Development Services, Department of Health and Human Services, Washington, D.C., 1987.

3. Administration for Children, Youth and Families. Head Start Bureau: "Head Start Program Performance Standards." U.S. Department of Health and Human Services, Washington, D.C., DHHS Pub No (OHDS) 84-31131.

4. Administration for Children, Youth and Families. Head Start Bureau: "Head Start Dental Health Curriculum." U.S. Department of Health and Human Services, Washington, D.C., DHHS Pub No. (OHDS) 86-31535.

5. Administration for Children, Youth and Families. Head Start Bureau: "Head Start Nutrition Education Curriculum." U.S. Department of Health and Human Services, Washington, D.C., 1987.

6. Administration for Children, Youth and Families. Head Start Bureau: "Head Start Nutrition Education Curriculum." U.S. Department of Health and Human Services, Washington, D.C., 1986.

7. Administration for Children, Youth and Families. Head Start Bureau: "The Status of Handicapped Chidren in Head Start Programs." U.S. Department of Health and Human Services, Washington, D.C.

SCHOOL HEALTH SERVICES

31

Philip R. Nader

Schools are a microcosm of society. Whatever health issues and concerns are utmost in the minds of people, these issues find themselves manifested in the schools. Current examples include prevention programs for child sexual abuse; mandatory reporting of child abuse cases; educational efforts to prevent smoking, alcohol, and drug abuse; and AIDS and AIDS-education issues. Historically, school health was an under-emphasized and neglected area of health care, dealing with "routine" issues such as immunizations, mandated sensory screening tests, and treatment for minor trauma. School health has become an increasingly important arena for attempting to deal with many of society's most difficult health concerns. This direction has created a marked imbalance in demands when compared to the resources usually allocated to schools. This signals that, in the future, school health programs are likely to undergo radical changes compared to their present configurations.

A new definition of school health is needed. Traditional conceptualizations restrict school health to school-based programs of services, curriculum, and school environment. A new definition will include the school as one locus of a range of health and educational activities carried out by a broad group of health and educational personnel, based both in schools and in the community. These activities will relate to either preventing disease, promoting health, or minimizing the complications of health problems of school-age children. It is important to note that "school-age" in many states now reaches from birth to majority, especially for children with health handicaps. The grouping together of younger and younger children will place increasing demands on school health services.

This chapter will review existing organization, staffing, and services offered by school health programs. It will then review unmet needs and future challenges for school health services.

I. ORGANIZATION

The organization of school health services is not standard. It varies qualitatively and quantitatively around the U.S. and the world. It may form a central arm of delivery of preventive health care to the school-age population or it may only be an adjunct to existing health service programs in the community.

It may be designed for specific purposes, such as to meet needs of a handicapped population or to attempt to bridge a gap in access to medical care for a specific group, such as adolescents.

The organization of school health services depends upon the definition which is derived from desired goals for the service. These goals and the subsequent definitions decided upon should be based upon the specific needs and resources of a given geographic or political division. School health often has been relegated to an "orphan" status. That is, nobody truly "owns" school health. In a recently published U.S. survey of School Health, 29 states indicated that the education department was responsible for school health, while 18 indicated that health was the responsible department. Four states did not respond.[1]

Various models of organization within either the health department or school (local education agency) exist, but often center on a key professional—the school nurse. Economic pressures on schools, a "return to the basics," and a lack of success of documenting the value of school health services has resulted in a recent trend toward replacement of the professional school nurse by less qualified nurse aides or licensed practical nursing personnel. This is likely to have a major impact on the quality and quantity of school health services available to children. The roles that various health and educational professionals play in school health will be considered below.

II. STAFFING

Many people influence school health, regardless of the bureaucracy under which the service operates. It is not unusual for a non-health trained individual to have administrative responsibility for the school health services. Table 1 illustrates some of these non-health-trained individuals and their role in relation to the school health services.

TABLE 1

NON-NURSING SCHOOL ROLES AND
RESPONSIBILITIES TO SCHOOL HEALTH

Position or Title And Activities	Decision Making Relevant To School Health
School Superintendent Chief administrator of school system; directly responsible to school board. Budgets and public relations are generally priority concerns; almost always has experience in teaching and administration in various schools, moves to new community to become superintendent.	Budgetary Personnel hiring and firing Represents "school" to parent Controls deployment of local school and district resources Controls teachers' time and distribution of effort
Assistant Superintendent Similar to superintendent, but may be more directly involved with other administrators in schools, eg, monitors principal's meetings, works closely with curriculum directors, personnel director.	
Principal Chief administrator of individual school. School is considered "his/her house," therefore guests are expected to greet principal as they enter and leave. Principal is of crucial importance in determining fate of change process in individual school.	
Classroom Teacher Works with children in regular educational program. Pupils receive most of their instruction from this team (many schools have "team teaching" at various grade levels so students may receive instruction from each teacher on the team).	Identification of students Referral of students Contacts parents Willingness to implement special programs for specific children
Special Educator, Resource Teacher a. Self-contained, works with special education pupils on a full-day basis. Pupils receive all instruction from this teacher.	Certification, individual investigation of need for services Carries out special or remedial instructional plan

(Continued on next page)

(TABLE 1 - Continued)

Position or Title And Activities	Decision Making Relevant To School Health
b. Resource room, teaches students who come from regular classroom to resource room as necessary for special instruction (small groups, sometimes individual tutoring).	Willingness to coordinate effort with regular teacher Personal assessment and interaction with child
Speech And Language Specialist Often administers screening test to students, provides individual and small group therapy.	Certification, individual investigation of need for services Carries out treatment programs for children with speech and/ or language problems
Counselor Roles of counselors vary depending on need and other resource staff in school Most are identified with certain responsibilities and areas, eg. vocational counselor monitors program and works with kids in this track, academic counselor is concerned with individual academic programs of children, coordinates program and often serves as liaison between student and teachers, special education counselor provides pupil and parent counseling, concerning problems arising out of child's handicapping condition.	Certification, individual assessment of need for services May coordinate special education resources for children May be liaison with parents, teachers in overall planning
School psychologist May provide same services as educational diagnostician and associate psychologist, but is likely more involved in a consultation role to teachers, supportive professional personnel, parents, and community agencies.	Certification, individual assessment of need for services May coordinate special education resources for children May be liaison with parents, teachers in overall planning
Associate Psychologist Role very similar to education diagnostician, however, can assess emotional and/or behavioral factors, may co-lead groups with social worker in school.	

(Continued on next page)

(TABLE 1 - Continued)

Position or Title And Activities	Decision Making Relevant To School Health
Education Diagnostician Serves on support services team (appraisal team); is the psychometrist in the school, often is involved in developing individual educational plans and talking with parents.	
Social Worker Generally more of an outreach worker with children and families, consults with school personnel and community agencies and parents, may do individual and group counseling in school context.	May be part of certification of need May coordinate liaison with parents and school staff May carry out direct counseling with children, parents
Outreach Worker May be paraprofessional from neighborhood of school, assist in obtaining services for families.	
Health Educator May have coordinating, classroom teaching, or combination role. Some districts and states combine health and physical education.	Coordinates, teaches health curriculum at all levels, K-12 Potentially could carry out educational programs integrated with school health services
Health Office Aide, Teaching Aide Usually a high school graduate, aide may be utilized in classroom or clinic to assist professional with clerical duties and individual supervision of children.	Provides direct services to children May act as gatekeeper for children's complaints Can facilitate record keeping, parent contacts

Used by permission from Pediatrics in Review

PHYSICIANS

Pediatricians and family physicians have shown interest in school health. Certain other specialists also have interests in the school-related aspects of care of their patients (e.g. orthopedic surgeons and the physically handicapped; allergists and children with asthma). In 1987, there were only 130 physician members of the national American School Health Association, and very few school districts employed either full-time or part-time physician consultants. Only one U.S. state requires special certification for school physicians.[1] This has resulted in increased need to involve community primary care physicians in school health programs.[2]

While there is extensive specialized knowledge and skill required to meet the many and varied demands of school health, many physicians are involved with aspects of school health or school sports programs with little specific graduate or continuing education in the field. The Academy of Pediatrics School Health Committee publishes, and regularly updates, a School Health Manual which can be useful to the physician with interests in school health.[3] Should the physician desire to become involved in school health, it would be wise to distinguish between a role as a caregiver for a given child and a role as a full- or part-time consultant to the school. Table 2 illustrates typical physician activities in relation to specific problems, and contrasts these roles.

NURSES

The level of professional preparation and patterns of care by nursing personnel in schools has been recently challenged by economic considerations, as previously mentioned. Thirty-eight U.S. states require school nurses to be registered nurses, while 19 states require the attainment of specific school nurse certification. In 15 states, certification is neither available nor required.[1]

There has been an interest in the role of the pediatric (school) nurse practitioner in expanding the traditional role of the school nurse. Their greater knowledge and enhanced clinical problem-solving skills should improve health care for children. Studies documenting these expectations have been difficult to carry out. In the few studies that have been done, the following results of utilizing school nurse practitioners have been noted: fewer children were sent home from school due to illness, there was better identification and follow-up of referred problems; and an initial increase in identification of problems in an adolescent population was noted after introduction of a school nurse practitioner to a high school.[4]

HEALTH AIDES/CLERKS

Schools frequently employ aides to assist the nurse to carry out triage or screening procedures (when allowable by law), or to assist with record keeping and to manage school health information. About half of states indicate that aides are

TABLE 2

PEDIATRICIAN'S ROLE IN SCHOOLS

Clinical Issue/ Problem	Examples Of Physician's Activities As Child's Primary Care Provider	Examples Of Physician's Activities As Consultnt To School or School System
Learning Disability	1. Requests teacher's perception of child's learning and behavior, results on individualized testing.	1. Serves on district committee to accomplish biannual review of handicapped children's progress.
	2. Shares results of medical evaluation of child with school.	2. Assists in setting up mechanism for providing follow-up behavioral and academic information to physicians who have placed students on psychoactive medication.
	3. Works cooperatively with school personnel and parent to develop educational and behavioral management plan for child (may include school visit).	3. Provides in-service session for classroom teachers on new concepts in attention deficit disorder.
	4. Sets up mechanism for follow-up on behavioral and educational progress of child.	4. Advises school board on need for movement training for children with learning disabilities.
Asthma (school-age)	1. Requests school information on absenteeism, visits to school nurse, evidence of nonparticipation in physical education activities.	1. Reviews absenteeism data to identify groups of students with excessive absences that might be amenable to some intervention.
	2. Sets up mechanism for regular administration of bronchodilator at school.	2. Assists curriculum director and nurse in developing educational program for children with asthma and their parents.
	3. Set up follow-up mechanism for continued monitoring of school attendance, medication-taking compliance, and participation in appropriate physical activities.	3. Helps publicize program and communicate directly with students' physicians' input and support for the educational program by reinforcing concepts in their patient visits.

Used by permission form Pediatrics in Review

employed, but there is no uniformity as to guidelines, supervision, or degree of autonomy permitted.[1]

Table 3 suggests advantages and disadvantages of various nursing patterns for a school health service.

III. SERVICES

A framework for approaching school health services[4] has been suggested to include at least four aspects: (1) ensuring access for the school child to a regular

TABLE 3

NURSING STAFFING PATTERNS FOR A SCHOOL HEALTH SERVICE

Model	Advantages	Disadvantages
Nurse Aide Alone	Cost; with appropriate back-up systems might be able to meet basic and required needs (eg. immunization records and first aid).	Requires outside resources; special education needs will not be met.
Aide With Nurse	Frees nurse to meet more important needs.	Increases costs if ratio too "rich."
Nurse/Teacher	Potential for increasing integration of health services and health education.	Costs may be difficult to justify; half of job usually sacrificed.
School Nurse	Readily available resource for children, teachers, parents.	Costs for services may be difficult to justify.
Public Health Nurse	Costs to district may be lower than district-supplied nurses.	Services to schools diluted by other tasks.
Nurse Practitioner	Cost for service obtained may be cost-effective; meets more special education needs on site (potentially decreases unnecessary referrals); better problem definition; potential for generating income for services provided.	Should have some form of MD back-up (may increase costs); role change difficult; requires time, training; potential exists for under-referral of complicated cases.

Used by permission from Pediatrics in Review

source of primary care; (2) provision of mandated health screening and health maintenance activities; (3) provision of health problem identification and problem-solving activities; and (4) consideration of additional optimal health maintenance or health promotion programs. A discussion of each aspect follows.

ACCESS TO PRIMARY HEALTH CARE

The school health service, because it has some regular contact with almost every school-age child, is relatively barrier-free when compared to the various bureaucratic and financial barriers to accessing a source of community primary care—whether it be for crises, episodic care, or for more comprehensive continuous care. Therefore, it makes sense to make attempts to connect, through formal and informal channels, the school health service to those community sources of primary care that serve a particular community.[5]

Recent demonstration projects in the U.S., such as those sponsored by the Robert Wood Johnson Foundation, have placed skilled nurse practitioners onsite in schools, backed up by physicians, to deliver direct primary care services to children and, in some instances, entire families. Such models have been especially attractive in sites where sources of routine primary health care are scarce, non-existent, or, for some reason, are not utilized. Another model of school health is more prevalent. In the more prevalent model, the emphasis is not on placing primary care services physically in schools but the emphasis is on improving, within the school, health services which identify problems or potential problems and work cooperatively with the family and community health care providers to solve the problems.

Both models have advantages and disadvantages. School-based primary health care services have immediate access to the population, at least to those children or adolescents who are in school. Because many presenting problems can be treated without an outside referral, the potential is present for reduction in cost of care. Financing of the service usually requires a special mechanism to be set up, since most school districts will be reluctant to assume fiscal or legal responsibility for direct health care services. Such services will also need to provide access into a back-up system of care for times when either school is not in session, or health problems require secondary or tertiary services.

The more prevalent model in which the school health service plays a more traditional brokerage role with regard to medical care services also emphasizes the educational aspects of school health within the school. Thus, attention is regularly given to the learning and behavioral problems of children; to development of specialized services for the handicapped; and to issues related to the healthy environment of the school. All these responsibilities are added to the routine health screening procedures and the monitoring/administration of required immunizations. It is not difficult to imagine, therefore, that one of the major problems with the traditional model has been the completion of medical referrals, especially if a portion of the population served is the urban poor, who may have difficulty accessing primary health care services. In such situations, it is often helpful for the school nurse to set up either formal or informal linkages with community physicians and clinics in order to facilitate the referral and feedback process.[6] Regardless of the model utilized, providing access to continuous high quality primary health care services is a legitimate, but often neglected, goal of school health programs.

PROVISION OF MANDATED HEALTH SCREENING AND HEALTH MAINTENANCE PROGRAMS

School Entry Requirements

Just as there is wide variation in ways of providing school health services, there is also wide variation in the range of currently mandated medical and health screening procedures. As an example of the acceptance of using required school entry to enforce a public health policy, note that all 50 U.S. states require immunizations for students entering school (Table 4). This table also lists the number and percentage of states with specific medical requirements for school entry.[1]

TABLE 4

**NUMBER AND PERCENTAGE OF STATES
WITH SPECIFIC MEDICAL REQUIREMENTS
FOR SCHOOL ENTRY**

Requirement	N	(%)
Immunizations:		
DPT	50	(98)
Measles	50	(98)
Polio	49	(96)
Rubella	46	(90)
Mumps	28	(55)
Hearing Test	22	(43)
Vision Test	21	(41)
Physical Exam	17	(33)
Tuberculosis Test	8	(16)
Height/Weight	5	(10)
Dental Exam	5	(10)
Developmental Evaluation	4	(8)
Speech Test	4	(8)
Scoliosis Evaluation	4	(8)

Used by permission from American School Health Association

Tables 5 and 6 provide information on the number of states with specifically stated policies for health screening activities, and the grade ranges in which they are required. In addition, some schools are now, or in the near future, being required to carry out screening for developmental, learning, and other handicapping conditions at the time of school entry. This will add significantly to the burden of work required from school health services.

TABLE 5

NUMBER AND PERCENTAGE OF STATES WITH POLICIES FOR SPECIFIC SCREENING ACTIVITIES FOR GRADES K-12

Activity		Mandated	Recommended	No Policy	No Response
Hearing	N	31	16	3	1
	%	(61)	(31)	(6)	(2)
Vision	N	29	17	4	1
	%	(57)	(33)	(8)	(2)
Sports Physical	N	20	17	8	6
	%	(39)	(33)	(16)	(12)
Scoliosis	N	17	28	5	1
	%	(33)	(55)	(10)	(2)
Health Appraisal	N	17	20	11	3
	%	(33)	(39)	(22)	(6)
Dental	N	10	26	10	5
	%	(20)	(51)	(20)	(10)
Tuber-culosis Test	N	9	6	26	10
	%	(18)	(12)	(51)	(20)
Health History	N	9	19	10	13
	%	(8)	(37)	(20)	(26)
Speech	N	8	19	12	12
	%	(16)	(37)	(24)	(24)
Height/Weight	N	5	22		14
	%	(10)	(43)		(28)
Sickle Cell	N	3	7	26	13
	%	(6)	(14)	(51)	(29)
Blood Pressure	N	2	17	19	13
	%	(4)	(33)	(37)	(26)
Lead Poisoning	N	2	4	31	14
	%	(4)	(8)	(61)	(28)

Used by permission from American School Health Association

Screening

Screening is defined as a process by which to separate from a large group of apparently healthy individuals those who have, or are at risk of having, a defined disorder. In relation to school screening programs, procedures that tend to yield a large number of false positives will only serve to overburden the community health system, plus it will undermine confidence in the school by community providers of care. On the other hand, the school health service would not wish to undertake a screening program with a significant false-negative rate, especially if the condition being screened for is very serious or if it has major implications to a child's ability to learn.

TABLE 6

NUMBER AND PERCENTAGE OF STATES WITH MANDATED SCREENING ACTIVITIES ACCORDING TO GRADE RANGES IN WHICH THEY WERE REQUIRED

	Grade Range						
	K-6		7-8		9-12		K-12	
ACTIVITY	N	(%)	N	(%)	N	(%)	N	(%)
Hearing	27	(53)	19	(37)	20	(39)	31	(61)
Vision	25	(49)	20	(39)	22	(43)	29	(57)
Sports Physical	1	(2)	9	(18)	10	(20)	20	(39)
Scoliosis	11	(22)	12	(24)	6	(12)	17	(33)
Health Appraisal	13	(25)	8	(16)	10	20)	17	(33)
Dental	6	(12)	3	(6)	3	(6)	10	(20)
Tuberculosis	1	(2)	–	–	–	–	9	(18)
Health History	6	(12)	2	(4)	3	(6)	9	(18)
Speech	1	(2)	–	–	–	–	8	(16)
Height/Weight	4	(8)	2	4)	3	(6)	5	(10)
Sickle Cell	1	(2)	–	–	–	–	3	(6)
Blood Pressure	1	(2)	–	–	1	(2)	2	(4)
Lead Poisoning	1	(2)	–	–	–	–	2	(4)

Used by permission from American School Health Association

When considering the value of school-based screening programs, it is important to keep in mind: (1) the seriousness of the problem, (2) the effectiveness of appropriate treatment or management, (3) the relative efficiency of the screening procedure, (4) the specificity and sensitivity of the procedure, and (5) the *most* important for school screening, the *availability* of the resources required to carry out the necessary remediation or treatment of the problem, once it is identified and confirmed. If these factors cannot be met satisfactorily, then serious doubt is raised about continuing or initiating the particular screening procedure.

A recent review (Cross) analyzed the current data supporting or raising questions about the screening procedures which are commonly undertaken in schools. The procedures reviewed included vision, hearing, scoliosis, dental, growth and nutrition, and blood pressure.[7,8]

Vision

Screening for strabismus and amblyopia should largely be accomplished in the preschool years, so the major aim of vision screening is to detect refractive errors, especially early, so that correction can occur. Mild hyperopia is normal in the early school years, but should not be confused with moderate hyperopia of >2.5D which may progress. Myopia prevalence increases from age six through age 16. Therefore, while no study has demonstrated a clear value of presymptomatic detection, many schools have elected to periodically screen children for distance vision, starting at kindergarten or first grade, through junior and senior high school. Standards for referral vary. The American Academy of Pediatrics recommends, for entering school children, referring any child with 20/40 in either eye, or with a one-line difference between the eyes, even if each eye passes independently. After age seven years, others have suggested referral if the child has 20/30 vision in either eye. Screening for strabismus and amblyopia might be considered, especially for populations who have not had previous access to medical care.

Hearing Testing

While persistent profound or significant hearing loss in infants and preschoolers has a documented influence on language development, the long-term effects of recurrent middle-ear disease/effusion, or mild intermittent hearing loss, are not completely known. Because of the relatively high (five to seven percent) percentage of children who will have demonstrable hearing losses at any one time, many schools have instituted a policy of one-to-two repeated abnormal screens before making a referral. The value of tympanography as a screening tool has not been established. Pure-tone sweep audiology of three frequencies (1000, 2000 and 4000 HZ) at kindergarten or first grade, with follow-up and communication between school personnel and physicians or specialists evaluating hearing loss, is mandatory. If the proposed screening concentrates on detecting those children with significant and persistent hearing losses, then schools should also learn to recognize the clinical signs of the child with a mild respiratory infection who may not be hearing the teacher well, and could benefit from an altered seat assignment or other classroom adjustments.

Scoliosis

Initially, scoliosis, screening by trained school paraprofessionals, was advanced as a cost-effective way to detect cases early, and initiate less costly and debilitating remedies such as surgical correction. Recent reviews have questioned the value, however, for several reasons, including poor predictive validity, and the problem of detecting a large number of mild curves for which the value of observation *vs* treatment was unknown. Also, since the problem is much more (ten times) common in girls, it definitely is not cost-effective to screen boys in schools. The value of such a screening program may also depend upon whether such programs have been present in the community. Some studies have documented fewer severe patients requiring surgery in areas where extensive screening has been in effect for several years. If screening is to be done, girls in the sixth and eighth grade will produce the highest yield. Screener training is crucial, as is upgrading the knowledge of the local community to current management strategies for mild cases of scoliosis likely to be detected.

Dental Screening

Dental disease: caries, malocclusion, and periodontal disease constitute a large unmet health need among U.S. school children. While slow progress is being made in the application of fluoride preventive strategies to preschool populations, dental disease is still prevalent among school children. Annual dental exams, which are comprehensive and include hygiene and education, are indicated because of the high incidence of dental disease in school-age children, and the prevalence of untreated caries. That portion of the school-age population with regular access to dental services does not require duplicated screening in the schools. However, a relatively large portion of the population, especially in rural and urban areas, have no ready access to dental services. It is for these populations that special efforts need to be developed. Demonstration projects have experimented with placing direct dental services onsite in schools. Cost-effectiveness analyses indicate difficulty in widespread dissemination of these models, except perhaps in highly dense urban-poor populations.

Problem Identification and Problem Solving

Aside from established screening programs, school nurses see children and their teachers on almost a daily basis and, therefore, are in a strategic position to identify problems and potential problems. At times these problems present themselves; at other times they need to be detected. A child with a crisis episode of asthma is not difficult to recognize. On the other hand, a child frequently visiting the nurse with minor trauma and stomach aches could be reflecting stress which is current in another part of his or her life, or he or she could be experiencing symptoms of peptic ulcer disease.

The frequent visitor to the school health room comprises a relatively small proportion of the school population, but a significant one with regard to associated difficulties in learning or adjustment. Ten percent of students, it will be found, contribute over half of the visits to a school nurse.[9] This population has been characterized as doing poorly academically, as well as more likely to be rated by teachers as having adjustment, behavior difficulties, or being excessively dependent.[10] Similarly, children who have been identified to be included in the category of the "new morbidity,"—that is, have school, family, or learning problems requiring special educational services—have also been shown to be higher users of *both* school *and* community health resources—not only for their specific new morbidity problems, but also for the more traditional, and common health problems.[11] Therefore, the school health service is in a strategic position to identify and remediate a broad range of problems.

The degree of successful resolution of identified problems can serve as a surrogate measure of the effectiveness of school-based health services. This requires first, however, that some system be set up which, at a minimum, records visits and/or referrals and their follow-up on a timely basis. The aim is to determine the level of care required and that which is achieved. In general, except for sites where resources are physically present in the school, the success of school health programs has not been bad—given the often obtained situations of lack of coordination of care and gaps in communication. Referral completion rates of 80 to 90 percent usually reflect special efforts on the part of school nurses to follow-up on the outcome of referrals.[12]

Using a defined "episode" of care for common health problems of school-age children, we traced the role of the school in obtaining necessary care.[6] In these studies, it was generally found that many health room visits were for minor and self-limiting conditions which could appropriately be handled solely by the school. Other problems required referral. It was discovered that a local M.D., E.R., or Pediatrics Department would have been able to contribute to the resolution of a more complex case, but too often there was a breakdown in communication between the school and the regular source of primary care for the child. On too many occasions, a child was being seen simultaneously by the school and by the family physician for a problem, yet there was no documented interaction between the school and the doctor. Certain families, who were targeted with special outreach services designed to bridge these gaps in accessing primary health care resources, showed improved care for health problems as a result of these efforts to connect the families with the sources of care in the community. These outreach services (home-school agents) were funded by a demonstration grant. When the outside funds were removed, the school district was unable to continue the program, except in a severely limited fashion.

Children with chronic illnesses and handicapping conditions comprise another special group within schools which are requiring more and more extensive and expensive school health services. In addition to the important overall health advocacy role played by the school nurse in special education settings, more specialized services are also required. Health care objectives are often included in mandated individualized educational plans for handicapped students. Tracheostomy care and urinary bladder catheterization are two procedures which are no longer unusual in schools. The expansion downward in age of mandated educational programs will result in grouping very young children—even infants—who are handicapped. This trend has major public health and communicable disease implications which will be expected to impact on school health services.

CONSIDERATION OF ADDITIONAL HEALTH MAINTENANCE OR HEALTH PROMOTION PROGRAMS

Schools can be an appropriate setting in which to carry out a wide variety of health education, health promotion, and health care activities, although it is only one of several avenues in which to carry out these functions.[13] A collaborative approach, in which the school is involved as a partner, is more likely to succeed, rather than assuming that the school should bear the entire responsibility for a program. The latter approach usually has the effect of increasing school resistance to the addition of new programs.

Several candidates for consideration as additional health programs can easily be identified, given a knowledge of current major health and educational concerns. Three of these would include: (1) AIDS education, (2) educational and screening programs related to cardiovascular disease prevention, and (3) educational and health programs for children with chronic handicapping conditions.

AIDS

It is likely that education will remain, for some time, the main preventive tool against this life-threatening sexually transmitted disease. It is imperative that young people become aware of the sexual and other behaviors that place them in jeopardy. This public health need has rapidly, and in a quantum leap, exceeded the capacity and ability of most community educational institutions to be able to respond effectively to this challenge.

Because of the salience of the topic, and the fact that certain legislatures are mandating that schools provide AIDS instruction, it is easy to predict that the issues of what should be taught, when, and by whom will be consuming-ones in the immediate future. At least five specific groups need to be targeted for educational efforts by school health programs: (1) school board members, (2) school administrators, (3) parents, (4) teachers and staff, and (5) students. School board members will need clarification of numbers of pupils and/or staff members likely to be affected by AIDS. Policies regarding home and school placement of AIDS pupils and staff will be needed. Issues of ethics, privacy, confidentiality, and public health safety will be prominent needs. School administrators, will need both information and skills training in daily management, policy implementation, and relationships with parents, staff, and students on the many emotional issues surrounding AIDS. Parents, teachers and staff are in need of factual material, as well as opportunities, to deal with fear and rumors, and of methods of keeping up-to-date on the latest scientific information on AIDS.

No greater public health urgency exists today than to inform students frankly and explicitly of all methods to avoid AIDS infection. They need to be aware of sexual and other behaviors that place them at risk of contracting infection. It is likely that the public health urgency of the problem will result in emphasis on this aspect of health education in the coming years. It is hoped that this emphasis on AIDS instruction will strengthen, and not replace, effects to implement *comprehensive* health education and sex education curricula in the nation's schools. A cooperative and collaborative approach should be the most productive in the long term.

Cardiovascular and Chronic Disease Prevention

School-based approaches to prevention of lifestyle behaviors thought to be precursors to increased cardiovascular risk have been receiving increasing attention from federal health agencies.[14] Many of these target dietary behaviors, physical activity, and prevention of smoking among late elementary and early adolescent school children. Some programs have also involved families and made attempts to alter the school environment in order to facilitate the adoption of more healthy habits early in life. It is likely that extensions of these projects, now largely in the research phase, will gradually become disseminated into schools. The school programs will mirror community based programs and federal initiatives with similar objectives.

One area which will be debated will be the screening of school children for cardiovascular risk indicators in order to identify families who are at high risk.[15] At present, data are not sufficient to determine predictive validity, reliability of measurements, nor efficacy of subsequent interventions—not to mention cost-effectiveness—to warrant wide-scale, school-based screening for cholesterol or blood pressure.[16,17] It is likely, however, that family history of cardiovascular disease will trigger more attention to this area by health care providers in primary care settings. It is also possible that improved technologies will overcome cost and reliability barriers that now contraindicate such screening programs.

Chronic Handicapping Conditions

Schools are being called upon increasingly to develop detection and treatment programs for a wide variety of handicapping conditions—beginning as early as shortly after birth and extending to age 21. In addition to those activities mentioned above, for major physical and mental handicaps, it is likely that more programs will be recommended in order to assist children and their families with the more common medical conditions, such as diabetes, seizures, and asthma.[3] Several projects have successfully engaged schools in such efforts.

Learning and Behavior Problems

The large arena of detecting and remediating learning and behavioral difficulties poses another challenge to educators and health professionals concerned with reducing the frequent outcomes of school failure: delinquency, drop outs, smoking, and substance abuse.

An approach other than the problem-oriented medical approach is needed in screening for the behavioral and educational problems of school children. Such an alternative is a profile-of-function approach, in which data collected on each entering school child detail the child's physical, cognitive, behavioral, and social strengths and weaknesses. This profile would provide parents and teachers with an estimate of the preferred learning style of children at each developmental level. This approach should match the educational environment to the needs of the child, involve parents at all steps in the process, and provide special programming for the exceptionally able student, as well as the potentially handicapped student.

Additional Programs Require Additional Resources

All of the above currently optional, or soon to be mandated, programs will require resources. Difficult analyses and decisions will have to be reached regarding allocation of scarce resources. It is possible that current school health mandates and programs will have to be revised in order to provide for additional new activities.

Future Challenge for the School Health Programs

Could one ever envision the school as a major initiator and promoter of health in a community? Schools are charged with education for life skills, and schools—as a microcosm of society—have the access to school personnel, students, and their families, which constitute a large portion of the nation's populace. Could the school become a place where every child could be assured of receiving basic preventive health services, and also have guaranteed access to regular and continuous health and dental care? Could the health services be designed to encourage self-care and responsibility for decision-making rather than promote dependency on a medical care system? Could the schools reach out to families to assist them to change basic health habits that tend to promote and model poor choices for children? Could the school, in concert with other agencies, provide an educational setting matched to the developmental needs and strengths of children?

School health has a ready-made historical structure and track record of attempting to meet many of society's educational and health desires. This structure is the school health council. Such councils or groups, if organized at each community level, could accomplish a great deal. They could identify needs and resources at the local level. Such a council should include all factions in the community: business, labor, government, financial interests, and student leaders; Parent-Teacher Associations; private and public health and welfare groups; and teachers and school administrators. Such a council, organized by the school, could promote health for all age groups in a community. In this sense, it could also promote good public relations for schools and perhaps overcome distrust and resistance to school initiatives.

Partners for Progress

The school is an appropriate setting in which to conduct health education, health promotion, and health care activities. These activities should not be the sole responsibility of the school; in fact, they can be more effective if carried out in partnership with other community agencies. Shared responsibilities and costs will enhance the effectiveness and continuity of school health programs.

REFERENCES

1. American School Health Association: School Health in America, 4th ed, 1987 Kent, Ohio.

2. Wright GF, Vanderpool NA. School and the pediatrician. Pediatr Clin North Am 28:643, 1981.

3. American Academy of Pediatrics: School Health: A Guide for Health Professionals. Illinois, Elk Grove Village, 1987.

4. Nader PR. A pediatrician's primer for school health activities. Pediatr Rev 4(3):82-92, 1982.

5. Nader PR, Gilman S, Bee D. Factors influencing access to primary health care via school health services. Pediatr 65:585, 1980.

6. Brink SG, Nader PR. Utilization of school and primary health care resources for common health problems of schoolchildren. Pediatr 68(5):700, 1981.

7. Cross AW. Health screening schools: Part I. J Pediatr 107(4):487, 1985.

8. Cross AW. Health screening schools: Part II. J Pediatr 107(5):653, 1985.

9. Nader PR, Brink SG. Does visiting the school health room teach appropriate or inappropriate use of health services? Am J Public Health 71(4):416, 1981.

10. Van Arsdell WR, Roghmann KJ, Nader PR. Visits to an elementary school nurse. J School Health 42:142, 1972.

11. Nader PR, Roy L, Gilman S. The new morbidity: Use of school and community health care resources for behavioral, educational, and social-family problems. Pediatr 67(1):53, 1981.

12. San Diego Unified School District Health Services: Referral Completion Study, 1986-7. San Diego, CA.

13. Bruhn JG, Nader P. The school as a setting for health education, health promotion and health care. Fam Com Health 4:57, 1982.

14. Stone E. School-based health research funded by the National Heart, Lung and Blood Institution. J School Health 55(5):168-174, 1985.

15. Fraser G. An approach to the child at risk for Ischemic Heart Disease, Ch. 16 in Preventive Cardiology. New York, Oxford Press, 1986, pp 219-236.

16. Berkowitz D, Cretin S, Keeler E. Cholesterol, children, and heart disease: An analysis of alternatives. New York, Oxford University Press, 1980.

17. Fixer DE, Laird WP. Validity of mass blood pressure screening in children. Pediatr 72:459, 1983.

CONTROL OF COMMUNICABLE DISEASES

32

Alan R. Hinman

Continued occurrence of communicable diseases is dependent on the interaction of the infectious agent, a susceptible host, and an effective means of transmission, all taking place in a favorable environment. Efforts to control communicable diseases may be directed at any part of this chain.[1,2]

Reducing the availability of the infectious agent can involve isolation of an infected patient or assuring that food or water does not become contaminated. Availability of a susceptible host can be modified either through removal of those at risk (e.g., exclusion of susceptibility) or through modification of the susceptibility of the host (e.g., through immunization).

Typically, four principal means of transmission are described: common vehicle, contact, airborne, or vector borne. Common vehicle transmission refers to contamination of some vehicle which subsequently comes in contact with several potential hosts. The typical examples are contamination of water supplies or foodstuffs, but drugs or intravenous fluids have also been contaminated.

Contact spread of disease may occur through direct physical contact (e.g., sexual intercourse), indirect contact (e.g., fecal-oral spread of enteric organisms), or through exposure to droplets of respiratory secretion which are inhaled by persons close to the infected party (e.g., the common cold, measles). The primary infectious diseases affecting children are spread by respiratory contact (the common cold, influenza, etc.) or fecal-oral contact (diarrhea, hepatitis A, enteroviral infections, etc.). It is difficult to control diseases spread by respiratory contact since patients are often infectious before they become symptomatic, and restricting face-to-face contact is often impractical. Diseases spread by fecal-oral contact are more amenable to control through strict attention to handwashing, etc.

The increasing proportion of young children who are attending day care facilities provides earlier points of congregation than previously was the case. As a consequence, many respiratory-spread illnesses are now seen in preschoolers whereas they previously were primarily problems of early elementary grades (e.g., varicella). Day care facilities also may provide opportunities for close contact between sizable numbers of children who either are not toilet-trained or not particularly oriented to personal hygiene, thus facilitating fecal-oral transmission.

Airborne transmission occurs when the infectious agent is contained in dust particles of droplet nuclei which can be transmitted over long distances. Airborne outbreaks of Q fever, tuberculosis, and smallpox have been described. Vector borne diseases are spread by insect vectors which may serve merely as physical transporters of the infectious agent or may play a critical role in its life cycle (e.g., malaria). Finally, the environment can be altered to make survival or multiplication of agents unlikely (e.g., chlorination of water supplies, refrigeration of foods).

Historically, communicable diseases have been the greatest cause of infant and childhood morbidity and mortality in the U.S.. Major advances in life expectancy have been brought about in the past century largely as a result of the control of communicable diseases. For example, in 1900, the life expectancy at birth for a white female in the U.S. was 51.1 years, infant mortality was more than 100/1,000 live births, and four of the ten leading causes of death were infectious diseases (pneumonia and influenza, tuberculosis, diarrhea and enteritis, and diphtheria, ranking first, second, third, and tenth, respectively). By contrast, in 1985, the life expectancy at birth for a white female was 78.7 years, infant mortality was 10.6/ 1,000 live births, and the only communicable disease in the top ten causes of death was pneumonia and influenza (ranking sixth).

Improvements in control of communicable disease began as part of the sanitary revolution of the mid- and late-nineteenth century, with provision of safe drinking water and proper disposal of waste. The next major impetus came with the development of effective toxoids and vaccines. The development of effective means of treating infectious diseases had a substantial impact on the mortality associated with these diseases but little impact on their incidence. This chapter will focus on the role of vaccines and toxoids in the control of communicable diseases of children. Space limitations do not allow discussion of the role of vaccines in preventing communicable diseases of adults.

CURRENTLY AVAILABLE VACCINES

Many safe and effective vaccines have been developed since Jenner first introduced the practice of vaccination in 1796, most within the past 50 years. Recommendations for use of vaccines are made primarily by the Public Health Service Immunization Practices Advisory Committee (ACIP),[3] the Committee on Infectious Diseases of the American Academy of Pediatrics (the "Red Book" Committee),[4] the Immunization Committee of the American College of Physicians,[5] and the Commission of Science and Public Health of the American Academy of Family Physicians.

Eight products are currently recommended for use in all infants and children, unless contraindications exist: diphtheria, tetanus toxoids, and pertussis vaccine (in combined form, as DTP); oral poliovirus vaccine (OPV); measles, mumps, and rubella vaccines (in combined form as MMR); and conjugated Haemophilus B polysaccharide vaccine. Table 1 shows the recommended schedule for administration of these vaccines to infants and children.

TABLE 1
RECOMMENDED IMMUNIZATION SCHEDULE
FOR INFANTS AND CHILDREN

Age	Vaccine/toxoid
2 Months	DTP (First)
	TOPV (First)
4 Months	DTP (Second)
	TOPV (Second)
6 Months	DTP (Third)
15 Months	Measles*
	Mumps*
	Rubella*
	DTP (Fourth)
	TOPV (Third)
18 Months	Hb (Conjugate)
At school entry	DTP (Fifth)
(4 through 6 years)	TOPV (Fourth)
14 Through 16 Years and every 10 years thereafter	Td

DTP:	Diphtheria and tetanus toxoids and pertussis vaccine adsorbed. 5 doses recommended)
TOPV:	Trivalent oral polio vaccine (live) (4 doses recommended; however, some physicians may elect to give one addtional dose of TOPV at 6 months of age)
TD:	Tetanus and diphtheria toxoids adsorbed (adult)
Hb Conjugate:	Haemophilus b Conjugate Vaccine

*May be combined as a single injection vaccine (MMR).

Widespread use of these vaccines has had a dramatic effect on the reported incidence of disease. Table 2 shows the maximum number of cases reported of each of these conditions (and the year in which that number was reported), as well as the provisional number of cases reported in 1987. Declines in reported incidence of more than 95 percent have occurred for nearly all of these diseases; comparable declines have been seen in deaths. In 1987, no cases of diphtheria or tetanus were reported in individuals less than 15 years of age. No cases of paralysis due to wild poliovirus acquired in the U.S. have been reported since 1979.

The success of the global smallpox eradication program and the striking reductions seen in morbidity due to measles and rubella led to the establishment of formal targets for the elimination of measles (by 1982)[6] and rubella (by 1990)[7] The strategy for elimination includes three components: achievement and maintenance of very high immunization levels (on the order of 95 percent or higher), effective surveillance to detect all suspected cases of illness, and aggressive response to the occurrence of cases. Implementation of this strategy has led to further declines in incidence. Although the target date for elimination of measles had not been met, progress on rubella is proceeding according to schedule.

TABLE 2

COMPARISON OF MAXIMUM AND CURRENT MORBIDITY VACCINE-PREVENTABLE DISEASES

	Maximum Cases (Year)		1987 Prov.	Percent Change
Diphtheria	206,939	(1921)	3	− 99.999
Measles	894,134	(1941)	3,588	− 99.60
Mumps*	152,209	(1968)	12,299	− 91.92
Pertussis	265,269	(1934)	2,529	− 99.05
Polio (paralytic)	21,269	(1952)	0	− 100.00
Rubella**	57,686	(1969)	329	− 99.43
CRS	20,000**	(1964-5)	5	− 99.98
Tetanus***	601	(1948)	40	− 93.34

*   First reportable in 1968
**   First reportable in 1966
*** First reportable in 1947

VACCINE SAFETY AND EFFICACY

Modern vaccines are safe and effective, but not perfectly so. Some persons who receive vaccines may not be protected; on rare occasions, some persons may be harmed by the vaccine. The goal in vaccine development is to maximize efficacy while minimizing the occurrence of adverse events. It is essential to consider the risks, as well as the benefits, of vaccine in balancing use of the vaccine against the risk and severity of disease. The balance may shift over time. For example, the rare complications associated with smallpox vaccination overbalanced the risk of disease in the U.S., several years before global eradication was achieved.

Adverse events associated with vaccines may be common and minor (e.g., fever ≥38°C occurs in approximately 45 percent of DTP recipients), or rare and severe (e.g., paralysis in a recipient of OPV or close contact occurs once for every 2.7 million doses distributed). Most of these events may occur in the absence of vaccination and it may be impossible, in an individual circumstance, to determine whether a given vaccine was responsible. It is important that patients (and parents) be aware of the potential adverse events associated with vaccination, as well as the benefits, so participation can be truly informed. The Centers for Disease Control has developed Important Information Statements for use with vaccines purchased using federal funds.

Section XXI of the Public Health Service Act (enacted by PL 99-660, the National Childhood Vaccine Injury Act of 1986), requires all vaccine providers to formally notify patients and parents of the risks and benefits of immunization. Development of the notification materials is presently under way. The Act also requires providers to record certain information on the patient's chart at the time of immunization, and requires reporting to the Department of Health and Human Services of compensable adverse events, as well as any adverse event considered a contraindication of administration of further doses of a particular vaccine.

Since vaccines are not perfectly effective, inevitably there will be cases of disease occurring in persons who have been vaccinated. Clinical vaccine efficacy is estimated typically by calculating the reduction in attack rate in vaccinated compared to unvaccinated individuals.[8] The formula used is: VE = (ARU - ARV)/ARU X 100, where VE is the vaccine efficacy (in percent), ARU is the attack rate in unvaccinated persons, and ARV is the attack rate in vaccinated persons. In general, the vaccines in use today are effective on the order of 90 percent or more; however, this means that up to ten percent of those who receive vaccines may not be protected and may develop disease following exposure.

IMMUNIZATION SERVICES

In the private sector, immunizations are given by pediatricians and family physicians, with the parent paying for the service. In the public sector, immunizations are given typically in local health departments (or community health center) and are either free or substantially cheaper than in the proportion of children receiving immunizations in the private and public sectors (Figure 1) but, nationwide, approximately one-half of children receive immunization in the private sector and one-half in the public sector.

Support for immunization in the public sector comes from local, state, and federal funds. Since 1963, federal grants have been given to state and local health departments to purchase vaccines and to support surveillance, investigation, coordination, and assessment. Figure 2 shows the levels of federal grant support from 1963-1988. The major increases in recent years have reflected the marked increases in vaccines prices, which have been attributed in part to the increasing number of suits brought against manufacturers claiming damage caused by vaccines. Table 3 summarizes the public and private sector prices of childhood vaccines in 1980, compared with 1988.

The major provisions of the National Childhood Vaccine Injury Act establish a mechanism for compensation of persons injured by specified vaccines (diphtheria and tetanus toxoids, pertussis, poliomyelitis, measles, mumps, and rubella vaccines). Table 4 lists the events which would be considered automatically compensable; other events are to be considered on a case-by-case basis. Injured parties are not allowed to file suit against a manufacturer or provider of vaccine until after going through an administrative review mechanism, which involves filing the claim in the U.S. Claims Court, after which a Special Master is appointed to review the claim. If the claimant is not satisfied with the outcome of this process, (s)he can make an irrevocable decision to reject the decision and then file suit against the manufacturer or provider.

It is hoped that implementation of the National Childhood Vaccine Injury Act will improve access to compensation for those injured by vaccines, reduce the number of suits brought against manufacturers, and lead to reductions in the prices of vaccines. Whether this will be the case is not clear.

IMMUNIZATION LEVELS

Due in part to the enactment and enforcement of school immunization laws in all 50 states, immunization levels in school-aged children are higher than they have ever been. Table 5 summarizes the immunization requirements in each state. For the 1986-1987 school year, 97 percent of all school entrants have received DTP, polio, and MMR. Since all children must attend school, these laws have the effect of ensuring that immunization levels are high among all levels of society and all ethnic groups. Unfortunately, they do not ensure that immunizations are received on time.

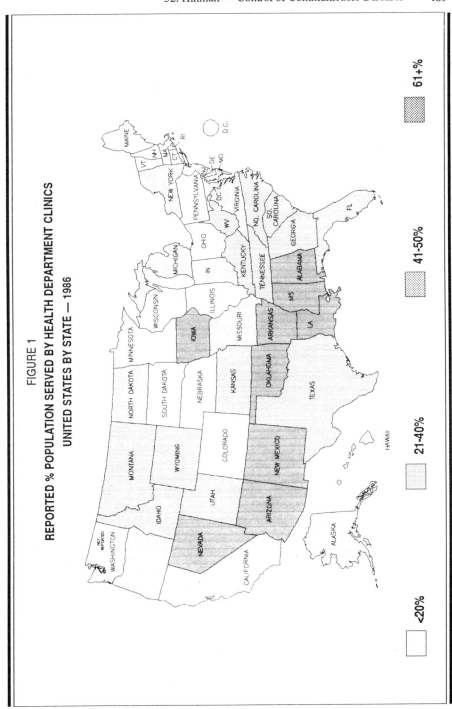

FIGURE 1

REPORTED % POPULATION SERVED BY HEALTH DEPARTMENT CLINICS
UNITED STATES BY STATE — 1986

<20%   21-40%   41-50%   61+%

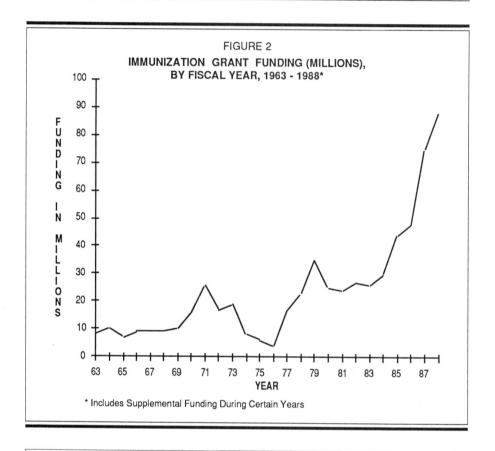

FIGURE 2
IMMUNIZATION GRANT FUNDING (MILLIONS),
BY FISCAL YEAR, 1963 - 1988*

* Includes Supplemental Funding During Certain Years

TABLE 3
U.S. VACCINE PRICES PRICE PER DOSE—1988 VS. 1980

Vaccine	Private Sector		Public Sector	
	1988	1980	1988	1980
DTP	$ 11.03	$ 0.30	$ 9.623	$ 0.15
DT	$ 0.78	$ 0.25	$ 0.193	$ 0.10
Td	$ 0.78	$ 0.25	$ 0.156	$ 0.10
OPV	$ 8.07	$ 1.60	$ 1.363	$ 0.354
IPV	$ 8.82	–	–	–
MMR	$ 27.23	$ 7.24	$ 15.11	$ 2.71
Me	$ 13.79	$ 2.73	$ 8.76	$ 1.15
Mu	$ 15.26	$ 3.57	$ 10.41	$ 1.63
Ru	$ 14.24	$ 3.05	$ 8.48	$ 0.94
MR	$ 19.55	$ 4.58	$ 10.99	$ 1.64
H Flu b (poly.)	$ 7.55	–	$ 2.17	–
H Flu b (conj.)	$ 13.75	–	–	–
Hepatitis B	$ 41.33	–	–	–
Influenza	$ 2.50	$ 1.78	–	–

TABLE 4

LIST OF COMPENSABLE EVENTS

Vaccine	Interval From Vaccination
1. DTP; PERTUSSIS.	
Illness:	
A. Anaphylaxis or anaphylactic shock	24 hours
B. Encephalopathy (or encephalitis)	3 days
C. Shock-collapse or hypotonic-hyporesponsive collapse	3 days
D. Residual seizure disorder	3 days
E. Any acute complication or sequela (including death) of above illnesses	Not applicable
2. MEASLES; MUMPS AND/OR RUBELLA VACCINES.	
DT; Td or Tetanus Toxoid.	
Illness:	
A. Anaphylaxis or anaphylactic shock	24 hours
B. Encephalopathy (or encephalitis)	15 days (for mumps, rubella, and/or measles vaccines; 3 days (for DT, Td or tetanus toxoid).
C. Residual seizure disorder	15 days (for mumps, rubella, and/or measles vaccines; 3 days (for DT, Td or tetanus toxoid).
D. Any acute complication or sequela (including death) of above illnesses	Not applicable
3. POLIO VACCINES (OTHER THAN INACTIVATED POLIO VACCINE).	
Illness:	
A. Paralytic Polio	
- in a non-immunodeficient recipient	90 days
- in an immunodeficient recipient	6 months
- in a vaccine-associated community case	Not applicable
B. Any acute complication or sequela (including death) of above illnesses	Not applicable
4. INACTIVATED POLIO VACCINE.	
Illness:	
A. Anaphylaxis or anaphylactic shock	24 hours
B. Any acute complication or sequela (including death) of above illnesses	Not applicable

TABLE 5

STATE IMMUNIZATION REQUIREMENTS
APPLICABLE TO ANY OR ALL OF GRADES K-12

State	Diphtheria	Tetanus	Pertussis	Measles	Mumps	Rubella	Polio
Alabama	K-12	K-12	K-6 yrs	K-12	K-12	K-12	K-12
Alaska	K-12	K-12	K-6 yrs	K-12	Not Required	K-11 yrs	K-12
Arizona	K-12	Not Required	Not Required	K-12	Not Required	K-12	K-12
Arkansas	K-12	K-12	K-6 yrs	K-12	Not Required	K-12	K-12
California	K-12	K-12	K-6 yrs	K-12	K-6 yrs	K-12	K-12
Colorado	K-12	K-12	K-6 yrs	K-12	K	K-6	K-12
Connecticut	K-12	K-12	K-6 yrs	K-12	K-12	K-12	K-12
Delaware	K-12	K-12	K-6 yrs	K-12	K-8	K-12	K-12
Dist. of Col.	K-12	K-12	K-6 yrs	K-12	K-12	K-12	K-12
Florida	K-12	K-12	K-6 yrs	K-12	K-12	K-12	K-12
Georgia	K-12	K-12	K-6 yrs	K-12	K-12	K-12	K-12
Hawaii	K-12	K-12	K-6 yrs	K-12	K-12	K-12	K-12
Idaho	K-5	K-5	Not Required	K-5	K-5	K-5	K-5
Illinois	K-12	K-12	K-5 yrs	K-12	K-12	K-12	K-12
Indiana	K-12	K-12	K-6 yrs	K-12	K-1	K-12	K-12
Iowa	K-12	K-12	K-6 yrs	K-12	Not Required	K-12	K-12
Kansas	K-12	K-12	K-6 yrs	K-12	K-12	K-12	K-12
Kentucky	K-12	K-12	Not Required	K-12	Not Required	K-12	K-12
Louisiana	New Enterers	New Enterers	New Enterers	New Enterers	New Enterers	New Enterers	New Enterers
Maine	K-12	K-12	K-6 yrs	K-12	K-8	K-12	K-12
Maryland	K-12	K-12	K-6 yrs	K-12	Not Required	K-12	K-12
Massachusetts	K-12	K-12	K-6 yrs	K-12	K-12	K-12	K-12
Michigan	New Enterers	New Enterers	New Enterers	New Enterers	New Enterers	New Enterers	New Enterers
Minnesota	K-12	K-12	K-6 yrs	K-12	K-6 yrs	K-12	K-12
Mississippi	K-12	K-12	K-6 yrs	K-12	Not Required	K-12	K-12
Missouri	K-12	Not Required	Not Required	K-12	Not Required	K-12	K-12
Montana	K-12	K-12	Not Required	K-12	Not Required	K-12	K-12
Nebraska	K-12	K-12	K-6 yrs	K-12	K-12	K-12	K-12
Nevada	K-12	K-12	K-6 yrs	K-12	Not Required	K-12	K-12
New Hampshire	New Enterers	New Enterers	New Enterers	New Enterers	New Enterers	New Enterers	New Enterers
New Jersey	K-12	K-12	K-6 yrs	K-12	K-14 yrs	K-12	K-12
New Mexico	K-12	K-12	K-6 yrs	K-12	Not Required	K-12	K-12
New York	K-12	Not Required	Not Required	K-12	K-12	K-12	K-12
North Carolina	K-12	K-12	K-6 yrs	K-12	K-12	K-12	K-12
North Dakota	K-12	K-12	K-6 yrs	K-12	K-12	K-12	K-12
Ohio	K-12	K-12	K-6 yrs	K-12	K-12	K-12	K-12
Oklahoma	K-12	K-12	K-6 yrs	K-12	Not Required	K-12	K-12
Oregon	K-12	K-12	Not Required	K-12	New Enterers	K-12	K-12
Pennsylvania	K-12	K-12	Not Required	K-12	K-12	K-12	K-12
Puerto Rico	K-12	K-12	K-6 yrs	K-12	K-12	K-12	K-12
Rhode Island	K-12	K-12	Not Required	K-12	K-6 yrs	K-12	K-12
South Carolina	K-12	K-12	K-5 yrs	K-12	Not Required	K-12	K-12
South Dakota	K-12	K-12	K-6 yrs	K-12	K-12	K-12	K-12
Tennessee	K-12	K-12	K-6 yrs	K-12	Not Required	K-12	K-12
Texas	K-12	K-12	Not Required	K-12	K-15 yrs	K-11 yrs	K-12
Utah	K-12	K-12	K-6 yrs	K-12	K-12	K-12	K-12
Vermont	K-12	K-12	K-6 yrs	K-12	Not Required	K-12	K-12
Virginia	K-12	K-12	K-6 yrs	K-12	New Enterers	K-12	K-12
Washington	K-12	K-12	Not Required	K-12	K1	K-12	K-12
West Virginia	New Enterers	New Enterers	New Enterers	New Enterers	Not Required	New Enterers	New Enterers
Wisconsin	K-12	K-12	K-6 yrs	K-12	K-4	K-11 yrs	K-12
Wyoming	New Enterers	New Enterers	K-6 yrs	New Enterers	New Enterers	New Enterers	New Enterers

No reliable information exists on national immunization levels in preschoolers, but studies in individual areas indicate that immunization levels in two-year olds are substantially lower than those in school entrants. A nationwide estimate of approximately 80 percent immunization levels in two-year olds seems reasonable. Nonetheless, in some central cities, it appears that only approximately 50 percent of children have completed the basic immunization series by the time of their second birthday (these data were obtained before Haemophilus b vaccine was introduced, and consequently do not reflect its uptake).

The reasons for this discrepancy apparently involve a mixture of lack of availability of acceptable services, competing priorities for parents' attention, and absence of effective systems to identify and recall children in need of immunization. It is also sadly true that health care providers may miss opportunities to provide immunizations to children who present for medical care either because they do not think of offering the vaccine, elect not to administer antigens simultaneously, or misperceive the existence of contraindications.

To improve immunization levels in infants and young children, it is imperative that every opportunity be taken to provide needed vaccines and that systems be established to identify and recall those in need of immunization. These systems can be as simple as postcards filled out by the parent at the time of one visit and stored in a file for the month when the next visit is due (an approach commonly used by dentists) or as complex as computer-generated telephone contacts or letters.

NEW VACCINES

The new techniques of biotechnology offer a wide array of possible vaccines for the future against continuing problems of infancy and childhood, as well as the possibility of improving existing vaccines to enhance efficacy or reduce adverse effects. In addition, traditional methods are still bringing forth new vaccines, such as a live attenuated varicella vaccine. Some of these vaccines may require multiple doses or may need to be administered at ages children do not currently receive vaccines. These factors make it even more important that systems be developed now to ensure that children receive needed vaccines on schedule.

Pre-licensure assessment of new vaccines poses some problems, since newer vaccines may well be targeted at relatively uncommon conditions (e.g., infections caused by *Haemophilus influenzae type b* occur in one of 1,000 infants and young children during the course of a year). Consequently, the sampler size necessary to demonstrate clinical efficacy in a field trial may be quite large, requiring enrollment and follow-up of several thousand children, a task that is both difficult and expensive. Use of serologic markers of immunity could reduce the sample size required; unfortunately, for many diseases (particularly bacterial infections), there is not yet a reliable correlation between presence of circulating antibodies and protection.

Nonetheless, the prospects are bright for the development and introduction of new vaccines which can further improve the health of mothers and children and ultimately lead to the eradication of other diseases.

REFERENCES

1. Last JM (ed). Maxcy-Rosenau Public Heatlh and Preventive Medicine. Twelfth edition. Norwald, Appleton-Century-Croft, 1986.

2. American Public Health Association: Control of Communicable Diseases in Man. Fourteenth edition. Washington, American Public Health Association, 1985.

3. Centers for Disease Control: Recommendations of the Immunization Practices Advisory Committee:

    a. General Recommendation of Immunization. MMWR 32:1-8;13-17, 1983.

    b. Diphtheria, Tetanus, and Pertussis Guidelines for Vaccine Prophylaxis and Other Preventive Measures. MMWR 34:405-414;419-426, 1985.

    c. Pertussis Immunization: Family History of Convulsions and Use of Antipyretics. MMWR 36:281-282, 1987.

    d. Measles Prevention. MMWR 36:409-418;423-425, 1987.

    e. Mumps Vaccine. MMWR 31:617-620;625, 1982.

    f. Rubella Prevention. MMWR 33:301-310;315-318, 1984.

    g. Poliomyelitis Prevention. MMWR 31:22-26;31-34, 1982.

    h. Poliomyelitis Prevention: Enhanced-Potency Inactivated Poliomyelitis Vaccine— Supplementary Statement. MMWR 36:373-380;385-387, 1987.

    i. Polysaccharide Vaccine for Prevention of Haemophilus influenzae Type b Disease. MMWR 34:201-205, 1985.

    j. Update: Prevention of Haemophilus influenzae Type b Disease. MMWR 35:170-174;179-180, 1986.

    k. Update: Prevention of Haemophilus influenzae Type b Disease. MMWR 37:13-16, 1988.

    l. Recommendations for Protection Against Viral Hepatitis. MMWR 34:313-324;329-335, 1985.

    m. Update on Hepatitis B Prevention. MMWR 36:353-360;366, 1987.

    n. Prevention and Control of Influenza. MMWR 36:373;385-387,1987.

    o. Update: Pneumococcal Polysaccharide Vaccine Usage—United States. MMWR 33:273-276;281, 1984.

    p. Meningococcal Vaccines. MMWR 34:255-259, 1985.

    q. Cholera Vaccine. MMWR 27:173-174, 1978.

    r. Plaque Vaccine. MMWR 31:301-304, 1982.

    s. Thyphoid Vaccine. MMWR 27:231-233, 1978.

    t. Yellow Fever Vaccine. MMWR 32:679-682, 687-688, 1984.

u. BCG Vaccine. MMWR 28:241-244, 1979.

v. Rabies Prevention. MMWR 33:393-402;407-408, 1984.

w. Rabies Postexposure Prophylaxis with Human Diploid Cell Rabies Vaccine: Lower Neutralizing Antibody Titers with Wyeth Vaccine. MMWR 34:90-92, 1985.

x. Rabies Prevention: Supplementary Statement on the Preexposure Use of Human Diploid Cell Rabies Vaccine by the Intradermal Route. MMWR 35:767-768, 1986.

y. Varicella-Zoster Immune Globulin for the Prevention of Chicken pox. MMWR 33:84—90;95-100, 1984.

4. American Academy of Pediatrics: Report of the Committee on Infectious Diseases. Twentieth edition. Elk Grove Village, American Academy of Pediatrics, 1986.

5. American College of Physicians: Guide for adult immunization, 1985. Philadelphia, American College of Physicians, 1985.

6. Hinman AR, Nieburg PI, Brandling-Bennett AD. The opportunity and obligation to eliminate measles from the United States. JAMA 242:1157-1162, 1979.

7. Orenstein WA, Bart KJ, Hinman AR, et al. The opportunity and obligation to eliminate rubella from the United States. JAMA 251:1988-1994, 1984.

8. Orenstein WA, Bernier RH, Dondero TJ, et al. Field evaluation of vaccine efficacy. Bull WHO 63:1055-1068, 1985.

CHILD ABUSE AND NEGLECT

33

Anne H. Cohn and Ruth A. Lee

Child abuse and neglect is a major social and health problem in the U.S. While the actual incidence of child abuse is hard to determine, in 1986 an estimated two million reports of child abuse were made to the responsible officials.[1] An estimated 1,200 children died in 1986 as a result of maltreatment. [2]

The long-term consequences of abuse are costly for all of us. Studies show that most juvenile delinquents, teenage runaways, and teenage drug and alcohol abusers are running away from abuse. We know most parents who abuse their children had poor childhoods themselves, characterized by serious abuse or neglect. The truth of the matter is that child abuse is the linchpin of so many other social problems.[3]

DEFINITIONS AND CAUSES OF CHILD ABUSE

What do we mean when we talk about child abuse? Definitions vary; professionals may define child abuse more broadly than a state law for instance. Typically though, child abuse includes physical abuse, physical neglect, sexual abuse, and emotional maltreatment, which can be defined as follows:

> Physical abuse is nonaccidental physical injury which may include severebeatings, burns, human bites, or strangulation with resultant bruises and welts, broken bones, scars or serious internal injuries, or death.

- Physical neglect is the withholding of, or failure to provide a child with, the basic necessities of life: food, clothing, shelter, medical care, attention to hygiene, or supervision needed for optimal physical growth and development.

- Sexual abuse is the exploitation of a child for the sexual gratification of an adult, as in rape, incest, fondling of the genitals, exhibitionism, or pornography.

- Emotional maltreatment is a pattern of behavior that attacks a child's emotional development and sense of self-worth. Examples include constant criticizing, belittling, insulting, rejecting, and providing no love, support, or guidance.

What are the reasons for child abuse? Who are the abusers? The answers to these questions are complex. Child abusers are usually ordinary people caught in situations that are beyond their control, and they do not know how to cope. Unemployment and related financial difficulties seem to be very significant factors; so are lack of access to the larger community, isolation from effective support systems, and simply having no one to turn to for help contribute to abuse. Being a single parent and being totally responsible for caring for a child, without supplementary caregivers, leaves a parent vulnerable to becoming abusive. The stresses of adolescent parenthood also can contribute to abuse.

There is evidence that many abusive parents were themselves abused as children; because abusive parenting is all they have known, they repeat it with their own children. Lack of knowledge of normal child development can be a contributing factor. Abusers tend to have unrealistic or inappropriate expectations of their children. They may set standards that are impossibly high. They may wrongly believe, for example, that children should always be quiet or never make a mistake.

Abusers often perceive a child as being "different" or having special needs that set the child apart from other children. Perhaps the child was unwanted or unplanned, or was premature or handicapped, causing special needs and stresses. Other factors associated with child abuse are alcohol misuse, legal problems, and inadequate living conditions. Although the problems and stresses of poverty can contribute to child abuse, it is a myth that child abuse is confined to the poor and minorities. Abusers come from all economic, racial, ethnic, and religious groups, and any of life's stresses can contribute to abuse.[4]

THE NATIONAL RESPONSE TO CHILD ABUSE

Organized efforts to respond to child abuse in the U.S. can be traced to 1874, when church workers found that Mary Ellen, a New York City child, had been chained to her bed by her guardians and repeatedly beaten. Because there was no precedent allowing for legal intervention in the case of child abuse, they were able to remove Mary Ellen from her home only on the grounds that cruelty to animals was illegal and Mary Ellen was a member of the animal kingdom. Thereafter, because of public outrage, societies for the Prevention of Cruelty to Children were organized in the U.S. and elsewhere. Recognizing a role for the federal government in children's issues, in 1912 the U.S. Children's Bureau was established and, in 1935, with the passage of the Social Security Act, government grants became available for the protection and care of homeless, dependent, and neglected children.

In the early 1960s, with help from the medical profession, the modern-day public got its first introduction to child abuse. Dr. C. Henry Kempe coined the term, *the battered child syndrome,* and spoke out about the atrocities he and his colleagues were seeing in their emergency rooms and private practices. The immediate public reaction seemed to be one of horror; the public recoiled. Some professionals and lawmakers did not. In 1962, the federal Children's Bureau prepared and disseminated a model child abuse reporting law. The Social Security Amendments of 1962 required each state to make child welfare services available to all children, including the abused child. Throughout the 1960s and into the early 1970s, states across the country passed or improved upon their child abuse reporting laws, and they developed or expanded their capacities to investigate and treat reports of child abuse. By the early 1970s, the rudiments of a nationwide response system were in place, but knowledge about the nature and extent of the problem was still scant.

In 1973, the first congressional hearing on child abuse was held, and established the gravity of the problem and the need for federal leadership. As a result, the federal Child Abuse Act (PL 934-247) was passed and signed into law early in 1974. The Act established a National Center on Child Abuse and Neglect (NCCAN) within the federal Department of Health and Human Services (at the time the Department of Health, Education and Welfare). Since 1974, NCCAN has had between $16 and $24 million-a-year to spend on research, demonstrations, training projects, and grants to states. Although NCCAN grants have been relatively small and short-lived, they have provided an incentive for local groups to become active in the child abuse area. NCCAN has distributed small grants across the country to all types of agencies, professionals, and communities. As a result of this small federal program, state and local professional organizations across the country have become involved in the problem, and our understanding of the problem has grown.

Responses to date in the U.S. are characterized by an emphasis on detection, intervention, and treatment. Research has concerned itself with "how much is there?" and "why does it happen?" and "what do you do once it happens?." Legal responses, the allocation of resources, and media coverage have followed suit. State reporting laws and court proceedings for alleged child abuse cases have been perfected. The deaths, the horrible beatings, the deprived children have been covered in newspapers and by television and radio stations. Professionals have sought expansion in dollars for protective service—so that more social workers could be hired and better counseling would be offered to parents who abuse their children. Training manuals for physicians, day care workers, and school teachers have been developed so that they can identify children who have been or are being abused.

The hallmark of responses to child abuse, since 1974 and through the early 1980s, has been *after the fact*. Politically and socially that has been the most obvious, and thus the most appropriate and acceptable, route to take. The legal system and the protective service system combined spend an average of over $2,000 (in 1985 dollars) per case of child abuse after the fact.[5] And studies show that rehabilitation success rates with these cases are less than 50 percent.[6] For all the dollars spent on treatment, most of the abused children will likely be abused again. Although the inclination of Americans is to respond to problems only once they occur, certainly it would appear worthwhile to take a look at the prevention of child abuse—stopping the problem before it occurs, before a child is hurt.

PREVENTION EFFORTS

Although research on the effectiveness of different programs in preventing abuse is scarce, we can begin to move from what we know about the underlying causes of child abuse and neglect to the design of promising prevention programs. It is clear that programs must be directed to all families, but on a voluntary basis. A comprehensive community-based approach to prevention begins with the following array of programs:[7]

Support programs for new parents The purpose of support programs for new parents, such as perinatal support programs, is to prepare individuals for the job of parenting. Such programs should include supports during both the pre- and postnatal periods. Prenatal programs can build on existing medical programs and educate about-to-be parents in child development, parent-child relationships, and adult relationships. Information on community resources available to new parents and to infants and children should be provided.

Education for parents Many parents know little about normal child development and may be poor observers of their children's behavior. Education for all parents, new parents, and even adolescents and young adults who one day will be parents, in child development and parenting techniques can go a long way in alleviating these problems.

Family support services Lacking anywhere to turn in times of crisis puts families at significantly greater risk for abuse or neglect. To provide immediate assistance to parents in times of stress, crisis care programs should be available on a 24-hour basis and should include the following services: telephone hot line, crisis caretakers, crisis baby-sitters, crisis nurseries, and crisis counseling. Through these programs, parents facing immediate problems could receive immediate support to alleviate the stresses of a particular situation. Help should be available over the phone or through in-person counseling.

Child care opportunities The purpose of child care or day care programs is to furnish parents with regular or occasional out-of-home care for their children. While child care is a necessity in households in which all adults are employed, such services are also beneficial for parents who do not work outside the home but who find continuous child care responsibilities very stressful. Child care programs also provide opportunities for children to learn basic social skills.

Prevention education for children and adolescents Prevention education for children and adolescents takes two forms: providing children with skills to help them protect themselves from being abused, and equipping them with interpersonal skills and knowledge that are valuable in adulthood, especially in the parenting role. Knowledge and skills can be imparted in a variety of ways through the school system and community centers.

Therapeutic services for victims and survivors It has been argued that prevention of abuse is, in part, tied to providing therapeutic treatment to children or young people who have been abused or neglected. To minimize the long-term effects of abuse, age-appropriate treatment services should be available to all maltreated children. For adult survivors of abuse, self-help groups should be available to help break the cycle. Treatment programs for abused children should include a thorough diagnosis of physical and developmental (social, psychological, and emotional) problems.

Will this array of programs solve the problem of child abuse? Certainly, if all of these prevention programs were in place all across the country, we should begin to make a dent in the amount of child abuse. However, because of the complex and systemic nature of child abuse, the problem must be fought on a number of fronts.

FUTURE DIRECTIONS

As we look to the future, we face some clear challenges. The first area for concern in the child abuse field is the increased number of reports of child abuse. The number of reported cases increased over 51 percent in the last five years.[8] This is probably due less to an increase in the amount of child abuse and more to increased awareness which has led to increased reporting. In either case, funding for child abuse programs has not kept pace, increasing only two-three percent in the same period.[9] Children's protective service agencies have been overwhelmed and unable to keep pace with the increased case loads. Thus, a critical need is to refine the children's protective service system so that reported families in need actually get help.

Along with the increased awareness of child abuse, interest in its prevention has grown. According to a Lou Harris poll conducted in 1987, 66 percent of the public stated that they could help prevent child abuse and 23 percent said they had actually done something in the previous year.[10] While this awareness is beneficial, even more needs to be done in the area of prevention. To make this possible, another need in child abuse is more funding for prevention. This need is being partially met by an innovation called the Children's Trust Fund. Conceived of by Dr. Ray Helfer, the idea of the Children's Trust Fund is to establish a fund in each state, with money generated through means other than annual legislative appropriations, to be distributed to local community groups for child abuse prevention activities. The first fund was established in 1980 and, by 1987, 44 states had funds with an estimated total of $28 million per year.

People have tended to view child abuse and neglect as a monolithic problem, when in fact physical abuse, physical neglect, sexual abuse, and emotional maltreatment are each distinct problems with their own unique causes and concerns. Another area of need then is to use our knowledge of the complexity of these problems to increasingly tailor our treatment and prevention programs to the specific type of abuse we are hoping to effect.

A fourth, and last, area that needs focus is the use of a more multidisciplinary response to child abuse. Social work or law-enforcement intervention alone are not the answer to this complex problem. There needs to be cooperation and integration of efforts with the public health, educational, and medical communities, as well as other professions. Only as we all work together in a multidisciplinary, community-wide effort will we be able to reduce and eventually end the problem of child abuse.

REFERENCES

1. American Association for Protecting Children, News Release, October, 1987.

2. Daro D, Mitchel L. Deaths Due to Maltreatment Soar: The Results of the 1986 Annual Fifty State Survey. Chicago, National Center on Child Abuse Prevention Research, National Committee for Prevention of Child Abuse, 1987.

3. Helfer RE, Kempe RS (ed). The Battered Child. Chicago, The University of Chicago Press, 1987.

4. Cohn A. An Approach to Preventing Child Abuse. Chicago, National Committee for Prevention of Child Abuse, 1983, pp 3-7.

5. Berkeley Planning Associates: Evaluation of the Joint OCD/SRS National Demonstration Program on Child Abuse and Neglect. Berkeley, CA, Berkeley Planning Associates, 1977.

6. Berkeley Planning Associates: Evaluation of the Joint OCD/SRS National Demonstration Program on Child Abuse and Neglect. Berkeley, Ca, Berkeley Planning Associates, 1977.

7. Cohn A. An Approach to Preventing Child Abuse. Chicago, National Committee for Prevention of Child Abuse, 1983, pp 3-7.

8. US House of Representatives' Select Committee on Children, Youth and Families: Abused Children in America: Victims of Official Neglect, Washington, D.C., US Government Printing Office, 1987, pp 1-9.

9. US House of Representatives' Select Committee on Children, Youth and Families: Abused Children in America: Victims of Official Neglect, Washington, D.C., US Government Printing Office, 1987, pp 43-49.

10. Daro D, Mitchel L. Public Attitudes and Actions Regarding Child Abuse and Its Prevention: The Results of a Louis Harris Public Opinion Poll. Chicago, The National Center on Child Abuse Prevention Research, National Committee for Prevention of Child Abuse, 1987.

11. National Committee for Prevention of Child Abuse: Fact Sheet No. 10: Children's Trust Funds. Chicago, National Committee for Prevention of Child Abuse, 1987.

CHILDHOOD INJURIES AND THEIR PREVENTION

34

Bernard Guyer and Susan S. Gallagher

The daily newspaper headlines are constant reminders of the tragedy of childhood injuries.

"8 KIDS IN DEATH CRASH HORROR"
"TAR CLEANUP IGNITES, BADLY BURNS 2 TOTS"
"PEDESTRIAN KILLED, 3 CHILDREN INJURED"
"WORKERS DRILLING IN EFFORT TO FREE TEXAS CHILD IN WELL"

While newspaper accounts often sensationalize events, in the case of childhood injuries, they merely provide the human drama behind the grim vital statistics; successful injury prevention rarely makes headlines. The purpose of this chapter is to describe the nature and magnitude of injuries in children and youth, review prevention strategies, and discuss future directions in the field.

THE EPIDEMIOLOGY OF CHILDHOOD INJURIES

INJURY, THE LEADING CAUSE OF YEARS OF POTENTIAL LIFE LOST

Injury, due to both unintentional (accidental) and intentional (violent and self-inflicted) causes, is the fourth leading cause of death in the U.S., surpassed only by heart disease, cancer, and stroke. In 1982, there were 147,884 deaths due to injury among all ages; 22,348 of these were homicides and 28,242 were suicides.[1] Because injuries occur predominantly in younger populations, however, their sig-

505

nificance is better measured by examining their contribution to premature mortality. Years of potential life lost (YPLL) is a measure of the total annual years of life, before age 65, that would have remained had these individuals not died from a specific cause. Unintentional injuries were the leading cause of YPLL in 1984, accounting for 2,308,000 years, or 19.6 percent of all YPLL.[2] Suicide and homicide together ranked fourth, accounting for 1,247,000 years or 10.6 percent of all YPLL.[3]

CHILDHOOD MORTALITY FROM INJURIES

Injury is the leading cause of death from the age of one to 44 years.[4] Among children and young adults, injuries surpass all other causes of death combined.[5] In 1984, 21,156 children and youth under age 20 died from injury (Table 1), resulting in an overall mortality rate of 30.0/100,000.[6] The major causes of fatal injuries in childhood can be described by age group.[7]

TABLE 1
INJURY DEATH, UNITED STATES, 1984 [1]

	Under 1 Year	1-4 Years	5-14 Years	15-24 Years	Total
Motor Vehicle Total	161	977	2,263	6,495	9,896
• Occupant	(115)	(349)	(709)	(3,596)	(4,769)
• Pedestrian	(14)	(502)	(809)	(536)	(1,861)
Unintentional (Non-motor vehicle)	737	1,893	2,010	2,153	6,793
• Drownings	(70)	(556)	(494)	(553)	(1,673)
• Burns	(136)	(606)	(466)	(169)	(1,377)
• Suffocation	(180)	(84)	(122)	(51)	(437)
• Poison	(21)	(77)	(56)	(184)	(338)
• Falls	(28)	(86)	(68)	(146)	(328)
Suicide	0	0	232	1,692	1,924
Homicide	237	341	429	1,536	2,543
TOTAL	**1,135**	**3,211**	**4,934**	**11,876**	**21,156**

[1]Source: National Center for Health Statistics. Data prepared by the Biometry Branch, Division of Injury Epidemiology and Control, Centers for Disease Control.

Infants Infants less than one-year old suffered 1,135 fatal injuries in 1984, a rate of 31.4/100,000. Surprisingly, the leading cause of death at this age is homicide, followed by suffocation and choking.

Preschoolers In the one-four age group, 3,211 children died from injuries in 1984, for a rate of 22.6/100,000. Burns, drownings, and motor vehicle pedestrian injuries are the leading causes of injury mortality at this age.

School age Children age five-14 are the healthiest age group in our population, yet 4,934 died of injury related causes in 1984, for a rate of 14.5/100,000. Pedestrian injuries are the major cause of death at this age, surpassing motor-vehicle occupant fatalities.

Adolescents and young adults Individuals 15-to 19-years old suffered the highest injury-related fatality rate, 63.2/100,000. Motor-vehicle related causes, including occupant, pedestrian, motorcycle, and bicycle, account for 55 percent of all injury-related deaths, followed by suicide and homicide.

RISK FACTORS FOR INJURY MORTALITY IN CHILDHOOD

Age and sex Age-group differences in the magnitude and type of injury deaths reflect differences in developmental level and exposure to hazards. Overall, males have nearly twice the injury-related mortality of females.

Poverty Black and low-income children suffer higher rates of mortality than affluent, non-minority children. While motor-vehicle occupant deaths do not follow this pattern and are directly related to income, mortality rates for other injuries, particularly burns and homicides, are higher for low-income children.[8]

Race and ethnic differences are related to the risk of injury death. Unintentional injuries affect American Indians at nearly twice the rate of the white population. Homicide among young black males is nearly twice as common as among whites.[9]

Alcohol Children are the victims of alcohol-related crashes as passengers, pedestrians, and bicyclists. In North Carolina, among child fatalities from alcohol related crashes, 56 percent were passengers in cars driven by drunken drivers, 23 percent were passengers in crashes where the other driver was drinking; and 21 percent were killed as pedestrians or bicyclists hit by drunken drivers.[10] In addition, approximately 40 percent of teenage victims of motor-vehicle crashes and 25 percent of victims of motorcycle crashes had detectable levels of blood alcohol. [11] Among non-traffic alcohol-related injuries, 38 percent of teenage drowning cases were found to have alcohol in their blood, at autopsy.[12] Finally, children of alcoholic parents, particularly sons of alcoholic fathers, experience more injuries than children of non-alcoholics.[13]

INJURY MORBIDITY

Deaths represent only a small fraction of the outcomes of serious injuries, the proverbial "tip of the iceberg." The 1981 National Health Interview Survey (NHIS) found that 332/1000 persons of all ages suffered an injury severe enough to require a medical visit or a day of restricted activity during the year.[14] Among children less than age 20, the Massachusetts Statewide Childhood Injury Prevention Program (SCIPP) found that 216/1000 annually suffered an injury resulting in an emergency room visit, and that another 7.7/1000 were admitted to the hospital.[15] For every injury-related death in the SCIPP population, there were 45 hospitalizations and 1300 emergency visits. Age-specific morbidity rates are shown in Table 2. These morbidity incidence data highlight frequent, but non-fatal, injuries from falls, sports, and product-related causes.

TABLE 2

ANNUAL INJURY SPECIFIC MORBIDITY RATES
(per 10,000 children), SCIPP, 1979-1982

EXTERNAL CAUSES	0 - 5 Years	6 - 12 Years	13 - 19 Years	Total
Motor Vehicle				
Occupant	33	37	194	98
Pedestrian	9	21	16	16
MV-pedal cycle	1	13	22	14
Motorcycle	0	0	10	4
Other transport	22	17	52	32
Unintentional (non-motor vehicle)				
Falls	810	568	361	548
Sports	15	344	703	402
Struck by object	279	396	407	370
Cutting, piercing	155	278	413	300
Overexertion	53	49	144	88
Bicycle	31	125	55	73
Foreign body	72	28	63	53
Burns	82	21	54	50
Poisonings	64	6	36	33
Choking	14	1	2	5
Explosives, arms	0.5	4	7	4
Electricity	2	1	1	1
Drowning	1	0.3	0.3	1
Other	126	130	176	147
Intentional				
Self-Inflicted	0.2*	3*	25*	9
Assaults	13	34	165	65

*Age groupings for intentional injuries are 0 - 4 years, 5 - 14 years, 15 - 19 years.

INJURY-RELATED DISABILITY

The National Safety Council estimates that, in 1984, there were 3.5 million non-fatal injuries related to motor vehicles alone, and that 1.7 million of these were disabling injuries.[16] Each year more than 80,000 people of all ages become permanently disabled through an injury to the brain or spinal cord.[1] It has been estimated that 100,000 children per year are admitted to a hospital for a brain injury; 93 percent of these cases are nonfatal, mild brain injury, but may suffer more long-term sequelae.[17]

One in every eight hospital beds is occupied by an injured patient.[1] Among Massachusetts children and youth age one-19, injuries accounted for more days of hospital care than any other disease and had an average hospital stay of over nine days.[18]

INJURY-RELATED COSTS

Injury in America identified injuries as one of the nation's most expensive public health problems, costing an estimated $75-$100 billion-a-year in direct and indirect medical costs.[1] It is estimated that $9-$11 billion-per-year of that amount is for injuries to children less than 15 years old.[19] The National Highway Traffic Safety Administration (NHTSA) estimated the total economic cost of motor vehicle collisions to be $69 billion, in 1984; these costs include property damage, productivity loss, and other costs as well as medical care.[20] In Massachusetts, the costs associated with childhood injuries seen at hospitals were estimated to be $186 million in 1982, or a minimum of $107 per year for every child in the state.[21]

THE PREVENTION OF CHILDHOOD INJURY

Injury-related deaths have declined 30 percent over the last 70 years, a relatively small change when compared to the major decreases in death related to infectious agents.[5] The Surgeon General identified injury as one of 15 priority areas in which further action was required to improve the health of Americans.[22] Fourteen objectives for injury prevention were designed to improve health, reduce risk factors, increase awareness, and improve protection and surveillance.[23]

Yet, the 1985 NHIS found serious gaps in injury-prevention knowledge and behavior.[24] Of persons in families with children younger than ten years, 88 percent had heard of poison control centers, but only 60 percent had a telephone number for such a center; only 45 percent had been advised by a health professional about the importance of using child safety seats; 40 percent of homes did not have a working smoke alarm.

While injuries can be described epidemiologically, the general attitude that injuries are random, chance events which cannot be predicted remains a barrier to control efforts. The purpose of this section is to provide a framework for injury control and some examples of efforts to prevent childhood injury. Although the field of injury control encompasses suicide and violence, the prevention of intentional injuries will not be discussed here; they are addressed in another chapter.

A MODEL OF INJURY CONTROL

The epidemiological model for describing diseases can be modified to describe injuries as well. The agent of injury is the excessive energy that damages body tissues; when discussing childhood injury, the host must be described in terms of developmental level; and the environmental factors include both the physical hazards and the human environment. Haddon conceptualized injuries in terms of three phases: the pre-event factors predisposing to injury; the event phase, when the impact and damage occur; and the post-event management that can determine the ultimate severity, long-term disability, or death.[25] Injury control is based upon a combination of efforts to make the environment and products within it safer through engineering design, to regulate hazards that cannot be modified, and to alter unsafe behaviors.

SUCCESSFUL CHILDHOOD INJURY PREVENTION EFFORTS.

Child passenger safety seats By 1985, all 50 states had passed legislation requiring the restraint of young children riding as passengers in cars. These laws vary from state to state but generally mandate approved automobile safety seats for children younger than four years. In Tennessee, which passed the first such law in 1978, observational surveys of child restraint use have shown an increase from eight percent before the law to nearly 50 percent five years later, and a decrease in fatal childhood occupant injuries associated with increased police enforcement.[26] An evaluation of the Michigan child passenger law found an increase in restraint use from 12 percent before to 51 percent after the law was implemented, and a 25 percent decrease in the number of children younger than four years injured in crashes.[27] The efficacy of child auto restraints serves to underscore the importance of expanding their use to the estimated 50-60 percent of children currently riding unprotected, assuring proper installation and use of these seats, and encouraging police enforcement of state laws.

Children's falls The severity of fall-related injuries is usually determined by the height of the fall and the nature of the impact surface.[28] Appropriate surfacing is essential to minimize the severity of playground falls. A New York program addressed this problem through playground inspections, training of professionals to purchase, install, maintain, and supervise playgrounds, and a public information campaign. An evaluation showed a significant reduction in hard surfaces beneath equipment and a 22 percent reduction in playground-related injuries requiring hospital treatment.[29] The incidence of fatal window falls from multi-story apartment buildings was dramatically reduced in a program initiated by the New York City Health Department. "Children Can't Fly" combined an intensive health education campaign, involving door-to-door counseling, mass media, and community organizing, with the provision of free window guards and follow-up to check for proper installation. A 50 percent reduction in window falls led to legislation requiring landlords to provide window guards to tenants with young children.[30]

Poisoning Aspirin ingestions and other poisonings in young children have been reduced dramatically since the enactment of the 1970 Poison Prevention Packaging Act (PPPA), which requires child-resistant closures for certain substances, including aspirin, prescription medicines, and household chemicals.[31] Pharmacist non-compliance with the PPPA is reported to be about 25 percent.[32] For regulated products, ingestions in children less than five years old have declined from 5.7/1000 to 3.4/1000, while the rate for unregulated products increased slightly.[33] Deaths from poisoning in this same group declined from 2.0/100,000 to 0.5/100,000.

Credit for the dramatic reduction in serious poisonings is also due to the establishment of regional poison control centers, which provide telephone access to consumers and health professionals on how to treat ingestions.[34] One study of the effectiveness of a regional poison center found that more than 63 percent of pediatric emergency room visits could have been averted through telephone triage.[35] Although the number and severity of poisonings have decreased in young children, significant numbers of cases continue to occur, especially in adolescents.

Burns The promulgation of strict federal and state standards of flammability of children's night clothing, in the late 1960s (the Flammable Fabrics Act of 1967, for example), resulted in a dramatic decline in sleepwear-related burns compared to other types of clothing related burns.[36] Childhood scald burns most commonly result from hot foods and drinks; unfortunately, little is known about their prevention. Scalds from hot tap water account for approximately 20 percent of scald burn admissions, however, and occur primarily to young children exposed to residential hot water heated to temperatures of 130°F, a temperature at which exposure for less than 30 seconds will result in a full thickness burn.[37] Efforts to inform the public about the risk of tap-water scalds and turn down the temperature of residential hot-water heaters to 120°F are an important part of public health programs.[38]

Evaluations of programs to make smoke detectors widely available in low-income urban areas,[39] and laws mandating smoke detectors be maintained operational, show they can decrease the risk of residential fire deaths.[40] Finally, a community-based comprehensive public education program for children, adolescents, and families found that knowledge of burn hazards could be increased through health education in the schools, but that education alone was not sufficient to reduce the incidence or severity of burns. Product modification and environmental redesign were proposed as essential additional activities.[41,42]

OTHER IMPORTANT INJURY PREVENTION EFFORTS

Injury prevention in pediatric anticipatory guidance   Health practitioners who provide care for children have a responsibility to counsel parents about deadly risks to their children. As recently as 1980, however, less than four percent of the approximately one minute spent in anticipatory guidance during the average pediatric well-child visit was devoted to safety.[43] Studies demonstrating a positive effect of counseling on injury-prevention behaviors are now available for a number of hazards, including car seat utilization,[44] purchase of smoke detectors,[45] reduction of tap water temperature,[46] reduction of falls,[47] availability of ipecac,[48] safer home environment,[49,50] and knowledge of poison prevention strategies.[51] Most of these programs have been conducted with well-educated, middle-class families who received care from private physicians or an HMO.

Developmentally oriented safety surveys are part of the American Academy of Pediatrics' (AAP) TIPP Program which aims to establish counseling on injury prevention as a routine component of well-child care.[52] The program includes specific injury prevention advice for pediatricians, a suggested counseling schedule, the Framingham Safety Surveys,[53] and educational materials for parents.

Injury in day care   The increasing proportion of mothers in the work force has led to concerns about the safety of children in day care and at home alone. While parents may assume that a regulated, licensed day care center is a safe environment, the extent to which current regulations governing day care result in reduced hazards is unknown. The *Safe Day Care* training module, developed by the Massachusetts Department of Public Health, is one attempt to equip day care facilities with safety checklists and other materials to evaluate the center's environment.

Injury in the home   Approximately half of all fatal injuries and 90 percent of nonfatal injuries to children under five take place in the home. The potential dangers of structural elements, furnishings, and commonly available household products are well-known. Home inspections in an urban area with substandard housing documented that most dwellings with young children lack safety items, such as fire extinguishers (79 percent), syrup of ipecac (78 percent), electric outlet covers (60 percent), smoke detectors (44 percent), and toddler gates for stairs where applicable (37 percent). An intervention was initiated that combined safety counseling in the home, distribution of safety devices, and enforcement of housing regulations. The program resulted in a ten percent reduction in overall household hazards. Although each strategy had some effect in reducing the number of hazards, the most significant reductions were achieved through the safety devices (53 percent) followed by code enforcement (17 percent) and education (seven percent).[54]

Teen drinking and driving   Youth are over-represented in automobile crashes and, in particular, in night-time crashes. Most efforts to reduce crashes related to teen drinking have used three approaches, which have had limited success:

deterrence through enforcement, arrest, and punishment; rehabilitation of those convicted of drunken driving; and education about the dangers of driving after drinking. Other approaches that show some effectiveness in reducing teen drinking and driving include curfew laws that limit night-time driving, increasing the age of licensing drivers, raising the legal drinking age, and increasing the price of alcoholic beverages.[55,56]

AREAS REQUIRING FURTHER RESEARCH

Pedestrian injuries The significance of pedestrian injuries has been obscured, often because they are grouped with other motor vehicle-related injuries. Demonstration projects to educate preschool and school-age children and youth about the hazards of traffic, and thereby reduce darting-out behavior, have been successful, but have not been widely applied.[57,58] In Western European countries, efforts have been directed to separating pedestrians from the flow of traffic.[59]

Bicycle helmets Less than two percent of school-aged bicyclists wear helmets.[60] Only six percent of physicians routinely include bicycle safety in patient education. [61] Although bicycle helmets have been proposed as a solution to the significant problem of head injuries and death in bicycle collisions, the relationship between helmet use and prevention of serious bike injuries has not been assessed directly in controlled studies.

Drowning Children and youth drown in a variety of settings—residential pools, public beaches, flooded quarries, bathtubs, boating accidents, and lakes and rivers. Pool fencing that eliminates direct access to backyard swimming pools has been proposed as an effective measure that could reduce 30-50 percent of drowning and near-drowning.[62,63] Few states or municipalities have requirements for such barriers around residential pools, where the majority of drownings occur in young children. Swimming instruction is often viewed as a factor in preventing drowning, but its effects have not been tested and may be mitigated by other factors, such as alcohol use and risk-taking behavior in adolescence.

ATVs and product regulation Three and four-wheel all-terrain vehicles (ATVs) are important hazardous products. As of early 1987, the U.S. Consumer Product Safety Commission had documented reports of 696 ATV-related deaths, with 45 percent of these occurring to children younger than 16 years, and 20 percent occurring to children younger than 12 years.[64] Emergency room visits for ATV-related injuries have increased from 2,984 cases in 1979 to an estimated 86,400 cases in 1986, with evidence of serious head and spinal cord injury.[65,66] Despite these data and the apparent unstable design of ATVs, there are few federal or state restrictors on their sale or use. [Ed. note: In 1988, agreement was reached prohibiting sales of three-wheel ATV's.]

FUTURE DIRECTIONS
IN CHILDHOOD INJURY CONTROL

In an effort to assess the current state of injury prevention, Rivara concluded that 29 percent of injury fatalities in childhood could be prevented by implementing 12 available strategies.[67] Unfortunately, most of these available interventions have not been applied at the state or local level. If children are to be protected from injury in the future, new coalitions of federal, state, and local agencies, with mandates in the areas of health, safety, child protection, education, highway traffic safety, and consumer protection, will need to work together.

Interventions must be initiated at the community level, based on locally identified needs and current data. However, state agencies must take a lead by providing a foundation upon which to build a statewide program of service provision, surveillance, and public policy.[68] States must develop resources, coordinate the multiple agencies and disciplines involved, and provide training and technical consultation at the local level. A federal commitment is required to direct funds to injury-prevention research and programming, and to re-invigorating the federal regulations concerning product safety.

State Maternal and Child Health (MCH) agencies and MCH programs have a special role in promoting childhood-injury prevention because of their ability to reach high-risk populations. In New England, the MCH units in the six state health departments have joined together to strengthen the injury-prevention programs region-wide.[69] As part of national efforts to increase injury-control programs, a National Committee on Injury Prevention has reviewed intervention efforts and made national recommendations for state and local health authorities. All of these efforts must be encouraged and supported if the prevention of childhood injury is to receive the priority it deserves.

REFERENCES

1. Committee on Trauma Research: *Injury in America*, Washington, D.C.: National Academy Press, 1985.

2. Centers for Disease Control. Premature mortality due to unintentional injuries - United States, 1983. Morbidity and Mortality Weekly Report. 1986;35(22):353-356.

3. Centers for Disease Control. Premature mortality due to suicide and homicide - United States, 1983. Morbidity and Mortality Weekly Report. 1986;35(22):357-360,365.

4. National Center for Health Statistics. *Health, United States, 1986.* DHHS Pub. No. (PHS) 87-1232. Public Health Service. Washington, D.C.: US Government Printing Office. 1986.

5. Baker SP, O'Neill B, Karpf RS. *The Injury Fact Book.* Lexington MA: Lexington Books, 1984.

6. National Center for Health Statistics. Advance Report of Final Mortality Statistics, 1985. *Monthly Vital Statistics Report.* Vol. 36, No. 5, Supplement, DHHS Pub. No. (PHS) 87-1120. Hyattsville MD: Public Health Service, August, 1987.

7. Guyer B, Gallagher SS. An approach to the epidemiology of childhood injuries. *Pediatr. Clin. North Am.* 1985;32:5-15.

8. Wise PH. Kotelchuck M, Wilson ML, Mills M. Racial and socioeconomic disparities in childhood mortality in Boston. *N Engl J Med,* 1985;313:360-366.

9. Baker SP, O'Neill B, Karpf RS. *The Injury Fact Book,* Lexington: Lexington Books, 1984.

10. Margolis LH, Kotch J, Lacey JH. Children in alcohol-related motor vehicle crashes. Pediatrics 1986;77:870-872.

11. Wagenaar AC. *Alcohol, Young Drivers and Traffic Accidents: Effects of Minimum-Age Laws,* Massachusetts, D.C. Health, 1983.

12. Wintemute GJ, Kraus JF, Teret SP, Wright M. Drowning in childhood and adolescence: a population-based study. *Am J Public Health* 1987;77:830-832.

13. Putnam SL, Rockett I. Parental alcoholism as a risk factor in children's illness and injury. Paper presented at the American Public Health Assoc Annual Meeting, New Orleans, October 1987.

14. National Center for Health Statistics: Current Estimates from the National Health Interview Survey: United States 1981. Series 10, Number 141. U.S. Dept. of Health and Human Services, October 1982.

15. Gallagher SS, Finison K, Guyer B, et al. The incidence of injuries among 87,000 Massachusetts children and adolescents: Results of the 1980-81 Statewide Childhood Injury Prevention Program surveillance system. *Am J Public Health.* 1984;74:1340-1347.

16. 1984 Accident Facts. Chicago, National Safety Council, 1985.

17. Kraus JF, Fife D, Conroy C. Pediatric brain injuries: the nature, clinical course and early outcomes in a defined United States population. *Pediatrics.* 1987;79:501-507.

18. Massachusetts Department of Public Health: *Injuries in Massachusetts: A Status Report,* Boston MA, 1987.

19. Robertson LS. Childhood injuries: knowledge and strategies for prevention. Background paper prepared for the Office of Technology Assessment, U.S. Congress, February 1987.

20. National Highway Traffic Safety Administration: The Economic Costs to Society of Motor Vehicle Accidents. DOT HS 806 342, January 1985.

21. Azzara CV, Gallagher SS, Guyer B. The relative health care and social costs for specific causes of injury. Paper presented to the American Public Health Assoc Annual Meeting, Washington, D.C., November, 1985.

22. Office of the Assistant Secretary for Health and Surgeon General: Healthy people. The Surgeon General's report on health promotion and disease prevention. DHEW Publication No. (PHS) 79-55071. U.S. Government Printing Office, Washington, D.C. 1979.

23. Department of Health and Human Services: Promoting health/preventing disease: objectives for the nation. U.S. Government Printing Office, Washington, D.C., 1980.

24. Thornbery OT, Wilson RW, Golden PM. Health Promotion Data for the 1990 Objectives, National Center for Health Statistics: *Advance Data from Vital & Health Statistics*, No. 126, DHHS Pub. No. (PHS) 86-1250, Public Health Service, Hyattsville MD, September 19, 1986.

25. Haddon W, Baker SP. Injury Control. In: *Preventive and Community Medicine*, Second Edition. Edited by Clark DW and MacMahon B. Boston, Little, Brown & Co. 1981, pp 109-140.

26. Decker MD, Dewey JD, Hutcheson RH Jr, et al. The use and efficacy of child restraint devices. *JAMA* 1984;252:2571-2575.

27. Wagenaar AC, Webster DW. Preventing injuries to children through compulsory automobile safety seat use. *Pediatrics*, 1986;78:662-672.

28. Garrettson LK, Gallagher SS. Falls in children and youth. *Pediatr Clin of North America.* 1985;32:153-162.

29. Fisher L, Harris VG, VanBuren J, et al. Assessment of a pilot child playground injury prevention project in New York state. *Am J Public Health.* 1980;70:1000-1002.

30. Spiegel C, Lindaman F. Children Can't Fly: a program to prevent childhood morbidity and mortality from window falls. *Am J Public Health.* 1977;67:1143-1146.

31. Clarke A, Walton WW. Effect of safety packaging on aspirin ingestion by children. *Pediatrics.* 1979;63:687-693.

32. Dole EJ, Czajka PA, Rivara FP. Evaluation of pharmacists' compliance with the Poison Prevention Packaging Act. *Am J Public Health.* 1986;76:1335-1336.

33. Walton WW. An evaluation of the Poison Prevention Packaging Act. *Pediatrics.* 1982;69:363-370.

34. McIntire MS, Angle CR. Regional poison control centers improve patient care. *N Engl J Med*, 1983;308:219-221.

35. Chafee-Bahamon C, Lovejoy FH. Effectiveness of a regional poison center in reducing excess emergency room visits for children's poisonings. *Pediatrics*, 1983;72:164-169.

36. McLoughlin E, Clarke N, Stahl K, Crawford JD. One pediatric burn unit's experience with sleepwear-related injuries. *Pediatrics*, 1977;60:405-409.

37. Feldman KW, Schaller RT, Feldman JA, McMillon M. Tap water scald burns in children. *Pediatrics*, 1978;62:1-7.

38. Katcher ML. Prevention of tap water scald burns: evaluation of a multi-media injury control program. *Am J Public Health*, 1987;77:1195-1197.

39. Gorman RL, Charney E, Holtzman NA, Roberts KB. A successful city-wide smoke detector giveaway program. *Pediatrics*, 1985;75:14-18.

40. McLoughlin E, Marchone M, Hanger SL, et al. Smoke detector legislation: its effect on owner-occupied homes. *Am J Public Health*, 1985;75:858-862.

41. McLoughlin E, Vince CJ, Lee AM, Crawford JD. Project Burn Prevention: outcome and implication. *Am J Public Health*, 1982;72:241-247.

42. MacKay AM, Rothman KJ. The incidence and severity of burn injuries following Project Burn Prevention. *Am J Public Health,* 1982;72:248-252.

43. Reisinger KS, Bires JA. Anticipatory guidance in pediatric practice. *Pediatrics*, 1980;66:889-892.

44. Reisinger KS, Williams AF, Wells JK, et al. Effect of pediatricians' counseling on infant restraint use. *Pediatrics,* 1981,67:201-206.

45. Miller RE, Reisinger KS, Blatter MM, et al. Pediatric counseling and subsequent use of smoke detectors. *Am J Public Health,* 1982;72:392-393.

46. Thomas KA, Christophersen ER, Hassanein RA. Evaluation of group well child care for improving burn prevention practices in the home. *Pediatrics,* 1984;74:879-882.

47. Kravitz H, Grove M. Prevention of accidental falls in infancy by counseling mothers. *Illinois Med J* 1973, 144:570-573.

48. Dershewitz RA, Posner MK, Paichel W. The effectiveness of health education on home use of ipecac. *Clin Pediatr* 1983:268-271.

49. Bass JL, Mehta KA, Ostrovsky M, et al. Educating parents about injury prevention. *Pediatr Clin of N America,* 1985;32:233-242.

50. Kelly B, Sein C, McCarthy PL. Safety education in a pediatric primary care setting. *Pediatrics,* 1987;79:818-824.

51. Woolf A, Lewander W, Fillippone G, Lovejoy F. Prevention of childhood poisoning: efficacy of an educational program carried out in an emergency clinic. *Pediatrics.* 1987;80:359-363.

52. Committee on Accident and Poison Prevention: *Injury Control for Children and Youth.* Elk Grove Village, IL, American Academy of Pediatrics, 1987.

53. Bass JL, Mehta KA. Developmentally-oriented safety surveys. *Clinical Pediatrics,* 1980;19:350-356.

54. Gallagher SS, Hunter P, Guyer B. A home injury prevention program for children. *Pediatr Clin North America,* 1985;32:95-112.

55. Insurance Institute for Highway Safety: Teenage Drivers. Washington, D.C., 1985.

56. Wagenaar AC. *Alcohol, Young Drivers and Traffic Accidents: Affects of Minimum-Age Laws,* Massachusetts: D.C. Heath, 1983.

57. Fortenberry JC, Brown DB. Problem identification, implementation and evaluation of a pedestrian safety program. *Accid Anal & Prev,* 1982;14:315-322.

58. Preusser DF, Blomberg RD. Reducing child pedestrian accidents through public education. *J Safety Research,* 1984;15:47-56.

59. Guyer B, Talbot AM, Pless IB. Pedestrian injuries to children and youth. *Pediatr Clin North America,* 1985;32:163-174.

60. Weiss BD. Bicycle helmet use in children. *Pediatrics,* 1986;77:677-679.

61. Weiss BD, Duncan B. Bicycle helmet use by children; knowledge and behavior of physicians. *Am J Public Health,* 1986;76:1022-1023.

62. Wintemute GJ, Kraus JF, Teret SP, Wright. Drowning in children and adolescence: a population-based study. *Am J Public Health,* 1987;77:830-832.

63. Pearn JH, Wong RVK, Brown J, et al. Drowning and near-drowning involving children: a five year total population study from the city and county of Honolulu. *Am J Public Health,* 1979;69:450-454.

64. Calhoun D. All-terrain vehicles: unsafe, unregulated and aimed at children. *Injury Prevention Network Newsletter,* San Francisco, The Trauma Foundation, 1987, pp 2-6.

65. Sneed RC, Stover SL, Fine PR. Spinal cord injury associated with all-terrain vehicle accidents. *Pediatrics,* 1986;77:271-274.

66. Kriel RL, Sheehan M, Krach L, et al. pediatric head injury resulting from all-terrain vehicle accidents. *Pediatrics*, 1986;78:933-935.

67. Rivara F. Traumatic deaths of children in the United States: currently available prevention strategies. *Pediatrics*, 1985;75:456-462.

68. Gallagher SS, Messenger KP, Guyer B. State and local responses to children's injuries: the Massachusetts Statewide Childhood Injury Prevention Program. *J Social Issues*, 1987;43 (2):149-162.

69. Molloy PJ. Childhood injuries. *Public Health Currents*, Columbus, Ross Laboratories, 1987;27(4):23-27.

SECTION V

HEALTH CARE OF ADOLESCENTS

HEALTH OF ADOLESCENTS

35

Mary Grace Kovar and Deborah Dawson

There are about 21 million people who are defined as adolescents, that is people who are ages 12-17, currently living in the U.S. This is far fewer than a few years ago, when the children born during the baby boom were adolescents, and fewer than there will be in the future; there will probably be about 24 million adolescents by the year 2000.[1]

Adolescents are so diverse that it is difficult to describe them as a group. Young men develop at a different rate from young women. The 12-year old who has not had an adolescent growth spurt, who lives at home, and who cannot legally drive, drink, or marry is in a different environment than the 17-year old. Even within an individual, different body systems do not develop at the same rate.

Nevertheless, it is critical to know something about adolescents as a group so that the individual adolescent can be placed in the context of his or her peers. The purpose of this chapter is to provide such a context.

Health is a concept that is difficult to define for people of any age. It is especially difficult for young people going through such a rapid and uneven physiological change in a society whose expectations are changing. It is made more difficult because the problems that can kill or cripple, or prevent the adolescent from becoming a fully functioning adult are not usually problems of disease or disability. They are problems that not many physicians have been trained to deal with; they are primarily social problems. Nevertheless, the search for solutions has been thrown back upon the medical care system, and physicians need to know all they can.

The data in this chapter are national data for the U.S. in the mid-1980s. Most are shown for males and females, and for Black and white adolescents. There are many other cultural and ethnic groups in this country. Adolescents in those groups may have different experiences and different problems. However, each adolescent must be considered in the context of what adolescence is like in the U.S. today because this is the society in which they must live, and hopefully, progress.

MORTALITY

The oldest and most universal measure of health is the complete lack of health, i.e., death. Despite our concerns about their death-defying behavior, few adolescents die. Of every 1,000,000 babies born alive, only 358 die during adolescence, according to the 1979-1980 life tables for the U.S.[2] Death rates have declined for both younger and older adolescents since then; and, in 1985, only 31.8 of every 100,000 12-14-year olds and 66.1 of every 100,000 15-17-year olds died (Table 1).

Three points need to be made: 1. Among adolescents, as among adults, death rates are higher for males than for females. 2. The death rates are significantly higher among the older than among younger adolescents. In both cases, the rates are higher primarily because of accidents and other external causes, but they are also higher for diseases. 3. Death rates for diseases are higher for Black than for white adolescents, but deaths from accidents and external causes are not. The reversal is almost entirely due to white adolescents having higher death rates from motor vehicles.

The chief threat to an adolescent's life is not disease; it is external. Death rates from external causes have declined so steadily (Table 2) that they comprise a smaller proportion of all deaths of adolescents than they did in the late 1970s, but even in 1985, about 48 percent of the deaths of 12-14-year olds and 54 percent of the deaths of older adolescents were from external causes. The single greatest threat is the motor vehicle; in 1985, motor vehicle accidents accounted for 27 percent of the deaths of adolescents age 12-14 years and 40 percent of the deaths of adolescents ages 15-17.

Suicide rates for adolescents are extremely low. However, in contrast with the general decline in death rates for adolescents, the suicide rates and the proportion of all deaths due to suicide have been increasing for both younger and older adolescents (Tables 1,2). In 1985, 258 children ages 12-14 and 883 youths ages 15-17 committed suicide. No one knows how many others may have attempted it.

TABLE 1

DEATH RATES FOR ADOLESCENTS
UNITED STATES, 1979-1984

Rates Per 100,000 Persons

| | All Causes | | | Adverse Effects And Accidents | | | | | | | | |
| | | | | Total (E800-E949) | | | Motor Vehicle E810-E825 | | | Suicide (E950-E959) | | |
Year	Total	Male	Female	Total	Male	Female	Total	Male	Female	Total	Male	Female
Ages 12-14												
1979	35.9	45.4	26.1	18.4	26.0	10.5	9.4	12.0	6.8	1.9	2.8	.9
1980	34.3	43.6	24.6	17.2	24.4	9.7	9.3	12.1	6.3	1.6	2.3	.9
1981	33.3	41.6	24.7	16.1	23.0	9.0	9.0	11.8	6.0	1.6	2.5	.7
1982	31.7	40.2	22.9	15.1	21.4	8.4	8.2	10.7	5.6	1.4	1.9	.9
1983	30.4	38.5	21.9	14.6	20.6	8.3	7.6	9.9	5.3	1.2	1.9	.5
1984	31.1	38.4	23.4	14.3	19.6	8.7	7.9	9.8	5.9	1.3	1.6	.9
Ages 15-17												
1979	79.9	111.5	47.1	48.1	69.7	25.8	35.4	48.7	21.5	7.1	10.8	3.2
1980	79.2	109.9	47.3	46.3	66.8	25.1	33.6	45.8	20.8	6.8	10.6	2.8
1981	72.2	99.4	43.8	40.8	59.1	21.9	30.0	41.1	18.5	6.2	9.7	2.6
1982	68.3	95.1	40.3	37.1	54.7	18.9	26.6	37.1	15.7	6.2	9.3	2.9
1983	65.4	89.9	39.8	34.8	50.0	19.0	25.1	33.9	16.0	6.0	9.6	2.2
1984	66.0	89.8	41.2	36.5	51.5	20.9	27.0	36.4	17.3	5.9	9.3	2.3

SOURCE: NCHS, National Mortality Registration System.

Notes: Population April 1 for 1980, July 1 for all other years. Numbers in titles are International Classification of Diseases codes.

TABLE 2
PERCENT OF DEATHS DUE TO ADVERSE EFFECTS AND ACCIDENTS. UNITED STATES, 1979-1984

| | Cause Of Death | | | | | | | | |
| | Adverse Effects and Accidents (E800-E949) | | | Motor Vehicle Accidents (E810-E825) | | | Suicide (E950-E959) | | |
Year	Total	Boys	Girls	Total	Boys	Girls	Total	Boys	Girls
Ages 12-14									
1979	51.3	72.4	29.2	26.2	33.4	18.9	5.3	7.8	2.5
1980	50.1	71.1	28.3	27.1	35.3	18.4	4.7	6.7	2.6
1981	48.3	69.1	27.0	27.0	35.4	18.0	4.8	7.5	2.1
1982	47.6	67.5	26.5	25.9	33.8	17.7	4.4	6.0	2.8
1983	48.0	67.8	27.3	25.0	32.6	17.4	3.9	6.3	1.6
1984	46.0	63.0	28.0	25.4	31.5	19.0	4.2	5.1	2.9
Ages 15-17									
1979	60.2	87.2	32.3	44.3	61.0	26.9	8.9	13.5	4.0
1980	58.5	84.3	31.7	42.4	57.8	26.3	8.6	13.4	3.5
1981	56.5	81.9	30.3	41.6	56.9	25.6	8.5	13.4	3.6
1982	54.3	80.1	27.7	38.9	54.3	23.0	9.1	13.6	4.2
1983	53.2	76.5	29.1	38.4	51.8	24.5	9.2	14.7	3.4
1984	55.3	78.0	31.7	40.9	55.2	26.2	8.9	14.1	3.5

Percent Of Deaths

SOURCE: NCHS, National Mortality Registration System.
NOTE: Numbers in titles are International Classification of Diseases code.

INJURIES

Most adolescents who are injured do not die of their injuries, and few of the injuries severe enough to cause restriction of usual activity or receipt of medical care are associated with motor vehicles (Table 3). Most adolescents who are injured suffer their injuries where they spend the most time—at home or at school. The most common place for an adolescent, whether male or female, to be injured is at school; the second most common is at home. The proportion of injuries suffered at school by young black people is especially striking; studies have shown that schools can be very dangerous. [3]

PREGNANCY AND CHILDBEARING

A major threat to the future well-being of adolescent men is injury or death from injury. A major threat to adolescent women is early childbearing. The birth rates for very young women (ages ten-14 years) have remained constant in the recent past. While birth rates for adolescent women went down during the 1970s,

TABLE 3

INJURIES TO ADOLESCENTS AGES 12-17 YEARS.
UNITED STATES, 1985-86

		Sex		Race	
	Total	Male	Female	White	Black
	Episodes Per 1,000 Persons				
Rates	369.3	468.7	266.7	374.5	243.1
	Episodes In Thousands				
Episodes	8,101	5,210	2,890	6,733	960
	Percent Distribution				
Total	100.0	100.0	100.0	100.0	100.0
School	37.0	37.5	36.1	34.6	46.5
Home	21.0	20.5	22.0	19.0	32.6
Street	10.5	10.3	10.9	11.2	10.6
Other & DK	31.5	31.7	31.0	35.2	10.3
Motor Vehicle	5.1	4.4	6.4	45.4	5.4

SOURCE: NCHS, National Health Interview Survey
NOTE: Only episodes severe enough to restrict activity for a day or to receive
               medical attention are included.

there has been little change in the rate since about 1976 (Table 4). However, because there are fewer adolescents, there were 168 thousand births to women age 15-17, in 1985, in contrast with 227 thousand a decade earlier.[4,5] As far as can be ascertained, there has been little if any change in pregnancy rates;[6,7] the decrease in the birth rate, most of which occurred before 1980,[8] is due to increased reliance on abortion to terminate the pregnancy.

Marriage rates have also decreased.[9] Premarital intercourse has increasingly become the rule for younger women,[10] marriage after conception but before the birth has become less common,[11] and young women are sexually active for a longer period of time before marriage.[10]

One result of these concurrent changes is that birth rates for unmarried adolescent women have increased, despite the overall decline in birth rates (Table 5). Young Black women historically have had high rates of out-of-wedlock births; their rate has decreased. The overall increase in out-of-wedlock birth rates is entirely due to the increased rates for white adolescents. As recently as 1975, there were 9.6 births for every 1,000 unmarried white women ages 15-17; by 1985, there were 14.2.

TABLE 4
LIVE BIRTH RATES FOR ADOLESCENT WOMEN.
UNITED STATES, 1970-1985

Year	Age In Years	
	10-14	15-17
	Births Per 1,000 Women	
1970	1.2	38.8
1971	1.1	38.2
1972	1.2	39.0
1973	1.2	38.5
1974	1.2	37.3
1975	1.3	36.1
1976	1.2	34.1
1977	1.2	33.9
1978	1.2	32.2
1979	1.2	32.3
1980	1.1	32.5
1981	1.1	32.1
1982	1.1	32.4
1983	1.1	32.0
1984	1.2	31.1
1985	1.2	31.1

SOURCE: MVSR 36(4) Table 4

Sexually active adolescent women risk having a child at an early age. Any adolescent who is sexually active is also at greater risk of sexually transmitted disease—including AIDS. The risk of HIV infection for adolescents, few of whom have settled into long-term monogamous relationships, is at present unknown.

HEALTH STATUS

Household surveys show that relatively few adolescents are in poor health (Table 6). In the mid-1980s, about three percent of all 12-17-year old adolescents were reported to be in only fair or poor health, seven percent were limited in activities usual for their age, and 13 percent had spent at least seven days in bed over the course of the previous year. Such measures of health are family, rather than clinical, evaluations, but it is the perception of health that influences behavior, such as seeing a physician or staying in bed. Adolescents reported to be in excellent health lost only 3.3 days from school and spent 2.8 days in bed, in contrast with 17 days lost from school and 16 days in bed for those in fair or poor health.[12]

TABLE 5

LIVE BIRTH RATES FOR UNMARRIED ADOLESCENT WOMEN
UNITED STATES, 1970-1985

Year	Ages 15-17		
	All races	**White**	**Black**
Estimated		Births Per 1,000 Women	
1970	17.1	7.5	77.9
1971	17.5	7.4	80.7
1972	18.5	8.0	82.8
1973	18.7	8.4	81.2
1974	18.8	8.8	78.6
1975	19.3	9.6	76.8
1976	19.0	9.7	73.5
1977	19.8	10.5	73.0
1978	19.1	10.3	68.8
1979	19.9	10.8	71.0
1980	20.7	11.7	70.6
Reported			
1980	20.6	11.8	69.6
1981	20.9	12.4	66.9
1982	21.5	12.9	67.6
1983	22.1	13.5	67.1
1984	21.9	13.5	66.8
1985	22.5	14.2	67.0

SOURCE: NCHS: MVSR 36(4)

USE OF MEDICAL CARE

Adolescents use less health care than any other age group except, perhaps, young adults (people ages 18-24). About 71 percent of the adolescents had had at least one contact with a physician during the preceding year; only four percent had spent as much as one night in the hospital (Table 7).

Adolescent women are more likely to have received medical care than adolescent men. Part of the reason is reproductive care, and the differences are apparent for hospitalization. However, even when hospitalization for delivery is excluded, young women were more likely than young men to have been hospitalized within a year. The impact of the high birth rates for adolescent Black women is seen when comparing the hospitalization rates with the rates-excluding-delivery.

There is no reason to believe that all adolescents need to make multiple contacts with a physician every year. Many are healthy. Those who are in poor health do use more medical care. For example, adolescents age 15-17 who were in excellent or good health had, on the average, 3.0 contacts with a physician during the year, in contrast with 8.4 contacts for adolescents in fair or poor health.[12]

However, failure to have any contact with a physician means that there is no opportunity for preventive care, and it appears that many adolescents are not receiving basic preventive care. Other data from the National Health Interview Survey show that about 30 percent of the 16-year old adolescents had not had a routine physical examination within two years; 18 percent had not had one within three

TABLE 6

HEALTH STATUS OF ADOLESCENTS
AGES 12-17 YEARS UNITED STATES 1985-86

	7 or More Beddays In Year	Limited In Activity	In Fair Or Poor Health
	Percent of Adolescents		
All Races	12.8	6.4	2.8
Male	10.2	7.3	2.5
Female	15.5	5.5	3.2
White	13.8	6.6	2.2
Male	11.0	7.6	2.0
Female	16.8	5.5	2.5
Black	8.7	6.3	6.0
Male	7.0	6.7	5.3
Female	10.4	5.9	6.6

SOURCE: NCHS, National Health Interview Survey

years; 11 percent had not had a routine physical within five years.[13] Twenty-seven percent had not had one within three years; seven percent had not had their eyes examined within five years.

SUMMARY

While death in adolescence is a rare event, there are indications from the death rates of these young people that carry warnings for the future. Young male adolescents are more likely than young females to die—primarily because of accidents and other external causes. By the time they move into young adulthood, the differences between the sexes are even larger, and it is this proclivity for violent death that accounts for so much of the loss of productive life of men.

The stress of adolescence is certainly reflected in the suicide rates, which are increasing. Despite the rarity of suicide, the death of any young people from suicide is profoundly distressing.

Because the birth of a child to a young woman who is not old enough to have graduated from high school severely limits her life opportunities, it is encouraging that birth rates are going down. The increased sexual activity of young women is not so encouraging—they are at greater risk of early pregnancy and of sexually transmitted disease. Whether the rise in birth rates for unmarried adolescent women is bad depends partly on values and partly on the kind of support there is for her. Certainly one prefers a child to be born into a family with a stable marriage.

TABLE 7

**MEDICAL CARE IN PAST YEAR OF ADOLESCENTS
AGES 12-17 YEARS UNITED STATES 1985-86**

	With			Number Of		
	Doctor Visit	Hospital Care Total Ex. Del.		Doctor Visits	Hospital Days Total Ex. Del.	
	Percent Of Adolescents			Per 100 Adolescents		
All Races	70.5	3.6	3.3	3.2	22.2	21.0
Male	68.7	2.8	2.7	3.0	17.6	17.6
Female	72.2	4.4	3.7	3.3	26.8	26.8
White	72.1	3.7	3.5	3.4	23.2	22.3
Male	70.6	3.0	3.0	3.3	18.5	18.5
Female	73.7	4.5	4.0	3.6	28.1	26.4
Black	63.6	3.2	2.4	1.9	20.1	17.5
Male	60.2	2.2	2.2	1.7	16.2	16.2
Female	67.0	4.3	2.7	2.1	24.0	18.8

SOURCE: NCHS, National Health Interview Survey

However, when pregnant adolescents were married before the child was born, the marriage often ended in divorce.

The lack of medical care may not be harmful for many adolescents, but there is evidence that some are not receiving the preventive care that is recommended. Problems are not being identified early. Glasses that might aid in school performance are not prescribed. Prenatal care that could help both the young mother and her child is either not received or is late.

By all of the traditional measures of physical health, most adolescents in the U.S. are healthy, and are perhaps healthier than the cohort ten years older were. The rates of smoking and illicit drug use have also leveled off or decreased. Their major problems are not problems of disease but of stress and change.

REFERENCES

1. U.S. Bureau of the Census: Projections of the population of the United States, by age, sex, and race: 1983 to 2080. Series P-25 no. 952, Washington, 1984.

2. National Center for Health Statistics: U.S. Decennial Life Tables for 1979-81, Vol. 1, No.1.

3. National Institute of Education.:Violent Schools - Safe Schools. The Safe School Study Report to Congress (Vol. 1. Washington D.C. U.S. Government Printing Office, 1978.

4. National Center for Health Statistics: Advance Report of Final Natality Statistics, 1985. Monthly Vital Statistics Report 36 (4) Supp. July, 1987.

5. National Center for Health Statistics by S.J. Ventura. Trends in Teenage Childbearing, United States, 1970-81. Vital and Health Statistics, Series 21 No. 41. U.S. Government Printing Office, 1984.

6. Ventura SJ, Taffel S, and Mosher WD. Estimates of pregnancy and pregnancy rates for the United States, 1976-81. Public Health Reports 100 (1), 1985 pp 31-33.

7. Ventura SJ, Taffel S, and Mosher WD. Estimates of pregnancies and pregnancy rates for the United States, 1976-84. American Journal of Public Health, in press.

8. Maciak BJ, Spitz AM, Strauss LT, et al. Pregnancy and birthrates among sexually experienced U.S. Teenagers 1974-1980-1983. JAMA 258:2069-71, 1987

9. National Center for Health Statistics: Advance Report of Final Marriage Statistics, 1984. Monthly Vital Statistics Report 36 (2) Supp.May, 1987.

10. National Center for Health Statistics by C.A.Bachrach and M.C. Horn. Married and Unmarried Couples: United States, 1982. Vital and Health Statistics, Series 23, No. 15, U.S. Government Printing Office, 1987

11. National Center for Health Statistics by S. Ventura. Trends in marital status of mothers at conception and birth of first child: United States, 1964-68, 1972, and 1980. Monthly Vital Statistics Report 36 (2) Suppl. May, 1987.

12. National Center for Health Statistics by P. Reis. Physician Contacts by Sociodemographic and Health Characteristics. Vital and Health Statistics, Series 10, No. 161, U.S. Government Printing Office, 1987.

13. National Center for Health Statistics by B. Bloom. Use of Selected Preventive Care Procedures. Vital and Health Statistics, Series 10, No. 157, U.S. Government Printing Office, 1986.

36 ADOLESCENT HEALTH CARE

Robert William Blum

INTRODUCTION

Adolescence is a dramatic time of rapid physiologic and emotional change. Puberty brings with it three primary alterations: assumption of mature physiologic capabilities, gender dimorphism, and adult reproductive capacity. Over the years 1860-1960, there was a progressive decline throughout the U.S. and Western Europe in the age of pubertal onset which has plateaued over the past 30 years to the point where females currently reach menarche on average at 12.6 years. The decline is most clearly associated with improved sanitation and nutrition.

The physiologic changes of puberty serve as a trigger for the cascade of emotional changes of adolescence. For most, this is a time of wonderment, with numerous experiences occurring for the first time. It is an age of experimentation, trying on new social roles and striving for a sense of self-identity established, in part, through reactions of others to the behaviors displayed. For most, it is a time when the intellectual and psychological structures of childhood give way to more complex perspectives of the adult, without the "storm and stress" erroneously associated with the age.

For others, adolescence is far more tumultuous, where risk-taking behaviors increase the likelihood of serious threats to health and well-being. For some, it is an age where the impact of poverty and social disenfranchisement becomes dramatically evident. For others, the stresses of the age have fatal consequences.

THE HEALTH STATUS OF YOUTH

MORTALITY

Over the past 40 years, there has been a dramatic shift in the causes of adolescent deaths, from primarily infectious illness to primarily social and environmental etiology. Currently, 77.1 percent of deaths among 15-to-24-year olds (Table 1) are the result of violence: unintentional injuries, homicides, and suicides. Homicides have risen over 300 percent since 1950, to 15.6/100,000 youths; and for Black males, the rate is 72.5/100,000. Suicide rates have increased 400 percent over the same period of time, to 12.3/100,000. This compares with 17.6/100,000 for Australia, 16.6 for Japan, and 28.8 for Austria. From a global perspective, juvenile suicide continues to rise dramatically; in the U.S., we have begun to observe a plateau among adolescent deaths under 19 years of age, while the young adult suicide rate continues to increase. [1]

Unintentional injuries kill more American youths than any other single cause. Motor vehicle deaths account for approximately 60 percent of fatal injuries, for which the case fatality rate of drunk driving is 58 percent. Adolescents continue to believe that drinking does not represent a significant risk in driving. A 1987 study of over 36,000 youths in Minnesota found that over one-fourth of males and one-in-six teenage girls believed that it is okay to drive after two or more drinks. In addition, less than 25 percent of youths surveyed indicated that they routinely wear seat belts. [2]

TABLE 1

MORTALITY AGES 15-24 YEARS N THE UNITED STATES, 1980

	Rate per 1000,000	Percent
ACCIDENTS	61.7	53.5%
HOMICIDES	15.6	13.5%
SUICIDES	12.3	10.7%
MALIGNANCIES	6.3	5.5%
CARDIOVASCULAR DISEASE	4.1	3.6%
CONGENITAL ANOMALIES	1.4	1.2%
INFLUENZA, PNEUMONIA	0.8	0.7%
ALL CAUSES	**115.4**	

SOURCE: Vital Statistics of the United States, U.S., DHHS,
        Pub. #(PHS) 85-1101, 1985.

MORBIDITY

1. Injuries Not only is unintentional injury the major cause of death during the second decade, it accounts for an estimated 15.2 million non-fatal injuries, in 1980, for six-to-14-year olds in the U.S. Data from the Massachusetts Department of Health indicate that the rate of injury for 18-to-19-year olds is nearly 2.5 times that for 12-to-15-year olds. For adolescents, the leading causes of accidental death and injury include vehicular injuries, drownings, poisonings, firearms, burns, and falls. [1]

2. Substance Use and Abuse While mass media portray a current crisis of substance abuse among America's youth, recent trends in the three major drugs of abuse belie that perspective. While there has been a slight decline in any use of cigarettes among high school students in the years 1979-1984, there was a marked reduction in daily use from 29 percent to 18 percent. While a greater proportion of adolescent females than males continue to routinely smoke cigarettes, the use of smokeless tobacco among adolescent males has risen rapidly in the last decade. In addition, for both males and females, there is a dramatic urban/rural split in cigarette smoking; nearly twice the percentage of urban female adolescents (18.8 percent) than rural (9.6 percent) report smoking daily. [1]

As with cigarettes, there has been a slight reduction of marijuana use and a marked decline in heavy use, from where 23 percent of high school seniors reported using marijuana daily in 1979 to five percent in 1984. What is most significant about marijuana trends in America is the ever earlier age of initiation. Alcohol use has not significantly changed over the last 30 years, with one-in-seven high school seniors reporting having been intoxicated in the last month, while five percent report getting drunk on a weekly basis.[1]

ADOLESCENT PREGNANCY

Since World War II, there has been a steady decline in adolescent childbearing to the 1983 rate of 51.7/1,000. Since 1980, both the pregnancy and abortion rates among teens have fallen nationally. The reasons for these trends remain conjecture, but most likely they are the result of growing use of more effective contraception among teenagers.[1]

For those who become pregnant during their teenage years, 36.5 percent are 17 years of age or younger. The physiological consequences of early pregnancy for both mother and infant, to a great extent, can be controlled through nutrition, public health. and health care services; however, for the adolescent mother 15 years of age or younger, perinatal risks persist: abruptio placentae, cephalopelvic disproportion, and toxemia. For many, the teens services still are either unavailable or underutilized; thus, the outcomes for young adolescent mothers and their offspring remain significantly worse than for older women.[3]

While many physiological sequelae can be managed with comprehensive prenatal care, profound social and developmental costs persist. Children born to young adolescent mothers appear to do less-well in cognitive development, school achievement, emotional development, and social skills. For the young mother, the social outcomes are equally costly. While school failure, for most, is antecedent to the pregnancy, failure to complete school is nearly assured with a young child. Once out of school, only 43 percent ever complete their high school education. The lack of such education, in turn, significantly increases the likelihood of unemployment; thus, the cycle of poverty is perpetuated. This cycle of adolescent childbearing, in 1986, had a public cost of 16.5 billion dollars.[4]

YOUTH'S CONCERNS

To understand the health problems of youth, we need also to understand their perspectives, as well as mortality and morbidity data. Repeatedly, studies have shown that the concerns of primary focus to public health and health care professionals are relatively low-level issues for youth. Primary adolescent concerns, on the other hand, include stress and anxiety, relationships (both with adults and peers), weight, acne, and feeling down or depressed. Stress, depression, nervousness, and health worries become translated by youth into somatic concerns (e.g., headaches, stomach aches, and fatigue), social problems (e.g., school concerns, getting along with teachers or parents), and psychological issues (e.g., eating/weight problems, and clinical depression). While youth indicate their concerns to be primarily social and psychological in nature, they appear reluctant to seek health services for problems they do not consider to be organic in nature, despite the fact that they indicate they would like help with these problems.[1]

FACTORS INFLUENCING ADOLESCENT HEALTH CARE SERVICES

PROVIDER LIMITATIONS

Barriers to teenagers seeking health care services stem not only from adolescent reluctance but from provider limitations, as well. Trained in the pathophysiology of disease, physicians describe themselves as ill-prepared to address the social and psychological concerns of youth. Specifically, in a national survey of primary health care physicians in 1985, major deficits identified included eating disorders (54.5 percent), gender identity issues (54.0 percent), school-based learning and behavior problems (50.0 percent), chronic illness (50.0 percent), and delinquent youth (55.1 percent).[5]

In the same survey, each health care profession identified comparable limitations. Nurses reported deficits related to gender identity, behavior problems (delinquency and drug use), and depression. While 90 percent or more of psychologists responses indicated adequate training in dealing with family conflict, school problems, and issues related to growth and development, one-third reported limitations in assessing the teenager at risk for suicide; over half reported deficits in managing concerns related to sexuality issues (homosexuality and pregnancy) and problems of drug use and obesity. Nearly two-thirds of psychologists reported insufficient training in managing problems of anorexia/bulimia and the psychological sequelae of chronic illness. Likewise, nearly half of the nutritionists surveyed acknowledged limitations in almost all adolescent concerns pertinent to the discipline. With nearly half of social workers reporting limitations in all pertinent issues, two-thirds reported deficits in problems of anorexia/bulimia and the management of social issues facing adolescents with chronic illness; half reported limitations with concerns related to teenage pregnancy, homosexuality, and alcohol/drug abuse.[5]

FINANCIAL LIMITATIONS

Repeatedly, the interrelationships between poverty and health status have been well-documented.[4] Between 1979 and 1984, childhood poverty rose 31.3 percent in the U.S. (41.2 percent for white children, 13.2 percent for Black, and 39.7 percent for Hispanic). By 1990, 20 percent of all youths will be living in poverty.

Poverty impacts health in a number of dramatic ways. Poor children experience more days of restricted activity and school lost due to illness. They experience more sequelae of chronic illness. Lead-poisoning and iron-deficiency anemias are disproportionally conditions of the poor, as are the long-term consequences of iron-deficiency anemia.

Not only is illness greatest among the most economically depressed, but their access to health care services is restricted as well. Disproportionately, children and youth in America are underinsured or uninsured. Medicaid recipients frequently lose coverage as family income fluctuates above state eligibility levels. As a consequence, among Medicaid recipients, 7.2 percent of 12-to-18-year olds have part year coverage only; for those with private insurance plans, the figure is 12.7 percent. An additional seven percent lack any insurance at all. Not only do family incomes fluctuate, but what is covered by Medicaid fluctuates from state to state, including eyeglasses, dental care, occupational therapy, and early periodic screening, diagnosis, and treatment.[6]

Given the greater likelihood of illness with poverty and the increased risk of the poor to more severe and persistent sequelae, what becomes clear is that while the health care needs of this segment of our population are greater than others, the poor and near-poor continue to make fewer medical visits and receive less preventive care than is warranted by their health status.[4]

LEGAL LIMITATIONS

Minor's rights within the health care system remain ambiguous, at best.[7,8] While few states have adopted a mature minor statute, common-law rule holds it very unlikely that parents could successfully sue a physician for "battery" for treating an older adolescent on his/her consent alone. On the other hand, where states do specify adolescent rights to confidential services, the services allowed are often narrowly and inconsistently defined both within and between states. For example, substance abuse counseling may be allowed for minors on their own consent, while other mental health services are denied. For other conditions where the public's health is at risk (e.g., venereal disease), all states provide for minor's consent to diagnosis and treatment. Other procedures, most notably abortion, are protected through judicial safeguards, nationally; thus states, to date, have been unsuccessful in mandating parental approval in such situations.

Complicating the picture of confidentiality and consent for minors is the issue of financial liability; here, too, states are inconsistent. Nebraska law, for example, allows minors to confidentially seek treatment for venereal disease; however, it also holds parents financially liable for such treatment. Minnesota statute, in comparison, holds the recipient of confidential services as financially responsible.

Legal confusion, coupled with provider reticence to intercede in areas which historically have been negotiated within the family system, have led to great discomfort on the part of not only the providers but consumers and their parents as well. Repeatedly, studies show that for youth, the *sine qua non* of health services is confidentiality; and one of the major barriers for seeking services for those concerns they define as "personal" is the anticipated breach of confidentiality. [9]

ORGANIZATION OF SERVICES

TRADITIONAL

Traditionally, adolescents receive the majority of their health care within mainstream medical services.[3,10] The National Ambulatory Medical Care Survey reported over 58 million physician visits by youths 15-to-21 years in 1975: family physicians (45.5 percent), obstetricians/gynecologists (14.6 percent), internists (6.3 percent), pediatricians (4.9 percent), and psychiatrists (2.4 percent).

In 1980, there were 1.67-per-thousand hospital discharges for youths 12-to-17 years of age, with females over-represented for every age except 12. Among females, the primary reason for adolescent hospitalizations included deliveries, pregnancy complications including abortion, gastrointestinal diseases, injuries, and poisonings. For adolescent males, injuries, poisonings, and gastrointestinal illnesses represented primary inpatient diagnoses. For mental health problems, adolescent inpatient treatment doubled during the decade 1970-1980. In 1975, the National Institute of Mental Health reported over 80,000 youths hospitalized, with a rate of 126.5 per 100,000 10-to-14-year olds rising to 433.4 per 100,000 youths 15-to-17 years of age.

COMMUNITY-BASED SERVICES

Paralleling the primary health care sector has been a host of community and alternative health services for adolescents, ranging from comprehensive service models to family planning, drug treatment, mental health, and school-based health care delivery. Whether condition-specific or comprehensive, effective adolescent clinical services appear to have the following characteristics in common: a) multidisciplinary teams; b) mid-level health professionals; c) patient monitoring, co-ordination and continuity; d) coordinated recordkeeping; and e) accessibility to all youths. In addition, true intersectoral coordination, which is rare, extends beyond health care services to include coordination with employment, housing, education, and social and legal services. [3]

DISEASE PREVENTION AND HEALTH PROMOTION SERVICE

Preventive health services for youth have gained increasing attention over the past decade. To a great extent, schools have been the primary target for these efforts. A number of innovative models have been developed and tested to address categorical issues. In smoking prevention programs, it has been shown that while traditional programs which emphasize health risks appear to increase knowledge, they have little impact on behavior. Those which have been most effective have focused on decision-making and social skills-building. Other successful programs have created a school environment where not-smoking has become the norm.[10]

In the areas of drug and alcohol abuse programming, while numerous inter-ventions abound, few have been shown to do more than increase knowledge. Recently, a multi-national study has shown the efficacy of peer-led over adult-led alcohol prevention programs on adolescent drinking behaviors. In addition, the creation of counter-cultures within schools, through efforts such as Students Against Drunk Driving, hold promise but their impact has yet to be well-documented.

For sex education, the primary objectives have tended to be reduction of adolescent pregnancy and the elimination of sexually transmitted diseases. School-based clinics, while being heralded by some as the methodology of choice for the 1990s, are unlikely to be successful by themselves. Innovative work/school incen-tive programs in New York schools, educational remediation/work/sex education programs in Philadelphia, and a community-school intervention program in South Carolina all hold promise for the future. In other Western cultures, where adoles-cent pregnancy rates are significantly lower than that in the U.S., contraceptive information and services are more widely available, discussion of sexual practices appears to be more public, and pregnancy prevention is an integrated effort of home, school, media, and community organizations.

To develop effective prevention programs, schools are unable to work in a vacuum. The issue is not just one of changing instructional methods to those more social-psychological in their orientation, but the broader social environments of school and community need to be supportive. In addition, to be effective, we must look beyond strategies of changing individual behaviors to those which provide system change, such as automobiles with passive seat-belt restraints or air bags.

REFERENCES

1. Blum R. Contemporary Threats to Adolescent Health in the United States, JAMA, 237(24):3390-3395, 1987.

2. Blum R, Resnick M, Geer L, et al. Health Status of Minnesota Youth. Unpublished monograph, Adolescent Health Program, University of Minnesota, 1987.

3. Klerman L, Stack M. Problems in the Organization of Health Services for Adolescents, Am J Public Health (in press).

4. Rosenbaum S, Starfield B. Poverty's Effects on Our Youth, Am J Public Health (in press).

5. Blum R. Physician's Assessment of Deficiencies and Desire for Training in Adolescent Health Care, J Med Educ 62:401-407, 1987.

6. Resnick M. The Financing of Health Care Services for Youth, Am J Public Health (in press).

7. Melton G, Schwartz I, Resnick M. Emerging Legal Issues in Children's Health Care in Richmond, J. (Ed.) Future Directions in Child Health. Cambridge University Press, 1987 (in press).

8. Bright W. Medical Treatment–The Legal Rights of Children. In Blum, R., Adolescent Health Care: Clinical Issues, Academic Press, New York, 1981.

| TEENAGE PREGNANCY: AN AMERICAN DILEMMA | 37 |

Janet B. Hardy

INTRODUCTION

Each year, more than one million American teenagers and preteens become pregnant; some as young as ten or 11 years of age. In 1985, almost 480,000 of these pregnancies produced a live infant; almost 400,000 were terminated electively by abortion; and, the remainder resulted in spontaneous fetal loss by miscarriage or stillbirth. It should be borne in mind that the great majority of these pregnancies were unintended and unwanted. Zelnik and Kantner,[1] in their national survey of metro area teenagers aged 15-19, reported that 82 percent of 312 teenage women experiencing a first premarital birth had not wanted to be pregnant. Hardy, et. al.,[2] found that 86 percent of Black and 60 percent of white urban adolescents (aged 17 or less at delivery) had not wanted to be pregnant.

The U.S. has the highest rates of teenage pregnancy, childbirth, and abortion among similar, developed Western countries,[3] even though age at first sexual experience and the frequency of sexual activity among teenagers is not different. Furthermore, the youngest (below age 15) American girls are five times as likely to bear a child as those in other Western countries. We appear to be much less open about discussing sex and contraception with our children.

Because of the high frequency of adverse pregnancy outcomes, both medical and social, for the young mother and her child, and because of the very large human and social costs involved, teenage pregnancy is a problem of major public health and social dimensions. The federal costs of welfare, food stamps, and Medicaid for families, where the mother had her first birth as a teenager, were an estimated $16.65 billion in 1985.[4]

Following a brief discussion of adolescent development, national and local statistics, with their somewhat conflicting trends, will be described and, where appropriate, comparisons will be drawn between teenagers, by age and race, and women aged 20-25 years, a group generally considered to be in an optimal age range for childbearing. A brief description of the social context in which the teenage pregnancy phenomenon has developed will follow.

ADOLESCENT DEVELOPMENT

The grouping of teenagers by ages 15 through 19 years, for statistical purposes, obscures the marked differences between the younger and older teens in physical, cognitive, and socio-emotional development. Understanding these differences is important to the planning of interventions to prevent pregnancy and/or to assure optimal outcome if it occurs. It has seemed useful to use the term adolescence to describe the period from the onset of puberty through age 17, and to consider those aged 18 and 19 as older teenagers. The adolescents, in general, are still growing physically, they are still in the stage of concrete operations, cognitively, and they are characterized by ego-centricity, impulsiveness, difficulty in planning ahead, and a feeling of invulnerability ("it can't happen to me"). Few have completed high school and even fewer are married. Pregnancy carries high medical and social risks in this age group. By contrast, most 18-19-year olds have finished growing; they are likely to be cognitively and socio-emotionally more mature. A large proportion has finished high school. Unless these young women have had a prior birth, their medical risks are not increased but, because of single parenthood and poverty, social risks may be high.

Thus, characteristics normal for the period of adolescence put these young people at high risk if they engage in premature sexual activity. They are likely not to have the information and services needed to protect them from unintended pregnancy. If they decide to bear and raise the child, they are likely to lack for the personal characteristics, knowledge, and resources for optimal parenting. Older teenagers are generally better equipped to cope with those and other problems.

TRENDS IN TEENAGE PREGNANCIES, BIRTHS, AND ABORTIONS

The picture which emerges from the examination of statistical data is both complex and confusing. As indicated by estimates developed by Hofferth,[5] the number of births to young women below age 20 has declined by over 25 percent, since 1972. However, the number of pregnancies steadily increased from 1972 to 1982 and was essentially unchanged in 1984. These changes were taking place during a period when the number of teenagers in the population was decreasing substantially. A 14-percent decrease occurred between 1975 and 1985, in females aged 15-19 years.[6] Pregnancy rates per 1000 females increased from 94, in 1972, to 110 in 1982. In 1984, the rate was 109. Examination of pregnancy rates among sexually active teens (15-19) during the 12-year period is somewhat encouraging; in 1972, the rate per 1000 was 272; in 1984, it was 233. The decreased pregnancy rate for sexually active girls during a period when rates for all teenagers were increasing is attributed to contraceptive use. During the period 1972-1982, the proportion of pregnancies among teenage women resulting in a live birth decreased dramatically, from 66.2 percent to 46.7 percent. Concomittantly with the legalization of abortion on a national basis in 1973, the proportion of pregnancies terminating in abortion among women under age 20 doubled, from 20.1 percent to 40 percent in 1984. The proportion of spontaneous fetal loss decreased slightly from 15.0 percent to 13.3 percent. It should be noted that, in general, the risks associated with early abortion, carried out by qualified personnel in appropriate clinical settings, are no higher for teenagers than older women. Also, these small risks are less than those associated with a live birth.

While overall birth rates among teenagers, 15-19 years, have declined quite substantially during the past ten years, those to non-white 18-and-19-year olds have not shared the decline, and those to white adolescents, below 15 years, have actually increased somewhat. In 1985, among young Americans who gave birth, there was wide disparity in frequency by race and by age at delivery (Table 1). Among white teenagers and preteens giving birth, 52 percent were adolescents less than age 18 years, as compared with 46 percent among Blacks; but among whites, only 12.7 percent of all births were to women under 20, as compared with 21.4 percent for Blacks. Hispanics were classified as white or Black on the basis of the perceived race of the child, however, their pregnancy and birthrates are intermediate between those of Black and white teens. American Indians, with 19 percent of all births to teenagers, ranked almost as high as Blacks. But, there were extremely low frequencies of teenage births among women of Asian or Pacific Island descent. Among almost 18,000 births to Chinese women, in the U.S., only 1.1 percent occurred among teenagers.

Table 2 shows the proportions of young mothers, in 1985, by age, race, and history of prior childbirth. Quite large proportions of these women had had one or more prior live-born children. Among 15-19-year olds, almost 21 percent of the white and 29 percent of the Black already had one or more prior live births. It is difficult for a teenager with one child to complete her education and become employed and self-sustaining; two or more children greatly compounds the problem.

TABLE 1

LIVE BIRTHS BY AGE OF MOTHER, RACE OF CHILD AND PROPORTION TO YOUNG WOMEN 10-19 YEARS OF AGE UNITED STATES, 1985.

Age Of Mother	All Races	American White	Black	Indian	Chinese	Japanese	Hawaiian	Filipino	Other
					Asian Or Pacific Islander				
All Ages	3,760,561	2,991,373	608,193	42,646	17,880	9,802	7,193	21,482	59,259
Under 15 Years	10,220	4,101	5,860	149	2	3	3	18	77
15 Years	25,002	13,276	11,001	425	5	11	58	54	157
16 Years	53,474	33,052	18,193	871	14	23	109	117	345
17 Years	89,313	59,714	26,895	1,564	30	51	185	213	610
18 Years	129,563	89,950	35,399	2,332	59	94	337	368	951
19 Years	170,133	122,733	42,062	2,791	88	106	450	483	1,317
15-19 Years	467,485	318,725	134,270	7,983	196	285	1,139	1,235	3,380
Percent Under 20 Years	12.7	10.8	21.4	19.1	1.1	2.9	2.0	5.8	5.8

SOURCE: Table 23 of the Monthly Vital Statistics Report, Advance Report of Final Natality Statistics, 1985. National Center for Health Statistics., Vol. 36, No. 4 Supplement, July 17, 1987.

Adoption

Adoption as an option for pregnancy resolution appears to be little-used by American teenagers, especially by those who are Black. As no overall national records of adoption are maintained, there is little precise information as to the proportion of teens who put their babies for adoption. Teenagers who use adoption as an option appear to hold more traditional attitudes about family life and adoption, and to be better students with higher educational objectives than those who elect to have a birth.[5] In the Johns Hopkins Adolescent Pregnancy Program,[7] which serves an inner-city and predominantly Black population, there were only five adoptions among some 2000 teenagers delivering between 1976 and 1982, with very few additional since 1982.

Pregnancy Risk

Data from the Kantner-Zelnik metropolitan area surveys suggest that half of all premarital pregnancies among girls 15-19 occur within six months, and over one-fifth within one month of first coitus.[8] The likelihood of pregnancy is affected by contraceptive use. Within two years of first intercourse, the risk of pregnancy is 50 percent for those using no contraceptive; 25 percent for those using a non-medical method, such as withdrawal or douche; and 15 percent for those using a medical

---

TABLE 2

DISTRIBUTION OF BIRTHS BY YOUNG MOTHER'S AGE AND RACE. UNITED STATES, 1985

Mother's Age Years	<15	15-19	20-24
White Births			
Total	4,101	318,725	894,195
1st Order	3,951	252,887	452,260
2nd Order Or Above	150	65,838	441,935
% 2nd Order Or Above	3.7	20.7	49.4
Black Births			
Total	5,860	134,270	207,330
1st Order	5,646	95,619	82,016
2nd Order Or Above	214	38,651	125,314
% 2nd Order Or Above	3.7	28.8	60.4

SOURCE: Table 2 of the Monthly Vital Statistics Report, Advance Report of Final Natality Statistics, 1985. National Center for Health Statistics, Vol. 36, No. 4 Supplement, July 17, 1987.

method (pill, IUD, diaphragm).[5] Calculations suggest that by age 20, 40 percent of white and 63 percent of Black women will have had a teenage pregnancy.[5]

Repeat Pregnancies

The rapid repetition of pregnancy is a serious problem among teenagers, as can be surmised from the relatively large proportions of second and higher-order births in this age group (Table 2). Data from the Kantner-Zelnik surveys of metropolitan women aged 15-19 indicate that half of premaritally pregnant teenagers who married while pregnant conceived again within 24 months of the termination of their first pregnancy. Among those who remained single, the risk of subsequent births was less, about 30 percent.. Among white metropolitan area women, the likelihood of a second pregnancy increased somewhat between 1971 and 1979, while that for Black teenagers declined. This decline appeared to be associated with increased contraceptive use.[9] Data from an 18-month follow-up of a random sample of Baltimore adolescents (< 17 years) giving birth in 1983 indicated that within a six-month period of delivery, 11 percent had conceived again and within 12 months, 22 percent. Those young women followed in comprehensive adolescent programs had somewhat lower risks than those who received more routine types of care: 11 percent had conceived in six months, 16 percent in 12 months. The relatively small number (n=37) followed in HMOs had the highest risk, 18 percent and 30 percent respectively.[2] Comparisons between primiparous mothers aged 17 or below at delivery, and those aged 20-25 in the same inner-city population and followed over a 12 year period, showed that the younger mothers had an average of 3.25 children each, as compared with 2.35 for the older mothers. Among the younger mothers, only three percent had no additional children and 46 percent had three or more, as compared with 14 percent and 21 percent respectively among older mothers.[10]

Contraceptive Use

One of the underlying causes of unintended teenage pregnancy is the failure of many teenagers to protect themselves adequately against pregnancy. Through ignorance, lack of motivation, or difficulty in obtaining contraceptive services and/or supplies, teenagers are inconsistent users of contraceptives. On a national level, 15 percent of sexually active girls report never using any method and 40 percent use them only sometimes.[3] Condoms unfortunately are not a preferred method among teenagers. Among adolescents (below 18) delivering a baby in Baltimore, in 1983, 55 percent of Black and 67 percent of white had never used a contraceptive method; 15 percent of Black and five percent of white girls were using a medical method, and 16 percent and five percent respectively were using a non-medical method around the time of conception.[10]

There is no sound published evidence that making information available about reproduction and contraceptives to adolescents leads to promiscuity. In fact, the Kantner-Zelnik surveys indicated fewer pregnancies among those exposed to sex education.[11] The provision of reproductive health education and services reduced the frequency of pregnancy among high school students in St. Louis.[12] The Johns Hopkins Pregnancy Prevention Program, which provided education and counseling in a values-oriented format in a junior and senior high school, and comprehensive reproductive health services in a special, nearby "store front" clinic, not only resulted in a significant decrease in pregnancies but also in an average delay of seven months in the age at onset of first intercourse.[13]

CHARACTERISTICS OF TEENAGERS WHO GIVE BIRTH

Marital Status

A matter for grave concern, because of its relationship with single parenthood, is the increasingly high frequency of non-marital births among teenagers (Table 3). The proportion of white mothers, aged 15-19, married at delivery has decreased from 85 percent in the mid-1960s to 64 percent in 1980. For Blacks, the decrease was even more marked, from 42 percent to 11 percent. Almost no Black and few white adolescents below age 15 at delivery were married.

TABLE 3

NUMBERS OF FIRST BIRTHS TO TEENAGERS AGE 15-19 AND PERCENT DISTRIBUTION OF MARITAL STATUS AT CONCEPTION AND DELIVERY BY RACE FOR 1980, 1972 AND 1964-66 (AVERAGED). UNITED STATES

	1980	1972	1964-66
Number Of First Births	305,000	294,000	340,000
White % Married At:			
Conception	30.5	52.0	50.0
Delivery	63.9	75.5	85.0
Black % Married At			
Conception	4.8	12.1	15.1
Delivery	10.6	20.7	41.9

SOURCE: Monthly Vital Statistics Report. Trends in marital status of mothers at conception and birth of first child. National Center for Health Statistics, Vol. 36, No. 2 Supplement May 29, 1987

Maternal Education

Table 4 shows the proportion of young mothers over 16 who have completed high school at the time of delivery, by age and race of child. With increasing age above 17 years, increasing proportions of young mothers have educational attainment of 12 years or more. Even so, only 61 percent of the white and 65 percent of the Black 19-year olds have competed high school, as compared with those who were 20-25 years at delivery. In this group, 74 percent of the white and 71 percent of the Black mothers had 12 or more years of schooling. It is interesting to note that, among teenage mothers, slightly higher proportions of Blacks than whites had completed 12 years or more. In work in progress,[2] among urban teenagers giving birth in Baltimore, in 1983, we are finding that at each age, Black adolescent mothers, on average, have higher educational attainment than white. Also, the Black teenagers were absent from school less than the white. Fewer were already drop-outs when they became pregnant (15 percent) as compared with whites (66 percent) and, of those in school at conception, a smaller proportion of Black (28 percent) than white (74 percent) dropped out during pregnancy. This is an interesting pattern, which suggests that white adolescents who drop out of school are at particularly high risk of pregnancy.

TABLE 4

PROPORTION OF YOUNG MOTHERS BY AGE AND RACE
WITH EDUCATIONAL ATTAINMENT OF 12 YEARS
OR MORE AT DELIVERY, 1985

Age In Years	12 Or More Years Of Education					
	White			Black		
	No. With Education Stated	Number	%	No. With Education Stated	Number	%
17	43,507	6,440	14.8	23,039	3,921	17.0
18	66,569	29,863	44.9	30,363	15,084	49.6
19	91,122	55,698	61.1	35,535	23,100	65.0
20-24	671,734	449,407	73.6	173,034	123,025	71.1

SOURCE: Calculated from data in Table 22, Advance Report on Final Natality Statistics, 1985, ibid.

Registration For Prenatal Care

Many teenaged pregnancies are compromised by inadequate prenatal care, in terms of both the late onset of care and a suboptimal number of prenatal visits. Table 5 shows the trimester of onset of care by age of mother and race of child. There is a well-recognized positive relationship between age of mother and time of registration for prenatal care. The younger the mother, the less likely is early registration for prenatal care and the greater the likelihood of no prenatal care at all. In general, these differences by age are greater for white women than Black. The proportions of Black women receiving care in the first trimester merit special attention because they are considerably lower than those of whites at each maternal age, (excepting the youngest). Even at age 20-25, only 60 percent of Black women, compared with 75 percent of white, are enrolled for care in the first trimester.

Complications of pregnancy, labor, and delivery are higher for teenage women than older women. However, these high rates appear to be primarily a

TABLE 5

LIVE BIRTHS BY TIME OF ONSET OF PRENATAL CARE, BY AGE OF MOTHER AND RACE OF CHILD
UNITED STATES, 1985

Mother's Age Years	Total No.	No. With Prenatal Care Stated	Trimester Care Initiated Percent Distribution*			
			First	Second	Third	None
White						
<15	4,101	3,947	58	40	15	7
15	13,276	12,887	45	40	10	5
16	33,052	32,169	52	37	9	4
17	59,714	58,234	54	35	9	3
18	89,950	87,628	57	33	8	3
19	122,733	119,770	62	29	7	3
20-24	894,195	875,717	75	19	4	2
Black						
<15	5,860	5,656	34	46	14	6
15	11,001	10,603	40	43	12	5
16	18,913	18,227	43	42	11	5
17	25,895	25,966	46	40	10	5
18	35,399	34,220	48	38	10	4
19	42,062	40,653	51	35	9	4
20-24	207,330	200,751	60	29	7	4

SOURCE: Calculated from figures in Table 25, Advance Report on Final Natality Statistics, 1985. National Center for Health Statistics, Vol. 36, No. 4 Supplement, July 17, 1987.
*Rounded percents may not add to 100

function of social class and quality of care rather than young age, per se.[14,7] Similarily, perinatal, neonatal, and infant mortality among the offspring of teenagers appear to be related to pregnancy factors, such as birthweight and maternal age, all of which are in turn strongly dependent upon the socio-economic background of the mother.[15]

Birthweight

The weight of the infant at birth and its relationship to the appropriateness of weight for gestational age are powerful predictors of the infant' survival and subsequent developmental course.[16,17] National statistics indicate a strong relationship between maternal age and birthweight for both white and Black women (Table 6). Among the youngest teens (<15 years), ten percent of white and 14.5 percent of Black delivered low birthweight infants (LBW). It is important to note that at each maternal age, including the 20-24-year old comparison group, the frequency of LBW, like delayed prenatal care, is higher for Blacks than for whites, and that the differential between the youngest and oldest (20-24 years) whites is much larger than Blacks and the decrease with age is less marked. Black women in the Collaborative Perinatal Study were noted to have an average gestational age which was more than eight days shorter than whites.[15] Data from resident, recorded births in Baltimore City, in 1983, suggest that a relationship exists between maternal age and

---

TABLE 6

**FREQUENCY OF LOW BIRTHWEIGHT (BELOW 2500 GRAMS)
BY AGE OF MOTHER AND RACE OF CHILD.
UNITED STATES, 1985**

	Race of Child					
	White		Black		Other	
Age Of Mother	No.	%	No.	%	No.	%
Under 15 Years	428	10.5	863	14.8	883	14.5
15 Years	1,265	9.5	1,537	14.0	1,603	13.7
16 Years	2,835	8.6	2,649	14.0	1,603	13.7
17 Years	4,759	8.0	3,673	13.7	3,874	13.1
18 Years	7,067	7.9	4,693	13.3	4,992	12.6
19 Years	8,393	6.8	5,341	12.7	5,714	12.1
20-24 Years	51,333	5.7	24,902	12.0	27,343	11.1

SOURCE: Monthly Vital Statistics Report, Advance Report on Final Natality Statistics, 1985.
                  National Center for Health Statistics, Vol. 36, No. 4 Supplement, July 17, 1987.

average length of gestation. Among teenagers, the frequency of preterm gestation (<37 weeks), which was higher for blacks than whites, decreased as maternal age increased.[2] In a large inner-city population of pregnant adolescents receiving comprehensive pregnancy care, including nutritional support, the youngest teens (≤15 years) had, on the average, the heaviest babies and lowest frequency of LBW.[7]

Maternal and Infant Health

The infants of mothers under 18 years at the time of birth appear to have more illness during the first year and greater rates of post-neonatal death than infants of older women. In a survey of a random sample of adolescent births in Baltimore City, in 1983, we found high frequencies of illness and accidents among infants followed 18 months. There were considerably higher frequencies of hospital admissions among white infant (31 percent) than Black (16 percent) [2] during the follow-up. Similarly, the white mothers had, on the average, more health problems, as indicated by hospital admission and out-patient visits, than Black.

Fathers of Babies Born to Teenagers

The fathers of babies born to teenagers have attracted relatively little attention, and available information comes, in the main, from vital statistics and small, non-representative samples. [21,22,23,24] National Natality Statistics for 1984 [25] indicate that, in actual fact, only a very small proportion (2.9 percent) of babies born to all women had fathers who were teenagers. Only 22.5 percent of babies born to women under 20 had teenage fathers. The proportion of all Black fathers who were teenagers, 3.8 percent, was considerably higher than among whites, where only 0.3 percent were below 20 years.

In our experience, [2] the age of fathers of babies born to adolescents ranged from 15 to 69. Black fathers tended to be closer in age to the mothers than white, where the age difference, on the average, was three to four years. More than half (57 percent) of the Baltimore adolescent mothers had known the father at least two years prior to conception. Even though only two percent were married, 65 percent of the fathers were having at least weekly contact with the child when he/she was approximately 18 months of age. At this point, 42 percent of Black fathers and 23 percent of the white were neither in school nor employed, and those who were employed tended to hold low-paying jobs, indicating the high degree of disadvantage experienced by the fathers involved in a teenage pregnancy, even though they may not themselves be teenagers. Longitudinal data from Project Talent [26] indicate that teenage fathers, like teenage mothers, suffer long-term educational, occupational, and economic disadvantage, as compared with classmates who were not involved in a pregnancy as a teenager.

The Children of Teenage Mothers

A number of studies suggest that, in addition to increased risks of LBW and perinatal and later infant mortality, accidents and illness, the children born to adolescents experience less-favorable development than those of otherwise comparable older women. Also, though the data are not clear cut, cognitive ability, as measured by IQ and tests of academic achievement, may also be compromised.[10,27,28,29] These findings are related to increased risk of academic difficulty, school drop-out and associated employment problems, and the repetition of the teenage pregnancy poverty cycle.

THE SOCIAL CONTEXT

During the past quarter century, a series of complex, interrelated changes have occurred concurrently within American society, setting the stage for the recent high rates of pregnancy, abortion, childbirth, single parenthood, and STDs among teenagers. As it is not possible to chronicle all the changes here, only a few major ones will be commented upon.

Two interrelated factors of major importance are: 1) the so-called "sexual revolution," with its marked increase in societal tolerance of premarital and extramarital sexual activity among adults and the widespread exploitation of implicit and explicit sexual themes by the media and press; 2) technological advances in contraception and the legalization of abortion have allowed women to control their fertility. However, unfortunately, sexually active teenagers tend to delay the use of contraceptives for an extended period after becoming sexually active.[30]

As part of these changes, the age at initiation of sexual activity has declined and the frequency of sexual experience has increased among teenagers.[1,31] However, since the late 1970s, the rapid increase has leveled off. In 1982, 53 percent of Black and 40 percent of white unmarried teenagers reported sexual activity.[32] Sexual activity has started earlier among Blacks than whites, and larger proportions of Black teenagers than whites have been sexually active and have borne children.[33] Among urban populations at high risk for teenage pregnancy, sexual experience begins very early and involves considerably larger proportions of both Black and white teens than the national data indicate.

Among Black females in the junior high school, 23 percent reported first coitus prior to age 13.[34] A random sample of pregnant adolescents delivering below age 18 yielded similar findings: 82 percent had experienced sexual intercourse prior to age 15 and 37 percent reported first coitus at age 13 years or below; 42 percent of the Black and 21 percent of the white adolescents.[2] In this study, an intergenerational pattern of early childbearing was identified. Over half of the mothers of the adolescents giving birth were themselves adolescents (below 18) at their first birth. Among the sisters, 30 percent were adolescent mothers. In a culture of poverty such as this, adolescent childbearing does not represent deviant behavior. It is the norm even though it is generally regarded as undesirable.

Changes in family structure, with the virtual disappearance of the extended family and erosion of the nuclear family through divorce, have resulted in less emotional support and supervision of children, particularly preteens and adolescents whose mothers may be working and forced to leave children unattended after school. The rates of marriage and remarriage have also declined while the frequency of divorce doubled between 1950-1983. As a result, the proportion of female-headed, single-parent families with children under 18 has almost doubled. Teenage, non-marital births have contributed to this trend. There has been an almost threefold increase in absent fathers. The majority of white and Hispanic children still live with two parents, but more than half of all Black children do not.[5] The proportion of children with working mothers has increased from 45 percent in 1960 to 62 percent in 1985. In female-headed households, the proportion is 66 percent.

During this 25-year period, economic conditions worsened as the result of inflation and stagnation. Beginning in 1979 and intensifying in 1982, reduction in the dollar value of public support contributed to the problems of the poor. Women and children suffered disproportionately. Today, almost one of every two Black, and one in six white children, live below the poverty level.[35] Appropriately 62 percent of all female-headed families with children under 18 received means-tested public assistance during the first quarter of 1984; 35 percent received cash assistance (AFDC or SSI) and 61 percent non-cash benefits, such as Medicaid, food stamps, and the like.[5,36]

While national figures paint a bleak picture for large numbers of women and children, they tend to dilute the relationships between poverty and teenage pregnancy and children among Blacks and whites living in congested inner-city areas. In a study of adolescent pregnancy and its outcome in relation to community characteristics, rates of pregnancy, births, and abortions reported among adolescents aged 15-17 years, between 1980-1985, in Baltimore City, were examined by Census Tract. Overall, during the five-year period, there were 1304 births and 1060 abortions (46 percent) among the white girls, and among Blacks, 5099 births and 3909 elective abortions (43 percent). Among whites, the risks of pregnancy and childbirth were significantly related to all six indices of poverty examined, but abortion was not related to poverty. Among Blacks, pregnancy and childbirth were also related to poverty but relationships with abortion rates were less clear. It appears that in more affluent areas the likelihood of pregnancy is less, and when it occurs among white girls abortion is an option frequently used to resolve the problem.[37]

CONCLUSIONS

Premature sexual activity and its consequences of STDs and unwanted pregnancy among unmarried teenagers, particularly those in young adolescents, is a social problem of major dimensions in the U.S. but it is one which is not evenly distributed by state and even within states.[38] It is urgent that high-risk areas be targeted for intervention on two levels.

The first and most urgent need is for pregnancy prevention. Effective prevention requires broadly based education aimed at developing personal responsibility and wise decision-making with respect to a number of interrelated risk-taking behaviors, including premature sexual activity, illicit drug and alcohol use, and cigarette smoking. This education should include specific information about puberty, pregnancy, contraception, the burdens of unintended parenthood, and STDs, including AIDS. Also required for pregnancy prevention, by those who choose to be sexually active, is ready access to confidential, comprehensive, reproductive health services and low-cost or free contraceptives. Few poor young people have discretionary funds to pay for these services.

Secondly, for those young women who become pregnant, unbiased and non-judgmental pregnancy option counseling, with referral for appropriate services, is indicated. It is unfair that inability to pay for an abortion may lead to the birth of an unwanted child. For those adolescents who decide to bear their children, comprehensive pregnancy services with follow-up of mothers and infants offer the best chances for healthy outcomes, including reducing the risk of early repeat pregnancies.[2,7] Efforts to promote and facilitate adoption are also indicated, but the most effective method of reducing abortion, legal or otherwise, is the prevention of unwanted pregnancy.

Far more difficult to resolve will be the societal changes and social and economic ills which form the backdrop for the single-parent, teenage-pregnancy phenomenon. Clearly, some very major changes in education, child day care, medical care and health education, and social support for poor mothers and children are needed to help our children become productive adults in today's technological society.

REFERENCES

1. Zelnik M, Kantner J. Sexual activity, contraceptive use and pregnancy among metropolitan area teenagers:1971-1979. Family Planning Perspectives 12:230-237, 1980.

2. Hardy JB, Flagle CD, Duggan AK. Resource Use by Pregnant and Parenting Adolescents, Final Report to the Office of Adolescent Pregnancy Programs on Grant Number APR 000906-03-0, June 1986.

3. Westoff CF, Calot G, Foster AD. Teenage fertility in developed nations. Family Planning Perspectives 15:105-110, 1983.

4. Burt MR. Estimates of Public Costs for Teenage Childbearing: A Review of Recent Studies and Estimates of 1985 Public Costs: Center for Population Options, 1986.

5. Hayes CD (ed). Risking the Future. Adolescent Sexuality, Pregnancy and Childbearing. National Academy Press, Volume 1, Washington D.C., 1987.

6. Bureau of the Census: Statistical Abstract of the United States: National Data Book and Guide to Sources, 1986, 106th Edition.

7. Hardy JB, King TM, Repke JT. The Johns Hopkins Adolescent Pregnancy Program: An Evaluation. Obstet Gynecol 69:300-306, 1987.

8. Zabin LS, Kantner JF, Zelnik M. The risk of adolescent pregnancy in the first months of intercourse. Family Planning Perspectives 1:215-222, 1979.

9. Koenig MA, Zelnik M. Repeat pregnancies among metropolitan area teenagers. Family Planning Perspectives 14:341-344, 1979.

10. Hardy JB, Welcher D, Stanley J, et al. Long-range outcome of adolescent pregnancy. Clinical Obstet Gynecol 21:1215-1232, 1978.

11. Zelnik M, Kim YJ. Sex education and its association with teenage sexual activity, pregnancy and contraceptive use. Family Planning Perspectives 14:117-126, 1082.

12. Edwards L, Steinman M, Arnold K, et al. Adolescent pregnancy prevention services in high school clinics. Family Planning Perspectives 12:6-14, 1980.

13. Zabin LS, Hirsch MS, Smith EA, et al. Evaluation of a pregnancy prevention program for urban teenagers. Family Planning Perspectives 18:119-126, 1986.

14. Strobino D, in Hofferth SL, Hayes CD (eds). Risking the Future: Adolescent Sexuality, Pregnancy and Childbearing. Working Papers and Statistical Appendixes, National Academy, Volume II, Washington, D.C., 1987.

15. Niswander KR, Gordon M. The Women and Their Pregnancies: The Collaborative Perinatal Study of the National Institute of Neurological Diseases and Stroke. Philadelphia, W.B. Saunders, 1972, pp 39.

16. Hardy JB, Drage JS, Jackson E. The First Year of Life: The Collaborative Perinatal Study (NINCDS). Johns Hopkins Press, July, 1979.

17. Hardy JB, Mellits ED. Relationship of low birthweight to maternal characteristics of age, parity, education and body size. The Epidemiology of Prematurity. Edited by D.M. Reed and F.F. Stanley. Baltimore, Urban and Schwarzenberg, 1977, pp 105-117.

18. Hardy PH, Hardy JB, Nell EE, et al. Prevalence of six sexually transmitted disease agents among pregnant inner-city adolescents and pregnancy outcome. The Lancet 2:333-337, 1984.

19. Lovchik JC. Chlamydial infections. Maryland Medical Journal 36:54-57, 1987.

20. Burke DS, Brundage JF, Herbold JR:, et al. Human immunodeficiency virus infections among civilian applications for United States Military Service, October 1985 to March 1986. N. Engl J Med 317:131-136, 1987.

21. Elster AB and Panzarine S. Teenage fathers: stresses during gestation and early parenthood.. Clinical Pediatrics 10:700-703, 1983.

22. Elster AB and Lamb ME. Adolescent fathers: the under studied side of adolescent pregnancy. Chapter 9 in "School-age Pregnancy and Parenting: Biosocial Dimensions". Lancaster JB and Hamburg BA (eds.) Aldine De Gruyter, New York, 1986.

23. Hendricks LE and Montgomery TA. Educational achievement and locus of control among black adolescent fathers. J Negro Education 53:182-188, 1984.

24. Rivara FP, Sweeney PJ, Henderson BF. Risk of fatherhood among black teenage males. Am J Public Health 77:203-205, 1987.

25. Advance Report of Final Natality Statistics, 1984. National Center for Health Statistics, U.S., DHHS, July 18, 1986.

26. Card JJ, Wise LL. Teenage mothers and teenage fathers: The impact of early childbearing on the parents' personal and professional lives. Family Planning Perspectives 10:199-205, 1978.

27. Baldwin W, Cain V. The children of teenage parents. Family Planning Perspective 12-34, 1980.

28. Belmont L, Cohen P, Dryfoos J, et al. Maternal age and children's intelligence. Teenage Parents and Their Offspring. Edited by K.G. Scott, T. Field and E.G. Robertson. New York, New York, Grune and Stratton, 1981, pp 177-194.

29. Broman SG. Long term development of children born to teenagers. Teenage Parents and Their Offspring. Edited by K.G. Scott, T. Field and E.G. Robertson. New York, New York, Grune and Stratton, 1981, pp 195-224.

30. Zabin LS, Clark, SD, Jr. Why they delay: A study of teenage family planning clinic patients. Family Planning Perspectives 13:205-217, 1981.

31. Zelnik M, Shah FK. First Intercourse among young Americans. Family Planning Perspectives 15:64-72, 1983.

32. Pratt WF, Mosher WD, Bachrach CA, et al. Understanding U.S. Fertility. Finding from the National Survey of Family Growth, Cycle III. Population Bulletin, 1984, 39:1-42.

33. Moore KA, Simms MC, Betsey CL. Choice and Circumstance, Racial Differences in Adolescent Sexuality and Fertility. Transaction Books, New Brunswick, U.S.A. and Oxford, U.K., 1986.

34. Zabin LS, Hardy JB, Streett RS, et al. A school, hospital and university based pregnancy prevention program. J Reproductive Medicine 29:421-426, 1984.

35. Edelman MW. Families in Peril. An Agenda For Social Change, Harvard University Press, 1987, pp 25-26.

36. Bureau of the Census: Money Income and Poverty Status of Families and Persons in the United States: Current Population Reports, 1984, Series P-60, Number 149

37. Duggan AK, Hardy JB. Relationships of urban adolescent pregnancies, births and abortions to six indices of poverty. Work in Progress, 1987.

38. Children's Defense Fund Data Book: Children's Defense Fund, 1985, Washington, D.C.

SEXUALITY EDUCATION

38

Douglas Kirby

BACKGROUND

Many people working with adolescents have viewed sexuality education as a partial solution to many of the numerous and sexual problems experienced by youth. As young people approach and attain puberty, many of them feel anxiety about their changing bodies and their changing relationships with members of the opposite sex and their families. Many feel vulnerable and succumb to peer pressure or exploitation; many also engage in sexual activity and then experience dissatisfaction and guilt; about a million become pregnant each year; many contract a sexually transmitted disease; and some are currently at risk of getting AIDS. Unfortunately, few teenagers feel comfortable turning to their parents or other adults for advice and help.

In response to these problems, sexuality educators have tried to increase knowledge about sexuality; to facilitate insights into personal, familial, religious, and societal values and behavior; to improve decision-making, communication, and assertiveness skills; to enhance self-esteem; to increase communication with parents and romantic partners; to reduce sexual exploitation; to reduce unprotected and irresponsible sexual activity; and to reduce unintended pregnancy and sexually transmitted disease.

PROVISION, TYPES, AND CONTENT OF SEXUALITY EDUCATION

For many years, the major providers of sexuality education have been those organizations primarily involved with educating youth (i.e. schools), and those organizations primarily involved with helping adolescents prevent or deal with pregnancy (i.e. family planning clinics). That is undoubtedly still true.

A 1982 survey of 200 school districts in large U.S. metropolitan areas revealed that 76 percent of the school districts offered sexuality education in their high schools and 75 percent offered it in their junior high schools.[1]

However, in more recent years, a number of youth-serving agencies have developed sexuality education programs. For example, the Girls Clubs, the Boys Clubs, the YWCA, and many churches—both liberal and conservative—offer sexuality education to their members.

Most programs in this country are relatively short. According to the same 1982 survey, about 48 percent last ten hours or less, and another 39 percent last 11 to 40 hours. These courses cover a variety of topics superficially, but they tend to focus upon the basics: anatomy and physiology, changes during puberty, decision-making about dating and sexual behavior, the consequences of sexual activity and parenthood, birth control, and sexually transmitted disease. The small number of sessions allow schools to fit this instruction into other courses, such as health and physical education.

A few schools offer comprehensive, semester-long programs. According to the 1982 survey, about 14 percent of school districts offered courses lasting longer than 40 hours, and 16 percent offered separate courses in sexuality education.

Such programs cover the basic topics in much greater depth than short programs, and cover a wider variety of topics. They typically include cognitive, affective, and skill components, and incorporate more group discussions and role playing. They devote more time to clarifying values, increasing decision-making and communication skills, improving self-esteem, and making behavior more responsible.

Some non-school organizations, and even a few schools, find it easier to provide the content of a short program in a single day, instead of dividing it over several days. Thus, they hold all day conferences. Sometimes they bring in outside resources (e.g. well-known personalities, student theater groups, or professionals in relevant health fields). Other times they combine the sexuality education component with health fairs.

Most sexuality education courses—especially those in the schools—are taught by the teachers within those schools. However, some are peer education programs. In these programs, selected youth leaders are often trained for 20 hours or more on both sexuality and on educating and counseling their peers. These peer educators then give presentations to school classes or other youth organizations, talk with their peers in the school, answer questions when stopped in the hallways or elsewhere, and refer students who need help to other resources.

For at least a decade professionals have recognized the important role of parents, and have tried to facilitate the parents' role as the primary sexuality educators of their children. For that reason, some programs offer classes for parents and their children together. During these courses, there are some didactic presentations, some films, and many games and activities that are designed to have parents and their children actually communicate with each other right there in the classroom. Although it is often difficult to get parents to come to these courses; those parents who do come rate them positively, and several different evaluations indicate that they do increase both parent/child communication and comfort with that communication.

During the early 1980s, a conservative movement began to have an increasing impact upon sexuality education. Consequently, nearly all sexuality education courses began placing more emphasis upon the advantages of abstinence. In addition, many courses were developed that were designed solely to promote abstinence. Many of them unabashedly stated that their only goal was to get adolescents to say "no" to sex. Some of these courses were simplistic and inaccurate in their presentation of facts, especially facts about contraception and sexual activity. Other courses were more balanced and more sophisticated and used peer educators to encourage younger teens to delay having sex.

Although many school districts and other organizations offer one or more of these types of sexuality education, not all adolescents take such courses, even when they are available. Estimates of the proportions of adolescents that have taken such courses vary. According to data from the National Longitudinal Survey of Youth—based on 12,069 young men and women in 1984—60 percent of the females and 52 percent of the males had taken a sex education course by age 19.[2] About half the respondents had taken courses covering the menstrual cycle and sexually transmitted diseases, while slightly lower percentages had taken courses which covered types of contraception (45 percent), where to obtain contraception (38 percent), and effects of contraception (40 percent). Other studies have indicated that as many as three-fourths of students receive at least a small amount of sexuality education.[3]

VALUES, CONTROVERSY, AND PUBLIC SUPPORT

For almost a century, school-based sexuality education has generated some controversy. At the turn of the century, the major purposes of sex education were to enforce premarital and extramarital abstinence and to eliminate venereal diseases. Social hygienists joined forces with anti-vice and anti-prostitution groups to mount the first national campaign to introduce sex education into all schools. They believed that biologically correct information would lead to abstinence before marriage, monogamy, and healthy sex within marriage. However, their religious fervor was not shared by all; they lost financial backing during the depression, and the movement remained only sporadically active for several decades. Its failure is believed to be at least partially due to the lack of social consensus on how to solve sexual problems, and what moral values to teach within the educational process.

During the late 1960s and 1970s, the sexual revolution in this country affected teens as well as adults. The number of sexually active teens increased substantially, and sexuality educators tried to avoid offending people with different values. Moreover, many professionals working with youth thought it was unwise and ineffective simply to encourage teens to say "no." Consequently, many sexuality educators developed a decision-making approach which taught the steps in the decision-making process and then laid out all the pros and cons of abstinence, sexual activity, and contraception.

When these programs were attacked for not giving sufficient emphasis to society's values, their promoters began to emphasize basic values in our society that are almost universal. These included the concepts that all people should be treated with respect and dignity, people should carefully consider the consequences before making important sexual decisions, no one should use either subtle pressure or physical force to get someone else to engage in unwanted sexual activity.

For the last two decades, sexuality education has appeared to be very controversial. In some communities, the introduction of sex education has, in fact, generated heated controversy. In those communities, there have been very vocal and active minorities of adults who believe that only abstinence should be taught, and that the decision-making approach to sexuality education essentially sanctions premarital sex and encourages teens to have sex. For example, these opponents often state that teaching about birth control is like teaching kids how to shop-lift so that they won't get caught.

However, these well-publicized controversies are misleading. In most communities, sexuality education programs are developed and taught with little opposition. Of course, when there is little opposition, there is little publicity, and thus media coverage provides a biased impression.

Moreover, there is a variety of national surveys and other evidence that demonstrate widespread support for sexuality education. In 1943, the Gallup Poll asked whether or not adults approved of sexuality education in schools—68 percent approved.[4] By 1977, this approval had increased to 77 percent.[5] A more recent poll, conducted by Harris in 1985, indicated that more than 80 percent of American adults believe sexuality education should be taught in schools.[6] Finally, in a 1986 national poll for *Time* Magazine, 86 percent of adults indicated their support.[7] Not surprisingly, adolescents also strongly support sexuality education programs.[8] In this country, few things receive such widespread support. In fact, the only disagreements are over what, when, and how topics should be taught, and not *whether* sexuality education should be taught.

Parents of students provide their support for sexuality education, as it is currently taught, in yet another way. When parents are given the option of excusing their children from sexuality education classes, less than one percent do so.[9]

This widespread support is increasingly manifested at the state level. By 1980, two states and the District of Columbia mandated sexuality education[10] and the number of states is continuing to grow. Moreover, many additional states encourage sexuality education, while no states prohibit it.

EFFECTS OF SEXUALITY EDUCATION

Numerous studies of sexuality education classes have measured the impact of sex education courses upon the knowledge of the students, and their findings are nearly unanimous—instruction in sex education does increase knowledge of sexuality.[9] In some cases, the increase in knowledge was quite small; in other cases, quite large. There is some evidence that younger students tend to learn more than older students.[9]

Evaluations which have measured the impact of courses upon attitudes have produced mixed results. In a national study of 14 sexuality education courses,[9] the author found that a few courses increased the clarity of students' values while many did not. Moreover, most of the programs did not measurably change the direction of the participants' attitudes toward premarital sex, birth control, or other issues in sexuality. Finally, the programs did not have a measurable impact upon self-esteem, satisfaction with social and sexual relationships, or comfort with a variety of social or sexual activities. Other studies[11,12,13] suggest that some sexuality courses increased the tolerance of the students' attitudes toward the sexual practices of others (when this was the explicit goal of the course), but the courses had little impact upon the students' beliefs about their own sexual behavior with others.

Three major studies have examined the impact of sexuality education upon sexual activity, use of birth control, and pregnancy. The first study employed a quasi-experimental design and evaluated 14 carefully selected sexuality education programs taught by highly trained teachers.[9] These programs included a variety of approaches, including short programs, all-day conferences, semester-long programs, and others. None of these programs had a measurable impact upon subsequent sexual activity, use of birth control, or pregnancy.

The other two studies are based upon data from two nationally representative samples of young people—the 1984 National Longitudinal Survey of Work Experience of Youth, and the 1982 National Survey of Family Growth.[2,14] Both had longitudinal data and both had very large sample sizes (12,069 and 1,888 respectively). Both of them included only a few questions about the nature and quality of the sexuality education programs in which the respondents participated, and thus little is known about those programs. Presumably they represent a cross-section of sexuality education programs in this country.

The first study found that among females 16 or 17-years old, sexuality education was not related to the subsequent initiation of sexual activity during the following year, but among females 15 or 16-years old, having previously taken sexuality education was slightly related to subsequent initiation of sexual activity. The importance of this should not be overemphasized, for other factors, such as race, parental education, and frequency of religious attendance were more strongly related to subsequent sexual activity. The second study found that among teenage females aged 15 to 18, there was no relationship between sexuality education and subsequent initiation of sex; for 14-year-old females, the results were mixed.

Both studies found that sexuality education was related to subsequent use of birth control—teens who had taken sex education were somewhat more likely to use birth control. Third, there were no measurable relationships between having had sex education and subsequent pregnancy.

Few of the programs which place primary emphasis upon abstinence have been carefully evaluated. However, a few of them which are designed for junior high school students, and which employ a skill-building approach, have reported preliminary and unpublished results which suggest that they may slightly delay sexual activity, especially among very young females. Nonetheless, thus far, the evidence is clearly too weak to reach any definite conclusions about their impact.

In sum, the research indicates that sexuality education courses are like other educational programs—they can substantially increase knowledge, but have relatively little impact upon behavior. Sexuality education programs do increase knowledge; may or may not affect initiation of sexual activity, depending upon the course content and the age and sex of the participants; may slightly increase the use of birth control; and don't measurably affect teenage pregnancy.

CURRENT AND FUTURE DEVELOPMENTS

Recognizing that increasing knowledge is not sufficient to change behavior,[14] sexuality educators are now trying different approaches or combinations of approaches with some evidence of success. Some programs are focusing more upon role playing and teaching situation-specific skills, i.e., having students practice saying "no" to sexual activity or insisting upon using birth control. Other programs are involving peers to help change the students' norms about having sex and using birth control. Still others are integrating sexuality education with other curricula or other programs. For example, a "Life Planning" curriculum[16] integrates sexuality education with career planning. Some school-based health clinics integrate sexuality education with the provision of reproductive health services and primary health care. Some communities integrate a school-based sexuality education program with community-wide sexuality education programs targeted at parents, churches, community leaders, and other groups. One such community-wide approach in South Carolina has demonstrated success in reducing pregnancy rates among 14-to-17-year-old teens.[16]

Sexuality education has also been affected by concerns about child abuse, date rape, and, most recently, AIDS. Although these concerns have generated greater support for sexuality education, they have also created a concern among sexuality educators that sexuality is being presented to young people in a negative light. As one teenager said, "From what we learn, first you get abused as a child; then you get raped by your date; and finally you die of AIDS." An important challenge for sexuality educators is to cover child abuse, rape, and AIDS, and also to give appropriate emphasis to the positive aspects of sexuality so that teens develop a more positive and balanced view of sexuality.

Another challenge to educators is encouraging young people both to delay having sex and to use birth control when they do have sex. In the past, some educators may have shied away from this "double message," but increasingly they recognize that many teens in their classes are not ready for sex and should be encouraged to wait, while others are having sex and should be encouraged to use birth control.

Finally, educators are increasingly recognizing or need to recognize that it is difficult to change behavior, particularly sexual behavior, and that a more reasonable goal should be to provide teens with the values, knowledge, and skills with which they can better make more responsible decisions. These goals are important and can be achieved.

REFERENCES

1. Sonenstein F, Pittman K. The availability of sex education in large city school districts. Family Planning Perspectives 16(1):19-25, 1984.

2. Marsiglio W, Mott F. The impact of sex education on sexual activity, contraceptive use and premarital pregnancy among American teenagers. Family Planning Perspectives 18(4):151-162, 1986.

3. Zelnik M, Kim Y. Sex education and its association with teenage sexual activity, pregnancy, and contraceptive use. Family Planning Perspectives, 16(3):117-126, 1982.

4. Gallup G. Gallup Poll Public Opinion 1935-1971, New York, Random House, 1972, p 387.

5. Gallup G. Teens want right to obtain birth control devices. Gallup Youth Survey. Princeton, NJ, news release, Sept 27, 1980.

6. Louis Harris and Associates, Inc. Public attitudes about sex education, family planning, and abortion in the United States. Planned Parenthood Federation of America, New York, 1985.

7. Leo J, Delaney P, Whitaker L. Sex and schools. Time, Nov 24, 1986.

8. Norman J, Harris M. The Private Life of the American Teenager. New York. Rawson Wade. 1981.

9. Kirby D. Sexuality education: an evaluation of programs and their effects. Santa Cruz, CA. Network Publications. 1984.

10. Kirby D, Scales P. An analysis of state guidelines for sex education instruction in public schools. Family Relations 229-237, 1981.

11. Parcel G, Luttman D. Effects of sex education on sexual attitudes. Jour of Current Adol Medicine 2:38-46, 1980.

12. Parcel G, Luttman D. Evaluation of a sex education course for young adolescents. Family Relations 30(1):55-60, 1981.

13. Hoch L. Attitude change as a result of sex education. Journal of Research in Science Teaching 8:363-367, 1971.

14. Dawson DA. The effects of sex education on adolescent behavior. Family Planning Perspectives 18(4):162-170, 1986.

15. Kirby D. Sexuality education: a more realistic view of its effects. JOSH 55(10):421-424, 1985.

16. Hunter-Geboy C, Peterson L, Casey S, et al. Life planning education. Center for Population Options, Washington DC, 1985.

17. Vincent M, Clearie A, Schluchter M. Reducing adolescent pregnancy through school and community-based education. JAMA 257(24):3382-3386, 1987.

SCHOOL-BASED CLINICS 39

Joy G. Dryfoos

The rapidity of social change in the U.S. is such that an entirely new system of health care can develop within the span of half a decade. In 1984, a first conference on school-based clinics (SBCs) was held in Houston, attended by representatives of ten school-based clinic programs, covering sites in 23 high schools. Despite the long and complicated history of health services in schools [1] these were the only agencies that could be identified that included contraceptive counseling and services in their definitions of comprehensive school health services for adolescents.[2] Two of the models, in St. Paul[3] and Dallas,[4] had been functioning since the early 1970s and both programs had produced reports showing reduced fertility rates among their student-clients.

By late 1987, according to Lovick,[5] 101 comprehensive health care clinics were operating in or near junior and senior high schools, as sites of 60 programs in 28 states, and another 100 were being planned. At least 26 states had taken actions to promote the initiation of SBCs and seven had actually allocated funds.[6] How could all of this occur, in light of the prevailing view in the early 1980s that "provision of such education and services in school is philosophically controversial and politically not possible in most U.S. communities today?"[7]

The emergence of SBCs as a potential system of health care for adolescents may be attributed to the convergence of a number of factors, such as deepening concern about increasing numbers of disadvantaged "youth-at-risk";[8] new documen-

563

tation of the powerful connection between school failure and early childbearing; [9] shifting public opinion that showed parents in support of the concept of linking public schools and family planning clinics; [10] search by school administrators for other institutions to share the role of "surrogate parents;"[11] and availability of support from local and state public sources and national foundations.

ORGANIZATION OF SCHOOL-BASED CLINICS

Initiation of a local SBC program either results from a spontaneous community-generated idea or as a response to a state or foundation Request for Proposal.[12] Whatever the path from concept to project, the process takes more than a year.[13] This involves consultation with, and approval from, school officials at system and school level; packaging services, usually from several agencies; formation of a community advisory board, including parents and community leaders; "needs assessment" surveys of students; remodeling of school space; securing funding (dollars and in-kind); hiring appropriate staff; establishing medical protocols; and obtaining parental consent.

Most, if not all, clinics require some form of written consent from the parents of each student before medical services can be provided.[14] Community Advisory Boards are frequently consulted on the design and implementation of parental consent forms and clinic policies regarding contraception. Generally, parents have the option of denying specific services on a check-off list. Laws in most states guarantee confidential family planning services to teenagers, but require consent for general medical services. Clinics have very explicit policies regarding confidentiality once consent is obtained: students' medical charts are not part of their school records, and access to a chart is not given without the students' permission.

While SBCs are by definition "school-based," they are almost all operated by agencies outside of the school system. A 1986 survey [15] of 61 sites revealed that among the sponsoring (grantee) agencies, 33 percent were hospitals, 23 percent health departments, 20 percent non-profit youth agencies, 17 percent health centers, four percent schools and three percent family planning agencies. However, the lead agency often contracts with other agencies for specialized medical and social services. All of these arrangements relieve school systems of fiscal responsibility; the outside agencies transfer their liability coverage to the clinics. They also deal with the thorny issues of parent involvement, community relations, and continuity of funding.

FUNDING

Federally supported, state-operated Maternal and Child Health Services Block Grants (MCHSBG) are the major source of funds for SBCs. However, most SBCs rely on a combination of public and private foundation funding. For example, medical services may be supported with local MCH funds and reimbursement from Early and Periodic Screening, Diagnosis and Treatment (EPSDT) and other Medicaid sources. Contraceptive services can be covered by Title X (family planning); mental health counseling by a local foundation; substance abuse counseling by the local drug prevention program or state funds; and infant care by Title XX (social services). A few clinics have a nominal enrollment fee (e.g., five dollars).

The seven states that directly fund SBCs include Connecticut, Illinois, Michigan, New Jersey, New York, Oregon, and Wisconsin.[6] Michigan's Statewide Adolescent Health Advisory Committee's five-year plan calls for the ultimate development of 100 clinics.[16] New Jersey's Youth at Risk initiative will fund 30 centers in schools that may address school dropout, youth unemployment, and adolescent pregnancy.[17] A severe limitation of these state funding initiatives is their treatment of family planning services. In some states, such as New Jersey, the center grant funds cannot be used to pay for contraception or abortion services. In Oregon, where the State Health Division funds five clinics, family planning is an optional service. Gurule found "startling" differences between modes: "In those clinics where a student can get a prescription for contraceptives, family planning services were requested 17 times more often than in clinics that did not offer prescriptions...it seems very clear that the clinics have to offer a viable service...to young people if we expect them to use it."[18]

Foundations have played a major role in initiating SBCs. The Robert Wood Johnson Foundation has recently awarded 20 five-year grants for school-based adolescent health care. Family planning is one of the required components.[19] Other foundations are supporting demonstration projects and evaluation research.

STAFFING

SBCs are typically staffed by a team of three, including a nurse-practitioner, physician, and social worker/counselor.[5] Arrangements are diverse, depending on the size and scope of the program and the amount of resources available. In many clinics, a full-time community aide provides the contact point with the student body, while the professional staff, such as nutritionists, health educators, dentists, and other specialists, are available part-time. People who work in SBCs suggest that staff be selected not only for their medical skills but also for their ability to communicate with young people. In Hispanic and other ethnic communities, bilingual personnel are essential.

School nurses have been integrated into SBC programs in almost half of the sites.[5] While nurses who work for school systems may be limited in the amount of direct medical care they are allowed to provide, experience has shown that they can complement the clinic team. School nurses are particularly effective in the areas of expediting school-clinic relationships and arrangements, and in fostering coordination with community agencies.[20] The cooperation of school personnel is essential to the operations of an SBC. The principal is considered the key factor;[13] decisions about space, maintenance, scheduling, policies, and involvement of other staff, such as guidance counselors, rest in the principal's office.

SERVICES

Although the St. Paul program is often described as "the model" SBC, each clinic reflects the needs of the community as well as its resources and the level of community acceptance. The service orientation of the provider agency may also determine the mix of services provided. SBC programs differ in the number of sites (one to six), the level of the school (junior and/or senior high school), the location of the clinic (in the school, next to the school, across the street), the efficiency of referral arrangements, hours open (school hours only to full-time including summer and weekends), and, most importantly, in the range of services provided. The variability in costs per student served, from about 100 to 200 dollars per year, reflects the diversity of the delivery system.

All clinics, however, have certain common elements. The most recent survey[5] showed that virtually all programs provide primary health care services, including physical exams, diagnosis and treatment of minor injuries, medications for treatment, laboratory tests, immunizations, and referrals. More than three-fourths conduct on-site gynecological examinations, diagnosis and treatment of sexually transmitted diseases (STD), and specific referrals for pregnancy and prenatal care. About half of the clinics directly prescribe contraceptives, and/or provide prenatal care on-site. More than one third provide pediatric care for infants of adolescents and/or dental services.

Counseling and educational services are also provided by the clinic staff. All report providing general health and nutrition education, mental health and psychosocial counseling, and sexuality and pregnancy counseling. Most clinics also have weight-reduction programs, drug and substance abuse prevention programs, and classes in parenting education. About a third of the programs offer employment and job counseling; organize school remediation and mentoring programs; and/or offer family counseling and social services.

Most of the visits to SBCs are for physical examinations and minor emergencies. This pattern is consistent in a variety of SBC models. While the media have focused on the provision of birth control in SBCs, only ten-25 percent of all visits are for family planning. Only about one-fifth of the clinics, following counseling and appropriate medical procedures, including pelvic examinations and Pap smears, distribute birth control pills and condoms on site; half give gynecologic exams and prescriptions, and refer to collaborating agencies for contraceptive supplies; and 30 percent counsel and refer only.[21] Abortion counseling and referral are considered too controversial to be included in the roster of services offered in schools.

In 85 percent of the SBCs, the clinic staff provides sex education in the classroom, usually integrated with individual and group counseling in the clinic. Emphasis is placed on decision-making and delaying first intercourse until the student is ready to assume responsibility. Compliance with medical protocols is emphasized. Students who use birth control are contacted routinely, usually once a month, including telephone calls to the home.[22]

Personal counseling in SBCs often reveals depression and severe family pathology, particularly sexual abuse and parental drug use. The staff attribute the unexpected prevalence of "confessions" of these very troubling problems to the previous absence of personal counseling prior to the opening of the clinic, and to the clinic's reputation for confidentiality and concern. Other problems that are frequently discovered through screening (e.g. heart murmurs, asthma, vision and hearing defects, respiratory diseases, parasites) require immediate referral for medical treatment. Because of the large number of students with either minor complaints or major problems, SBCs are heavily utilized and often have difficulty keeping up with the demand.

EVALUATION

Because SBCs are controversial, measuring impact is important. Since the St. Paul model was identified as one of the few pregnancy prevention interventions that had been proven to decrease fertility rates, it has been assumed that SBCs hold great promise for reducing teen childbearing in areas with high rates. This position was recently supported by the Panel on Adolescent Pregnancy and Childbearing of the National Research Council, which recommended that "school systems, in cooperation with various health care and youth-serving agencies, should further develop and refine comprehensive school-based clinics for implementation in schools with large high-risk populations."[23]

A number of major studies are underway that are designed to evaluate the effectiveness of SBCs in preventing pregnancy and school dropout, and improving health status. The methodology for measuring changes in fertility is complex and costly, requiring longitudinal data and control groups.[24] SBC providers believe that the one-on-one individual attention they are offering is making significant differences in the lives of the young people they treat. However, given the low utilization of the clinics for family planning, aggregate data may not be sensitive enough to document these effects.

A summary of available data provides preliminary evidence of positive outcomes in selected programs. More recent data from the St. Paul SBCs show a continuing decrease in fertility rates, from 79 births per 1,000, in 1972-1973, to 35 births per 1,000 in 1985-1986.[25] A recent three-year school-related clinic demonstration project in Baltimore reported that pregnancy rates dropped by 30 percent in program schools compared to an increase of 58 percent in control schools.[26]

Sexual activity among the students does not appear to increase after a clinic opens. A two-year follow-up in Kansas City [27] revealed almost no change, while in the Baltimore study researchers found a seven-month average postponement of first intercourse among program participants. Among students who were already sexually active, clinic patients in Kansas City showed higher rates of contraceptive use than non-patients, and a striking increase in use of condoms among males. In Baltimore, younger female students and males in the program schools were much more likely to use birth control than those in the control schools. And in St. Paul, female contraceptive users had an extremely high rate of continuation; 91 percent were still using the method (mostly the pill) after a year and 78 percent after two years of use.[25] This is much higher than for adolescent users of free-standing family planning clinics; one study reported a 12-month program dropout rate of close to 50 percent.[28]

The sheer volume of services provided by SBCs and the amount of health screening is one type of evidence of effectiveness. Almost all programs report utilization rates of 70 percent or higher. In Dallas, 85 percent of the student body is enrolled in the program.[29] In a recent year, a total of 11,000 clinic visits were recorded by the Dallas clinic; one of the impacts reported from Dallas has been a 62 percent lower rate of hospitalization for youngsters from the target area. Clinics reported an average monthly caseload of 204 students with a total of 372 visits, but there is wide variation ranging from 20 to 400 students served per month.[5]

The Kansas City program reported a substantial drop in substance use among clinic clients during a two year period. Never-use of alcohol went from 59 percent to 64 percent, never-use of marijuana from 69 percent to 79 percent, and non-smokers increased from 87 percent to 95 percent.[27] The Kansas City SBC also reported changes in mental health outcomes, including reductions in hopelessness, suicidal ideation, and low self-esteem.

Almost three-fourths of New York City students who used SBCs thought that the clinic had improved their health, and more than a third stated that the clinic had improved their school attendance. Most (91 percent) stated that the clinic had improved their ability to get health care when they needed it, and 88 percent stated that the clinic had improved their knowledge of and ability to take care of their bodies.[30]

LIMITATIONS OF THE SBC MODEL

While there are many advantages to the placement of medical services within a school building, there are also a number of disadvantages. At the clinic level, only a few programs serve out-of-school youth, many of whom are the most needy. Few of the programs operate in schools or make arrangements for medical backup through the summer months and during school vacations. Budgetary limitations do not allow for the necessary outreach to make home visits and involve parents, particularly those who fail to complete parental consent forms. In many schools, the space allotted to the clinic is too small for the volume of demand and privacy is inadequate.

At the community level, the opposition to SBCs has centered on the birth control issue. The label "sex clinic," created by the media and promoted by conservative organizations, has been used to try to influence school boards and community groups.[31] In several places where clinics have proliferated in inner cities, the issue of genocide has been raised.[32] In other areas, church leaders, educators, and parent group leaders have expressed apprehension about the pre-emption of the parental role by providing any form of social services in schools. One educational leader stated, "Schools are not a substitute for city and county health departments."[33] Concern has been expressed about the future role of private pediatricians, if health services proliferate in schools.

In regard to the adequacy of the reproductive health care component in SBCs, one limitation may be the lack of effective family planning services in many programs. Some practitioners have backed away from the pregnancy prevention objective and present their programs entirely in the context of "comprehensive health." Adolescents who need family planning are referred back to the free-standing clinic system which they were not adequately utilizing.

SBCs clearly have limitations both in terms of the quality of care they can provide and the amount of controversy they generate in the community. However, the most pressing obstacle to further development may be the lack of long-term funding. Although there is Congressional support for demonstration projects in adolescent health, no new funds are expected in the near future. The separate state initiatives will be useful but they are not being launched in the states with the greatest needs, and many have restrictive policies that limit the provision of family planning. As long as state programs remain in their current forms, as demonstration projects dependent on year-to-year funding, the development of a stable system of school-based health care for needy adolescents will be fragmented.

OUTLOOK FOR THE FUTURE

SBCs appear to be one of the battlegrounds on which the endless conflict over conservative and liberal definitions of "morality" will be fought. Despite the heavy opposition, support for SBCs has been growing among national organizations, including the American Academy of Pediatrics, the Society for Adolescent Medicine, the National Education Association and the Committee for Economic Development.[34]

Despite the amount of negative publicity and harassment that SBCs have received at the community level, programs have continued to progress from the conceptual stage to implementation, with few exceptions. Advocacy by parents and school personnel have been important factors in advancing the cause of SBCs.[35] Students want to get much-needed health services, including family planning, in a convenient place from people who care about them. If the social development and critical health needs of young people are compelling-enough reasons to convince decision-makers to ignore the critics, these services will expand.

REFERENCES

1. Cronin G, Young W: 400 Navels. The Future of School Health in America, Blooming-ton, IN, Phi Delta Kappa, 1979.

2. Dryfoos J. School-based health clinics: A new approach to preventing adolescent preg-nancy? Family Planning Perspectives 17:70-82, 1985.

3. Edwards LE, Steinman ME, Hakanson EY. An experimental comprehensive high school clinic, American Journal of Public Health 67:765, 1970.

4. Ralph N, Edginton E. An evaluation of an adolescent family planning program, Jour-nal of Adolescent Health Care, 4:158, 1983.

5. Lovick SR. The School-Based Clinic Update 1987, Washington, DC, The Center for Population Options, 1987, pp 4-5.

6. Center for Population Options: School-based Clinic Policy Initiatives Around the Country: 1986, Washington, 1987.

7. Rogers KD, Young FH. Health services in schools, Maternal and Child Health Practices. Second edition. Edited by H. Wallace et al. New York, H. Wiley, 1982, p 633.

8. Research and Policy Committee: Children in Need: Investment Strategies for the Educationally Disadvantaged, New York, Committee for Economic Development, 1987, pp 5-10.

9. Pittman K. Preventing adolescent pregnancy: What schools can do, Washington DC, Children's Defense Fund, 1986, pp 3-15.

10. Harris L. Inside America, New York, Vintage Press, 1987, p 84.

11. Altback PG. Underfunded and oversold, Education Week, Oct 15, 1986.

12. Hadley EM, Lovick SR, Kirby DK. School-Based Health Clinics: A Guide to Imple-menting Programs, Washington, DC, Center for Population Options, 1986.

13. Futterman R, Dryfoos JG. Process evaluation of a comprehensive school-based clinic program, Paper presented at Annual Meeting of American Public Health Association, New Orleans, Oct, 1987.

14. Tereszkiewicz L, Brindis C. School-based clinics offer health care to teens, Youth Law News, Vol VII No 5, pp 1-5.

15. Lovick SR, Wesson WF. School-Based Clinics: Update 1986, Washington, DC, The Center for Population Options, 1986, p 7.

16. Michigan Department of Public Health: Final Recommendations on School-based Teen Health Centers, Adolescent Health Advisory Committee, Jan 9, 1987.

17. State of New Jersey Department of Human Services: School-based Youth Services Program, Request for Proposals, Aug 6, 1987.

18. Gurule D. School-based clinics in Oregon: The first year, Paper presented at annual meeting of American Public Health Association, New Orleans, Oct, 1987.

19. The Robert Wood Johnson Foundation: The School-Based Adolescent Health Care Program, 1986.

20. Edwards L. The school nurse's role in school-based clinics, Journal of School Health, 57:4, 157-159, 1987.

21. Dryfoos JG, Klerman LV. School-based clinics: Their role in helping students meet the 1990 objectives, Health Education Quarterly, 1988 (in press).

22. Shirley A. Testimony regarding Jackson-Hinds Comprehensive Health Center's school-based clinics, The United States Senate Children's Policy Forum, Washington, DC, June 5, 1985.

23. Hayes C (ed). Risking the Future: Adolescent Sexuality, Pregnancy and Childbearing. Washington, DC, National Academy Press, 1987.

24. Dryfoos J. Preventing teen pregnancy: What works? Planned Parenthood Review, 6:6-8, 1986.

25. Healthstart Inc: Information about the St. Paul school health clinics, Report, St. Paul, MN, 1987, p 10.

26. Zabin L, Hirsch M, Smith E, Streett R, Hardy J. Evaluation of a pregnancy prevention program for urban teenagers. Family Planning Perspectives 18:119-126, 1986.

27. Kitzi J. Presentation at Third Annual Conference of the Support Center for School-Based Clinics, Denver, Oct, 1986.

28. Shea J, Herceg-Baron R, Furstenberg F. Clinic continuation rates according to age, method of contraception and agency. Paper presented at the Annual Meeting of the National Family Planning and Reproductive Health Association, Washington, DC, March, 1982.

29. Dallas Children and Youth Project: Sixteen years of comprehensive health care..., Report, May, 1984.

30. Welfare Research Inc: Health services for high school students. Short-term assessment of New York City High school-based clinics. Report to New York City Board of Education, June 3, 1987.

31. Glascow R. Abortion and the rise of school-based clinics (Part III). National Right-to-Life News, Oct 9, 1986.

32. Clinics' birth control efforts aim to control growth in black population, some charge. Education Week, Nov 12, 1986.

33. At-risk children seen turning to schools for basic health care. Education Week, Dec 17, 1986.

34. Warren C. Improving Student's Access to Health Care: School-Based Health Clinics, New York, Center for Public Advocacy Research, Inc., 1987.

35. A school's RX for sex: A controversial clinic at DuSable High divides Chicago on birth control in -the schools, People, Oct 28, 1985.

40 | SUBSTANCE ABUSE

Donald Ian Macdonald

Illegal drug use by young people is a major public health concern. Prior to the late 1960s, the illegal use of drugs other than alcohol was limited, for the most part, to a readily defined, deviant segment of the adult population. By 1979, however, use pervaded all sectors and age groups of society; in any given month, more than one in three high school seniors used marijuana and nearly three of every four used alcohol. One in four seniors were daily cigarette smokers.[1,2]

The 1980s have been marked by intensive efforts to reduce and eliminate illegal drug use by all Americans. The movement advocating "zero tolerance" for the use of illicit drugs has benefited immensely from the sustained leadership and commitment of President Reagan and First Lady Nancy Reagan; from the burgeoning involvement of families in grassroots anti-drug organizations; and from a continuously expanding, research-based awareness of health and development risks associated with psychoactive drug use.

Despite the changes in attitude and knowledge, probability is high that contemporary health care workers in the MCH field will regularly encounter either the use or the direct and/or indirect effects of illegal drug use during the course of their practice. Failure to observe such phenomena is less likely to indicate a non-using client or patient population than to suggest that the worker is unable or unwilling to acknowledge the problem.

This chapter first will discuss the role of MCH personnel in assisting families and youth in resisting illegal drug use. Later portions of the chapter will review several of the key illegal substances which today threaten the healthy development and function of young people and their families; describe the current emphases and foci of prevention strategies; and cite recent developments in anti-drug legislation and funding.

ROLE OF MCH WORKERS

How seriously the MCH professional views adolescent drinking and other drug use will be influenced by one's understanding of the extent and causes of drug abuse and familiarity with the user's characteristic clinical course. It is important to recognize that persons currently between the ages of 20 and 40—i.e., who grew up in the 1960s and 1970s—are the principal users of illicit drugs, accounting for the majority of the 23 million Americans who use these substances regularly. Of greater concern, perhaps, is that many of these users now are parents themselves. Continued drug involvement on their part strongly influences the likelihood that their offspring will see few sanctions against the use of illicit drugs and will become and remain involved themselves. In the absence of unequivocal anti-drug education and awareness, what began as an epidemic of drug use in past decades will become an endemic, with patterns involving regular use entrenched within growing segments of the society.

Among the most effective primary preventive strategies to which MCH workers can contribute is that of helping parents to be good role models, guides, and protectors of their children. Parents must be encouraged to appreciate the primacy of the responsibility for building a child's self-image and bonding the child to family and society. Parents must teach their children skills of communication and assertiveness; the importance of deferment of gratification and separating needs from wants; young people who have given up, or see no hope for their futures, tend to want and seek regular gratification immediately through dangerous means. Also, children must be taught a respect for the consequences of their actions. The child's education should continue in an environment sufficiently protected to allow the building of these assets. With these in place, environmental and peer factors which increase the risk of susceptibility to illegal drug use are more readily countered.

Parents and other caretakers must recognize that, during adolescence, a relationship exists between drug use and other problem behaviors. Precocious sexual activity, for example, often is a function of intoxication, which leads to a decrease in normal—and protective—inhibitive and judgment on the part of teens. One of the clearest indicators of impending trouble is a change in a younger's peer group. As deviant activity begins, old friends who do not engage in such behaviors are seen as boring, and positive peer pressure—a profoundly important protective barrier—is weakened and lost.

It is particularly important that personnel in the MCH field understand how experimentation with drugs may progress to moderate use, to immoderate use, and finally to dependency, in a pattern many have likened to a disease process. The standard public health model considers many diseases to be caused by: 1) interaction of a susceptible host, with 2) a harmful agent (drugs), in 3) a suitable environment. Prevention and treatment must address each of these three factors. Too often, efforts focus on just one, such as changing the environment or helping the young patient to build up resistance skills, while omitting considerations of others, such as the progressive and contagious nature of chemical dependency; risk factors extending from genetic to parental and family attitudes and practices to community standards; and critically, peer group experiences.

THE EXTENT AND EFFECTS OF ILLEGAL DRUG USE

Today's youngsters—and young parents—have been prepared for drug use by growing up in a world where there seems to be a drug for relief of every problem, from minor aches and pains to "night cough" and "tired blood". Television, magazines, movies, and music strongly influenced the popularization of drugs, but only recently have begun to be used effectively to educate and deglamorize the use of these substances.

Illegal drug use persists in the late 1980s as a profound threat to the well-being of young people and their families. Despite significant continuing reductions in rates of use of some types of substances, the 12th National High School Senior Survey[3] revealed that slightly more than half of the Nation's 1986 senior class members had, at some time in their lives, used illicit drugs. Approximately 27 percent of the seniors were "current users," that is, had used illegal drugs within the month prior to the survey (Table 1). Reductions in the use of certain drugs, such as marijuana, moreover, have been partially offset by the exposure of young people to dangerous and highly addictive substances, such as cocaine and a variety of illicitly synthesized drug analogs.

Alcohol Abuse Alcohol remains the most popular drug among adolescents. The 1986 survey found that 85 percent of all 12th graders used alcohol at least once during the year; two-thirds used it in the month prior to being interviewed; 37 percent admitted having five or more drinks in a row in the two weeks prior to interview; and five percent reported daily or near daily use in the month prior to interview.

The consequences of drinking by the young are often tragic. Teenagers and young adults, aged 16-25, account for only some 22 percent of the population but are responsible for 44 percent of fatal night-time crashes. About half of all teenage homicides are associated with alcohol and drugs. Adolescent suicides, which have increased an estimated 150 percent since 1960, frequently are committed under the

TABLE 1

TRENDS IN DRUG USE AMONG HIGH SCHOOL SENIORS, 1975-86**

	Percent Using Drug, Class Of						
	1975	1977	1979	1981	1983	1985	1986
Marijuana							
Used In Past Year	40	48	51	46	42	41	38.8
Used In Past Month	27	35	37	32	27	26	23.4
Daily Use	6	9	10	7	6	5	4
Alcohol							
Used In Past Month	68	71	72	71	69	66	65.3
Daily Use	6	6	7	6	6	5	4.8
Cigarettes							
Used In Past Month	37	38	34	29	30	30	29.6
Daily Use	27	29	25	20	21	30	18.7
Stimulants							
Ever Used	22	23	24	32	35	26*	23.4*
Used In Past Month	9	9	10	16	12	7*	5.5*
Cocaine							
Ever Used	9	11	15	17	16	17	16.9
Used In Past Month	2	3	6	6	5	7	6.2
PCP							
Used In Past Year	NA	NA	7	3	3	3	2.4
Used In Past Month	NA	NA	2	1	1	2	1.3
Inhalants (Glue/Aerosols)							
Ever Used	NA	NA	19	17	19	18	20.1*
Used In Past Year	NA	NA	9	6	7	7	8.9*
Illicit Drugs							
Ever Used	55	62	65	66	65	60.6	57.6
Used In Past Year	45	51	54	52	49	46.3	44.3
Perceived As Harmful							
Marijuana (Reg. Use)	43	36	42	57	63	70.4	71.3
Cigarettes (Pack/Day)	51	58	63	63	62	66.5	66.0
Cocaine (Regular Use)	73	68	70	71	74	80	82.2
Cocaine (Occasional)	43	36	32	32	33	36	54.2
Friends Disapprove Of Use							
Marijuana (Occasional)	55	49	48	56	60	64.2	64.4
Marijuana (Regular)	75	69	70	75	78	81	82.3
Cigarettes (Pack/Day)	64	68	73	74	72	73.7	76.2

*   Adjusted rate

**   Compilations from <u>National Trends in Drug Use and Related Factors Among High School Students and Young Adults, 1975-1986.</u> National Institute on Drug Abuse, 1987. (DHHS Publication No. (ADM) 87-1535.)

influence of alcohol or drugs. The provision of information regarding the risks of excessive alcohol use is critical, particularly as it pertains to persons of childbearing age. Fetal alcohol syndrome (FAS) is of special concern, though other illicit drugs also carry negative effects.

Tobacco Following a 25 percent to 33 percent decline in the late 1970s, in the number of adolescent cigarette smokers, the slope of the curve of reduced use flattened; since 1981, the proportion of young people who are daily smokers has remained constant, at approximately 20 percent. In light of what is known with certainty of the extensive health consequences of tobacco use, failure to achieve further reductions in cigarette smoking among adolescents is a cause of added concern, given the finding that 60 percent of smokers start by the age 13 and 90 percent before their 20th birthday.[4]

Gateway Drugs Despite modest progress in reducing the use of cigarettes and alcohol by young people, the frequency of use remains unacceptable—all the more so in light of research demonstrating these as "gateways" to a broad array of illegal substances.[5] Longitudinal studies of drug use suggest that if a person uses one drug, he or she is likely to use other drugs. Use of legal substances, such as alcohol and tobacco, often leads to marijuana use and, eventually, to other illicit psychoactive drugs or combinations of drugs. Conversely, use of drugs, such as cocaine and heroin, are unusual in those who have not previously used alcohol and tobacco and/or marijuana.

Marijuana Although it remains the most widely used illicit drug among adolescents, current (i.e., within a given month) and daily use of marijuana has declined significantly since the late 1970s, when 37 percent of seniors used the substance monthly and 11 percent used it daily. In 1986, 23 percent of seniors reported current use and less than five percent, daily use. In real numbers, that percentage drop means that 194,000 fewer members of a much smaller 1986 graduating class were seriously involved in drugs than would have been had rates remained the same.

The adverse physiological effects of marijuana, which extend from chronic cough and emphysema to endocrine system disruption and immune system compromise, are increasingly well-documented. Of greater concern, however, are the effects of marijuana on brain and behavior. Even if use eventually stops, an educational or developmental window will have been lost. If a student is "stoned," or absent from school or life, can he or she make up for lost time? Also among the behavioral effects frequently is a deleterious change in the adolescent's routine peer contacts.

Cocaine By the mid-1980s, cocaine—the "glamor" drug of the prior decade—had become accessible to every widening groups of users. By 1986, it was among the drugs most widely used by adolescents, following cigarettes, alcohol, and marijuana; one senior in six (17 percent) had tried cocaine, 13 percent had used it within the past year, and six percent within the prior month. The rapid increase in cocaine use among young adults is attributable in large part to the introduction of "crack," a potent, smokable form of the drug. The popularity and inexpensive unit price of this highly addictive form of cocaine explains its sudden popularity during the late 1980s, when many students reported using crack, as well as difficulty in discontinuing use. Moreover, while rates of initiation to most drugs decline after high school, recent longitudinal studies have indicated that the prevalence of cocaine use increases with each year, into early adulthood.[6]

Other drugs   The popularity of other drugs fluctuates over time and geographically; it is useful for MCH workers to familiarize themselves with the array of substances available and their current, local prevalence. LSD, for example, continues to be used in some areas. Taken orally on a sugar cube, cookie, or blotter paper, or injected, it often is used in a group setting. Hallucinogenic effects last eight-12 hours, with possible recurrence of a "trip" even after a prolonged period of abstinence. LSD tends to intensify existing psychosis and may trigger suicidal tendencies. PCP, first developed as an animal tranquilizer, also has prolonged hallucinogenic effects and can result in violent, psychotic behavior, which may last several days or weeks after one "hit" of the drug. Seizures, coma, and death may occur.

PREVENTION OF ILLEGAL DRUG USE

While enforcement of anti-drug laws, in this country and abroad, is necessary and accounts for the largest portion of federal expenditures in this area, enforcement alone will not solve the nation's drug problem. In recent years, increasing attention has been paid to the prevention of illegal drug use through the reduction of demand, by users, for illicit substances. Demand reduction requires different messages and strategies to maintain non-use or to discourage use among different population groups. Recognizing this, the Prevention and Health Coordinating Committee of the National Drug Policy Board, the entity established by President Reagan to oversee all federal anti-drug activities, has segmented users and potential users on the basis of age and "accessibility" to preventive interventions, measured by one's extent of risk for, or actual, drug-taking behavior.

The model employed for this purpose thus may be conceptualized as a two-by-two matrix consisting of "easy" and "hard-to-reach" groups and "young" and "older" persons.

- For easy/young and easy/older target audiences, for whom the primary problem is drugs, per se, preventive strategies focus on education and clearly articulated "no use" school and work-place policies. Also effective is the notion that the user will be held accountable for disregarding strictures against use. These groups comprise the vast majority of the U.S. population, do not use drugs for the most part, and are well-positioned to influence and otherwise help others avoid drug use.

- "Hard-to-reach" groups, young and older, are characterized by confounding, serious underlying problems and factors that exist along with drug use. Among youth, factors typical of adolescence—e.g., immaturity, curiosity, willingness to take risks, and need for peer acceptance—may be compounded by problems of truancy, delinquency, familial discord, early sexual activity, and other risk factors. Individuals falling within the older/hard group are subject to a variety of co-morbidity factors, such as psychiatric disorders, illiteracy, poverty, and lack of skills; they are at high risk for criminal involvement, as well as for severe physical illness, including AIDS incurred through IV needle-sharing.

In contrast to enforcement efforts, strategies to reduce demand are not typically a federal responsibility. The challenge is to mobilize local organizations and individuals committed to making drug use unacceptable.

LEGISLATION AND FUNDING

Warning that in the absence of efforts to eliminate drug abuse, the nation risks "losing a great part of a whole generation," President Reagan has assigned high priority to the national anti-drug program.[7] In August 1986, he launched a national campaign against drug abuse, outlining six specific goals:

1. drug-free work places for all Americans;
2. drug-free schools, from elementary to university level;
3. expanded treatment for drug abusers;
4. improved international cooperation to cut off the production and transport of illegal drugs;
5. strengthened drug law enforcement; and
6. public awareness and prevention.

In response to the President's proposal, Congress enacted the Anti-drug Abuse Act of 1986 (PL 99-570), which authorized $1.7 billion in FY 1987 for a sweeping new program to reduce both the demand, for and the supply, of drugs.

With $163 million of these funds, the Alcohol, Drug Abuse, and Mental Health Administration (ADAMHA) awarded a new Alcohol and Drug Treatment and Rehabilitation block grant to each state to expand the availability of treatment resources.

The law also directed that an Office for Substance Abuse Prevention (OSAP) be established in ADAMHA to provide national leadership to prevent alcohol and other drug problems through public education; support of public, private, and community-sponsored prevention activities; and intervention demonstration programs targeted at high-risk youth.

In 1987, OSAP, in cooperation with the National Institute on Alcohol Abuse and Alcoholism, launched a multi-media campaign—"Be Smart! Don't Start! - Just

Say "No"—directed at youth eight to 12 years old, and involving all 50 states. The campaign was developed in partnership with parent and community groups, business, industry, and state and local governments.

OSAP also operates the National Clearinghouse for Alcohol and Drug Information (NCADI), formed through a merger of the former National Clearinghouse for Alcohol Information and the National Clearing house for Drug Abuse Information. NCADI provides printed and audiovisual materials, reference and referral services, and state clearinghouse network support. NCADI can be reached at P.O. Box 2345, Rockville, MD 20852.

CONCLUSION

The role of MCH workers in controlling the illegal use of drugs is one of the most critical issues affecting the health of America's children and families. Sustained effort will be needed to correct the nation's problem with illegal drug use. Much of the necessary impetus for such efforts now exists, and a variety of methods are being utilized to encourage, assist, and promote attitudes intolerant of illegal drug use. One, for example, is work-place drug testing; broad public support of these programs is evidence of a growing social consensus regarding the severity of the problem and the necessity of intervention. In the future, continued government efforts, paired with increased awareness of, and cooperation on the part of, parents, professionals, communities, and state and local governments ultimately will yield drug-free schools, communities, and work places to the benefit of today's youth and all future generations.

REFERENCES

1. Johnston LD, O'Malley PM, Bachman JG. Drug use among American high school students, college students, and other young adults, national trends through 1985. DHHS Publication No. (ADM) 86-1450. Washington, DC: US Government Printing Office, 1986.

2. Macdonald DI. Prevention of adolescent smoking and drug use. Pediatric Clin NA 33(3):995-1005, 1986.

3. Johnston LD, Bachman JG, O'Malley PM. 12th Annual high school senior survey. Ann Arbor: University of Michigan, Institute for Social Research, 1987.

4. Tye R. "R.J. Reynolds targets teens with sophisticated marketing campaign. In Tobacco and Youth Reporter, 2(1):1, Summer, 1987. Article cites data gathered through the "Health Information Survey, 1978-1980, compilations. National Center for Health Statistics, U.S. Public Health Service, Department of Health and Human Services.

5. Rounsaville B, Weissman MM, Wilber CH, et al. Pathways to opiate addiction: An evaluation of differing antecedents. Br J Psychiatry 141:437-446,1982.

6. O'Malley PM, Johnston LD. Cocaine use among American adolescents and young adults. National Institute on Drug Abuse, 1985.

7. National Strategy for Prevention of Drug Abuse and Drug Trafficking: Washington, DC: U.S. Government Printing Office, 1984.

SUICIDE AND HOMOCIDE*

41

Patrick W. O'Carroll and Jack C. Smith

The scope and definition of maternal and child health (MCH) services have evolved and grown, just as the scope and definition of public health itself have evolved and grown. Traditionally, efforts to ensure optimal MCH have gone beyond the provision of personal health services to include social and environmental health considerations as well.[1] In pursuit of the goal of healthy mothers and children, MCH professionals must now draw on this tradition to face other threats to the health of mothers and children: suicide and homicide, and their morbid counterparts, attempted suicide and nonfatal injuries from assault.

Suicide is not a new problem, but its prevention among the young has become increasingly urgent. Although suicide rates among persons 35 years of age and older generally declined from 1950 to 1980,[2] the suicide rate among persons 15-to-19-years of age more than tripled during the same period.[3] Suicide rates are much higher among 15-to-19 year olds than among younger children, but marked increases in the rate of suicide have also been reported for those 10-to-14 years of age; from 1960 to 1984, the suicide rate doubled for males and tripled for females in this age category.[4,5] At present, we do not know what factors are responsible for these trends.

---

* Note that homicide is considered in this chapter as a cause of death, not as a criminal act. In this context, the homicide rate denotes the rate of death from homicide—that is, the rate of homicide victimization, expressed as the number of homicide deaths per 100,000 persons at risk.

Likewise, homicide as a cause of death among children is not new, but only recently have public health professionals recognized the legitimacy of addressing homicide as a health (as opposed to a criminal justice) problem. Although homicide rates* are typically highest among persons 20-to-44 years of age, the rates of homicide victimization among children and adolescents have increased alarmingly in the past 25 years. From 1960 to 1984, homicide rates among both males and females increased in every childhood age category.[4,5] Partly because of these increases in the homicide rate, and partly because of success in decreasing childhood mortality from other causes, homicide has steadily climbed the list of leading causes of death in childhood. In 1980, homicide was the second leading cause of death among persons 15-to-24 years of age and the fourth leading cause of death among children one-to-14 years of age. [2] Among Blacks, homicide is actually the leading cause of death for those 15-to-24 years of age and the third leading cause of death for children one-to-14 years of age.[6]

In this chapter, we will describe the extent and nature of suicide and homicide among children and adolescents, with reference to MCH where appropriate. We will also discuss present obstacles to prevention, as well as the potential role of MCH professionals in preventing suicide and homicide. By reviewing the epidemiology of suicide and homicide, we hope to encourage MCH professionals at all levels to consider the prevention of these violent and tragic deaths as an appropriate part of their mission.

SUICIDE

THE EXTENT OF THE PROBLEM

It is generally agreed that a child less than five years of age cannot commit suicide, although the age at which a child understands the finality of death and the implications of suicide certainly varies from child to child.[7,8] In any case, the rate of suicide is very low during early childhood and does not really increase significantly until after age ten. After the first decade of life, age-specific suicide rates climb dramatically, increasing a hundredfold during the course of the teenage years (Table 1). For the period 1980 to 1984, the average annual suicide rate for 19-year olds was 12.8 per 100,000,** which was higher than the total suicide rate for all ages in 1982 (12.2). Furthermore, although suicide rates generally increase throughout life, the steep increase during the teenage years is such that, by age 19, the suicide rate has risen to almost 70 percent of its maximum lifetime level.

** Average annual rates for single-year-of-age are calculated by the following: 1) summing the deaths for persons of that age during the five-year period 1980 to 1984; 2) dividing this sum by five to get the average annual number of deaths for that age; and then 3) dividing by the population of that age in 1982, the middle year of the five-year period. This procedure lends stability to rates for single-years-of-age.

After age ten, male suicide rates are greater than female rates at every age, a pattern that continues throughout life but which is especially strong during adolescence and young adulthood (Figure 1). Male suicide rates are from three to five times greater than female suicide rate during the teenage years. A racial pattern also emerges during the teenage years and also persists throughout life: white suicide rates are consistently 1.5 to two times greater than Black suicide rates. Rates for non-Black minorities are generally quite similar to rates for Blacks.

The methods by which suicide is committed vary by age during the teenage years. Among ten-to-12-year olds, more than half (55.9 percent) of the victims commit suicide by hanging. With advancing age, however, firearms increasingly be-

TABLE 1

AVERAGE ANNUAL SUICIDE AND HOMICIDE RATES* FOR PERSONS 0-19 YEARS OF AGE, BY SEX AND SINGLE YEAR OF AGE UNITED STATES, 1980-1984

	Suicide			Homicide		
Age	Male	Female	Both	Male	Female	Both
0	–	–	–	6.24	5.76	6.01
1	–	–	–	4.08	3.26	3.68
2	–	–	–	3.17	2.70	2.94
3	–	–	–	1.60	1.98	1.79
4	–	–	–	1.68	1.30	1.50
5	0.01	0.01	0.01	1.24	1.24	1.24
6	0.04	0.01	0.03	1.08	0.86	0.97
7	0.02	0.03	0.02	0.92	0.92	0.92
8	0.05	0.00	0.03	0.85	0.98	0.91
9	0.13	0.01	0.07	0.83	0.77	0.80
10	0.22	0.00	0.11	0.97	0.85	0.91
11	0.51	0.10	0.31	0.91	0.88	0.89
12	1.07	0.28	0.68	1.21	0.98	1.10
13	2.16	0.57	1.39	1.58	1.46	1.52
14	3.63	1.51	2.59	3.07	2.04	2.57
15	5.93	2.08	4.04	5.52	2.78	4.18
16	10.03	2.83	6.51	8.80	3.36	6.14
17	13.97	3.29	8.75	13.94	4.16	9.16
18	17.70	3.36	10.64	19.15	5.72	12.54
19	20.79	4.69	12.79	21.65	6.10	13.92

SOURCE: National Center for Health Statistics detailed mortality tapes, and U.S. Bureau of the Census Current Population Reports.

* Rates per 100,000 population.

come the preferred method of suicide. The proportion of suicides committed with firearms increases from 30 percent at age ten to over 60 percent by age 19. This pattern is somewhat more pronounced for male than female adolescents.

TRENDS

As noted previously, suicide rates among teenagers increased markedly in the 25-year period of 1960 to 1984 (Table 2). The suicide rate doubled among males ten-to-14 years of age and among males and females 15-to-19 years of age. Among females ten-to-14 years of age, the suicide rate increased threefold. The magnitude of the suicide rates in these age groups is quite low when compared with rates during later life. Nevertheless, as Table 2 indicates, this trend of increasing suicide rates is quite consistent from one period to the next, and thus merits concern.

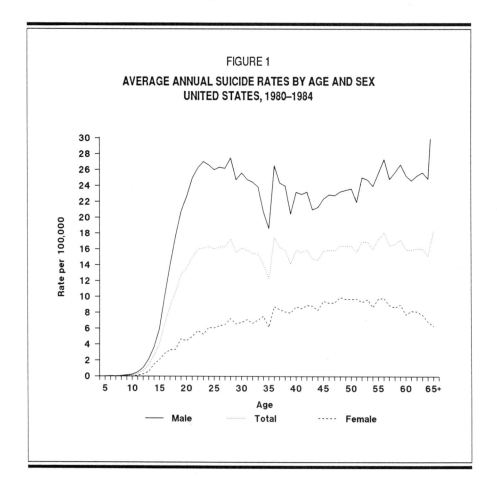

FIGURE 1

AVERAGE ANNUAL SUICIDE RATES BY AGE AND SEX
UNITED STATES, 1980–1984

TABLE 2

SUICIDE AND HOMICIDE RATES* FOR PERSONS 0-19 YEARS OF AGE, BY AGE GROUP AND SEX FOR VARIOUS YEARS, UNITED STATES, 1960-1984

SUICIDE

Both Sexes Age Group	1960	1965	1970	1975	1980	1984
<1	—	—	—	—	—	—
1-4	—	—	—	—	—	—
5-9	0.0	0.0	0.0	—	0.0	0.0
10-14	0.5	0.5	0.6	0.8	0.8	1.3
15-19	3.6	4.0	5.9	7.6	8.5	9.0

Males Age Group	1960	1965	1970	1975	1980	1984
<1	—	—	—	—	—	—
1-4	—	—	—	—	—	—
5-9	0.0	—	0.0	—	0.0	0.1
10-14	0.9	0.9	0.9	1.2	1.2	1.9
15-19	5.6	6.1	8.8	12.2	13.8	14.3

Females Age Group	1960	1965	1970	1975	1980	1984
<1	—	—	—	—	—	—
1-4	—	—	—	—	—	—
5-9	0.0	0.0	—	—	—	0.0
10-14	0.2	0.2	0.3	0.4	0.3	0.6
15-19	1.6	1.9	2.9	2.9	3.0	3.5

HOMICIDE

Both Sexes Age Group	1960	1965	1970	1975	1980	1984
<1	4.8	5.5	4.3	5.8	5.9	6.5
1-4	0.7	1.1	1.9	2.5	2.5	2.4
5-9	0.4	0.6	0.6	0.8	0.9	0.9
10-14	0.5	0.7	1.2	1.2	1.4	1.6
15-19	4.0	4.3	8.1	9.6	10.6	8.3

Males Age Group	1960	1965	1970	1975	1980	1984
<1	4.7	6.2	4.5	6.3	6.3	7.2
1-4	4.7	6.2	4.5	6.3	6.3	7.2
5-9	0.4	0.6	0.6	0.7	0.9	0.8
10-14	0.7	0.9	1.5	1.4	1.6	1.7
15-19	6.1	6.5	12.8	13.9	16.2	12.3

Females Age Group	1960	1965	1970	1975	1980	1984
<1	4.9	2.6	4.1	4.9	5.6	5.8
1-4	0.7	4.8	1.9	2.0	2.2	2.4
5-9	0.4	1.1	0.6	0.9	0.9	1.0
10-14	0.4	0.6	0.9	1.0	1.3	1.5
15-19	1.9	0.4	3.2	4.9	4.9	4.2

SOURCE: Vital Statistics of the Untied States, Vol II - Mortality (various years).
*Rates per 1000,000 population.

There have also been trends, over time, in the methods of suicide. Among teenagers 15-to-19 years of age, there has been a steady increase in the proportion of suicides committed with firearms. In 1970, 47.9 percent of all suicides in this age group were committed with firearms. By 1980, this proportion had increased to 63.3 percent.[3] The same pattern was noted for both males and females, but the increasing proportion of firearm suicides was most evident for females. In 1970, only a third (34.2 percent) of suicides among females aged 15 to 24 were committed with firearms. By 1980, over half (55.7 percent) of these suicides were committed with firearms.

MATERNAL HEALTH CONSIDERATIONS

In 1983, suicide was the fourth leading cause of death for women 15 to 44 years of age. For this reason alone, one might add suicide prevention to the list of appropriate maternal health services. But there are particular reasons why suicide prevention efforts should be considered for pregnant women and new mothers. For example, it has been estimated that 20 percent to 40 percent of all women may experience emotional or cognitive disorders in the early postpartum period.[9] It is only reasonable to assume that, during the postpartum period, women may be at increased risk of suicide or attempted suicide compared with women in the same age group who are not in the postpartum period. Further, it may be appropriate to inquire about thoughts of suicide with pregnant women or new mothers who appear to be having any emotional difficulty during this stressful period of life.

PAST APPROACHES TO PREVENTION

For many years, the typical suicide victim was an older, depressed white male. It was reasoned, therefore, that doing a better job of diagnosing and treating depression was the most appropriate way to prevent suicide. This may well have been true, and the decreases that have been recorded in the suicide rates of persons in older age groups may be due in part to this approach. Unfortunately, it does not appear that this strategy is as appropriate for preventing suicide among the young.[10] Depression, as clinically defined by psychiatrists, remains an important risk factor for suicide in this age group. However, suicides attributable to clinical depression seem to account for a much lower proportion of suicide among the young than among persons in older age groups.[11] New approaches to identifying adolescents at high risk of suicide are urgently needed, and a great deal of research is under way in an effort to identify and evaluate the importance of a number of putative risk factors.

Other approaches to suicide prevention are based on the notion that many suicides could be prevented if suicidal individuals just had someone to talk to. Suicide crisis centers and suicide hot lines represent two logical manifestations of this reasoning. Despite the intuitive appeal of these approaches, however, there is very little scientific evidence demonstrating their effectiveness. It may be that hot lines and crisis centers are used primarily by those who would have attempted—but not completed—suicide, whereas those intent on committing suicide eschew these potential avenues of aid. Evaluating crisis centers, hot lines, and other intervention modalities is another urgent priority for suicide prevention research.

OBSTACLES TO PREVENTION

One of the most fundamental theoretical obstacles to suicide prevention is the validity, or lack thereof, of the data used to calculate the magnitude and trends of suicide rates.[12] It is widely recognized that many suicide deaths are misclassified by coroners and medical examiners, usually as deaths due to unintentional injuries ("accidents").[13,14] It is not clear, however, what proportion of all suicide deaths are so misclassified. It is generally believed that the magnitude of misclassification is not such that it threatens the validity of conclusions drawn from general analyses of existing suicide data.[15] Nevertheless, various social, religious, financial, and political factors may make coroners and medical examiners reticent to arrive at a determination of suicide in equivocal cases. These factors may be especially influential in cases of suicide among children and adolescents. In response to these concerns, a group of individuals from an array of professional organizations related to death certification has developed Operational Criteria for the Determination of Suicide.[16] It is hoped that the use of these criteria during the investigations of equivocal deaths will increase the validity of suicide mortality data.

Another difficulty in preventing suicide among the young is that our knowledge of risk factors for suicide for this group is quite limited. Many potential risk factors have been suggested,[17] including mobility, coming from a broken family, substance abuse, and depression and other mental illness. Unfortunately, very few of these potential risk factors have been confirmed in studies where suicide cases have been compared with a control population. If we are able to identify risk factors that distinguish young persons at high risk of suicide from all other persons, these comparisons must be rigorously performed. In other words, it is of little use in focusing suicide prevention resources to say that most teenaged suicide victims have had problems in school, with their parents, or with that girl friend/boy friend. Such a description might fit most teenagers.

It is well-documented, however, that persons who have attempted suicide once are more likely than others both to attempt suicide again and to complete suicide.[18,19,20] This risk factor—history of a past suicide attempt—might be very useful in bringing those at high risk of suicide in touch with existing suicide prevention resources. For example, a system for identifying suicide attempters might be established in emergency rooms. These individuals could then be referred for special counseling and could be advised of the resources available in their community (hot lines, crisis centers, etc.). At present, most communities are doing very little to systematically identify and refer suicide attempters, although such a system represents a logical and appropriate first step in maximizing the effectiveness of existing prevention activities.

Focusing resources on suicide attempters raises an issue that has yet to be resolved: the relationship between suicide attempters and suicide completers. It appears that these two groups are composed of different, but overlapping, populations. In other words, not all suicide attempters go on to complete suicide, but many suicide victims have had previous suicide attempts. From a prevention standpoint, however, this is a moot point. Attempted suicide is an injury event that should be prevented in its own right. Moreover, attempted suicide may be an indicator of other problems that need to be addressed, such as alcoholism, depression, spouse abuse, or child abuse.

The most formidable obstacle to suicide prevention may well be the prevailing assumption among many health professionals that either nothing can be done to prevent suicide (except perhaps among those presently suicidal) or that suicide prevention can only be accomplished by mental health professionals. There is no reason to accept either assumption; indeed, the experiences of MCH professionals with past, seemingly intractable problems, would argue otherwise. A substantial reduction in mortality from infantile diarrhea, for example, has been accomplished in many places, largely through providing clean water and educating mothers about proper techniques for countering dehydration in their children. Suicide may not yield as readily to such social and environmental interventions, but it would be uncharacteristically fatalistic for public health professionals to presume form the outset that nothing can be done in this regard to prevent suicide.

HOMICIDE

THE EXTENT OF THE PROBLEM

Unlike suicide, children of all ages can and do die from homicide. Indeed, homicide victimization rates are quite high during the first year of life. Rates then decline with increasing age until about age ten, when the homicide rate rises precipitously (Table 1). During the teen years, the homicide rate increases by a factor of 15. By age 19, the homicide rate for both males and females has risen to at least 75 percent of its maximum lifetime level. Unlike suicide rates, homicide rates peak during the third or fourth decade of life, and then decline with increasing age (Figure 2).

After the first decade of life, male homicide rates are greater than female rates at every age. By age 19, male rates are more than 3.5 times greater than female rates. Another consistent pattern emerges when homicide rates are examined by the race of the victim. At every age, Blacks are at much higher risk of death from homicide than whites (Figure 2). During the first few years of life and during the teen years, the rates of homicide among Blacks are about four times greater than those among whites.

The weapons with which homicide victims are killed vary with age. Over half of all children two years of age and younger are killed by assailants using "personal weapons," that is, by blows with hands or feet. [21] As with suicide, the proportion of child firearm homicide deaths increases steadily with age. By age 11, more than half of the victims are killed with firearms; by age 17, more than two-thirds of the victims are killed with firearms.

The relationship between the victim and the assailant also varies with age. Most homicide victims less than age three are killed by family members. This pro-

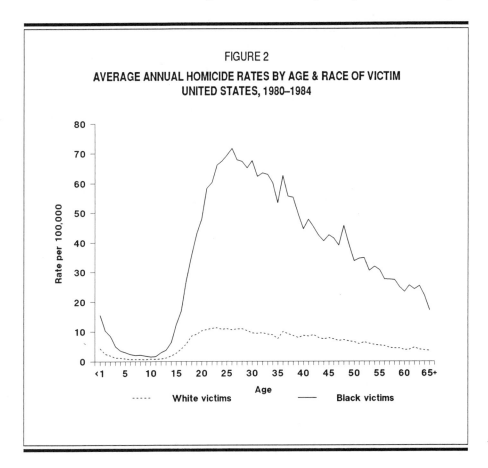

FIGURE 2

AVERAGE ANNUAL HOMICIDE RATES BY AGE & RACE OF VICTIM
UNITED STATES, 1980–1984

portion decreases with age until, by age 19, family homicides account for less than ten percent of the total. During the first decade of life, about 20 percent of all homicide victims are killed by acquaintances; during adolescence, this proportion increases to about 40 percent. Only a minority of childhood homicide victims are killed by strangers.

Homicides may also be considered according to the circumstances under which they occur. In other words, homicides committed during the perpetration of other felony crimes (e.g., robbery or rape) may be considered separately from non-felony-associated homicides that occur in the context of an argument or fight. The highest proportion of non-felony-associated homicides is seen among children less than three years of age (about 70 percent). After age three, non-felony-associated homicides account for 40 percent to 60 percent of all homicides.

TRENDS

Homicide rates among persons less than 20 years of age have increased fairly steadily during the past 25 years (Table 2). This increase has occurred among both males and females. Increases in the homicide rates, over time, are relatively more pronounced for whites than Blacks. This pattern of increasing homicide rates for persons less than 20 years of age may be compared to that for the population as a whole. From 1970 to 1983, overall Black homicide rates decreased by 21 percent, while white homicide rates increased by 30 percent.

MATERNAL HEALTH CONSIDERATIONS

Homicide is considered by many to be primarily a "male" problem. This is not the case. The homicide rate for Black females is in fact higher than that for white males in all age groups less than 50 years of age.[22] Moreover, there are indications that pregnancy may be a time when women are at particularly high risk of battering.[23] In addition to the obvious physical and mental suffering caused by such assaults, spontaneous abortions and miscarriages are reportedly increased among battered women.[24] One of the most important risk factors for battering during pregnancy is being previously battered. This raises the question of whether pregnancy is a risk factor for battering or whether women who are repeatedly battered simply continue to be victimized during pregnancy. Further study is needed to clarify this issue. In the meantime, we should make every effort to identify battered women—pregnant or otherwise—who come into contact with the health care system and to help them take whatever steps are necessary to prevent any further abuse.

PAST APPROACHES TO PREVENTION

Homicide has traditionally been considered a criminal justice problem. For this reason, the focus for prevention has been on the assailant, not the victim. The mechanisms of homicide prevention under this approach are deterrence (the threat of imprisonment) and incapacitation (imprisonment, per se). To a large extent, these mechanisms are designed to prevent criminal homicide—that is, premeditated homicide or homicide committed during the commission of some other felony crime (such as robbery or rape). Such an approach has, of course, proved woefully inadequate for dealing with the types of childhood homicide that we have described. The root causes of these tragic details are social and environmental, not criminal, and thus it is no surprise that sanctions designed to punish and incapacitate criminals have not been effective in preventing family and acquaintance homicide.

We are not suggesting that public health interventions must be directed only toward victims. Indeed, homicide among infants and young children can only be prevented by intervening with the parents or others who care for the child. For these homicides, we must find ways to help parents "at risk" of hurting or killing their children find a way to avoid such tragedies. Our efforts in this regard have centered on better identifying nonfatal child abuse and intervening so as to prevent further abuse. Unfortunately, this strategy is easier to describe than it is to carry out. For many reasons, physicians and other health personnel are still reticent to diagnose child abuse except in obvious cases, and most health professionals are not adequately trained to make such a diagnosis in subtle cases. As to intervening to prevent further abuse, what constitutes the "best" intervention is still hotly debated. Careful evaluation of the intervention strategies being employed in different areas of the country is urgently needed.

On the other hand, for homicides among adolescents, as with so many other health problems, victims must share in the responsibility for their own health. We do not mean to say, of course, that homicide victims are to blame for their own deaths, if by this it is meant that the assailant is somehow exonerated of responsibility. Rather, we suggest that the distinction between homicide victim and assailant is not a particularly productive one for many homicides committed by family members or acquaintances. When two adolescents engage in a physical fight, for example, who becomes the victim and who the assailant is based on the outcome—not on the distinction of who was "to blame" for the fight. That distinction, again, derives from a criminal justice point of view that one party must be responsible for the assault and that the other party must be an innocent victim. In fact, there must be many such altercations for which the combatants are mutually responsible, and where action—or inaction—on the part of either person might have defused the situation. As public health professionals, we must discover what techniques can be used by adolescents and others to avoid situations where they are at risk of either dying from, or committing, homicide and to prevent the escalation of minor arguments into homicidal violence. We must also find ways to teach these techniques to our children.

OBSTACLES TO PREVENTION

The main obstacle to public health efforts to prevent homicide and assaultive violence is the prevailing belief that homicides are committed by criminals in the course of their criminal activities. Clearly this is not the case. An equally discouraging belief holds that even if some portion of the homicide problem is not criminal in nature, nothing can be done to prevent such homicides short of a radical alteration in society itself. This belief stems from the conclusion that the root causes of homicide are often social and environmental in nature. This latter point is certainly true, but as we indicated above for suicide, it is no reason for discouragement. Certainly many things short of radical societal changes might be done to prevent homicide.

A more technical obstacle to homicide prevention is our ignorance of specific risk factors for victimization at the individual level. Risk factors suggested by past research include poverty,[25] the experience of racism and discrimination,[26] and a subculture of violence.[27] Much of the research supporting these risk factors has been done at the aggregate level. Studies are needed at the individual level to identify those specific mechanisms that increase the risk of homicide victimization and that are potentially subject to preventive interventions.

THE ROLE FOR MCH PROFESSIONALS IN PREVENTING SUICIDE AND HOMICIDE

The causes of suicide and homicide are clearly multifaceted, and neither of these public health problems is likely to be solved by any single approach or any single discipline. But this has been true of many causes of childhood mortality and morbidity. Indeed, because MCH professionals have traditionally addressed the health problems of mothers and children through a multidisciplinary approach, they are uniquely prepared to address the problems of suicide and homicide among the young. A further strength of the MCH approach lies in its tradition of health promotion at the social, environmental, and cultural levels, as well as through the provision of personal health services. Finally, MCH professionals are trained to recognize and address childhood behavioral problems during their early—and potentially modifiable—stages. Addressing such problems during early childhood may well be among the most effective approaches to the primary prevention of homicide and suicide later in life.

A number of potential avenues for intervention are suggested by the previous review of the epidemiology of suicide and homicide among the young; some have already been alluded to. For example, that most homicides occur among acquaintances in the course of arguments suggests that the participants probably do not anticipate the possibility of a lethal outcome to such confrontations. Educating adolescents to the potential lethality of such conflicts may prevent some homicides, while teaching appropriate conflict resolution skills may prevent others. The pattern of weapon use for both suicide and homicide also suggests some possible intervention strategies. The ready availability of lethal weapons, such as handguns, may be the final ingredient that turns an impulsive decision to harm oneself or another into an irrevocable tragedy. There are clearly contentious political, as well as public health, dimensions to any consideration of limiting access to firearms. Nevertheless, this should not prevent us from exploring the hypothesis that the ready availability of lethal weapons increases the risk of suicide and homicide. Careful scientific research in this regard is necessary if we are to advocate any such interventions.[28]

But what role, in particular, can MCH professionals play in preventing homicide and suicide? There are several possibilities. One important role would obviously be the identification, proper treatment, and referral of those who are currently suicidal or at risk of assaultive injury (e.g., victims of child abuse). But MCH professionals should also seek to address patterns of behavior early in a child's development that might later put that child at increased risk of death from suicide or homicide. Withdrawn children might be helped to share their feelings with others, for example, and combative children might be taught more appropriate ways to resolve conflicts.

MCH professionals might also actively explore attitudes and beliefs regarding suicide with adolescents and their parents. Many may not know or believe that occasional thoughts of, or impulses toward, suicide are normal—and transient. Such assurances may increase the chances of communication between parents and adolescents, should suicidal feelings arise. Similarly, both parents and adolescents, should be alerted to the risks attendant to seemingly trivial altercations. Both must be informed that whether one should respond to violence with more violence is not simply an ethical issue but a health issue as well. Finally, we should educate parents about simple environmental modifications that may decrease the likelihood of homicide or suicide. Potentially lethal doses of medications should not be readily available to adolescents, especially if they appear depressed. Similarly, if firearms are present in the home, they might be stored in such a manner that they are not immediately accessible in the event of an impulsive wish to die or kill.

Clearly, none of the aforementioned measures will prevent all suicides or homicides. We are still a long way from being able to prescribe proven preventive interventions for either suicide or homicide. Nevertheless, MCH professionals cannot and should not ignore these important causes of injury and death among the population whose health they are dedicated to improving. In the absence of definitive answers, we should do whatever seems reasonable and appropriate to prevent these violent deaths. In the meantime, it is reassuring to consider that progress has been made in recognizing suicide and homicide as public health problems. The inclusion of a chapter on suicide and homicide in this textbook is evidence to that effect.

REFERENCES

1. Haggerty RJ, Darney PE. Maternal and child health services. In: Last, JM, ed. Maxcy-Rosenau Public health and preventive medicine. 11th ed. New York: Appleton-Century-Crofts, 1984, pp 1753-86.

2. Centers for Disease Control: Suicide surveillance, 1970-1980. Atlanta: Centers for Disease Control, April 1985.

3. Centers for Disease Control: Youth suicide in the United States, 1970-1980. Atlanta: Centers for Disease Control, November 1986.

4. U.S. Department of Health, Education and Welfare, Public Health Service: Vital Statistics of the United States, 1960. Vol. II - Mortality, Part A, Washington, D.C.: U.S. Government Printing Office, 1963.

5. National Center for Health Statistics: Unpublished final data. U.S. Department of Health and Human Services, Public Health Service, National Center for Health Statistics, Hyattsville, Maryland.

6. Centers for Disease Control: Homicide surveillance: high risk racial and ethnic groups - Blacks and Hispanics, 1970 to 1983. Atlanta: November 1986.

7. Paulson MJ, Stone D, Sposto R. Suicide potential and behavior in children ages 4 to 12. Suicide and Life-Threatening Behavior 8(4):225-69, 1978.

8. Rosenthal PA, Rosenthal S. Suicide among preschoolers: fact or fallacy. Children Today 12(6):22-4,1983.

9. Freedman AM, Kaplan HI, Sadock BJ. Modern synopsis of comprehensive textbook of psychiatry/II. 2nd ed. Baltimore: Williams and Wilkins, 1976, pp 523-525.

10. Eisenberg L. Adolescent suicide: on taking arms against a sea of troubles. Pediatrics 66:315-20, 1980.

11. Shaffer D, Gould MS, Phillips D, Stanley M, Trautman T. Developments in teen suicide research. Presented at the 33rd Annual Meeting of the American Academy of Child Psychiatry, Los Angeles, California, October 1986.

12. Hopper K, Guttmacher S. Rethinking suicide: notes toward a critical epidemiology. International Journal of Health Services 9(3),1979.

13. Sainsbury P. Validity and reliability of trends in suicide statistics. World Health Statistics Quarterly 36:339-48, 1983.

14. Litman LE. Psychologic-psychiatric aspects in certifying modes of death. Journal of Forensic Sciences 13(1):46-54, 1968.

15. Sainsbury P, Jenkins JS. The accuracy of officially reported suicide statistics for purposes of epidemiologic research. Journal of Epidemiology and Community Health 36:43-8, 1982.

16. Rosenberg ML, Davidson LE, Smith JC, et al. Operational criteria for the determination of suicide. Journal of Forensic Sciences 1988, in press.

17. U.S. Department of Health and Human Services: Report of the Secretary's Task Force on Youth Suicide. Vol II: Risk factors for youth suicide. Washington, D.C.: U.S. Government Printing Office, in press, February 1988.

18. Tuckman J, Youngman MA. Suicide risk among persons attempting suicide. Public Health Reports 78:585-7, 1963.

19. Motto JA. Suicide attempts: a longitudinal view. Archives of General Psychiatry 13:516-20, 1965.

20. Dahlgren KG. Attempted suicides—35 years afterward. Suicide and Life-Threatening Behavior 7(2):75-9, 1977.

21. Federal Bureau of Investigation: Uniform crime report program, supplemental homicide master files, 1980 to 1984.

22. O'Carroll PW, Mercy JA. Patterns and recent trends in black homicide. In: Hawkins DF. ed. Homicide among Black Americans. Lanham, MD: University Press of America, pp 29-42, 1986.

23. Helton AS, McFarlane J, Anderson ET. Battered and pregnant: a prevalence study. American Journal of Public Health 77:1337-9, 1987.

24. Richwald GA, McCluskey TC. Family violence during pregnancy. In: Jelliffe DB, Jelliffe EFP, eds. Advances in international maternal and child health. Oxford: Clarendon Press, pp 87-96, 1985.

25. Flango VE, Sherbinou EL. Poverty, urbanization, and crime. Criminology 14:331-46, 1976.

26. University of California at Los Angeles, Centers for Disease Control: The epidemiology of homicide in the City of Los Angeles, 1970-79. Atlanta, GA: U.S. Department of Health and Human Services, August 1985.

27. Wolfgang ME, Ferracuti F. The subculture of violence: toward an integrated theory in criminology. London: Tavistock, 1967.

28. Wright JD, Rossi PH, Daly K. Under the gun: weapons, crime, and violence in America. New York: Aldine, 1983.

SECTION VI

CHILDREN
WITH
SPECIAL
NEEDS

DESCRIPTION OF THE POPULATION

42

Henry T. Ireys

The category of children with special needs encompasses infants, children, and adolescents with a wide range of disabilities, chronic illnesses, and sensory impairments. No precise boundaries can be drawn around this population, in part because the definition of "special need" varies with the purpose for classification. In this chapter, the category is understood to be far-reaching. Children with special needs—regardless of the particular diagnosis applied—constitute a group because their "specialness" places them and members of their family at risk for emotional distress and social isolation. This specialness has two particular consequences. First, the nature of the childrens' needs usually requires them to depend on health and education services to a far greater extent than children who have no such special needs; if these services are poorly organized or inadequate, then the child and family will face additional problems. Second, from the perspective of many communities, being special means being different. As a result, these families may be socially isolated and victims of unwarranted myths about chronic conditions. The application of a diagnostic label for the purposes of securing special services may have unfortunate mental health consequences for the child and family.

POPULATION ESTIMATES

Estimates of the number of children with disabilities and chronic illness have varied between one percent and 20 percent of the nation's children, depending on the particular definitions used, the measurement strategies, and the population under study. The lower estimates include only children with severe chronic illnesses, such as spina bifida or muscular dystrophy; these conditions are generally associated with high levels of functional impairment. The larger estimates of the rate of children with special needs are based on broader definitions of disability. For example, if the population is defined as those children identified by schools as handicapped under The Education for All Handicapped Children Act, then an estimate of 11 percent is typically cited as the prevalence rate for school-aged children. The highest estimates incorporate children with relatively mild functional impairments, such as uncomplicated asthma, minimal sensory deficits, or minimal emotional disturbance.[1,2]

A recent review of available evidence suggests that the *incidence* of children with chronic childhood disorders (i.e., the frequency of occurrence of these disorders in the general population) remained the same over the last several decades, but *prevalence* rates for many disorders (i.e., the number of children affected by the disease at any given time) are increasing. For example, one study found that the number of children with functional impairments has doubled over the past two decades.[3] The rise in prevalence rates can be attributed to several factors, including 1) enhanced survival of children who would have previously died at a young age, and 2) increased detection and labeling, at young ages, of children with relatively minor conditions that would have remained undetected or undiagnosed in earlier decades. Gortmaker and Sappenfield also note that most of the increase has already occurred and further increases are likely to be marginal.[2]

Some studies suggest that the increasing survival rates of low birthweight and very-low birthweight infants have contributed to higher prevalence of children with diverse kinds of developmental disabilities.[4] For low birthweight infants (i.e., infants born between 1500 and 2500 grams), prognosis for normal development appears to be excellent, with only minimally higher rates of chronic neurological or developmental problems, in comparison to children born at normal weights. Rates of severe impairment among *very*-low birthweight infants are estimated to be less than 20 percent. Furthermore, because the birth of a very-low birthweight infant is relatively rare in a given year (about 10 per 1000 births), improvements in neonatal survival rates will contribute in only a minor fashion to higher prevalence of children with special needs.[2]

EXTENT OF THE PROBLEM

Although children with special needs constitute a relatively small percentage of the nation's child population, they consume a disproportionately large percentage of the health and educational services provided to children. These services are provided through community institutions that are familiar to the general public—such as pediatrician's offices and local schools—and through special programs established by state and federal law.[5] The Education for All Handicapped Children

Act (PL 94-142), and its recent amendment (PL 99-457), are examples of national legislation that have sought to assure the availability of a free and appropriate education to children with special needs. The national program for Children With Special Health Care Needs is an example of health care legislation which seeks to assure that some of these children have access to needed medical care and related services.[6]

Despite these important legislative acts, the services available to these children and their families are frequently unavailable, poorly coordinated, and capricious in eligibility criteria. For example, with respect to the implementation of PL 94-142, Butler and Stenmark note, "The extent and pattern of compliance have varied substantially from state to state and school district to school district. Differences in part reflect the varying prevalence of handicapping conditions but more importantly a variety of other factors, such as lack of uniformity in identification and diagnostic procedures, differing approaches to the formulation of IEP's, differing conceptions of the 'least restrictive environment,' variations in the availability of services and placements, differing financial constraints on placement choices exercised by school districts, and different incentives to define children with minor problems as handicapped."[7] Access to special health care services through the program for Children With Special Health Care Needs is also known to be extremely variable, depending on such factors as residential location, family income, and the child's particular diagnosis.[6]

For children with special health care needs, the array of providers involved with the child and family may be quite large, depending on the child's condition. For example, a child with spina bifida may require the services of a neurologist, urologist, orthopedist, and physical therapist, in addition to a general pediatrician and social worker. When a child with a major health condition also requires special education services, the health and education teams must work together. The development of such interdisciplinary, inter-institutional collaboration has been extremely difficult.[8] Special problems also arise for children whose health condition does not interfere with learning but does require special services to be provided at school. These children need "related services," as defined under PL 94-142, but may not be in need of "special education." In many school districts, the only way to get the necessary services is to be classified as needing special education, a classification which itself may have undue negative consequences.[9]

In general, the problems raised by children with special needs have grown more urgent over the last several years. Parents have become more knowledgeable and insistent on having access to both educational and health services of high quality. As Lynch[10] notes about the area of special education, "Many parents have become exceedingly successful advocates and are taking roles of importance in the service delivery system." A similar trend can be found in the health care system as well.[11]

TRENDS IN SERVICES AND CARE

In 1987, the Surgeon General of the U.S. developed a report on children with special health care needs that established a national agenda for services to these children and their families.[12] This report emphasized family-centered, community-based, coordinated care, and suggested that the following elements should form the foundation of the system of care for these children:

- Recognition that the family is the constant in the child's life, while the service systems and personnel within those systems fluctuate.

- Facilitation of parent/professional collaboration at all levels of health care—care of an individual child; program development, implementation, and evaluation; and policy formation.

- Sharing of unbiased and complete information with parents about their child's care on an ongoing basis in a supportive manner.

- Implementation of comprehensive policies and programs that provide emotional and financial support to families.

- Recognition of family strengths and diversity, and respect for a variety of methods of coping.

- Encouragement of normal patterns of living in the home and community.

- Understanding and incorporation of the developmental needs of infants, children and adolescents, and their families into the health care delivery system.

- Encouragement and facilitation of parent-to-parent support.

- Assurance that the design of health care delivery systems is flexible, accessible and responsive to families.

The Surgeon General's report underscores several important trends in services and care for children with special health needs. These trends include enhanced communication among providers, increased emphasis on comprehensive care, and active incorporation of the family into health and education programs. Numerous demonstration projects have been supported by the Department of Education and the Bureau of Maternal and Child Health to investigate how these elements can be translated into workable programs.[12] Recently passed amendments to the Education for All Handicapped Children Act, contained in PL 99-457, mandate educational services for handicapped infants and toddlers, thereby bringing greater uniformity to previously disparate and uneven services throughout the states. This legislation also contains progressive guidelines for parent-provider partnerships, individualized family service and case management plans, and programs for public awareness.[13] To a great extent, future trends in services for children with special needs are embedded, in and will emerge from, the language and stipulations of PL 99-457.

Despite these promising efforts, other developments in the health and education fields bode poorly for children with special needs. Many school districts have witnessed a retrenchment in support for resources in special education, and in many quarters there is reluctance to implement PL 99-457 vigorously. Perennial efforts to assure minimum health services for all children and adolescents typically fail to account for the circumstances of children with special needs. Most health care arrangements, especially prepaid group practices and health maintenance organizations, have few incentives to provide the comprehensive, resource-intensive services that are required by children with complex health problems.[9] Furthermore, the current atmosphere of "crisis," regarding the nation's budget deficit, can easily serve to justify curtailment of programs that provide care to groups of children who are seen as marginal or potentially unproductive. No solace can be found in the promise of a change in the administration of the political affairs of this country; so-called "economic realities" can lead to powerful bipartisan arguments for misplaced efforts to balance a budget. The case for reduction in special programs can be made regardless of the political party in power. Hence, the need for advocacy for improved services for these children and their families is likely to remain strong.

ISSUES IN PRIMARY PREVENTION

For the purposes of this chapter, primary prevention efforts are conceptualized as falling into either of two categories: prevention of the occurrence of the conditions that give rise to a child's special needs; and prevention of the negative consequences of the condition, especially the negative consequences for the child's emotional development and for the family's well-being.

The simplest issue in preventing the occurrence of serious health or developmental problems involves the relatively few conditions that result from single gene mutations or defects. Under these circumstances, prevention is possible because parents who are known to be "carriers" of genes that result in children with specific defects can elect to have no children, or no further children. These choices are possible for such conditions as hemophilia, sickle cell anemia, or muscular dystrophy. In most instances, however, prospective estimates of risk for the occurrence of a defect in any given fetus are extremely difficult to make. Extraordinary progress in understanding the genetically based dysfunctions of many chronic health problems and developmental conditions has brought improved efficacy in the intrauterine detection of serious problems. For example, high levels of alpha-fetoprotein in amniotic fluid indicate the presence of major problems in the development of the fetus' spinal cord. The enhanced capacity to detect problems prenatally, and to terminate pregnancies that are likely to lead to the birth of a child with a defect, continues to provoke intense debate and suggests that this nation has yet to resolve the difficult ethical issues that biomedical technology has brought.

Many chronic impairments result, at least in part, from environmental causes. For example, motor-vehicle injuries leave many children and adolescents seriously impaired and in continuing need of special services. High levels of environmental toxins have also been implicated in increasing the rates of selected chronic health conditions. Thus, for these conditions, primary prevention depends on changes in the environment in which children live and grow.

For most conditions that give rise to a child's special needs—conditions such as learning disabilities, orthopedic problems, or asthma—primary prevention remains a distant possibility because the etiologic factors are unknown or rest on very complex interaction of genetic predisposition, environmental "triggers," and individual behavior. For these children, the prevention of negative mental health problems and family disruption becomes a compelling goal. Although most families and children appear to cope well with the presence of a serious health or developmental problem, they nevertheless face extraordinary stress and must deal with problems generally unknown to the broader public. In many instances, this stress can overwhelm available resources. Evidence from several studies suggests that rates of mental health problems are twice as high for children with serious health conditions. Other studies have documented higher rates of mental health problems among siblings and increased stress and tension between parents of a child with special needs. Prevention of these problems are likely to be successful if efforts can enhance the available supports for these children and families, promote effective responses to the challenges of raising or being a child with special needs, and build service programs that are serious in accounting for family life and child development.[9,14]

FUTURE NEEDS

Much has been accomplished in creating health and education programs for children with special needs and for their families, but many challenges remain ahead and new difficulties will surely arise. Children with AIDS, for example, represent a growing population whose needs will severely test the resources of many communities, schools, and health providers. The population of children with special needs and their families have suffered in part because relatively little is known about them. A comprehensive national data base is urgently needed, one that combines prevalence figures with information on service utilization, mental health status, and educational achievement.

Except for an occasional movie or front-page story, the general public remains largely uninformed about the extent of the problem and what might be effective solutions. The translation of available knowledge into effective policies and community-based programs that integrate these children and their families into ongoing community events is essential. To date, only modest attention has focused on the development of the older adolescent and young adult with special needs. Yet, as children with special needs grow into adolescence and face the tasks of adulthood, they may find few services responsive to their needs, few providers or employers willing to create a niche for them, and few communities that view them as valued members. Here again, more information about the issues and difficulties that they face is urgently needed.

REFERENCES

1. Butler J, Rosenbaum J, Palfrey J. Ensuring access to health care for children with disabilities. NEJM 317:162, 1987.

2. Gortmaker S, and Sappenfield W. Chronic childhood disorders: Prevalence and impact. Ped Clin of N Am, 31:3, 1984.

3. Newacheck P, Budetti P, and McManus P. Trends in childhood disability. AJPH, 74:232, 1984.

4. Ross G. Mortality and morbidity in very low birthweight infants. Ped Ann, 12(1):35, 1983.

5. Wallace HM. Organization and provisions of public programs. Handicapped Children and Youth. Edited by H. Wallace et al. New York, Human Sciences Press, 1987, pp 50-70.

6. Ireys H, Hauch R, and Perrin J. Variation among state crippled childrens service programs: Pluralism thrives. AJPH, 75:375, 1985.

7. Butler J, Stenmark S. Evaluating effects of P.L. 94-142. Working paper. Institute for Health Policy Studies, San Francisco, 1982.

8. Klerman L. Interprofessional issues in delivery services to chronically ill children and their families. Issues in the Care of Children with Chronic Illness. Edited by N Hobbs and J Perrin. San Francisco, Jossey Bass, 1985, pp. 420-440.

9. Hobbs N, Perrin J, and Ireys H. Chronically Ill Children and Their Families: Problems, Prospects, and Proposals from the Vanderbilt Study. San Francisco, Jossey Bass, 1985.

10. Lynch E. Special education. Handicapped Children and Youth. Edited by H. Wallace et al. New York, Human Sciences Press, 1987, pp. 213-222.

11. Shelton T, Jeppson F, and Johnson B. Family-centered care for children with special health care needs. Association for the Care of Children's Health, Washington, D.C., 1987.

12. Koop CE: Surgeon General's report on children with special health care needs. U.S. Department of Health and Human Services (HRS/D/MC 87-2), Washington, D.C., 1987.

13. Gilkerson L et al. Commenting on P.L. 99-457. Zero to Three, 7(3):13, 1987.

14. Stein R, Jessop D, and Ireys H. Prevention of emotional problems in children with chronic illness. Family In Transition: Primary Prevention Programs That Work. Edited by L. Bond, B. Wagner. Beverly Hills, Sage, 1987.

SYSTEMS OF CARE FOR CHILDREN WITH SPECIAL HEALTH CARE NEEDS 43

Allan C. Oglesby

Services to meet the needs of children with special health care problems and the needs of their family have developed in several major federally supported programs, state service agencies, private voluntary agencies, and the private health care system in the U.S.

Organized efforts began in the first-half of the twentieth century with voluntary health agencies and the passage by Congress, in 1935, of the Social Security Act, which established Crippled Children's Services. However, in the 1960s and 1970s there was evidence of increased public concern and national programs emerged to provide health, educational, and rehabilitation services for children with special health care needs.

PROGRAMS FOR CHILDREN
WITH SPECIAL HEALTH CARE NEEDS (CSHC)

These programs were formerly known as Crippled Children's Programs. They were started in the states when the Social Security Act was enacted in 1935. Title V, Part 2, provided federal funds to the states "to extend and improve" services for diagnosing, treating, and providing other needed care "for children who are crippled or who are suffering from conditions leading to crippling". The programs developed, using federal and state funds, with an emphasis on improving availability and accessibility of services, especially to children in rural areas. Each state defines the diagnostic and eligibility criteria for services within broad federal guidelines. The programs serve children from birth to 21 years of age.

The state programs for CSHC are located in state agencies. Sixty percent are in the state health agency, 20 percent are in broader state agencies that include the responsibility for public health, and 20 percent are in other state agencies (e.g., education, welfare, state university, and a commission).[1]

Federal funds were made available through "grants-in-aid" to the states until 1981, when the Omnibus Reconciliation Act created block grants to the states for Title V funds, giving the states more discretion in the expenditure. In 1987, the law was amended to change the Crippled Children's Program to Programs for Children with Special Health Care Needs.

Eligible conditions, while initially focused on orthopedic conditions and the residual effects of poliomyelitis, have gradually been expanded to include a variety of congenital anomalies, genetic conditions, chronic illnesses, and children dependent on newer technology and life-sustaining equipment. There is increasing concern with prevention and identification of children at risk for disabilities and handicapping conditions.

The programs from the early beginnings have emphasized comprehensive, multidisciplinary, quality care, and family support. Many of the programs have developed case management services which have been formalized and recognized in an amendment to the Title V legislation that defines case management. A recent survey showed that all but four state CSHC agencies provide case management or similar activities.[1]

Services are provided through clinics by the CSHC agency in most states. Some programs use vendors to provide care. Most agencies use a combination of direct services and vendors to meet the child's health care needs. There has been a growing trend under the MCH Block Grant to utilize other services, when feasible, through multiple funding, Medicaid reimbursements, third party payment, and interagency agreements. This has led to improved coordination of services, family support, and community participation in care plans. With rising cost of health care and declining funds available, services require the maximum use of resources, with elimination of overlaps and duplication in community-based programs.

Federal funds appropriated for FY 1987, for the MCH Block Grant, were $496.75 million, which include both the MCH and CSHC programs in this amount.

Children with special health care needs have received increasing attention at the national level, in the 1980s. As definitions have broadened, so has the concern for integration of resources through such approaches as case management. The Surgeon General's Report on Children with Special Health Care Needs,[2] in 1987, took a strong national position as reflected in the call for action by the Surgeon General. He stated:

I am asking:

FAMILIES - to actively participate in caring for their children and to help shape health care policy and programs.

STATES - to implement systems of care which support the strengths and needs of families, to assure the input of families at all levels of care, and to assure the adequate preparation of professionals for new collaborative roles.

PRIVATE HEALTH CARE PROVIDERS - to develop systems which meet the needs of families and which encourage their independence, by forging strong linkages between primary, secondary, and tertiary levels of care (physicians' offices, community health services, clinics, community hospitals, health maintenance organizations, children's hospitals, other teaching hospitals).

THE HEALTH CARE FINANCING SECTOR - to assure that all children with special health care needs have access to quality health care, and that support services are adequately funded to enable families to care for their children in their own homes and communities.

DEVELOPMENTAL DISABILITIES

Until the 1960s, services for persons with mental retardation were generally limited to state supported care, most often in institutions, and those provided by voluntary agencies. The federal Children's Bureau earmarked funds from Title V of the Social Security Act to develop a network of multidisciplinary diagnostic clinics in the states,, in the late 1950s. In 1963, Congress enacted amendments to the Social Security Act that were the first categorical program for the mentally retarded. The program was intended to stimulate the states to build community facilities, to construct facilities for research, and to build facilities in universities that would provide clinical services that would be used to train professional personnel to provide services to mentally retarded persons. Further amendments, in 1965, to the Social Security Act expanded these facilities by supporting personnel for research and training.

The Developmental Disabilities Services and Facilities Construction Amendments of 1970 brought a new emphasis on state planning and services. It provided for state Developmental Disability Councils to serve as planning bodies, and expanded the forces from mental retardation to include other developmental disabilities (DD), such as cerebral palsy, epilepsy, autism, and other neurological conditions that require similar long-term care and services. The Developmental Disabilities Assistance and Bill of Rights Act, enacted in 1973, provided a new and separate statutory base for services and changed the categorical definition to a functional one which expanded those eligible for services. Also, it provided for state Protective and Advocacy agencies and for demonstration projects to demonstrate new and more effective ways of providing care. The training programs continued as the University Affiliated Programs (UAF), for providing services that would be model programs and serve as a base for training professional personnel to work in an interdisciplinary approach. [3]

The overall purpose of this legislation is to assist the states in appropriate planning for DD persons, to assist in providing comprehensive services to DD persons, especially those whose needs are not met through other health, education, or welfare programs—to make grants to states and public or private agencies for model programs, to provide grants to states for the support of a system to protect the rights of all persons with DD, and to make grants of university-affiliated facilities for the administration and operation of model service programs and interdisciplinary training for personnel who will provide specialized services.

UAFs had their beginnings in the 1960s. Today they are organized nationally as the American Association of University Affiliated Program (AAUAP). There are 49 programs which operate at 55 sites throughout the U.S. Six do not receive any federal funding. Of those remaining, 35 are supported by the Administration on Developmental Disabilities; seven are satellites of these programs, and 21 receive funds from Title V through the Bureau of Maternal and Child Health.[3]

The programs of the UAFs serve the needs of the developmentally disabled populations through:

- interdisciplinary training of personnel,
- model comprehensive service program,
- Technical assistance and dissemination of information to the state, regional, and community service programs, and,
- Applied research in the prevention, diagnosis, treatment, management, and remediation of developmental disabilities.

In FY 1985, interdisciplinary training was provided for 10,137 trainees. A total of 62,421 individuals received services; of these, 46,186 were children.[3]

SPECIAL EDUCATION FOR HANDICAPPED CHILDREN

Educational services provided by state and local education agencies were permissive and not well-developed in the U.S. until the late 1970s. The Elementary and Secondary Education Act, which was enacted by Congress in 1965, provided federal funds to the states for a variety of services to children in school, including deaf-blind and handicapped children. This legislation set the scene for the Education of All Handicapped Children's Act, PL 94-142, which was passed in 1975.

This landmark federal legislation provided for a free, appropriate education for all handicapped children ages three through 18 years. It emphasized special education in "the least restrictive environment" and also provided for the development of an individualized education program (IEP) for each child, parent participation in the planning process, due process, and related services. The related services were those deemed necessary for the child to receive maximum benefit from the educational program, and included transportation, medical evaluation, and professional services related to psychology, counseling, occupational therapy, physical therapy, speech pathology, audiology, and recreational therapy.[4,5]

The Act required that the state education agency should attempt annually to identify and enroll all eligible children in the special education program.

The IEP must be updated annually to meet the changing needs for each child. The parents must agree with the IEP and sign-off on it. To protect the rights of each child, the family has the right to appeal if they do not agree. Independent persons were trained as hearing officers to assure due process in protecting the rights of the child and the parents. If children cannot be served appropriately in the school setting, they receive educational services in private school or institutions.

Federal funds were made available to assist the states in implementing the provisions of PL 94-142. The required services were initially focused on children of mandated school age, which in most states began at five or six years of age and ended at age 17 or 18 years. Trends have been for states to gradually extend special education to the three-to-five year olds and upward to 21 years of age. There have been increasing interests in programs for youths that are transitional from school age to adulthood, that go beyond vocational education and training. As the younger child has been included in educational services, the field of early childhood education has grown rapidly.

In 1986, PL 94-192 was amended by Congress with the enactment of PL 99-457, the Education of All Handicapped Children Amendments, which provides for early childhood developmental and educational services from birth to three years of age. This law requires that states develop coordinating councils will assure the maximum utilization of existing resources and develop new resources to serve the infant and younger child. The programs may be administered by an agency designated by the governor of the state. Many of these programs are in state health and social agencies, rather than in the state education agency.

VOLUNTARY HEALTH ORGANIZATIONS

Voluntary health organizations have developed in the U.S. in the twentieth century. They have evolved around specific diseases, disabilities, and conditions. The first voluntary health care in America was the National Tuberculosis Association, which was founded in 1904 and later became the American Lung Association. From this demonstrated success, hundreds of voluntary agencies have been founded at the national, state, and local levels. However, there is a group of these that are national in scope and are the most-widely known, such as the National Easter Seal

Society, National Association for Retarded Citizens, March of Dimes Birth Defect Foundation, Epilepsy Foundation of America, American Cancer Society, Cystic Fibrosis Foundation, United Cerebral Palsy Association, National Society to Prevent Blindness, and others. There are 25 voluntary organizations that account for the major part of support of services, education, and research, from more than 100 national organizations. In 1985, the support of the 22 member voluntary agencies of the National Health Council was more than $1.8 billion. Voluntary health organizations have focused their resources in three major areas for children with special needs: services for children and the family, education, and research and advocacy.[6]

The voluntary health agencies have national organizations that determine the agency policy and raise funds. Some have regional or state organizations that provide fundraising, implement national policy, assist in the development and monitoring of grants and programs, and serve as advocates. Services are provided at the community level, where there are chapters of the organization. Individuals and families are the recipients of services which are based on national policy.

Services have been made available in various ways. They have filled gaps in needed services that cannot be provided through the publicly supported programs and are not available through the private sector, often because of funds limitations. The rapidly developing technology in the medical care field and the decrease in public funds or third party coverage have often left the voluntary health agency as the only source of support for needed services.

Family-support services, when there is a child with special health care needs, have often been inadequate or unavailable. Voluntary agencies have been able to meet many of these needs through programs that are aware and sensitive to the family issues such as financial help, education, emotional support, guidance, and the need for in-home care.

Educational efforts have been directed to the child and family, the community, and the professional who provide care for children with special health problems and needs. Family and patient education assist in understanding the condition, identifying needs, finding appropriate resources, and coping with family stress and adjustment.

Community awareness is usually focused on prevention, genetic services, understanding the condition, and volunteerism. As the U.S. has moved toward family-centered, community-based services for children with special health care needs, the voluntary health agencies have played a major role in community understanding and acceptance of handicapped and chronically ill children.

Significant contributions have been made in professional education through scholarships and fellowships to prepare many professional disciplines to work effectively with these special children and the family. Specialty training related to specific conditions has helped to develop the highly specialized care that is often needed over long periods or throughout the life span.

Research has been specific and targeted at many diseases or conditions that have inadequate funding support from public or other sources. Many areas of effective prevention, diagnosis, treatment, and rehabilitation have been supported through voluntary health agencies.

A role of voluntary agencies that has had increasing importance is advocacy. The national agencies have been a deciding force in achieving national legislation that makes possible new and needed resources for children with special health care needs. Lobbying for legislation nationally and at the state level has been a broadly accepted and effective role. The Developmental Disabilities Act of 1970 was moved through Congress primarily due to the effort of several voluntary agencies.

HEAD START

In 1964, the Economic Opportunity Act provided federal assistance for community action programs. Head Start was developed from this statutory base. The program is administered by the Office of Human Services. Recently, responsibility for the Head Start health program has been delegated to the federal Bureau of Maternal and Child Health.

The Head Start programs provide preschool services to four-year old children from low-income families to prepare them for entry into the school system. The philosophy was stated in the 1975 Head Start Performance Standards: "A child can benefit most from a comprehensive interdisciplinary program to foster development and remedy problems as expressed in a broad range of services. The overall goal of the Head Start Program is to bring about a greater degree of social competence in children of low income families."

This philosophy is broadly interpreted to include the individual child, the family, the community, and the environment, and involves education, health services, social services, and parent involvement.

In 1974, it was mandated that the Head Start Program enrollment include ten percent handicapped children. Most of the handicapped children served have been mildly or moderately involved and have received a full range of services, including referrals as needed. Head Start serves as a valuable resource for early interdisciplinary services and is the entry point into other systems for many of these handicapped preschool children.

VOCATIONAL REHABILITATION

Vocational rehabilitation services have a history dating back to World War II, when the federal Office of Vocational Rehabilitation was established in 1943, under the Vocational Rehabilitation Act, to administer a grant program to the states. Currently, the basic legislation is the Rehabilitation Act of 1973 (PL 93-112).[7] There is not only support for vocational rehabilitation services but this legislation also includes provisions for independent living programs, state planning and evaluation of services, studies of services, construction, training of personnel, development and application of new and innovative methods of vocational training, and the rights of the handicapped to access to all programs and facilities that have federal support.

Vocational rehabilitation programs are administered in the states through a separate or designated agency. These programs have been one of the leading service systems that work with handicapped youths in the transition to adult living.

Vocational rehabilitation services may include: [5]

- medical services, such as diagnosis, care, and equipment and devices
- comprehensive vocational evaluation
- counseling
- training
- reader services for the blind
- interpreter services for the deaf
- attendants
- case management
- independent living training and support
- assistance with housing
- transportation

Special education and CCHS programs usually refer clients to vocational rehabilitation services when they reach the eligible age (which may vary in the state programs), to prepare handicapped adolescents and young adults for the transition to adult roles and more independent living.

REFERENCES

1.   Colton M, and Gittler J. The Title V programs and the provision of case management services for children with special health care needs. University of Iowa, Iowa City: National Maternal and Child Health Resource Center, 1986.

2.   Koop CE. Surgeon General's report on children with special health case needs. U.S. Department of Health and Human Services (HRS/D/MC 87-2). Washington, D.C., U.S. Government Printing Office, 1987.

3.   Eberly S, Eklund E, and Simon R. (Eds):. Profiles in excellence. Silver Spring, Maryland: American Association of University Affiliated Programs for Persons with Developmental Disabilities, 1986.

4.   Wallace HM, Gold EH, and Oglesby AC (Eds.). Maternal and child health practices (2nd ed.). New York: John Wiley & Sons, 1982.

5.   Wallace HM, Biehl RF, Taft L, and Oglesby AC (Eds). Handicapped Children and Youth. New York, Human Sciences Press, 1987.

6.   Lierman TL (Ed).   The role of voluntary health organizations.   Building a Health America, Washington, D.C., Mary Ann Liebert, Inc. pp 49-53, 1987.

7.   Wilson FA and Neuhauser D.   Health services in the United States (2nd ed.).   Cambridge, Massachusetts, Ballinger, 1985.

PREVENTION OF MENTAL RETARDATION AND RELATED DISABILITIES*

44

Raymond M. Peterson and James O. Cleveland

INTRODUCTION

More than six million American of all ages are mentally retarded. One out of every ten persons in our country has a family member who is mentally retarded. Every five minutes, another child is born with mental retardation. Mental retardation presents a major social, education, health, and economic problem for our nation. More than 50 percent of all cases of mental retardation can be prevented through known intervention strategies, such as proper nutrition, immunization, control and early treatment of disease, management of maternal illness, genetic counseling, identification and treatment of inborn errors of metabolism, high-risk pregnancy identification and care, early identification and treatment of learning problems, early childhood stimulation, child abuse prevention, childhood injury prevention, and avoidance of harmful drugs and environmental chemicals. Effective prevention programs will reduce the personal loss, grief, and anxiety to the individuals and their families who are affected by this disability, and will result in cost savings to our nation.

---

* Adapted from A Guide for State Planning: for the Prevention of Mental Retardation and Related Disabilities, President's Committee on Mental Retardation, DHHS Publication No. (OHDS) 87-21034.

619

SOCIO-ECONOMIC FACTORS

Socio-economic factors are major causes of mental retardation and related disabilities. These factors are emphasized in subsequent sections; however, because of their importance, socio-economic factors are also presented in this section. Society has frequently failed to acknowledge the importance of poverty and social disadvantage as determinants of developmental outcomes. More than 85 percent of persons with mental retardation are classified as being mildly retarded. An organic origin will not be identifiable for the majority of these individuals. Persons with low socio-economic status (SES) and from sociocultural minorities are over-represented in this group.

Persons living in poverty are more vulnerable to the multiple variables that cause mental retardation and related disabilities. Some of the variables are:

- Poor nutrition
- Improper sanitation
- Unsafe and substandard housing
- Poor medical care
- Inadequate immunization
- Delayed or absent prenatal care
- Delayed medical treatment or intervention
- Use of walk-in emergency care, rather than anticipatory health care
- Lack of stimulation and education
- Limited parenting
- Limited developmental/educational opportunities
- Unemployment or underemployment
- Limited resources of all types
- Abuse or neglect
- Lack of access to services
- Depression or other mental disability
- Lowered expectations
- Poor synchrony with the surrounding cultural system
- Mis-diagnosis of low intelligence
- Ignorance toward good health practices and the need for prevention/intervention

Recent reports show that low-income pregnant women, who did not receive regular prenatal care, had three times as many infant deaths as those who did receive care. Studies have revealed that women who have limited financial resources have been shown to have a significantly increased risk of having a child with low birthweight, and neonatal mortality rates are almost double for poor infants. Infant mortality rates are also disproportionately increased, reflecting complications of management in the first year of life. Early and repeated pregnancies often result in limited education and depression, combining to create added disability and limitations in the individual's ability to cope with stress. Parental time and energy for child training can be diverted, the mother may be young or single, and she may, herself, have had jeopardized development. In this setting there are often reduced opportunities for incidental learning and broader experience. Such families may use language and play less effectively, and place less value on intellectual curiosity and achievement. Neglect or abuse can sometimes occur. Intervention can provide support to the whole family constellation to help break this vicious poverty cycle.

An aggressive approach must be taken to resolve the socio-economic problems that cause mental retardation and related disabilities. Services need to be provided to all residents regardless of the individual's socio-economic status. Many of the existing federally assisted support programs are incompletely utilized or undersubscribed. Outreach efforts to SES disadvantaged populations, supported by an adequate level of funding, may be needed. Programs that should be available are: MCH services, including prenatal and obstetrical (OB) access for low-income families, transients, and other populations at risk; immunization programs; nutritional programs, including WIC (Special Supplemental Food Program for Women, Infants, and Children); early intervention and parent-training services; educational programs; day care; comprehensive medical care; social services; and housing assistance.

PRENATAL AND PERINATAL CARE

The infant mortality rate in the U.S. dropped almost 50 percent during the fifteen years between 1965-1980 (from 24.7 to 13.1/1000 live births). The decline in infant mortality (especially neonatal mortality) can be attributed to increased survival of low birthweight infants, in large part due to specialized hospital-based management through regionalized perinatal care programs. The success in saving the lives of low birthweight infants has not increased the burden of babies with severe handicaps. The proportion of infants with severe congenital malformations or severe retardation remains approximately the same, and there has been a decrease in the proportion of survivors with severe problems relating to birth. Concern remains about the effects of increased survival of the smallest infants (weighing less than 1000 grams). To further decrease the mortality (and morbidity) rate will require new direction and emphasis in preparing for childbearing, including pregnancy planning, increased accessibility to obstetrical services, and continued emphasis on improving pre-pregnancy, pregnancy, delivery, and follow-up care. Following are some basic strategies that should be considered.

Pre-pregnancy

Numerous opportunities exist before pregnancy to decrease the risk of a poor-pregnancy outcome. Healthy pregnancies begin before conception, as heralded in the *HEALTHY MOTHERS/HEALTHY BABIES* national campaign. Every woman should be aware of, and have access to, pre-pregnancy risk identification, counseling (including genetic counseling), risk-reduction health education, relating to pregnancy outcome, and should have full access to family planning services. This is particularly important for underprivileged SES women and adolescents.

Some of the areas for pre-pregnancy risk identification and reduction are:

- Chronic disease
- Hypertension
- Anemia
- Diabetes mellitus
- Poor nutritional status
- Inadequate weight for height
- Maternal (very young or older)
- Previous problems during pregnancy
- High parity
- Short interval between pregnancies
- Susceptibility to infectious diseases, such as rubella
- Presence of sexually transmitted disease
- Smoking
- Alcohol or other drug use

Health education in schools should include information about reproduction, including facts about the principal factors that place a woman at risk for a poor-pregnancy outcome. This should include information about specific risks and the ways of reducing them. Information should emphasize the importance of early pregnancy diagnosis and early prenatal care, with continued care throughout the pregnancy. Information should be provided about resources that are available within the community and how these services can be obtained.

Pre-pregnancy counseling, as part of parenting skills, should be made available to all through health education curricula. Assisting women to have pregnancies by "choice, not by chance" will help the individual to be ready to assume the responsibilities of childrearing. Without this intervention, we will continue the ever-increasing problem of "children having children," a national dilemma. Improper planning for childbearing results in increased poverty for the parents, due to limited education and employment opportunities, isolation, potential child abuse, and other problems causing, or significantly contributing to, mental retardation and related disabilities. This issue is addressed in more detail in the section on socioeconomic factors.

Pre-pregnancy counseling should be available to all women, using resources within the community. Information can be provided by a variety of professionals in many different settings: physicians, nurses, nurse-midwives, health educators, public health and family planning clinics, through personal contact, and public media and educational systems. Everyone should be made aware of the importance of pre-pregnancy risk identification.

Family planning services should be an integral part of the overall strategies to prevent unwanted pregnancies and to reduce the incidence of mental retardation and related disabilities.

Pregnancy (including prenatal care and obstetric care)

Each year in the U.S., approximately 6,000,000 women become pregnant. More than half of these pregnancies are unintended. Some studies report that unintended pregnancies have resulted in 46 percent abortion, 13 percent miscarriage and 41 percent live births. The American College of Obstetricians and Gynecologists (ACOG) and others have developed informational materials about sexual responsibility and contraception, which are available without charge. Toll-free telephone numbers are available to assist women to obtain information about services in their communities.

Neonatal outcomes will be improved when early prenatal care is provided. All women who have been identified as being at significant risk of having a poor-pregnancy outcome, due to medical or other high-risk factors, should be referred to a medical center for necessary care.

Those factors that may increase a woman's risk for problems during pregnancy include:

- Maternal hypertension and/or history of eclampsia or preeclampsia
- Maternal illness, including anemia, diabetes mellitus, or malnutrition
- Maternal epilepsy
- Metabolic disorders, such as phenylketonuria (Maternal PKU)
- History of repeated fetal loss
- Multiple fetuses
- Exposure to toxic substances
- Obesity
- Eating disorders
- Early adolescence
- Advanced maternal age
- Alcohol and other drug abuse
- Presence of a developmental disability
- Family history of a genetic disorder

Labor and Delivery

Regionalization of high-risk obstetrical care has been shown to be an effective method of improving pregnancy outcome. A regional plan provides coordination and oversight of service provision for highly specialized and/or highly technical services. It should focus on specific geographical areas, where local resources (economic, technical, and professional) are scarce and the problems to be addressed cross political lines (states, counties, etc.).

Special Considerations

Low Birthweight Low birthweight is a major determinant of infant mortality and is one of the leading factors causing mental retardation and related disabilities. In 1982, 6.8 percent of infants born in the U.S. weighed less than 2500 grams (5 lbs. 8 ozs.) and approximately one percent were considered to be very-low birthweight (1500 grams or less). There are certain risk factors that are associated with premature birth and with intrauterine growth deficiency. There is considerable variation in the percentage of infants with low birthweight among various ethnic groups (approximately 5.7 percent white, 5.4 percent Hispanic, 5.6 percent Asian, nine percent Puerto Rican, and 12.5 percent Black). The difference between the various ethnic groups may be due to a number of factors, including poverty, lack of prenatal care, and drug exposure (including alcohol, smoking), and undetermined genetic factors. Prevention programs must be developed that consider the needs of the population served.

Preterm prevention programs have been successful in decreasing the incidence of preterm delivery in high-risk women. These programs focus on various measures that will prevent the onset of preterm labor. Tocolytic treatments and the treatment of infection may be of assistance in stopping premature labor. Every state should develop a program for preventing preterm delivery to decrease costs of medical care and to assist in the prevention of mental retardation and related disabilities.

Rh Blood Disease One out of eight women in the U.S. has RH negative blood. Despite the knowledge about the treatment and the prevention of Rh blood disease, there are still infants who develop neurological deficits, including mental retardation, because of hyperbilirubinemia associated with Rh disease. Rh immune globulin has been widely accepted as an effective method for reducing Rh immunization for women at risk of becoming sensitized because of an Rh positive fetus. This cost-effective treatment should be available and information about the risks and treatment should be included in every public and professional education program.

Maternal Diabetes The combination of diabetes mellitus and pregnancy presents a special challenge. Diabetes mellitus or gestational diabetes mellitus are associated with three-four percent of all pregnancies. Until recently (last ten years), strategies for the prevention of adverse outcomes in offspring of women with established diabetes were unknown. Effective strategies are currently available and have been shown to reduce the frequency of adverse perinatal events to that seen in the general population of offspring of women without diabetes. Identification, referral for appropriate treatment, and follow-up of women of childbearing age, with established diabetes, should be the major focus for intervention.

A program for improving pregnancy outcomes for women with diabetes should include: 1) identification and appropriate referral of women of childbearing age with established diabetes, and screening and diagnosis of gestational diabetes; 2) resources for referral and care, to include patient education, nutrition counseling, and management by a specialized team; 3) careful maternal and neonatal treatment and follow-up; and 4) professional education. Guidelines for care have been developed by the Division of Diabetes Control, Center for Prevention Services, CDC, in collaboration with the federal Bureau of Maternal and Child Health.

The management of pregnancy in women with diabetes mellitus is best accomplished by a specialized and experienced team, including obstetricians skilled in high-risk pregnancies, diabetologists, and neonatologists. The team should have available to it the services of a modern laboratory and inpatient facilities to meet the needs of the mother and the newborn infant. The primary health care provider is an important member of the team, and provides counseling, pregnancy planning assistance, and support to other members of the team.

Maternal Epilepsy Special care must be taken to assist women who must take medications, which have been shown to be, or are potentially, teratogenic. The incidence of epilepsy has been estimated to be approximately one percent in the population, and many women must take anticonvulsant medications during their pregnancies. Fetal malformation has been associated with maternal ingestion of several of the antiepileptics, including the hydantoins, valproic acid, and the diones. The treatment of epilepsy with drugs has greatly improved due to an increased knowledge of pharmacokinetics and drug interactions, and the widespread use of monitoring of the serum concentrations of the antiepileptic drugs. A woman who is being treated for a seizure disorder (epilepsy) requires close follow-up during pregnancy. Close collaboration between the obstetrician and other health professionals is required to assure the best possible pregnancy outcome.

GENETIC FACTORS

It is estimated that approximately 250,000 children are born in the U.S. each year with major hereditary conditions and disorders that will seriously impair their health. Some of these conditions are immediately apparent at birth, others are not manifested until later in life. Genetic diseases and related disorders account for approximately 25 percent of all inpatient hospital admissions and placements in long-term care facilities. Many of the genetic conditions are associated with mental retardation and many can be detected during uterine life or during infancy. The apparent increase in the incidence and prevalence of these inherited genetic disorders may be related to advances in obstetrical management and in improved health care.

It is essential to educate the public about the prevention and treatment of genetic conditions. This can be accomplished through public awareness campaigns, by including information in curricula at all educational levels, and through professional sources, such as physicians' offices, health clinics, etc. Information regarding the risks of genetic diseases, methods of detection, and treatment should be available for all persons, and provided at an appropriate level of understanding for each person. Genetic counseling should be required as a part of the curriculum for all health professionals and should be available as a standard of medical practice within each community. A significant cost-benefit of screening programs has been demonstrated for certain genetic disorders, where early treatment can prevent mental retardation. Recent discoveries have provided new information about genetic disorders, and it is expected that in the near future we will be able to identify many additional genetic factors that are responsible for disabling conditions. Additional research in the field of molecular genetics, gene mapping, etc., will result in expanded and improved genetic services for our nation.

Genetic Counseling

Genetic counseling is the process by which information is provided regarding the risks of occurrence and recurrence of genetic disorders within the family. The purpose of genetic counseling is to provide factual information to assist the individual in making rational decisions and to provide support in relation to the information provided. The counselor assists the individual in making the decision and is not in a role of advising or telling the person what to do or how to act. Supportive counseling and follow-up are essential components of every genetic counseling program and may be provided by many resources within the community.

Genetic Screening Programs

Prenatal diagnosis (amniocentesis/chorionic villus sampling)   A prenatal diagnosis is a method of detecting virtually all chromosome abnormalities, many inborn errors of metabolism, and some important structural abnormalities during early pregnancy. Specific indications for prenatal diagnosis are:

- Advanced maternal age
- Previous child with chromosome abnormality
- Parent(s) has/have an unusual chromosome arrangement
- Both parents are carriers of a gene causing an inherited metabolic disorder for which a prenatal test is available
- Mother is a known carrier of an X-linked gene that causes a genetic disorder in male offspring
- Family history of a neural tube defect

Amniocentesis can be done at approximately the 16th week of pregnancy, to obtain a small sample of amniotic fluid to be analyzed for chromosomal abnormalities, neural tube defects, and certain other genetic and infectious conditions. Chorionic villus sampling (CVS) sometimes is an alternative to amniocentesis and can be done between the 9th and 12th week of pregnancy. The limitations, safety, and reliability of CVS are being evaluated, under the auspices of the National Institute of Child Health and Human Development.

Resources should be identified within each community to offer prenatal diagnostic services. Provision of services through the use of regionalized laboratories is a method of assuring quality control and cost-effectiveness.

Newborn Screening   Screening for certain disorders can be done early in life, prior to identification of symptoms. Large-scale screening of newborns for certain disorders was made possible in the early 1960s by the development of a simple, reliable, inexpensive screening test for the detection of phenylketonuria (PKU), using bacterial inhibition techniques. Newborn screening has been expanded so that screening programs are not in place throughout the U.S. Most states currently test for PKU and hypothyroidism, and many states test for other genetic metabolic disorders, such as galactosemia, homocystinuria, maple syrup urine disease, and biotinidase deficiency. Some states are also screening newborns for hemoglobinopathies, such as sickle cell disease, as a part of their prevention program.

The following criteria should be considered before newborn screening for a specific metabolic disorder is initiated:

- Affected children do no exhibit symptoms at birth
- The disease, if untreated, is expected to have serious consequences
- The treatment is unquestionably effective and requires early detection for optimum results
- There is adequate knowledge about the natural course of the disorder
- The screening test has acceptable low rates of false-negative and false-positive tests
- The incidence of the disorder is sufficiently high and the costs of the test reasonably priced to assure that the cost-benefit of the screening is acceptable

Newborn screening can identify some significant inherited disorders, resulting in information that can be provided to families for assistance in planning treatment and intervention, as well as for planning future pregnancies.

The success of the newborn-screening programs has resulted in large numbers of infants who have been identified early and treated so that they are not disabled. There is a need for flexibility within the program to make certain that the testing program can be modified to include additional disorders, as they are identified. The cost of collecting the blood specimen and transferring it to the screening laboratory is much greater than the cost of the laboratory procedure. It is important and cost-effective to obtain the maximum benefit from the specimen that has been obtained. Cooperative programs are needed to pool resources to reduce costs and to improve quality assurance. Any program must take into consideration ethical issues and have an effective educational and public information component.

Heterozygote Detection   We have developed a technical ability to detect heterozygote carriers for certain genetic diseases that are associated with mental retardation and related disorders. The Tay-Sachs heterozygote screening program is an example of an effective program where persons at high risk for having a child with Tay-Sachs disease can be identified by carrier detection. This information is then used to assist in genetic counseling. The identification of certain abnormal genes by the use of "gene probes" and recombinant DNA technology has increased the number of detectable genetic disorders for which the carrier and affected states can be detected—for example, phenylketonuria (PKU).

Other Population Screening

Screening for specific genetic disorders in the general population has been attempted with limited success. Routine karyotype analysis of newborns has been helpful in providing information about the incidence of specific chromosomal abnormalities, but is not a cost-effective method for population screening. Programs for analysis of a blood sample, obtained from a pregnant woman between the 16th and 20th weeks of pregnancy, have been expanded to include women who have either an elevated or lowered level of alpha fetoprotein in the maternal serum (MSAFP). Follow-up studies, including sonography and amniocentesis for further evaluation, can identify a number of birth defects, including neural tube defects and anencephaly (associated with a high MSAFP) and various chromosomal problems, such as Down syndrome (when the MSAFP is found to be abnormally low). Many states are not offering MSAFP testing on a voluntary basis. It is expected that, in addition to the detection of certain birth defects, these screening programs will result in improved pregnancy care.

There is much to be learned and there will continue to be a rapid growth in knowledge within the field of genetics. The efforts of universities, medical centers and other research centers, and the government and private (including the nonprofit) sectors of society must be coordinated to assure that 1) genetic services are available; 2) quality control is maintained; 3) there is outreach and assistance to populations who need these services; and 4) there is adequate data collection.

INFANTS AT RISK

Many infants, because of biological, environmental, or established risk factors, or a combination of these factors, may be at risk for becoming mentally retarded or having related disabilities. Infants in the biological risk group may include those who have experienced prematurity or perinatal insult to the developing central nervous system. Infants in the environmental risk group may include those who are biologically sound, but experience poor health care, lack of physical and social stimulation, poor parent-infant bonding relationships, and/or inadequate parenting. Many of these infants have parents who, due to medical or mental conditions, or limitation of resources, are unable to fulfill parental responsibilities. Infants in the established risk group include those with syndromes or situations known to have developmental liability, such as chromosomal aberrations or complex birth defects.

Early intervention programs for infants, who are at risk for becoming mentally retarded or having related disabilities, have become increasingly recognized as extremely important service components in the fields of health, education, and child development. Early intervention services are essential in order to reduce the incidence and severity of mental retardation and related handicaps, improve the development of each child, and decrease future costs related to infant/child services.

Comprehensive intervention would include, but should not necessarily be limited to:

- Linkage to medical services
- Physical and occupational therapy
- Audiology, speech, and language therapy
- Social work services/crisis intervention
- Developmental/educational services, e.g., infant stimulation
- In-home support
- Parent education/counseling
- Respite care

Individualized care plans for the infants at risk and their families are based on the assessment findings. These plans should include needed intervention services for the infant, and education and counseling for the family members regarding infant development. Services should be provided for the "family unit," expecting that the family unit will be involved in the development and the implementation of the infant's individual care plan.

The child and the child's environment need to be monitored in order to assure that care plans are appropriate and to track the effectiveness of early intervention services provided. Many states have initiated "statewide" tracking systems in an effort to follow children whose parents do not complete the intervention plans developed for their children.

An outreach and educational component, to inform health care providers, appropriate community agencies, and parents concerning the services, must be provided to identify infants who are at risk for becoming mentally retarded and disabled.

ENVIRONMENTAL FACTORS

Accidents

Injuries are the leading causes of death in young children and are major factors in causing mental retardation and other handicapping conditions. More children are killed in traffic accidents than by any other cause. Eighty-five percent of the deaths could be prevented by the use of car safety seats and safety belts. All states now have enacted laws requiring the installation and use of restraint systems to protect infants and children, under five years, who are passengers in automobiles. Forty-seven states had at least one bill making seat-belt use mandatory introduced into its legislature during 1985.

Non-accidental injury, including child abuse, is well-recognized as a cause of mental retardation and other disabilities, and is found in all social strata of our society. Child abuse is being reported throughout the country with increasing frequency. Children who have developmental deviations are particularly vulnerable to being abused, resulting in mental retardation and related disabilities. Effective reporting and intervention programs are essential for protection of all children.

Drowning is a significant cause of death in many states. Arizona, the state with the highest per-capita number of backyard swimming pools, reports drownings as the leading cause of death for children under age five years. Most drownings in this age group occur in the family's own backyard pool. Near-drowning victims frequently have severe neurological and intellectual impairment and require an ongoing high level of care. The cost of care and the loss of productivity of the individual are major problems. Although drowning occurs at a high frequency in "sunbelt" states, it is a problem in all. Local, statewide, and regional public education programs directed at preventing drownings and near-drownings can significantly change the incidence of this tragedy. Prevention campaigns need to be carefully evaluated for their effectiveness. It is unlikely that infants can be made "water safe," and in fact parents may develop a false sense of security if they believe that their infant can "swim" a few strokes.

Poisons also contribute as causes of mental retardation in infants and young children. It is expected that, this year, as many as 130,000 children under the age of five will ingest some type of poison. The number of poison-related deaths among children under five years of age decreased from 450 in 1961 to 55 in 1983. This 88 percent decline was thought to be due largely to an extensive public awareness campaign facilitated by PL 87-319, passed in 1961, which designates the third week of March each year as National Poison Prevention Week.

Lead Poisoning   Lead poisoning continues to be a factor causing mental retardation. Although often associated with poor inner-city children who have eaten paint from decaying walls, it is actually found in all populations within our society. Lead-based paint is still on an estimated 30 to 40 million homes in the U.S. Renovation of older homes is a common cause of lead poisoning in middle-class families. Combustion of leaded gasoline continues as an important source of environmental contamination, although this has decreased significantly in recent years. Other less common lead sources include Hispanic and Asian folk remedies for childhood illness, improperly glazed pottery, and some arts and crafts materials. Many children who have significantly elevated blood-lead levels have subtle clinical symptoms. Simple inexpensive screening tests are available to detect elevated lead levels so that treatment can be initiated even before clinical signs are observed. Public awareness has been the most effective prevention activity in decreasing the incidence of lead poisoning.

Infections   Infectious diseases have been major factors in causing mental retardation and related disabilities. Despite the many advances in diagnosis and treatment, there continue to be many cases where disability due to infectious diseases could have been prevented. Progress is being made through the development of safe, effective immunization measures, and new treatments are becoming available which will improve the outcome from diseases due to infectious agents. Efforts must be made to increase awareness, acceptance, and utilization of these preventive measures, in order to be truly effective in our efforts to reduce the incidence of mental retardation due to infective agents.

Immunizations   Routine immunizations for children have resulted in only rare occurrences of diphtheria, tetanus, and poliomyelitis, and significant decreases in the incidence of pertussis, measles, mumps, and rubella. Immunization for specific infectious agents can be an effective primary prevention strategy. A schedule for immunization of infants and children is recommended by the American Academy of Pediatrics (AAP).

An example of the effectiveness of an immunization program is the experience in the U.S. following the licensure of rubella vaccine in 1969. Over 130 million doses of rubella vaccine have been distributed in the U.S. during the past sixteen years, with a decrease of rubella cases by 90 percent or more in all age groups. Because the major risk of rubella infection is the teratogenic effect on the fetus (Congenital Rubella Syndrome—multiple congenital malformations involving many organ systems resulting in visual and hearing impairment, cardiovascular defects, microcephaly and mental retardation), prevention efforts need to be directed toward protecting women from developing rubella infection during pregnancy. Since 1979, the decline in incidence rates for persons 15 years of age or older has been associated with a significant decline in the occurrence of Congenital Rubella Syndrome (CRS).

Despite the progress that we have made, there were still two cases of CRS reported to the National Congenital Rubella Syndrome Register (NCRSR) in 1985 (as compared to two in 1984; six in 1983; 12 in 1982; ten in 1981; 14 in 1980; and 57 in 1979). Immunization of women of the childbearing age should be based upon documentation of vaccination after one year of age, or documentation of protection through serologic studies. Women who do not meet these criteria can be vaccinated without serologic screening, or can be tested prior to immunization. There is no harm in vaccinating a woman of unknown status, should she already be immune.

Women should be advised of the theoretical risks of the rubella vaccine to the fetus, and pregnancy should be avoided for three months following rubella vaccination. Vaccination should not be undertaken in women who are pregnant.

Haemophilus influenzae, type b, is the leading cause of bacterial meningitis in the U.S., accounting for some 12,000 cases annually. Neurological sequelae are found in 19 percent to 45 percent of survivors. A polysaccharide vaccine for prevention of Haemophilus influenzae b disease is now available (HBPV) and should be given to children at two years of age, routinely. Vaccination should be considered for children as young as 18 months of age in high-risk settings, such as day care. As the vaccine currently available is not immunogenic in most children younger than eighteen months, many young infants will remain unprotected from this serious disease. (Haemophilus influenzae rates peak between six months and one year of age and decline thereafter.) Efforts are being made to develop a safe effective vaccine for the younger population. It is important to educate persons about the risk, particularly for infants who are exposed to groups of children in locations such as day care.

Common infectious diseases, such as measles and chickenpox, may cause significant disability, including mental retardation. An effective immunization is available to prevent measles (rubeola), and it is expected that a safe effective vaccine will be available for chickenpox (varicella) in the near future. Despite the availability of measles vaccine, we still see cases of measles causing disability in the U.S. The first 26 weeks of 1986 saw an increase of over 100 percent in the number of cases reported, as compared to the same period in 1985. The nearly 4,000 measles cases reported during the first half of 1986 exceed the total number of reported cases in any year since 1980. At least one third (35.8 percent) of the cases reported were considered to be preventable.

Other Infections of Significance Cytomegalovirus infection is the most common viral infection that causes mental retardation during the intrauterine period. This is an ubiquitous organism that is endemic throughout the world. The cytomegalovirus most often causes mild symptoms in the infected person except during the intra-uterine period. It is expected that a vaccine will be available in the near future to assist in preventing this significant cause of mental retardation and related disabilities. Herpes simplex and other common viruses may cause infections resulting in significant disability. Efforts must be continued to develop effective measures of prevention and treatment.

Sexually transmitted diseases (STD) are important factors in the causation of mental retardation and related disabilities, and should be considered in the development of any prevention plan. Syphilis is still the third most frequently reported communicable disease in the U.S. exceeded only by chickenpox and gonorrhea. Despite decades of experience and knowledge regarding congenital syphilis, problems still arise in case definition, diagnosis, treatment, and follow-up. Genital herpes infection is a major public health problem, and the infected mother can pass the virus to her baby during the birth process. It is important that women be aware of the signs and symptoms of genital herpes, and that they seek appropriate medical care when it is suspected. A fetal infection with the AIDS virus (T-cell lymphotropic virus type III-[HTLV-III]) has been reported to cause a congenital dysmorphic syndrome consisting of growth failure, microcephaly, and other malformations. Factors contributing to a sustained level of sexually transmitted diseases include an increase in the number of infections among pregnant women, the lack of availability of prenatal care, and the failure of the prenatal-care system to provide timely evaluation and prompt follow-up. Screening programs during pregnancy should be fully utilized as an important prevention strategy, particularly in those areas where the prevalence of sexually transmitted infections is high.

Parasitic infections, such as toxoplasmosis, may infect the fetus in utero, causing severe disability. Prevention strategies should include awareness of the sources of infection and proper health practices to avoid excessive risk from becoming infected.

Teratogens

The teratogenicity of various infectious agents, such as rubella, has been known for many years and is now being followed by increasing knowledge about the importance of exogenous causes of congenital malformation. Chemicals of several categories, including substances found within the general environment, medicines, and substances used because of personal habits and predeliction, may act as teratogens. Environmental chemicals, including additives, contaminants, and pollutants, are a major public concern because of their ubiquity and insidiousness, and, most important, because persons have little say as to whether they want to be exposed to them.

The use of alcohol by pregnant women may result in a pattern of irreversible abnormalities, including mental retardation, in their offspring. The number of persons in the U.S. with Fetal Alcohol Syndrome (FAS) is unknown; however, the prevalence appears to be in the range of one-two per 1,000 births. This disorder is one of the most common types of diagnosed mental retardation. The FAS is preventable by abstinence during pregnancy. Smoking during pregnancy is clearly associated with birthweight deficits of up to 250 grams in full-term newborns. A clear dose-response relationship exists between the number of cigarettes smoked and the birthweight deficit. Mothers who smoke have increased rates of premature delivery and their newborns are also smaller at every gestational age. Women who are pregnant consume numerous "over-the-counter" drugs, which may be potential teratogens.

Occupational exposure to antineoplastic drugs and certain anesthetic gases has been shown to result in increased fetal losses in women exposed during pregnancy, which emphasizes the need for caution in the handling of these agents.

Recent studies have shown that pregnant women will reduce or cease their alcohol intake, if they are made aware of the deleterious effects of alcohol on their babies. It is likely that the avoidance of other teratogens can be accomplished by increasing public and professional awareness of the preventability of mental retardation and related disorders due to exposure to teratogens during pregnancy.

Professionals who are involved in the care of pregnant women are in a key position to intervene; however, the most effective prevention strategy will be information provided to the general public and to all health professionals.

SPECIAL CONSIDERATIONS

Each geographic area may have specific populations or problems that will need special consideration. Some of these will be unique to the area and many will affect all parts of the country in a greater or lesser degree. Population density, climate, poverty level, pregnancy rates, the special needs of minorities and of immigrants, and other factors, need to be considered. Issues, such as adolescent pregnancy, and the problems experienced by parents who are themselves mentally retarded are problems found throughout the country. There are other problems that may be unique to only one locality.

Adolescent Pregnancy

Adolescent pregnancy is one of the major medico-social crises facing the U.S. in this decade. Forty percent of female teenagers will have conceived by the age of 19 years, and 50 percent of these women will have delivered a baby. The effect of a pregnancy on the mother (and father) will significantly impact the development of the infant and subsequent offspring. For many teenagers, pregnancy is a one-way ticket to poverty. A number of innovative program models are available for consideration as a part of the prevention effort. The U.S. must work to stem the tide of one million teenage pregnancies each year by providing sex education and information regarding the prevention of unwanted pregnancies.

Parents Who Are Mentally Retarded

Infants who are born of parents who are mentally retarded or mentally handicapped may have significant developmental delay due to a number of factors. Many mothers who are mentally retarded will be unable to provide the care that is needed by the infant or young child, resulting in developmental delay and mental retardation in later ages. A number of innovative projects located throughout the U.S. have demonstrated the positive effects of intervention.

The recent changes in the care for the disabled, which allows greater freedom and protection of the rights of persons with mental retardation, have resulted in a new set of problems relating to relationships, including marriage and childbearing. Many mentally retarded parents are further disadvantaged by socio-economic factors, including poverty and limited support systems. Some of these persons have significant medical problems that affect childbearing, such as endocrine dysfunction and physical malformations, which can influence the pregnancy and/or delivery. Certain inherited metabolic/genetic factors, which have caused the individual's disability, may result in the offspring also being disabled.

There is a need for outreach and intervention to affect social change. The lack of follow-up for medical care and other needed services may be due to unavailability of transportation, a fear of agencies or professionals, an inability to read instructions or even the appointment card, a lack of understanding legal barriers, and/or poor judgement about how to provide care.

Other Populations at Risk

The special needs of selected populations within the state or region will need to be considered to determine priorities for prevention programs. Problems affecting Native Americans, such as poverty, isolation and alcoholism, all are associated with an increased incidence of mental retardation. There is a high incidence of the fetal alcohol syndrome (FAS) in some Native American populations. Various ethnic groups have an increased incidence of certain rare inherited disorders, such as Tay-Sachs disease among Ashkenazi Jews.

Immigrants, including refugees, may have special needs associated with limited knowledge of resources, cultural, and language differences, and limited family and financial resources. The undocumented alien is faced with additional problems, being ineligible for certain health and welfare programs and also hesitant to request services or utilize resources due to a fear of legal reprisals. Non-English speaking persons may not be aware of resources and may not use the services because of a lack of knowledge of the types of services available and knowledge of how to access these services.

Persons who are migrants have special problems due to their inability to establish stable relationships with community resources. This problem is frequently compounded by poverty and language and cultural barriers.

EDUCATION/PUBLIC AWARENESS

Education and public information pertaining to the prevention of mental retardation and related disabilities must be provided to all people, and especially to adolescents, prospective parents, and all practicing professionals. Education and public information on prevention will encourage self-awareness, informed decision-making, and appropriate action. Effective educational prevention/intervention programs can, and do, make a dramatic difference in decreasing the incidence of persons with mental retardation and related disabilities.

The goal of the education and public awareness programs should be to ensure that all people will have an understanding and acceptance of persons with mental retardation and related disabilities, as well as the knowledge and awareness of factors which contribute to mental retardation and related disabilities, and the prevention of these conditions.

Mental retardation is one of America's major concerns affecting children and adults, and is a significant health, social, educational, and economic problem. Young people must be made aware of the vital link between their health and the eventual health and well-being of their own children. Prevention education can assist in ensuring that all students will have the knowledge, awareness, and attitudes necessary for responsible parenthood and preventive health care. A comprehensive prevention curriculum should be a permanent part of the community's educational program for students of all ages, in public and private schools. Prevention information should be included in the curricula for continuing education. Efforts to prevent problems before they occur are necessary components of a systematic approach to promoting good health, which in turn greatly assist in the prevention of mental retardation and related disabilities.

Dissemination of current information must be tailored for many different high-risk target populations, such as adolescents, prospective parents, certain ethnic groups, and low socio-economic populations. Written and audiovisual materials, along with professional training programs, workshops, seminars, professional publications, journals, public service announcements, and media talk shows are extremely useful in educating all people about prevention of mental retardation and related disabilities. Materials and presentations should be available to meet the needs of non-English speaking populations.

Topics suggested for prevention education and public awareness include:

• Human Development	• Prevention of Birth Defects
• Nutrition	• Alcohol and Drug Abuse
• Parenting	• Environmental Hazards
• Safety	• Family Planning
• Immunization	• Acceptance of Difference
• Local Resources	• Maternal Health and Birth Defects
• Child Abuse	• Developmental Disabilities
• Family Roles	• Mental and Physical Health
• Human Genetics	• New Genetic Technologies
• Bioethics	

Classrooms and various public mass-media systems offer excellent channels for dissemination of innovative prevention efforts. Prevention education is a major vehicle for improving the quality of life for all people and for decreasing the incidence of mental retardation and related disabilities, as well as its emotional and financial burdens. Television and radio are excellent vehicles for reaching the general public as well as targeted populations. These public media should be considered for use in disseminating information through regular programming during the daytime and the "prime time" hours.

PERSONNEL DEVELOPMENT

For any prevention plan to be effective, knowledgeable and capable individuals must be available to develop, implement, and maintain that plan. The number of individuals (professionals, para-professionals, and parents) currently trained in the area of prevention/intervention is limited. Personnel development resources must be identified and encouraged to provide necessary training.

Resources for the development of trained personnel in the area of prevention include the institutions of higher learning, university affiliated programs, mental retardation research centers, schools of public health, and regional networks and consortia which operate beyond state boundaries. Information should be included in curricula to educate students about the causes and prevention of mental retardation and related disabilities. Other resources for personnel development include the health, education, and social service agencies at the federal, state, and local level. These service agencies should offer training opportunities for their staff, as well as for community providers and consumers.

Existing personnel resources should be evaluated to determine current and future needs. Individuals already in the delivery system need to be recognized for their contributions and should be provided with the means to update their skills and to incorporate the knowledge being learned through rapidly advancing technologies and research findings.

Under-represented minority groups should be targeted for personnel development to make certain that ethnic, cultural, socio-economic, and other special situations are addressed. Prevention programs will only be effective if they are accepted, utilized, and supported by person to be served.

Advocacy and support groups are an essential part of the personnel pool and provide a link between the community and the service delivery system. Orientation, training, inservice seminars, and assistance in designing and delivering public education programs are important contributors to the maintenance and expansion of the personnel pool.

DATA COLLECTION/EVALUATION

Over the years, the reporting from the CDC through the *Morbidity and Mortality Weekly Report* (MMWR) has attempted to reflect the changing panorama of national public health concerns. The current focus of the CDC is on a number of diseases of importance, as well as environmental situations and other problems that impact the nation's health. Since 1980, the reporting has included an emphasis on the 15 areas of priority, published in *Promoting Health/Preventing Disease:*

Objectives for the Nation. This landmark report from the Surgeon General sets the national health objectives for 1990. The fifteen areas of priority include:

- high blood pressure control,
- family planning,
- pregnancy and infant health,
- immunization,
- sexually transmitted diseases,
- toxic agent control,
- occupational safety and health,
- accident prevention and injury control,
- fluoridation and dental health,
- surveillance and control of infectious diseases,
- smoking and health,
- misuse of alcohol and drugs,
- nutrition,
- physical fitness and exercise, and
- control of stress and violent behavior.

The majority of these priority areas are associated with, or cause, or contribute to the problems associated with mental retardation.

Individual states collect data from birth and death certificates. Information from the birth certificate is commonly obtained from the labor-and-delivery log and includes such information as date and time of birth, sex, plurality, birthweight, presentation, mode of delivery, etc. Vital statistics information should be available from state health departments. The accuracy of the information will vary based upon a number of factors. Other more specific data-base systems may be available in some states and/or regions to provide information about the incidence and prevalence of specific disorders, such as phenylketonuria (PKU), Down syndrome, or more general information about mental retardation and birth defects.

Data may be obtained from local and state education departments, health departments, and departments of social welfare and mental hygiene. Data from other states and countries may also be helpful in determining priorities for program development and implementation, for data collection, research, and evaluation.

Private and nonprofit groups often have valuable information that can be used in planning and evaluating the prevention effort. Special interest groups, including organizations of parents and other interested persons representing low-occurrence disorders, may be able to contribute information that is not found in any other data system.

RESEARCH

Many of the major gains in the prevention of mental retardation and related disabilities have been due to basic and applied research, resulting in discoveries regarding the causes and effective methods of treatment and intervention. These gains have been evidenced in biological, social, educational, and other fields. Research must be encouraged in the biological field, including basic and applied research relating to neurotransmitters, molecular genetics, cellular biology, electrophysiology, nutrition, the environment, and other areas.

The National Institutes of Health (NIH) each year fund intramural and extramural research to improve our nation's health. In 1984, the NIH budget of approximately $4.5 billion represented more than half of the total annual budget allocation for the Public Health Service. The National Institute of Child Health and Human Development (NICHD) supports research in mental retardation in specialized Mental Retardation Research Centers throughout the country, and also funds studies with a broad focus regarding human development. NICHD has investigated questions relating to preconception, conception, intrauterine development, in-utero treatment, the birth process, physical and mental disabilities, and investigation about neonates and older children, including nutrition, normal growth and development, and developmental deviations. Some recent studies have focused on the reasons for low birthweight and methods of intervention, problems associated with teenage pregnancy, and risks associated with births to older mothers. Many of these research efforts have had a significant impact on the incidence of mental retardation and related disabilities.

Many of the discoveries made in university centers have been possible only through joint efforts and cooperation with community programs, and through collaboration with institutions which have congregated populations of persons with disabilities caused by low-incidence etiological factors. The current trends in the provision of care, including the depopulation of large institutions, make it essential to ensure that data are kept and information is coordinated and shared by all segments of the delivery system. We must look to the future by encouraging basic and applied research in state institutions, universities, and in community-based programs. Effective research, resulting in important new discoveries in the prevention and treatment of mental retardation and related disabilities, will be facilitated through careful data collection, information sharing, and collaboration to ensure effective research.

SUGGESTED READINGS

1. Report to the President, Mental Retardation Plans for the Future. President's Committee on Mental Retardation, U.S. Department of Health and Human Services, Office of Human Development Services, Washington, D.C., March 1985.

2. National Open Forum on Prevention of Mental Retardation from Environmental and Psychosocial Causes, Conference Proceedings. Boca Raton, FL, President's Committee on Mental Retardation, U.S. Department of Health and Human Services, Office of Human Development Services, Washington, D.C., May 16-18, 1984.

3. Assessment of the National Effort to Combat Mental Retardation From Biomedical Causes, Conference Proceedings. Washington, D.C. President's Committee on Mental Retardation, U.S. Department of Health and Human Services, Office of Human Development Services, Washington, D.C., November 14-16, 1983.

4. National Prevention Showcase and Forum, Technical Proceedings. Atlanta, GA. President's Committee on Mental Retardation in Cooperation with the Atlanta Association for Retarded Citizens. U.S. Department of Health and Human Services, Office of Human Development Services, Washington, D.C., September 15-17, 1983.

5. Report to the President, Mental Retardation: Prevention Strategies That Work. President's Committee on Mental Retardation, U.S. Department of Health, Education and Welfare, Office of Human Development Services, Washington, D.C., December 1980.

6. Report to the President, Mental Retardation: The Leading Edge. President's Committee on Mental Retardation, U.S. Department of Health, Education and Welfare, Office of Human Development Services, Washington, D.C., May 1979.

7. International Summit on Prevention of Mental Retardation from Biomedical Causes, Conference Proceedings. Wingspread, WI. President's Committee on Mental Retardation, U.S. Department of Health, Education and Welfare, Office of Human Development Services, Washington, D.C., December 15-16, 1977.

8. Report to the President, Mental Retardation: Century of Decision. President's Committee on Mental Retardation, U.S. Department of Health, Education and Welfare, Washington, D.C., March 1976.

9. Developmental Handicaps: Prevention and Treatment. American Association of University Affiliated Programs, Washington, D.C., August 1983.

10. Developmental Handicaps: Prevention and Treatment II. American Association of University Affiliated Programs, Silver Springs MD, September, 1984.

11. Fotheringham JB, Hambley WD, Haddad-Curran HW. Prevention of Intellectual Handicaps. Ontario Association for the Mentally Retarded, Toronto, 1983.

12. Crocker AC. Current Strategies in Prevention of Mental Retardation, Pediatr Annals 11:450-457, 1982.

13. Kalter H, Warkany J. Congenital Malformations, Etiologic Factors and Their Role in Prevention. N Engl J Med 308:424-431; 308:491-497, 1983.

14. Preventing Mental Retardation. Report to Congress by the Comptroller General of the United States, October 3, 1977.

15. Klein DC, Goldstein SE (eds). Primary Prevention: An Idea Whose Time Has Come. U.S. Department of Health, Education, and Welfare, Public Health Service; Alcohol, Drug Abuse and Mental Health Administration; National Institutes of Mental Health, Washington, D.C. 1977.

45

EARLY IDENTIFICATION

Raymond M. Peterson

There are many reasons for the early identification of children who have special health care needs. Early identification facilitates the development of an effective treatment plan and assists in providing counseling and guidance for the child, parents, and other care providers. Future care needs can be anticipated to assist in planning for needed resources. Early identification will result in the prevention* of disability which may persist for a lifetime.

Identification techniques must be planned and implemented, taking into consideration the resources available and the sources and types of care within the community or geographical area. Although some national, state, regional, and local

---

* PRIMARY PREVENTION—represents the attempt to eliminate the occurrence of the problem in the individual and to reduce the prevalence in the community. Classical examples of this include: addressing the medical and social factors, including poverty, which predispose to child disability; improving prenatal and perinatal care; and prevention of catastrophic illnesses, accidents, poisonings, abuse, and neglect.

SECONDARY PREVENTION—attempts to identify a problem early so that intervention at the outset will eliminate the potential for abnormality or alter the circumstances which create the condition. Traditional examples of these include early identification of high-risk conditions and early medical, social, and educational, or other therapeutic interventions, such as the dietary treatment of the child with phenylketonuria (PKU).

TERTIARY PREVENTION—aimed at minimizing the long-term disability, or at least mitigating some of its effects. This usually takes the form of case-finding and provision of specific and/or comprehensive services for individuals or populations at large. An example would be early intervention services for a child with cerebral palsy or Down syndrome.

jurisdictions have registries for specific conditions, there are no comprehensive risk registries available for all areas of the U.S.

Significant risk reduction can be achieved by identifying persons who are at high risk for parenting a child who will require special health care.[1,2,3] Some of the risk factors relating to pregnancy outcome are:

- maternal illness, including hypertension, anemia, epilepsy;
- metabolic disorders;
- extremes in maternal age;
- poor nutritional status;
- inadequate weight for height;
- exposure to toxic substance;
- exposure to infectious agents, including sexually transmitted disease (STD);
- use of tobacco, alcohol, or other drugs;
- high parity;
- short interval between pregnancies;
- multiple fetuses;
- previous problems with pregnancy;
- history of repeated fetal loss;
- significant physical, mental, or developmental disability; and
- family history of a genetic disorder.

Early intervention services, including medical, social, and developmental interventions for handicapped and "at-risk" infants have been shown to decrease the incidence and the severity of disability.[4,5] Some of the criteria for identifying infants who are at high risk are:

- prematurity/low birthweight;
- small for gestational age (SGA);
- postterm (greater than 43 weeks);
- perinatal asphyxia with documented low Apgar scores, or a need for prolonged resuscitation after delivery;
- prolonged assisted ventilation;
- significant neonatal jaundice;
- sepsis/meningitis;
- symptomatic hypoglycemia;
- neonatal drug addiction;
- neonatal neurological abnormalities;
- major congenital anomalies;
- poor maternal-infant attachment;
- extended hospital stay; and
- other risk factors identified by care providers.

There are a number of congenital disorders that can be identified during pregnancy and/or early in life. Maternal serum alpha fetoprotein (MSAFP) screening, the widespread use of ultrasound imaging during pregnancy, and genetic amniocentesis have resulted in the early identification of infants who will have or are at significant risk of having long-term special health care needs.

Screening of newborn infants for genetic metabolic disorders, hearing loss, and other disorders has allowed the identification and initiation of treatment before symptoms are identified. Most states provide screening of newborns for PKU and hypothyroidism, and many states include screening for other genetic disorders, such as galactosemia, homocystinuria, maple syrup urine disease, biotinidase deficiency, and the hemoglobinopathies.[6,7] The successes in preventing disability by early identification and early treatment have been encouraging and support proposals to expand the screening programs to include additional disorders. Important criteria to be considered before developing new programs are: 1) the effectiveness of early treatment and the degree of disability if untreated; 2) the ability to test at an optimum time to ensure detection and to allow initiation of early treatment; 3) acceptable low rates of false-negative and false-positive test results; and 4) a known and acceptable cost-benefit as a result of the testing.

Screening is also available for the identification of persons who are heterozygous for certain genetic disorders.[8] Technology is rapidly expanding, with the use of desoxyribonucleic acid (DNA) probes, so that persons who are carriers of rare genes can be identified and counseled regarding genetic risks. Gene therapy may soon be available for the treatment of many inherited diseases.

The identification of problems in young children in the U.S. is achieved primarily during periodic health supervision visits which focus on biomedical, developmental and psychological issues. Health assessments should be arranged at scheduled intervals, in addition to the physical and neurodevelopmental examination, and should incorporate history about developmental achievements, identified problems or concerns, an observation of parent-child interaction, and anticipatory guidance discussions. The frequency and timing of the health supervision visits will vary, as will the substance and length of the visits.

The Early and Periodic Screening, Diagnosis and Treatment (EPSDT) program was enacted in 1967 as an amendment to the Medicaid provisions of Title XIX of the Social Security Act. The intent of Congress was to provide screening for children ages zero-21 years, who are eligible for medical services under Medicaid, in order to identify and treat problems that can cause disability. States are required to inform Medicaid recipients about the availability of the EPSDT program and must assist families to participate. Screening tests that are recommended from birth through adolescence include, in addition to the history and physical examination, a developmental history and assessment; dental assessment; nutritional assessment;

vision and hearing screening; and laboratory studies, including hematocrit or hemoglobin, urinalysis, and screening for elevated lead blood levels, if health history warrants.

Childhood disabilities are frequently identified through assessment at the time the child enters school, and through periodic screening of vision, hearing, developmental progress, and general health. The school can be a very important focal point for the evaluation of disabilities that may present at various ages, as demonstrated in the effectiveness of the scoliosis screening programs. Children and young adults who have musculoskeletal problems that are identified early will benefit from treatment initiated during the growing years.

Health professionals, educators, and others who have regular contact with the child and/or the family play a major role in the early diagnosis of disabilities. Early identification leads to early treatment and intervention, resulting in a decrease in the incidence and degree of childhood and adult disability. Screening is the application of simple techniques to identify children who are likely to need special services. Screening procedures must not be confused with diagnostic procedures, and are used only to differentiate persons who are at risk from those who are most likely unaffected. Screening procedures determine which persons should be referred for more extensive comprehensive diagnostic studies. Treatment should not be initiated until after a clear diagnosis is confirmed. Effective early identification tools will improve the health of our pediatric population, reduce the costs of care, and significantly impact the level of human suffering.

REFERENCES

1. Freeman JM (ed). Prenatal and Perinatal Factors Associated with Brain Disorders. National Institute of Child Health and Human Development; National Institute of Neurological and Communicative Disorders and Stroke; U.S. Department of Health and Human Services, Public Health Service, National Institute of Health, NIH Publication No. 85-1149, April 1985.

2. Johnson KG. The Promise of Regional Perinatal Care as a National Strategy for Improved Maternal and Infant Care. Pub. Health Reports 2:134-139, 1982.

3. McCormick MC, Shapiro S, and Starfield BH. The Regionalization of Perinatal Services. JAMA 253:799-804, 1985.

4. Cross L, Goin K (eds). Identifying Handicapped Children: A Guide to Casefinding, Screening, Diagnosis, Assessment and Evaluation. New York, Walker & Co., 1977.

5. Kearsley RB and Sigel IE (eds). Infants at Risk. Lawrence Erlbaum Associates, Publishers, Hillsdale, New Jersey, 1979.

6. Andrews, L.B. State Laws and Regulations Governing Newborn Screening. American Bar Foundation, Chicago, 1985.

7.   Guthrie R. Mass Screening for Genetic Diseases. Hospital Practice 7:93-100, 1972.

8.   Screening and Counseling for Genetic Conditions: The Ethical, Social and Legal Implications of Genetic Screening, Counseling, and Educational Programs. The President's Commission for the Study of Ethical Problems in Medicine and Biomedical and Behavioral Research, Superintendent of Documents, Government Printing Office, Washington, D.C., 1984.

EARLY INTERVENTION

46

Jean F. Kelly and Kathryn E. Barnard

INTRODUCTION

In recent years, interventionists have developed many programs for infants who are handicapped or at risk. Although all of these programs share the common goal of optimal infant development, they approach this goal in different ways. Some programs are home-based models, others are center-based models, and others are a combination of those two approaches. As discussed in this chapter, intervention programs also differ with respect to their program philosophy and goals, the population that is served, team composition, program content, and program evaluation.

Federal law is significantly influencing the development of early-intervention programs. The most applicable law was enacted in October 1986, and is called Title I, or Part H, Handicapped Infants and Toddlers, of PL 99-457, Education of the Handicapped Amendments of 1986. That law provides incentive grants to states to assist in developing comprehensive early-intervention services for infants (zero-35 months) and their families. The law outlines the requirements to which states must adhere when developing a statewide plan for services, and describes individual elements of the required service plan. The law is important to consider when discussing the components of early-intervention programs, for several reasons: 1) states choosing to participate in the grant incentive program must develop specific program components, as outlined in the law; 2) program planners in each state should recognize the federal government's positions on early intervention; and 3) the law and its guidelines may well be used by funding agencies as a measure of program appropriateness.

This chapter discusses the various components of early-intervention programs and the impact of federal law on the development of these programs. For the purposes of this chapter, the term *early intervention* refers to any organized treatment that supports the developmental progress of children, birth to 36 months, and is aimed at ameliorating or eliminating a current or anticipated deficiency. The concept of early intervention has taken on dimensions that encompass the entire family.

PROGRAM PHILOSOPHY AND GOALS

An intervention program's goals and objectives must be based on the program's philosophy of intervention, and the philosophy, in turn, should be validated by the literature and research in the field. Research shows that parents and families critically influence the development of the child.[1-9] The presence of a handicapping condition in infancy can complicate parent-infant interaction and jeopardize the successful functioning of the family unit.[10-18] This suggests than an early-intervention program should focus on the quality of interaction between parents and infants and should be attentive to individual family needs.

Parents' knowledge of their child's capabilities and knowledge of specific activities and environmental conditions that enhance development contribute to their competence in providing an environment that fosters social and emotional growth. This suggests that another major focus of an intervention program should be accurate assessment of infant needs and the development of specific growth-fostering activities.

Suggested Program Goals

The suggested program goals should be to maximize a child's development within the existing family structure by:

a. responding to the personal and family needs expressed by the individual family;

b. fostering quality parent-infant interactions; and

c. developing and implementing appropriate and specific growth-fostering activities for the individual child.

These goals are responsive to the requirements outlined in Part H of PL 99-457, under the Individualized Family Service Plan. That plan requires that the handicapped infant or toddler be assessed in all areas of child development, and that the family's strengths and needs relating to the enhancement of the child be specified. Further, the plan must include statements of major outcomes and specific early-intervention services necessary to meet the unique needs of the child and family.

POPULATION TO BE SERVED

In developing intervention programs, program planners must first decide what population of infants and their families to serve. A possible criterion for involvement in a comprehensive intervention program is to include those infants (and their families) who will not be able to achieve close to their potential unless they receive intervention, and who will most likely be in need of more extensive medical, educational, or institutional services if intervention is not provided.[19] There are three groups of infants most commonly identified as likely to benefit from early intervention: 1) infants who have a diagnosed handicapping condition; 2) infants who are disadvantaged and therefore at risk for developmental delay; and 3) infants who are medically at risk.

INFANTS WHO HAVE A HANDICAPPING CONDITION

Although it is generally accepted that infants who have a diagnosed handicap should receive early intervention services, there remains a need to research the long-term benefits of such intervention. White[20] points out that the question of whether early intervention with handicapped infants produces long-term results is largely unaddressed and unanswered. The decision to provide services is currently based on an understanding of the available research on the harmful effects of handicapping conditions on development and the importance of early experiences on later development, the evidence that early intervention is important to the immediate development of the child and to family functioning, and the belief that a responsible society must respond to a diagnosed need. Our society has generally agreed that it owes a child with a handicap early-intervention services that will ameliorate the immediate effects of that condition, and possibly alter the long-term effects.

Part H, Handicapped Infants and Toddlers, of PL 99-457, provides financial incentives for those states that decide to provide early-intervention services for infants and toddlers with diagnosed delays.

INFANTS WHO ARE ENVIRONMENTALLY AT RISK (DISADVANTAGED)

It is more difficult to identify infants who are not diagnosed as having a handicapping condition but who are, because of environmental factors, at risk for developing later delays. Much research over the past decade has been devoted to identifying and serving these "disadvantaged" infants.[21-23] White and Casto[24] observe that, with the notable exception of the Perry Preschool Project, the preponderance of the currently available evidence shows very few long-term benefits that can be directly attributed to early intervention disadvantaged children. Because of the conclusive evidence to support the relationship between deprived environments and depressed child functioning, however, researchers continue to investigate why this relationship exists [25] and to explore types of intervention that could prevent or mitigate later harmful effects.[26]

Federal law currently leaves to individual states the discretion to decide whether to broaden the legislative definition of children who qualify for early-intervention services under Part H of PL 99-457 to include those at risk for developmental delay.

INFANTS MEDICALLY AT RISK

Due to medical advances, many infants now survive with more severe conditions than in the past.[27] The conditions range from prematurity to conditions resulting in life-long chronic illness. These infants and families require varying amounts of intervention and support. Generally, children with chronic illnesses are cared for in the home. The ability of families to keep children in their homes and continue to function well despite the stresses of coordinating complicated health care plans might well depend on the success of supportive intervention programs.

States are now encouraged to include chronically ill infants, and infants requiring frequent or extended hospital stays, in their definition of infants qualifying for intervention services under Part H of PL 99-457.[28]

PROGRAM SETTING

There are three alternative settings for providing services to infants: the home, the center (e.g., school, university, hospital, daycare center), and a home-center combination. There is debate over the relative advantages of the three settings, and there is little evidence on which a program developer can base a choice of one setting over the other. White and Casto's [24] review of early intervention efficacy studies reports no substantial advantage for home or center-based programs.

Proponents of the three different settings for early-intervention programs generally list the following advantages for the particular model they advocate:

Home-based:
1. Parents feel more comfortable in their own home, and therefore act more like themselves and feel more in control.
2. Children perform better in their own homes.
3. The health of the child is better protected.
4. Family and child routines are not disrupted.
5. There is more likelihood of being able to include other members of the family in intervention efforts.
6. Sessions are more regular; there is not as great an attendance problem.
7. Suggestions for modifying the natural environment of the child and family may be made to facilitate development.

Center-based:

1. The parents and child have access to a larger staff and more services.
2. Parents have the opportunity to share experiences with other parents and seek and provide support.
3. Parents of children in the program serve as additional role models for one another.
4. Children have the opportunity to receive additional stimulation from other children.
5. A special learning environment can be developed and provided.

Home-center based combinations:

Proponents of this setting contend that it maximizes most of the advantages found in both center-based and home-based programs.

Suggested Settings for Birth to Three:

- zero-six months—Home-based weekly visits;

- seven-18 months—A flexible program that provides services dependent on the assessed needs of the child and family;

- 19-36 months —Home-center combination. The center program could offer a group setting. Choice of this approach would still depend on individual needs of child and family.

THE TEAM APPROACH

The term *transdisciplinary* has come into vogue as a suitable expression for team functioning. The transdisciplinary approach, as described by Haynes,[29] markedly reduces the number of one-to-one interventions by professionals. Following evaluation, one or two members, based on the child and family needs, serve as team facilitator(s). This approach is similar to the intent of Part H of PL 99-457, that requires the assignment of a "case manager" from the profession most immediately relevant to the infant's or toddler's, and family's, needs who will be responsible for the implementation of the family service plan. The facilitator or case manager can reduce family and staff confusion, serve as a supportive advocate for families in coordinating interagency services and implementing the family service plan, and encourage competence and parent-infant attachment by reducing the number of professionals dealing with the family.

There are several professions, each with unique skills, prepared to give early-intervention services. The law states that available intervention services include family training, counseling, special instruction, speech services, physical therapy, psychological services, case management services, medical services for diagnostic or evaluation purposes, early-identification services, and health services.

It goes on to specify that these services must be provided by qualified personnel, including nurses, special educators, speech and language pathologists and audiologists, occupational therapists, physical therapists, psychologists, social workers, and nutritionists. This is a fairly exhaustive list of possible personnel, and certainly the needs identified by the family and the assessment team would determine what services are appropriate for an individual family and child.

In addition, the law requires that each state participating in the incentive program to provide services for handicapped infants and toddlers, under Part H, PL 99-457, must have a lead agency designated by the governor to develop, among other things, "procedures to ensure that services are provided to infants and families in a timely manner pending the resolution of any disputes among public agencies or service providers." This section of the law speaks to the need for specific role descriptions that allow for coordination and cooperation among service providers. Instead of competing for a role in the arena of available services, a lead agency must seek to determine how each group of service providers fit in most advantageously for the family and child.

Finally, a statewide system for providing comprehensive early-intervention services should address the issue of certification. State planners should consider the development and regulation of standards in all participating professions to ensure high quality and appropriate services to children and families. Pre-service and inservice training requirements must coordinate the efforts of colleges and universities to include early-intervention preparation programs in or across all related disciplines.

PROGRAM CONTENT

If a program considers the unique needs of each child and family, then program content will be individualized and vary according to assessed needs. A program should have a specific set of procedures and guidelines. In addition, each discipline should have specific activities and materials available to meet the designated objectives outlined by families and staff in the individualized service plan.

The first step in developing program content is to specify the procedures to be followed in determining the individual service plan. According to Part H, PL 99-457, these procedures should include the following: 1) a statement of the child's present levels of physical development, cognitive development, language and speech development, psycho-social development, and self-help skills, based on acceptable objective criteria; 2) a statement of the family strengths and needs related to enhancing the development of the child; 3) a statement of the major outcomes expected to be achieved by the child and the family, and the criteria, procedures, and timelines used to determine the degree of progress; 4) a statement of specific early-intervention services necessary to meet the unique needs of child and family; 5) the projected dates for initiation and duration of the services; and 6) the name of the case manager most relevant to the child and family needs.

In addition to specific procedures, program planners should develop guidelines for assessment and delivery of services. These guidelines could include the following:

1. Concentrate on family priorities as perceived by the families.
2. Respect parents' goals for the infant.
3. Include parents as primary members of the infant's assessment team.
4. Include parents in the planning of specific objectives and activities.
5. Develop activities to share knowledge about normal and delayed child development when appropriate.
6. Reinforce the observational skills of family members.
7. Explain all suggested activities and procedures so that families can generalize from specific knowledge.
8. Deal positively, not judgmentally, with all family members, and encourage them to deal positively with the child.
9. Give positive feedback to families about specific achievements and encourage family members to recognize small increments of child success.
10. Recognize and respect the diversity of cultural values.

Team members representing each discipline should have valid and reliable assessment procedures for determining child and family needs. The procedures used by various disciplines will depend on the area of assessment. In addition, each team member should have available curriculum materials and activities for meeting the specified child and family needs. See Bagnato and Neisworth[30] for descriptions of several packaged curricula designed to enhance child skill development. Personnel can choose from one of the published curricula or compile their own curriculum resources. There is very little packaged curriculum material available designed to meet family needs or foster parent-infant interaction. Activities for responding to these areas must be designed by the staff, with the assistance of program activities reported in the literature.[31-39]

PROGRAM EVALUATION

There are two types of program evaluation: formative evaluation and summative evaluation. *Formative evaluation* is an ongoing process of information-gathering used for the purposes of feedback and giving a program direction. It is generally conducted by internal staff. The users of the information are the program developers and staff. *Summative evaluation* occurs at the end of a program and provides information as to whether the program was effective in reaching its goals. It can also be used to judge the relative desirability of different program procedures or components. It is usually conducted by outside personnel, and the information is used by outsiders such as funding agencies. A rigorous summative evaluation employs control groups.

Olds[40] suggests that process or formative evaluations are the most realistic and helpful for local programs. Properly designed and implemented, process evaluations can be used to improve program quality and thus the lives of the children and families being served. Olds goes on to describe the elements of a good process evaluation:

> A good process evaluation should include the following features: a clear statement of goals and objectives for the children and families served; a clear statement of what is done and why; accurate record keeping for families (based on program goals and objectives); a statement of who is served, why, and what proportion of the target population is reached; a description of the contexts in which service is provided; documentation regarding the services actually performed; an assessment of the relationship between service provider and family; and an examination of those categories of infants and families who made the most progress and those who failed to progress.

CONCLUSION

This chapter has considered the following components of intervention programs for infants who are handicapped or at risk, and their families: 1) philosophy and goals; 2) population to be served; 3) program setting; 4) team approach; 5) program content, and 6) program evaluation. All of these components are interrelated, and program developers should not make decisions about one component without considering the other related parts.

There are several requisites in developing these components: a detailed assessment of the needs of the community as a whole, a careful examination of the available literature and expertise from many disciplines, flexibility in program development and implementation, and finally involvement of families in the planning, implementation, and evaluation efforts.

This last consideration—the involvement of families in intervention—is perhaps the newest focus of intervention efforts. The emphasis in early intervention has moved from a child-centered approach to a family-centered approach. The term, *ecological* intervention—that is, intervention planned around the relationship between the child and the environment—is greatly influencing the development of what are considered appropriate and effective intervention services. With this relatively new emphasis, intervention efforts could be more comprehensive and prove to have broader and longer-lasting results.

REFERENCES

1. Barnard KE. *Instructor's learning resource manual.* NCAST, University of Washington, Seattle, 1979.

2. Gallagher J (ed). *Final report: 1977-82 Carolina Institute for Research on Early Education for the Handicapped.* Chapel Hill, NC: CIREEH Project at the Frank Porter Graham Child Development Center, 1983.

3. Lillie D, Trohanis P. (eds). *Teaching parents to teach.* New York: Walker and Company, 1976.

4. Mahoney G, Finger I, & Powell A. Relationship of maternal behavioral style to the development of organically impaired mentally retarded infants. *Am Journal of Mental Deficiency,* 90:296-302, 1985.

5. Moore, C (ed). *Preschool programs for handicapped children.* Eugene, OR: Regional Resource Center (RRC) of the University of Oregon, 1974.

6. Olson SL, Bates JE, Bayles K. Mother-infant interaction and the development of individual differences in children's cognitive competence. *Developmental Psychology,* 20:166-179, 1984.

7. Stern G G, Caldwell B M, Hersher L, Lipton E L, Richmond J B. Early social contacts and social relations: Effects of quality of early relationship. In L. J. Stone, H. T. Smith, & L. B. Murphy (ed). *The competent infant.* New York Basic Books, Inc,1973.

8. Wachs TD, Uzgiris IC, Hunt J McV. Cognitive development in infants of different age levels and from different environmental backgrounds: An exploratory investigation. *Merrill-Palmer Quarterly,* 17, 283-317, 1971.

9. Yarrow LJ, Rubenstein JL, Pederson FA. *Infant and environment: Early cognitive and motivational development.* New York, John Wiley & Sons, 1975.

10. Berger J, Cunningham CC. Development of early vocal behaviors and interactions in Down's syndrome and non-handicapped infant-mother pairs. *Developmental Psychology,* 19, 322-331, 1983.

11. Dunlap W R. How do parents of handicapped children view their needs. *Journal of the Division for Early Childhood,* 1:1-10, 1979.

12. Eheart BK. Mother-child interactions with nonretarded and mentally retarded preschoolers. *American Journal of Mental Deficiency,* 87:20-25, 1982.

13. Farber B. *Family organization and interaction.* San Francisco, Chandler Publishing Company, 1964.

14. Farber B. *Mental retardation: Its social context and social consequences.* Boston, Houghton Mifflin Co, 1968.

15. Gath A. Parents' reaction to Down's Syndrome. *Journal of the Division for Early Childhood,* 1:11-17, 1979.

16. Klaus MH, Fanaroff AA. *Care of the high risk neonate.* Philadelphia, London & Toronto, W. B. Saunders Company, 1973.

17. Olshansky S. Chronic sorrow: A response to having a mentally defective child. *Social Casework,* 43:190-193, 1962.

18. Stone NW, Chesney B H. Attachment behaviors in handicapped infants. *Mental Retardation,* 16:8-12, 1962.

19. Kelly JF. *Analysis of service delivery to children, birth to three years, and their families.* Developed for the Washington State Education Agency as a WESTAR Search. Monmouth, Oregon, 1980.

20. White K. *Evaluating the effectiveness of early intervention.* Paper presented at a Child and Youth Research Luncheon Forum, Washington, D.C. Sponsored by Research Resources for Children, Youth, and Families, and organized by the National Center for Clinical Infant Programs, November 5, 1985.

21. Bronfenbrenner U. Is early intervention effective? In U. Bronfenbrenner & M. A. Mahoney (Eds.) *Influences on human development.* Hinsdale, IL: The Dryden Press, 1975.

22. Lazar I. *Preliminary findings of the developmental continuity longitudinal study.* Paper presented at the Office of Child Development Conference, "Parents, Children, and Continuity." El Paso, TX, May 23, 1977.

23. Weber CU, Foster PW, Weikart D P. An economic analysis of the Ypsilanti Perry Preschool Project (*Monographs of the High/Scope Educational Research Foundation, No. 5*). Ypsilanti, MI: High/Scope Press, 1978.

24. White K, Casto G. An integrative review of early intervention efficacy studies with at-risk children: Implications for the handicapped. *Analysis and Intervention in Developmental Disabilities,* 5:7-31, 1985.

25. Bee HL, Barnard KE, Eyres SJ, Gray CA, Hammond MA, Spietz AL, Snyder C, Clark B. Prediction of IQ and language skill from perinatal status, child performance, family characteristics, and mother-infant interaction. *Child Development,* 53:1134-1156, 1982.

26. Ramey CT, Sparling JJ, Bryant DM, Wasik BH. Primary intervention of developmental retardation during infancy. In HA Moss, R Hess, C Swift (eds.), *Early intervention programs for infants* (pp. 61-82). New York, Haworth Press, 1982.

27. Gruenberg EM. The failure of success. *Millbank Memorial Fund Quarterly,* 3:24, Winter 1977.

28. Johnson BH. Executive Director, Association for the Care of Children's Health, Washington, D.C. Memo regarding recommendations for the regulations pertaining to Part H of the Education for the Handicapped Act Amendments of 1986, December 23, 1986.

29. Haynes UB. The national collaborative infant project. In TD Tjossem (ed), *Intervention strategies for high risk infants and young children.* Baltimore, University Park Press, 1976.

30. Bagnato SJ, Neisworth JT. *Linking developmental assessment and curricula.* Rockville, MD, Aspen, 1981.

31. Affleck G, McGrade BJ, McQueeney M, Allen D. Promise of relationship focused early intervention in developmental disabilities. *Journal of Special Education,* 16:413-430, 1982.

32. Barnard KE, Hammond MA, Sumner GA, Kang R, Johnson-Crowley N, Snyder C, Spietz A, Blackburn S, Brandt P, Magyary D. Helping parents with preterm infants: Field test of a protocol. *Early Child Development and Care,* 27:255-290.1987.

33. Barnard KE, Hammond M, Mitchell SK, Booth CL, Spietz A, Snyder C, Elsas T. Caring for high-risk infants and their families. In M. Green (ed), *The psychosocial aspects of the family.* Lexington, MA, DC Heath, 1985.

34. Barnard K, Kelly JF. Infant intervention: Parental considerations. In *Guidelines for early intervention programs.* Based on a conference, Health Issues in Early Intervention Programs. University of Utah, Salt Lake City, May, 1980.

35. Bromwich R. *Working with parents and infants: An interactional approach.* Baltimore,

University Park Press, 1981.

36. Dunst CJ, Lesko, JJ, Holbert KA, Wilson LL, Sharpe KL, Liles RF. A systematic approach to infant intervention. *Topics in Early Childhood Special Education,* 7:2, Summer, 1987.

37. Foster M, Berger M, McLean M. Rethinking a good idea: A reassessment of parent involvement. *Topics in Early Childhood Special Education,* 1: 55-65, 1981.

38. Honig AS. Working in partnership with parents of handicapped infants. *Early Child Development and Care,* 14:13-36, 1984.

39. Kelly JF. Effects of intervention on caregiver-infant interaction when the infant is handicapped. *Journal of the Division for Early Childhood,* 5:53-63, June, 1982.

40. Olds D. *Evaluating the effectiveness of early intervention.* Paper presented at a Child and Youth Research Luncheon Forum, Washington, DC. Sponsored by Research Resources for Children, Youth, and Families and organized by National Center for Clinical Infant Programs, Nov 8, 1985.

CASE MANAGEMENT FOR CHILDREN WITH SPECIAL HEALTH CARE NEEDS

47

Josephine Gittler

Case Management* has emerged as an important, even critical, service for children with special health care needs (i.e., children with disabilities, handicaps and chronic illnesses).

DEFINITION

Although case management is a widely used term, there is considerable confusion as to its meaning.[1] Having surveyed the literature, two noted authorities concluded that the simplest way to define case management is as "a set of logical steps and a process of interaction within a service network which assure that a client receives needed services in a supportive, effective, efficient and cost-effective manner."[2] The central thrust of case management is organization of resources for a client in a systematic fashion, and a key element of case management is the fixing of responsibility for such organization of resources in either an individual case manager or a case management team.

HISTORY AND DEVELOPMENT

The origins of case management can be traced to the social work profession during the early twentieth century. Historically, it was viewed by the social work

---

* Terms, such as care coordination, managed care, service coordination, and service integration have come to be employed more or less interchangeably with the term case management.

profession as a means of mobilizing and coordinating services for the poor. [3] As case management has evolved, it has come to be used not only in the social work field but also in such other fields as mental health, developmental disabilities, geriatrics, and MCH. Case management has recently received a great deal of attention, specifically in relation to the population of children with special health care needs.

A major impetus for the recent development of case-management programs for children with special health care needs has come from the federal level. Initiatives by both the U.S. Congress and the U.S. Department of Health and Human Services have had the effect of encouraging the creation, expansion, and upgrading of case-management services for this population.[1]

The current focus upon case management for children with special health care needs and their families is attributable in part to the comprehensive service need of this population and the complexity and fragmentation of existing service systems. The majority of these children need multiple health and health-related services of varying degrees of intensity, from a variety of professionals over a considerable period of time. They frequently also need other types of services, including special education, vocational, social, mental health, and recreational services. Moreover, their families may need various types of services. Since the 1960s, there has been a proliferation of public and private programs serving this population. These programs have differing mandates, eligibility requirements, and policies that sometimes overlap and are inconsistent, and, as a result, there are gaps and duplications in services. Because of the complexity and fragmentation of service systems, children with special health care needs and their families are likely to encounter significant difficulties in obtaining access to needed comprehensive services and coordinating these services. Case managers who assist these children and their families in negotiating service systems have come to be seen as a solution to the problems stemming from the complexity and fragmentation of service systems.

The current focus upon case management for children with special health care needs and their families is also attributable in part to efforts to contain rising health care costs. One response to the inflation in health care costs has been the spread of health maintenance organizations and other forms of prepaid or capitated health care plans, which have a built-in financial incentive to control the costs of services by preventing unnecessary utilization of services. In such health care delivery systems, a case manager generally acts as a "gatekeeper" and must approve all health services received so as to eliminate or reduce unnecessary utilization. Even in more traditional fee-for-service health care delivery systems, a case manager may monitor provision of services for cost-containment purposes. Since many children with special health care needs are relatively heavy users of high-cost health services, case management for this population has come to be seen as promoting health care cost-containment, at least by some private insurers and public programs that finance such care.

CASE-MANAGEMENT PROCESS

While there is tremendous diversity in case-management programs, the case-management process in different programs tends to have similar components, with the core components being: (1) assessment, (2) service planning, and (3) implementation of the service plan. [3,4,5,6]

Assessment

The first core component of the case-management process is an individualized assessment of a client, involving a determination of the client's problems, resources, and service needs. The assessment produces information that furnishes the basis for subsequent planning of services and implementation of the service plan.

The assessment component of case-management programs vary widely in scope. The assessment of a child with special health care needs has traditionally focused upon diagnosis of the child's medical problems and determination of the child's medical care needs. However, there has been an increasing emphasis on assessment of the child's overall functioning, as well as medical status. There is also a growing awareness of the importance of an assessment of the child's family, inasmuch as the child's parents and other family members are usually the primary source of care for the child and create the child's home environment. In short, an optimal assessment of a child with special health care needs should be broad-based.

Assessment may be done by an individual or a team. However, a broad-based assessment of a child with special health care needs and the child's family usually requires the knowledge and skills of more than one discipline. Hence, it has long been recognized that a team approach to assessment is preferable. The team may be multidisciplinary, with team members from various disciplines functioning more or less independently, or the team may be interdisciplinary, with team members from various disciplines functioning in a collaborative fashion. The composition of the team depends upon the child's disease or condition and may also depend upon the availability of professionals from various disciplines in particular settings. The case manager should be, but is not always, a member of the team.

Service Planning

The next core component in the case-management process is service planning. Service planning refers to the development of some type of individualized plan of services, or plan of care for the client, based upon the information generated by the assessment.

There is wide variation in the service-planning component, as well as the assessment component of the case-management process. Service plans may be informal or formal, and formal plans differ in specificity and format. Ideally, service planning should result in a written plan delineating the specific problems to be addressed, services needed, existing resources, the service providers to whom referrals will be made, potential barriers to service delivery and utilization and proposed steps to overcome these barriers, and expected or desired outcomes and time frames for achievement of those outcomes. In some instances, the assessment team may do the service planning and, in other instances, the case manager may do the service planning. Active participation of the child's family is essential to good service planning.

Service planning is a dynamic process and does not end with the development of a service plan. Since children with special health care needs and their families tend to have long-term service needs that change over time, these children and their families should be periodically reassessed and the service plan should be modified to reflect changes in service needs.

Service Plan Implementation

After the service plan is completed, the next component in the case-management process is the implementation of the plan. The term, *case management*, is often used to refer to only this component of the process. Since there are pronounced differences among case-management programs, as to the activities that occur at this stage, precise statements about the functions performed by case managers cannot be made. However, there are a series of functions that should be considered to be an integral part of case management.

1. Case managers typically perform the function of linking the client with providers of the services specified in the service plan. Such client-provider linkage activities may range from the simple referral of a child and the child's family to a service provider, to making an appointment with the provider for the child and the child's family, and then accompanying them when they meet with a provider.

2. Case managers also typically perform the function of coordinating services specified in the service plan. Case-management coordination activities are aimed at assuring the proper sequencing and continuity of services and at assuring that delivered services are complementary. As it has been pointed out, the need for coordination of services exists because needed services often must be obtained from a number of providers. Coordination is particularly important when the providers of services are associated with several different institutions, agencies, or organizations.

3. Another typical function performed by case managers is the monitoring of services provided to the client in accordance with the service plan. Monitoring involves various forms of follow-up to assure that the child

and the child's family do, in fact, receive all of the services which have been agreed upon and for which arrangements have been made. Monitoring may also involve assuring that the child and the child's family are able and willing to comply with the recommendations of service providers. In addition, monitoring may involve oversight of the utilization of services so as to assure that they are neither under-utilized nor over-utilized, and evaluation of services so as to assure that their quality is appropriate and their cost is appropriate. In connection with monitoring, the case manager should measure the progress of the child and the child's family, and identify changes in service needs.

4. Another function sometimes performed by the case manager is individual client advocacy. At the client level, advocacy may be characterized as efforts directed at securing financial and other types of assistance and services to which the child and the child's family are entitled. It also may be characterized as efforts directed at removing barriers may interfere with linkage, coordination, and monitoring activities, client advocacy may be necessary for successful case management.

5. Case managers may also engage in activities that benefit not only an individual client but also the target population as a whole. Case managers can, and do, promote formal and informal collaboration between agencies, institutions, and organizations in the service system, and they can, and do, work to overcome inadequacies that they have identified in the service system. Thus, the efforts of case managers can contribute to the overall rationalization of service systems for children with special health care needs and their families.

CASE-MANAGEMENT PERSONNEL

The performance of case-management functions by paid professionals is the prevailing pattern in the delivery of case-management services to children with special health care needs and their families.[4,5,7] Both primary care physicians and specialist, and subspecialist physicians, regularly engage in certain case-management activities in relation to the health service needs of these children. In formally organized case-management programs, the professionals most likely to be designated as case managers are nursing personnel, followed by social work personnel. Many of these professionals provide clinical services, as well as case-management services. There appears to be a trend towards the use of interdisciplinary or multidisciplinary teams for case management, at least for some categories of children with special health care needs, albeit a member of the team usually acts as the primary case manager or the coordinator of case-management services.

It is difficult to generalize about the qualifications that case-management personnel should possess. The staffing appropriate for a particular case-management program will depend upon the client population, the tasks assigned case managers and the service system or systems within which the case managers work, and the staffing must be consistent with the program's resources and organizational structure.

The prevalence of health professionals as case managers for children with special health care needs reflects the fact that case management for this population has had a medical orientation, which in turn reflects the fact that this population, by definition, has significant health problems. However, case management should address the service needs of the child and the child's family as a whole, and these needs may dictate a psycho-social model, or some other model requiring a knowledge basis and skills not normally associated with health professionals. The team approach to case management has the advantage of making available individuals with a variety of professional backgrounds to provide case-management services. A related approach is to assign, as case manager, the individual with the professional background most relevant to the service needs of the child and the child's family.

FUTURE DIRECTIONS OF CASE-MANAGEMENT SERVICE

Family-Centered Case Management

There is a growing commitment to a philosophy of family-centered services,, including case-management services for children with special health care needs. [9] Basic to this philosophy is that families and professionals should be equal partners and collaborate in the care of these children, and underlying this philosophy is the recognition that the family is generally the child's primary caretaker and is the constant in the child's life.

Incorporation of the philosophy of family-centered services into case management requires that the parents of a child with special health-care needs fully participate in all aspects of decision-making with respect to the provision of case-management services for their child. It also requires that families be involved in the planning, design, and implementation of case-management programs.

It must be stressed that not all families require case-management services. Among families that do need such services, there is great variation in the nature and extent of the services needed. At one end of the spectrum are families in need of short-term minor services, and at the other end of the spectrum are families in need of long-term extensive and intensive services. Whatever the nature and extent of the services needed, the aim of the case manager should be to empower the family to assume, to the extent possible, the responsibility for performing case-management functions.

Community-Based Case Management

Just as a child is part of a family, a family is part of a community, and the philosophy of community-based services is closely related to the philosophy of family-centered services. The U.S. Surgeon General has enunciated, as a national goal, the building of systems of community-based services for children with special health-care needs, which involves giving these children and their families access to needed services in or near their home. [9]

Community-based case management is directed at assisting families to obtain access to needed services, and coordinating these services. An essential element of community-based case management is the fostering of linkages between the tertiary medical center and community health providers, and the fostering of linkages between community health providers and other community-service providers.[10,11]

One characteristic of community-based case-management programs is that they are geographically decentralized. Community-based case-management requires knowledge on the part of the case manager both of the problems confronted by a child and the child's family and knowledge of the resources available to them in or near their home community; it also entails personal interaction between the case manager and community-service providers. Therefore, the case manager must be located close to the children and families being provided case-management services. [10,11]

Community-based case-management programs are also usually generic in nature, rather than disease-specific or condition-specific, because it is simply not feasible from the standpoint of personnel availability and costs to conduct separate programs for children with different diseases or conditions in every community.[10,11]

CONCLUSION

There is a developing consensus that contemporary case management should be family-centered and community-based. The concept of family-centered, community-based case management is not complicated, but its implementation will require changes in, and expansion of, existing services. However, this type of case management has the potential of providing needed support to families and improving the care of children. This type of case management also has the potential of improving service systems, as a whole, through the establishment of networks of integrated services at the community level.

REFERENCES

1. Gittler J. Future directions of case management services for children with special health care needs: an overview, *National Conference Proceedings: Future Directions of Case Management Services For Children With Special Health Care Needs*, Edited by J. Gittler & M. Colton, Iowa City, IA, University of Iowa, National Maternal and Child Health Resource Center, 1987, pp 7-13.

2. Weil M, Karls JM. Historical elements and recent developments, *Case Management in Human Service Practice*, Edited by M. Weil and J. M. Karls, San Francisco, CA, Jossey-Bass Publishers, 1985, pp 1-28.

3. Weil M. Key components in providing efficient and effective services, *Case Management in Human Service Practice*, Edited by M. Weil and J M Karls, San Francisco, CA, Jossey-Bass Publishers, 1985, pp 29-72.

4. Gittler J, Colton M. *Community-Based Case Management Services for Children with Special Health Care Needs: Program Models,* Iowa City, IA, University of Iowa, National Maternal and Child Health Resource Center, 1986.

5. Gittler J, Colton M. *Alternatives to Hospitalization for Technology Dependent Children: Program Models,* Iowa City, IA, University of Iowa, National Maternal and Child Health Resource Center, 1987.

6. Levine IS, Fleming M. *Human Resource Development: Issues in Case Management,* Baltimore, MD, Center of Rehabilitation and Manpower Services, University of Maryland, 1984.

7. Colton M, Gittler J. *The Title V State Programs and the Provision of Case Management Services for Children with Special Needs,* Iowa City, IA, University of Iowa, National Maternal and Child Health Resource Center, 1986.

8. Shelton JL, Jeppson ES, Johnson BH. *Family-Centered Care for Children with Special Health Care Needs,* Washington, D.C., Association for the Care of Children's Health, 1987.

9. U.S. Department of Health and Human Services, Public Health Service, *Surgeon General's Report: Children with Special Health Care Needs, Campaign '87,* Washington, D.C., U.S. Government Printing Office, 1987.

10. Gittler J. *Community-Based Systems of Comprehensive Services for Children with Special Health Care Needs and Their Families,* Iowa City, IA, University of Iowa, National Maternal and Child Health Resource Center, 1988.

11. MacQueen JC. *Community-Based Case Management, National Conference Proceedings: Future Directions of Case Management Services for Children with Special Health Care Needs,* Edited by J. Gittler and M. Colton, Iowa City, IA, University of Iowa, National Maternal and Child Health Resource Center, 1987, pp 17-26.

INSTITUTIONAL CARE FOR CHILDREN WITH SPECIAL NEEDS

48

Elhamy F. Khalil

For many centuries children with severe handicapping conditions were looked after by their families at home. During the 19th century and up to the 1950s, many such children, who were increasing in number, were admitted to state run facilities for custodial care. The last two decades have witnessed an increasing emphasis on de-institutionalization. The goal is to place most children in home-like settings to approximate the environment in which non-handicapped children of the same age would be residing.

There remains, however, a small percentage of children whose medical and nursing needs are so great that small foster homes are not able to provide the needed care. Less than ten percent of known developmentally disabled children in California now reside at state facilities, compared to approximately 20 percent only a decade ago.

The basic criteria for admission of developmentally disabled children to institutions is the level of fragility of their health. Those admitted are usually children with unstable medical conditions who require nursing care 24 hours per day, as well as the need for the immediate availability of medical personnel to handle life-threatening situations. These children may have tracheostomies and are in need of respiratory therapy several times daily. Others might require assisted respiration and are connected to ventilators requiring frequent changes of equipment settings and ongoing monitoring. Still others may need to be monitored frequently, even daily or more often, by medical specialists. Most community care facilities are not equipped or staffed to handle the constant possible occurrence of life-threatening situations. Children who have severe or even profound mental retardation, but have no serious health problems, are not admitted to state facilities in California.

The diagnostic categories of children admitted to Lanterman Developmental Center, which is one of seven state-run institutions in California, have changed over the last five years. Many such children are in a state of irreversible coma. The highest category is now due to postnatal accidental, rather than perinatal, conditions or congenital malformations.

The etiological factors of the last 100 children under 18 years of age, admitted to Lanterman Developmental Center, are as follows:

Status post near-drowning	24 cases
Severe and multiple congenital malformation	22 cases
Perinatal hypoxia and prematurity	11 cases
Post central nervous system infection	10 cases
Post trauma head injuries	9 cases
Postnatal cerebral anoxia due to other causes	6 cases
Degenerative and metabolic disorders	4 cases
Prenatal exposure to drugs	3 cases
Other causes	11 cases
	100 cases

The increasing number of admissions to institutions of the post near-drowning children is a reflection of the increasing number of backyard swimming pools in California, where 90 percent of these incidents occur. Most of the children in this category are two-four-years of age at the time of admission. Ninety percent of near-drowning victims either die, or recover without brain damage or with minor sequelae. However, ten percent survive with severe and irreversible brain damage. Such children almost always have difficulty in swallowing and frequent aspiration pneumonias. Tracheostomy and gastrostomy are usually required to facilitate breathing and maintain nutrition. A large number of these children have severe spasticity and temperature instability. They may have periods of neurogenic fevers or hypothermia. Many suffer from frequent seizure activity and diabetes insipidus. The latter requires frequent monitoring of fluids and electrolytes. Recently a number of adolescents with severe brain damage due to post hanging, in attempted suicide, as well as infants of drug-addicted mothers, have been admitted.

The responsibility of placement of developmentally disabled children in out-of-home facilities rests with 21 Regional Centers in California. Admission to a state institution is initiated only after exhaustive search for a less restrictive placement has proven fruitless. The admission has to be approved by the parent or legal guardian. The child is assessed by professionals in the fields of pediatrics, nursing, social services, dietetics, occupational therapy, physical therapy, audiology, developmental psychology, and education. Other disciplines may be involved as needed. An individual program plan is formulated by an interdisciplinary team. The goal is to improve or maintain health, enrich the child's life, and promote developmental progress and life skills up to the child's highest potential. Parents are integral members of the team. They are encouraged to visit and participate in all decisions related to their child's program. With proper training and support, some families take their child home for a few hours, a day, or a short holiday.

Support groups are available for families, especially in their grieving period. These are conducted by parents, with a social worker acting as a facilitator. Specialists in most fields are available for consultation. Physicians are in the institutions 24 hours a day, seven days a week. Respiratory therapists are assigned to children on assisted ventilation, at all times. Children requiring intensive care are usually transferred to tertiary-care facilities in the community. Special transport systems, staffed by highly trained personnel, are available for the transfer.

Some children remain at the institution for life, while others are discharged either to a small family care home or to their parents' care. Certain preparation is required to assure the success of the placement.

If, at the interdisciplinary conference, the child's condition seemed to be appropriate for discharge to the community, the Regional Center representative would search for a suitable facility. Once located, several staff members, from the unit on which the child resides at the institution, visit the prospective home or small facility and discuss the child's needs with the care providers. The child and his/her family participate in the discussion and decision. If found suitable, and all concerned are agreeable, the staff from the institution transmits detailed reports of the child's condition, needs, and program. To avoid any interruption in the type of service the child requires, the child is discharged only after all the training programs, medical, and nursing services, as well as school programs, are available. After discharge to the community, the Regional Center staff in that geographical area will be responsible for monitoring the placement and the programs for that child.

Occasionally the child's family request caring for their child at home. An elaborate preparation is set in motion, with a large number of individuals and agencies involved. This can be summarized as follows:

1. Initial planning conference to identify the level of need in the areas of health and training in great detail.

2. Middle stage of discharge planning. In that session, the following is usually discussed:

   a. Living home arrangements during day and night.
   b. Equipment needed—methods of obtaining, maintenance, and repair.
   c. Supplies—type, amount, and availability, e.g. oxygen.

    d. Availability of medical care and emergency care.

    e. Training of family members in specific areas of care, e.g., tracheostomy, gastrostomy, the use of oxygen, suction machines, etc.

    f. The need for in-home nursing care, and the number of hours required in conjunction with the family members.

    g. "Trouble shooting" of equipment, training in CPR and management of emergencies and life-threatening situations.

    h. Availability and strength of family-support system.

    i. Funding for all the required services, equipment, and supplies.

    j. Treatment needs e.g., occupational and physical therapy, usually in home.

    k. Schooling in- or out-of-home, if child's medical condition permits.

    l. Transportation.

    m. Other services or needs peculiar to that child's condition.

    n. Charting methods done after discharge.

3. Final stage. A meeting is held with all concerned in attendance. A checklist of all items mentioned above is discussed to assure proper implementation. Team members give their final recommendations and a date for discharge is agreed upon. A summary of all the above is transmitted to the Regional Center and family. The medical summary is sent to the local physician who would be responsible for the child's care. School reports, physical therapy, etc., are sent to their counterparts by various professionals, to arrive prior to the day of discharge.

4. Post Discharge Follow-up. The family is encouraged to call the institution during the first few days for advice. The social worker calls on the family to assure that all plans are in operation. The Regional Center's staff then takes over the monitoring and ongoing support for the family. If at any given time the family is unable to cope with the child's needs, a readmission to the state facility may be requested. Well-planned discharges rarely result in readmission to the institution.

The cost of care of children with special needs depends on the level of staffing required since staff salary and benefits usually account for 70 percent to 80 percent of the total cost in most health care facilities. The present cost varies from $150 to $200 per-day per-child in institutions. The cost is comparable, or even higher, for those who are cared for at home, if the same level of nursing care is given. For children who need frequent visits by physicians and who require frequent acute hospitalization, state institutions would be less costly when all the expenses are included. There are, however, many children who can be appropriately placed in the community, either small care homes or in their own homes, if suitable supportive measures are available.

There are unmet needs in the following areas:

1. Expanding in-home services, such as nursing and various therapy professionals and improvement of methods of funding.

2. Making available respite care, either in the home or for short-term admission to state institutions, through simplifying procedures for temporary admission.

3. Encouraging partnership between community and state facilities in the utilization of expertise of individuals and services in state facilities, e.g., mobility engineering for the design, fabrication, and repair of specialized equipment for children in the community, where often no such services exist.

4. Training of care providers in the community in specialized procedures and care of children who have tracheostomies, gastrostomies, and other nursing needs.

5. Joint support groups for families who have children with similar conditions, such as post near drowning and post head injury, through attendance of parents of children both in institutions and at home.

6. Increasing public awareness of preventive measures, such as water safety, as well as promoting legislation to make swimming pools less hazardous for children.

7. Improving funding for small family-care homes, and offering incentives for families to care for their children at home.

The need for institutional care will probably remain for some time to come for the following reasons:

1. There are more children surviving with multiple and severe congenital malformations, as a result of the recent tendency to treat severely affected babies, as well as the ability to salvage smaller and smaller premature babies.

2. Children whose condition is unstable and who are dependent on ventilators and other equipment for survival. Some of them can be cared for at home when their condition becomes stable; however, many require almost constant attention by respiratory therapists and physicians not available elsewhere.

3. The argument that cost will be decreased in home care compared to institutional care is invalid, if we compare the same type of child with the same needs and the same level of professional involvement. In fact, the opposite may be true.

4. Care in institutions is continuously scrutinized by various licensing and accreditation agencies. Such quality control is more difficult to attain in small facilities, for logistics reasons. The quality of care, to a large extent, in small care providers' homes depends on the persons in charge, which can vary from excellent to poor.

5. De-institutionalization of the mentally ill from state mental hospitals leaves a great deal to be desired. Such actions have sometimes resulted in many homeless individuals incapable of taking care of themselves, and who do not use even the inadequate local mental health services.

Various legislations at the federal and state levels are in the discussion phase, to find out the most economical methods of funding and caring for the severely handicapped and technologically dependent children. Also, individual cases are being looked into through the courts. It would be counterproductive to eliminate one type of facility before a viable alternative is tested for adequacy and quality. Institutions need to remain as a part of a continuum of facilities serving the disabled. Integration between community services and institutional services would close many gaps and assure the availability of various options as to the best type of placement for each individual child.

HOME CARE OF CHILDREN ASSISTED BY HIGH-TECH MEDICAL SUPPORTS

49

Kathryn A. Kirkhart and A. Joanne Gates

INTRODUCTION

Medical technology can be used to sustain or promote life for children with a multitude of conditions. Technology can accompany a child out of the hospital into the home post-discharge. The technology is increasingly more available, cost-contained, efficient, and portable. The specialized medical community is comfortable with its uses, both in and out of the hospital. However, community-based medical, financial, psychosocial, and educational supports are not developed to meet the needs of the child and family who live at home. The focus of efforts has been on the technology rather than on the child.

A workshop convened by Surgeon General Koop of the U.S. Public Health Service, in 1982, has examined the problems of service delivery and funding mechanisms for community-based services, focusing on the ventilator-assisted child as the prototype.[1] Dr. Koop has identified a new category of disability—a group of individuals defined by the use of medical technology. The Surgeon General's 1987 conference on children with special health care needs is a call to action for family-centered, community-based, coordinated care.[2] The report of the conference is an action plan for the provision of better services and service systems for children and their families, with an emphasis on home care.

Quality-of-life concerns are often raised regarding the uses of medical technology. In the Hastings Center guidelines,[3] quality-of-life is promoted as an "ethi-

673

cally essential concept that focuses on the good of the individual, what kind of life is possible given the person's condition, and whether that condition will allow the individual to have a life he or she views as worth living." A better quality-of-life can be achieved by most technology-assisted individuals in a home setting rather than in a medical institution. Home care is desirable for all medically stable, technology-assisted children. Goldberg [4] asserts that "community-oriented care can be safe and cost-effective and can result in healthier lives for ventilator-dependent people."

EXTENT OF THE CONCEPT

Two national task forces have been authorized by Congress to define the scope of the concept and to identify the populations who are technology-assisted. The report of the Office of Technology Assessment,[5] published in 1987, defines the technology-dependent child "as one who needs both a medical device to compensate for the loss of vital body function and substantial and ongoing nursing care to avert death or further disability." OTA identifies four separate populations as 1) ventilator-users, 2) children who require prolonged intravenous administration of nutritional substances or drugs, 3) children who use other devices for respiratory or nutritional support, such as tracheostomies or tube feedings, and 4) children with prolonged dependence on other medical devices, such as apnea monitors or urinary catheters. This report estimates that, in the U.S., there are 2,300-17,000 children in the first three groups, and even larger numbers in the fourth group—maybe 81,000 or more.

As authorized by Congress, the Task Force on Technology Dependent Children, of the U.S. Department of Health and Human Services,[6] reports on its two-year study in April 1988. Their working definition is as follows, "A technology dependent child is a person through 21 years of age who has a chronic disability; requires the routine use of a particular medical device to compensate for the loss of use of a life sustaining body function; and requires daily ongoing care or monitoring by trained personnel."

The needs of children who are technology-assisted vary across individuals and their unique circumstances. Commonalities include 1) a family willing to assume responsibility for the care of their child's medical, developmental, and psychosocial needs; 2) access to a medical service system, which includes tertiary health care specialists who provide acute care and stabilization interventions, as well as prepare the child, family, and community providers for home care through planning and training activities; 3) case management for service coordination and monitoring; 4) a home community, which is supportive of planning and providing for emergency responsiveness, the child's education in a least-restrictive environment, accessible resources, primary care, and family support; and 5) stable financial support of service needs.

CONTENT OF CARE

The care provided to a child with high-tech medical supports is based on the child's individual needs, as well as the sophistication of the health care team. Care routines established by hospital personnel must be extended to home care, modified to normalize daily living within a family setting and to utilize available resources.

The family is central to the child's routine care management. Adult caregivers must be thoroughly trained in routine care and emergency procedures, which have been individualized to their child's unique characteristics (e.g., baseline functioning, signs and symptoms of distress, type of equipment). *Getting It Started and Keeping It Going* [7] is a combination videotape and workbook designed by the Ventilator Assisted Care Program at Children's Hospital, New Orleans, for instruction of respiratory care procedures for children at home. Videotapes and manuals on clean intermittent catheterization, positioning, home oxygen use, CPR, and emergency procedures for infants and young children have been developed for training in home care at the University of Colorado Health Sciences Center.[8] These and other tools can be useful adjuncts to hands-on-training.

Home care plans should include developmental, as well as medical interventions. Ahmann [9] provides comprehensive coverage of the process of planning by nurses, for various conditions requiring home care. Jones [10] provides a resource manual for parents, with attention to some high-tech interventions and thorough discussions on child and family needs of home care. *Homeward Bound: Resources for Living with a Chronically Ill Child at Home* [11] uses the child with ventilator-assistance as a prototype and describes how to access various community resources. Initial home-care planning and training of caregivers must be completed during the hospital stay. A hospital trial and overnight pass are recommended prior to a discharge home with high-tech medical supports.[12]

Once home, the care plan is supervised by a physician who provides intermittent direct services. Direct-care providers of routine care in the home include parents, trained extended family members, trained respite or attendant care personnel, and/or trained licensed/certified professionals (nurses, respiratory therapists, etc.). Home or outpatient clinic-based services are intermittently provided by nurses, equipment vendors, therapists of allied health services, educators, mental health professionals, and/or others. The child should travel to community settings for education, socialization, and recreation, as possible. Historically, home-care services have been fragmented.[13] Case managers should assist the family in continuously coordinating home care and community services.

CONTENT OF SERVICES

Services to families and children with high-tech medical supports at home are based on child health-care needs, developmental needs, and family needs. Only a few families have the benefit of local service systems which help them to locate, coordinate, maintain, and advocate to meet their care needs. Five programs described by Gittler and Colton [14] as model systems include, specifically, Illinois, Iowa, Louisiana, Maryland, and Pennsylvania programs located within both public and private service organizations. The Bureau of Maternal and Child Health was instrumental in the initial funding of four of the five programs. The Iowa and Illinois programs are primarily sponsored by statewide Title V Crippled Children's Services Programs. The Louisiana and Pennsylvania programs are located at children's hospitals and include Title V funds. The Maryland program is community-based and also is sponsored by Title V. Funds from Title XIX, in the form of Medicaid waivers or optional, targeted case-management services, are available to the Illinois, Maryland, and Louisiana programs, while Pennsylvania's program includes state funds secured through legislative action. In most areas of the country, such organized service systems for high-tech populations do not exist; home care services are unavailable or inadequate.

National legislation has been introduced to Congress which would impact on the child who requires high-tech home care. During 1985, plans were introduced to establish funds for services and programs for ventilator-dependent children,[15] to establish high-risk insurance pools for the under-insured/uninsured children with catastrophic conditions,[16] and change the focus from institutional to community-based service systems for Medicaid recipients with disabilities/chronic conditions.[17] No such legislation has been approved to date.

Current sources of funding for individual home-care packages can include private insurance and managed care systems; public funders, such as Medicaid and Crippled Children's Services; disease-oriented organizations, such as Easter Seal and the Muscular Dystrophy Association; and civic and religious groups. Families incur many out-of-pocket expenses. Services approved for purchase by the various funders can vary by individual, community, and state; and a combination of funders is usually involved to meet all of a child's service needs.

No national agenda yet exists for children who use high-tech home care. The DHHS Task Force on Technology Dependent Children has been directed to recommend in its 1988 report ". . .changes in the provision and financing of health care in private and public health care programs (including appropriate joint public-private initiatives) so as to provide home and community-based alternatives to the institutionalization of technology-dependent children."[18] These recommendations are forthcoming.

STANDARDS OF CARE

Although the Surgeon General has recommended model guidelines and standards for high-tech care at home,[1] no comprehensive standards package has been available nor accepted by the community. Attempts have been made to improve planning for home care through the development and utilization of general discharge planning standards, by such groups as the Joint Commission on Accreditation of Hospitals, American Hospital Association, American Nurses Association, and others.[20] Pediatricians have published a position statement on *Transition of Severely Disabled Children from Hospital or Chronic Care Facilities to the Community.*[21] Guidelines are still needed which will define minimal acceptable limits for home care to provide for the child's best interest in a variety of community settings.

EVALUATION RESULTS

Goldberg[4] summarizes that "when a child returns home to the community, positive influences such as an improved family situation, appropriate education, developmental interaction and stimulation from friends, and spiritual growth result in a wellness that cannot be realized in the setting of the hospital." Research results indicate that this philosophy has merit.

Burr, Guyer, Todras, et al[23] report the success of six children at home with ventilation. Schreiner, Donar, and Kettrick[24] describe the outcomes of 101 children who lived at home on ventilation. They found fewer and less serious infections, surveillance equal to or better than in the hospital, better nutrition, more rapid socialization, facilitation of gross motor skill development, and increased mobility post-hospitalization. When looking at the problems faced by this same population in home care, Schreiner, Downes, Kettrick, et al[25] report that 30 out of the 101 children had died, most commonly as a result of progressive pulmonary insufficiency and cardiac failure, with complications of airways, stenosis of the trachea, tracheomalecia, and accidental disconnections or trach accidents. Families identified additional problems of sustaining financial burdens and the stress of having a child with a chronic condition.

Goldberg, Fauvre, Vaughn, et al[26] describe a home care sample of 18 ventilator-assisted children, and have determined that a change in thinking and roles needs to occur for health caregivers to successfully work with families to manage these children at home. This study reported a 70 percent cost savings, with improvements in both the child's medical condition and psychosocial development, once at home.

The largest national evaluation of children with ventilator-assistance at home is the Ventilator Assisted Children Programs Evaluation Project (VACPEP). This sample includes 121 children from three sites. Aday, et al[27] identifies issues regarding programs, patients and families, policy needs, and research needs. They indicate that children from all sites were reported by parents to be doing better at home, compared to when they were hospitalized. Higher functional adaptation at home was realized by children with stable prognoses, primary conditions other than traumatic injuries, fewer needs for non-parent caregivers, and who had shorter initial hospital stays.

NEEDS OF FAMILIES

VACPEP has isolated six conditions which affect home care of ventilator-assisted children, including 1) not all children have the same needs, 2) caregivers think it is better for the child to be at home, though it often makes it hard on the family, 3) full-time nursing care has its "pros and cons," 4) caregivers need "T.L.C.," too, 5) the needs of the child and family are different at different points in time, and 6) the financial burden adds additional stress.

Providers and families are striving to create a model of care that is family-centered and community-based. Thomas [29] notes that parents and health care providers struggle for control of the care of the child and aspects of the family's lifestyle, as a result of turf issues which arise between the domains of home and hospital. These control issues are difficult to resolve. Shelton, Jappson, and Johnson[30] have defined elements of family-centered care, including recognizing that the family is the constant in the child's life, facilitating parent-to-parent support, facilitating information sharing and collaboration by parents and professionals, designing and implementing responsive health care services/systems/policies, and others. A national parent-professional organization, SKIP,[13] provides education, support, and advocacy for technology-assisted youth and their families.

UNMET NEEDS

Major needs for successful provision of home care remain. Outstanding needs are for:

1. National data bases of incidence or definitive estimates of cost for various conditions and home care alternatives: both the OTA Report[5] and McManus, Melus, Norton, et al [33] have summarized issues regarding incidence and cost from existing data. Long-range planning needs to include initiatives in which incidence and cost can be well-described.

2. Nationally accepted guidelines for the delivery or financing of care: children and their families receive services which vary in composition, quality, and quantity. Children in some hospitals may not survive the acute phase, may be retained because there is no/inadequate financing for home care, may be discharged to long-term care or step-down facilities, or may be discharged home without a thorough home-care plan and monitoring package.

3. Education policies: in some locations, children receive related services so that they are educated in integrated, academically appropriate class-

rooms.[34] In other education districts, they may be required to be educated in segregated settings or at home.

4. Supportive/relief services to families who care for their children at home: for most families, there remains a need for relief from 24-hour care duties by competent, trained personnel in the form of nursing, respite, or attendant care services. Other support is needed in the form of case management, counseling, or parent-to-parent support services. With more support, there would be more natural, foster, and adoptive family units capable of providing quality of care and nurturance to these children.

5. Community-based, non-specialist pediatricians: Pierce, Freedman, Frauman, et al[35] speculate that such physicians are reluctant to get involved because of the low incidence of the conditions, uncertainty about how routine primary care affects chronic care, and feared increased liability. Some pediatricians are unable to change their attitudes from experiences of high-tech in intensive care settings to acceptance of the technology in the community.

For most children with stable medical conditions and high-tech needs, home care is the best living arrangement. This arrangement requires that the child's medical and developmental needs be managed by a local team of family members and professionals who know how to access community resources to provide ongoing safe care, assistance, and support.

REFERENCES

1. US Public Health Service: Report of the Surgeon General's Workshop on Children with Handicaps and their Families, Washington, D.C., US Government Printing Office, 1983, p 1.

2. US Public Health Service: Surgeon General's Report: Children with Special Health Care Needs, Washington, D.C., US Government Printing Office, 1987, p 5.

3. The Hastings Center: Guidelines on the Termination of Life-Sustaining Treatment and the Care of the Dying: A Report by the Hastings Center, Bloomington, IN, Indiana University Press, 1987, p 134.

4. Goldberg AI. Home care for a better life for ventilator-dependent people. Chest 84:4, 1983.

5. US Congress, Office of Technology Assessment: Technology-Dependent Children: Hospital v. Home Care - A Technical Memorandum, Washington, D.C., US Government Printing Office, 1987, pp 3-4.

6. Unpublished Manuscript. Task Force on Technology Dependent Children: Draft Definition, Washington, D.C., Department of Health and Human Services, 1987.

7. Whitesal E, Carlin P, Cimo D. Getting it Started and Keeping It Going: A Workbook, New Orleans, LA, Children's Hospital, 1987.

8. Learner Managed Designs, Inc: University of Colorado Health Sciences Center: Videotape Instructional Units, Lawrence, KS, 1988.

9. Ahmann E: Home Care for the High-Risk Infant, Rockville, MD, Aspen, 1986.

10. Jones ML. Home Care for the Chronically Ill or Disabled Child, New York, NY, Harper & Row, 1985.

11. Ventilator Assisted Care Program: Homeward Bound: Resources for Living at Home with a Chronically Ill Child, New Orleans, LA, Children's Hospital, 1985.

12. Steele NF, Harrison B. Technology assisted children: Assessing discharge preparation. J Pediatr Nurs 1:3, 1986.

13. Haddad AM. High Tech Home Care, Rockville, MD, Aspen, 1987, p 209.

14. Gittler J, Colton M. Alternatives to Hospitalization for Technology Dependent Children: Program Models, Iowa City, IO, National Maternal and Child Health Resource Center, 1987.

15. Kennedy E, Hatch O. Alternatives to Hospitalization for Medical Technology Dependent Children Act of 1985, Washington, D.C., US Congress, 1985.

16. Kennelly B. Health Insurance Availability Act of 1985 (HR 1770), Washington, D.C., US Congress, 1985.

17. Chafie J. Community and Family Living Amendments of 1985 (S 873 and HR 2902), Washington, D.C., US Congress, 1985.

18. US Congress: Omnibus Reconciliation Act of 1985: Charter-Task Force on Technology-Dependent Children, Washington, D.C., Department of Health and Human Services, 1985, p 1.

19. Zarle NC. Continuing Care: The Process and Practice of Discharge Planning, Rockville, MD, Aspen, 1987, pp 4-6.

20. Committee on Children with Disabilities, American Academy of Pediatrics: Transition of severely disabled children from hospital or chronic care facilities to the community. Pediatrics 78:3, 1986.

21. Burr BH, Guyer B, Todres ID, et al. Home care for children on respirators. N Engl J Med 309:21, 1983.

22. Schreiner MS, Donar ME, Kettrick RG, et al. Pediatric home mechanical ventilation. Pediatr Clin North Am 34:1, 1987.

23. Schreiner MS, Downes JJ, Kettrick RG, et al. Chronic respiratory failure in infants with prolonged ventilator dependency. J Am Med Assoc 258:23, 1987.

24. Goldberg AI, Fauvre EAM, Vaughn CJ, et al. Home care for life-supported persons: An approach to program development. J Pediatr 104, 1984.

25. Aday LA, Aitken MJ, Wegener DH. Results of a National Evaluation of Programs for Ventilator-Assisted Children, Chicago, IL, Pluribus Press, 1988, pp 251-252.

26. Thomas R. Family adaptation to a child with a chronic condition, Children with Chronic Conditions. Edited by MH Rose and RB Thomas. New York, NY, Grune & Stratton, 1987, p 48.

27. Shelton TL, Jeppson ES, Johnson BH. Family-Centered Care for Children with Special Health Care Needs, Washington, D.C., Association for the Care of Children's Health, 1987.

28. McManus MA, Melus SE, Norton CH, et al. Guide to National Data on Maternal and Child Health: With Special Emphasis on Financing Services for Chronically Ill Children, Washington, D.C., McManus Health Policy, Inc, 1986, pp 10-20.

29. Sicotte S, Kirkhart K. Helping parents and teachers cope with technology for care of chronically ill children at home and at school, Interventive Strategies in Infant Mortality, Morbidity, and Childhood Handicapping Conditions. Edited by EL Watkins & LR Melnick. Chapel Hill, NC, University of North Carolina, pp 47-55.

30. Pierce PM, Freedman SA, Frauman AC, et al. Reducing costing with a community outreach program, Pediatr Nurs 11:5, 1985.

REPRODUCTIVE HEALTH CARE NEEDS FOR THE DEVELOPMENTALLY DISABLED

50

David Muram

INTRODUCTION

In the past two decades, the field of developmental disabilities underwent significant changes. During that time, patients were removed from hospitals and chronic care institutions and were integrated into the community. As these former patients were released into the community, a major effort began in the areas of rehabilitation and training services. The rehabilitation effort no longer focused on vocational training alone, but attempted to address the social and emotional needs of these individuals. Placement of these previously institutionalized persons within the community has resulted in an improvement in their quality of life. With special education, the handicapped acquired new skills and became entitled to education and employment opportunities which previously were unavailable to them. All these changes enabled individuals with disabilities to lead as normal a life as possible. The health care system must adjust to these changes as well. The care provided in an institution may be very different from the care provided in the community. Most institutions had provisions for preventive care, routine examinations, immunizations, and facilities to provide for minor illness. Contracts with other hospitals provided acute care for serious illness. The patients' health care needs were met, with minimal involvement on the part of the patients or their families. In contrast, patients who live in the community must now seek their own care, participate in the decision-making, and be partially responsible for compliance with prescribed treatment. Some communities may not be equipped to provide medical services that are as accessible or as comprehensive as needed, especially for those with complex conditions.

One cannot generalize about the health care needs of persons with developmental disabilities. Some are physically handicapped only while others may be both physically and mentally disabled. Those with minor impairments have similar health care needs to people in the general population and thus may not require special consideration. At the other end of the spectrum are persons with significant disabilities which require highly sophisticated and specialized care. The health care delivery system must be responsive across that entire range to be able to provide not only the basic level of care, but also the highly specialized services required for those with severe disabilities.

Furthermore, the health care needs of individuals with disabilities are constantly changing. With improved medical technology and care, life expectancy for people with disabilities is greater today than ever before. Many of these persons are now elderly, and their age necessitates changes in the kinds of services and medical care which they require. Many persons in this older population are multi-handicapped and present an even greater challenge to the community service system.

ACCESSIBILITY TO CARE

How health care is paid for shapes how care is delivered more directly than any other force. Many disabled persons rely upon Medicaid to defray their health care costs. The disincentives to the integration of these individuals into the "mainstream" are compounded by inefficient payment mechanisms.[1] Fees-for-service must be fair and set at the prevailing market level. In addition, reimbursement schedules must take into consideration the special requirements of persons with disabilities. Otherwise, one can expect that:

1. periodic examinations for prevention, screening, and health maintenance programs would be curtailed.

2. choices among providers would be restricted.

3. the quality of health care services attained would be inferior to the modal quality of services in the community.

4. health care would become increasingly crisis-oriented.

Availability of medical and mental health services is essential to assure the delivery of appropriate care. Health care professionals are expected to be not only competent but also understanding, sensitive, and emphatic. They should be skilled in listening to the family members and willing to include them in the decision-making process. Above all, professional services delivered by various specialists and agencies must be well-coordinated.

As in the general population, individuals with disabilities require the services of an identified primary health care provider who assumes longitudinal responsibility for their overall well-being, furnishes general medical and preventive care, and makes referrals to specialty care when needed. In such a setting, the person's health status is well-known, an up-to-date and comprehensive medical record exists, and a long-term relationship can be developed with the patient and the family.

Reproductive Health Care Needs

In general, the reproductive health care needs of a disabled individual are the same as those of the general population. However, the disability creates difficulties for the health care provider. Individuals with disabilities often suffer from multiple health problems which may require consultations with multiple specialists and continuing medical attention. In one study[2] the investigators have found associated medical conditions in 80 percent of children with mental retardation. Children with lower IQs had more complicated medical problems, resulting in a more significant disability. Other investigators found that adults with mental retardation had a complex set of chronic, often multiple, health-related problems which required frequent medical attention.[3]

From a medical perspective, individuals with severe physical disabilities also have specific areas of concern which require constant monitoring and frequent intervention:

1. Seizure disorders are common and may be complex. More than one anticonvulsant may be required for optimal management, which may cause medication interactions, interfere with the menstrual cycle, and may even impair the ability of that person to interact with others.

2. Multiple joint contractures, which often preclude ambulation, cause impaired sitting posture, and predispose to the development of decubitus ulcers.

3. Nutrition is often complicated by feeding difficulties. The presence of gastroesophageal reflux, with vomiting, further aggravates the situation.

4. Recurrent respiratory problems are a major health concern and are the most common cause of death in this group.[4] These are often the result of aspiration secondary to either gastroesophageal reflux, or to incoordinate swallowing.

To further complicate the picture, many of these patients have only a limited ability to communicate. Sometimes the only sign of a physical ailment may be an alteration in behavior. Many care providers are attuned to this fact, particularly if they have known the person for some length of time. However, the severity of the problem may not be recognized and can result in a delay in bringing the patient to appropriate medical attention. This is a serious issue and needs to be addressed regularly in training and supervision.

THE GYNECOLOGIC EXAMINATION

The gynecologic examination of any adolescent girl may create significant anxiety. The mentally handicapped person may have only limited understanding of the examination and its purpose, and may refuse to be examined. Obtaining a cervical smear for cytology may become an impossible task. However, such periodic examinations are required as part of the routine disease prevention care we recommend for all patients.

Patients with disabilities are sensitive to a physician's attitude. They tend to withdraw if he/she is hurried, brusque, or indifferent, but they react positively to someone who is kind, warm, and patient. Many patients would like the mother to be present in the examination room, as she provides them with a sense of security. The patient should be asked to help with the examination. By helping the physician, she receives a sense of control over the examination and her apprehension diminishes. Palpation of the pelvic organs can often be accomplished by performing a rectal examination. A rectal digital examination often can be accomplished and should not cause pain. Samples for cytosmears may be obtained by inserting Q–tips into the vagina. When the vagina requires evaluation, special instruments, e.g., vaginoscope, Huffman-Graves Virginal Speculum, etc. may be required. Prior to inserting the instrument, one must show it to the girl in order to decrease apprehension. She is allowed to touch the lubricated instrument with her index finger, and it is pointed out to her that it feels strange, slippery, and cool. Then the instrument is placed against the inner thigh and she is reminded that it feels cool, slippery, and unusual. Only then is the instrument passed through the hymenal orifice. If the aperture is too small for an instrument to be passed without discomfort, or if the patient is uncooperative, vaginoscopy should not be attempted without sedation or general anesthesia. Periodic sonograms may be utilized in selected patients for routine pelvic assessment.

SEXUALITY

Many physicians are now familiar with the unusual medical requirements of the developmentally disabled, but some are still uncomfortable dealing with issues of sexuality. It is well-accepted that every individual needs to develop his or her sexual feelings and be able to express these feelings freely. As these disabled individuals now live within the community, the emergence of their sexuality is no longer a hidden phenomenon. Although the accepted socio-sexual model is to find a partner, marry, and have children, many perceive it as abnormal when a disabled person expresses or acts out these desires. Lack of proper education has caused even people who approve of sexual expression to voice concerns that such sexual activity may result in an increase of handicapped offspring.

Physicians and other health care professionals undertook responsibility for all their patients' needs while they were in an institutional setting. A high standard of behavior was expected from all patients, and any expression of sexuality was regarded as a potential public scandal which could damage the image of the institution. Sexual expression was regarded as a problem for which a solution must be found. The solution often was the cessation of the behavior and thus suppression of sexual expression. Obviously, such control cannot be exerted on patients residing within the community. The staff must accept the fact that disabled people are sexual individuals and have the right to express their feelings. While nobody can actually control their sexual behavior, these patients must be helped to channel their sexual behavior into accepted social norms.

Even parents of disabled children are uncomfortable discussing sexuality. Although they would very much like their child to be "like everyone else," many do not wish their child to receive sex education. Some may feel that ignorance makes the children innocent and therefore less likely to have sexual experiences in the future. Some are convinced that the child has no interest in sexual expression, and would have a sexual experience only because somebody would take advantage of his/her disability.

The concerns of parents vary, as the child grows. Parents of a young girl with disabilities wish to learn how to prepare the girl for the physical changes which occur at puberty. As the child matures, the major concerns are menstruation, hygiene, dating, possible sexual activity, and contraception. Parents of older patients are more concerned with potential reproduction, and many request that the girls be surgically sterilized. Over half the patients referred to the Reproductive Health Clinic at the University of Tennessee, Memphis, requested surgical sterilization for their daughters; either tubal interruption or hysterectomy. Some even requested that a gonadectomy be performed prior to pubertal development, to prevent sexual development altogether.

CONTRACEPTION

Options for contraception continue to be quite limited. Barrier methods are highly effective when used properly by a highly motivated patient. In addition, condoms provide protection against sexually transmitted diseases. These methods may be well-suited for certain physically disabled individuals, and are particularly suited to a patient who may have infrequent sexual experiences. The use of barrier methods requires motivation and a supportive partner, and even among non-disabled adolescents there is a tendency to use this method haphazardly. The relationship is sometimes casual, and the long-term consequences are not a deterrent to contraceptive failure.

Most intrauterine contraceptive devices (IUCD) were recently withdrawn from the U.S. market. Although the Progestasert is still available, IUCDs are probably not suitable for use in mentally disabled individuals. Once inserted, the IUCD is quite effective, has a low-failure rate, and requires no patient compliance. But mentally disabled individuals may not recognize symptoms of the potential complications, e.g., pelvic inflammatory disease and ectopic pregnancy. Failure to seek early medical attention may prove to be fatal.

The oral contraceptive pill is highly effective, with a failure rate estimated to be less then 0.5 percent. The patient is required to take the medication on a daily basis. In most instances, the parents are supportive and can be trusted to ensure compliance. The oral contraceptives are obviously not suitable for individuals who cannot swallow pills, for patients who live alone and, therefore, may be non-compliant, or for patients who have severe side effects.

Long-term injectable contraceptives have been developed and are in use throughout the world. The drug most commonly used is depot medroxyprogesterone acetate (DMPA). Although this preparation has not been approved for general use as a contraceptive in the U.S., it may be used in certain situations. This method is highly effective, with a failure rate of 0.7 per 100 women-years for 12 months of use. The medication is associated with a low incidence of side effects. Breakthrough bleeding, which may become quite disturbing, is the most common complaint.[5]

Other injectable contraceptives. using various combinations of estrogen and progestins. are now being tested in clinical trials. Some of these have been reported to provide adequate contraception for up to five years. If approved for clinical use, these injectable contraceptives may provide long-term contraception. with minimal reliance on patient compliance.

MENSTRUATION

The first menstrual period is often a startling and scary thing for any girl, and for a mentally disabled girl who is not adequately prepared it can be a traumatic event. This prompts many parents to seek medical advice as pubertal changes become apparent. Almost all patients seen at the Reproductive Health Clinic at the University of Tennessee, Memphis, were seen either just prior to menarche or immediately following the initiation of the menstrual cycles. In some instances, menarche sounds alarm bells in the family. It raises fears of initiation of sexual activity and, with it, the potential for unintended pregnancy. When the parents feel that the child's supervision may be insufficient, e.g., the child is in school, special programs, etc., the parents often request contraceptive advice. The older individuals are more likely to request contraception. Like all school-age children, developmentally disabled individuals should be offered sex education programs appropriate for their level of understanding. Similar programs should be offered to the parents. Patients who are considered able to manage their own hygiene during menstruation should be provided with menstrual hygiene classes, and those who are sexually active should be given contraception.

Severely handicapped girls may not be able to keep themselves clean during periods. In these girls, the menstrual blood may cause significant hygiene problems and, therefore, they are often isolated from their normal environment during menstruation. Some of these patients who have had difficulties in mastering toilet control may decompensate at this time. Others who are not toilet-trained have an added problem to cope with. Many parents become frustrated and request that a hysterectomy be performed to abolish the menstrual cycle. In some clinic facilities, menstrual hygiene is a leading indication for hysterectomy in severely disabled girls.

Anovulation and dysfunctional uterine bleeding are common in young adolescents following menarche, and developmentally disabled adolescents are no exception. Many present with complaints of irregular, and often heavy, menstrual flow. Anovulatory cycles are common for the first year following menarche. Periods are often irregular, and the bleeding may be heavier than the flow in ovulatory cycles. Irregularity and heavy flow create further difficulties for the patient and her family. The menstrual cycle may cause other problems, as well. Some patients who suffer from epilepsy or emotional instability may notice a significant increase in the frequency of seizures, or a marked impairment of social behavior. Some are sent home from school during menstruation. This disrupts special education efforts and increases isolation. To address this problem in our clinic, a team of social workers is utilized to conduct home–training sessions for menstrual hygiene. This behavior modification program is often successful when the parents are supportive and when the patient is toilet–trained. When properly prepared, many parents are willing to let the menstrual cycle establish its own pattern.

Abolishing the menstrual cycle altogether, either medically or surgically, would alleviate these problems. Menstrual control can often be achieved using DMPA. This agent has been used in our clinic in 23 patients. Adequate menstrual control was achieved in 21 of the 23. Two patients failed to respond to all hormonal manipulation, and a hysterectomy was deemed necessary.

STERILIZATION

Performing sterilizations for mentally disabled individuals is almost impossible. U.S. Public Health Service regulations, which govern sterilization programs supported in whole or in part by federal financial assistance, state that these programs shall not perform or arrange for the performance of a sterilization of any mentally incompetent individual or institutionalized individual.[6] Although some feel that sterilization of the mentally handicapped is a decision for the courts,[7] successful litigation by the handicapped have made the practice of sterilization, based upon court order, highly debatable.[8-10] However, such limitations may be frustrating to a physician who wishes to perform a hysterectomy or tubal sterilization for a patient in whom such a procedure is reasonable or even essential. Any facility which cares for mentally handicapped patients must establish its own procedures which would allow for the delivery of appropriate care, but also take into consideration legal precedents, ensure "due process," and the rights of the disabled. These obstacles do not exist when the patient is physically disabled but otherwise mentally competent. However, similar guidelines for the physically disabled are desirable.

SEXUAL ABUSE

Sexual exploitation is a major problem for this patient population and their families. While the actual incidence of sexual abuse is unknown, it now appears that sexual abuse of children is widespread. The National Center on Child Abuse and Neglect estimates the number of child-victims to be more than 200,000 per year.[11]

Children of all ages, from infancy to young adulthood, have been victims of sexual abuse, with an average reported age at-first-incident ranging between eight and 11 years.[12,13] A more recent report suggests that younger children, ages four-nine, may be at a higher risk due to a naive and trusting approach to adults and a vulnerability to being misled regarding the meaning of various sexual activities.[14] Developmentally disabled individuals are also victims of sexual abuse. Many parents believe that the severely retarded girl is at the greatest risk and that the assailant is often a stranger or another retarded individual. However, studies have shown that mildly retarded patients are, in fact, at greatest risk and assailants are more likely to be family members or persons well-known to the victims.[15] Special effort is required for the development of effective prevention programs in the community, if the sexual exploitation of the disabled is to be controlled. In addition, there is a need for educational programs specially designed for the level of understanding of the disabled individuals.

THE FAMILY

Although the crucial role of the family is beyond dispute, the needs of the family members are often forgotten. Most parents do well with their disabled children, but they require a variety of support mechanisms. They need training and advice concerning management of daily problems without creating a crisis. Common examples are mismanagement of masturbation through punitive measures, or overprotection which leads to isolation, low self-esteem, and depression. It is important to help these families learn to foster their children's success and to achieve gratification from them.

REFERENCES

1. Master RJ. Medicaid after 20 years: Promise, problems, potential. Mental Retardation 25:211-214, 1987.

2. Smith DC, Decker HA, Herberg EN, Rupke LK. Medical needs of children in institutions for the mentally retarded. American Journal of Public Health 8:1376-1384, 1969.

3. Hagberg B, Kyllerman M. Epidemiology of mental retardation - A Swedish survey. Brain and Development 5:441-449, 1983.

4. Herbst DS, Baird PA. Survival rates and causes of death among persons with non-specific mental retardation. Perspectives and Progress in Mental Retardation.Vol 2 - Biomedical Aspects. Berg JM, DeJong JM (Eds). University Park Press, Baltimore, 1984.

5. Fraser IS, Holck S. Depot Medroxyprogesterone Acetat. Long Acting Steroid Contraception. Mishell DR Jr. (Ed). Raven Press, New York, 1983.

6. 42 C.F.R. 50:201-210, 1979.

7. Annas GJ. Sterilization of the mentally retarded: is a decision for the courts. The Hastings Center Report, 18-19, August 1981.

8. Stump vs. Sparkman, 435 U.S. 349, 1978.

9. Downs vs. Sawtelle, 574 F. 2d 1 (C.A.1,) 1978.

10. In re: Gloria Sue Lambert 1976.

11. National Center on Child Abuse and Neglect (NCCAN) "Child Sexual Abuse: Incest, Assault and Exploitation" Special Report, HEW,Children's Bureau, August 1978.

12. Kemp CE. Sexual abuse, another hidden pediatric problem. Pediatrics 62:382-389, 1978

13. Kemp CE. Incest and other forms of sexual abuse in The Battered Child. Kemp CE, Helfer RE (Eds). University of Chicago Press, Chicago, 1980.

14. Gelinas DJ. The persisting negative effects of incest. Psychiatry 46:312-332, 1983.

15. Chamberlain A, Rauh J, Passer A, McGrath M, Burket R. Issues in fertility control for mentally retarded female adolescents: I. Sexual activity, sexual abuse, and contraception. Pediatrics, 73:445-450,1984.

SECTION VII

A
GLOBAL
OVERVIEW
OF
THE
HEALTH
OF
WOMEN
AND
CHILDREN

A GLOBAL OVERVIEW OF THE HEALTH OF WOMEN AND CHILDREN*

51

Mark A. Belsey and Erica Royston

INTRODUCTION

The health of women and children forms a continuum from one generation to another. It reflects not only the vulnerabilities inherent in the biological and behavioral aspects of reproduction, growth, development, and maturation, but also the social, ecological, and historical situation of societies. The successful and healthy transition from one critical stage of life to the next is enhanced in societies that have made a commitment to social justice, and provide a minimum level and appropriate distribution of resources for health and social development. The health of women and children is threatened by imbalances in the distribution and access to resources by discrimination against women and illiteracy. Social changes, such as urbanization, economic crises, and natural and man-made disasters, all leave an imprint on the health of women and children.

Women's life-long health can be compromised by discriminatory treatment in childhood. Traditionally, many cultures prefer male children. Sons are perceived as an economic asset to the family, contributing productive labor. Girls, on the other hand, are seen as a burden, who often have to be provided with a costly dowry and whose economic productivity will benefit their husband's family rather than that of their parents. Sons usually have the main responsibility for the care of their parents

---

* There are a large number of tables in this chapter. They are placed at the end of the text in order to facilitate the ease of reading.

695

in old age. Girls may get less food, be sicker before they are taken for curative health care, and receive less preventive health care. Evidence of such practices includes poorer nutritional status of girls than boys, fewer girls than boys immunized, higher case fatality among girls brought to hospital, and higher mortality overall (Table 1). Significantly, where women's economic productivity is high the preference for sons is less-pronounced.

Women's education is also an important determinant of their own health and that of their children. In every economic setting, the children of literate women have a better chance of survival than those of illiterate women. Educated women tend to marry later, delay the onset of childbearing, and are more likely to practice family planning. They generally have fewer children with a wider spacing between births. Women with no schooling, on average, have almost twice as many children as those with seven or more years schooling.[1]

MATERNAL MORTALITY

Each year at least half a million women die from causes related to pregnancy and childbirth.[2] All but about 6,000 of these deaths occur in developing countries (Table 2). Maternal mortality rates are highest in Africa, with community rates of up to 1000 per 100,000 live births reported in several rural areas. The risk of dying from maternal causes is somewhat lower in the urban areas of Africa, but rates of over 500 have been reported in several cities. High maternal-mortality rates are compounded by high fertility.

Very-young age is an added risk in childbearing the world over. Teenage marriage is widespread in the developing world, with the highest recorded incidence in Bangladesh, where 90 percent of women are married before they are 18-years old. By the age of 17, almost half of all women in Bangladesh are mothers and by the age of 19, one-third have at least two children.[3] In Bangladesh, girls aged ten-to-14 had a maternal-mortality rate five-times higher, and women aged 15-to-19 two-times higher, than women aged 20-to-24.[4] Even in the U.S., girls under 15 have a maternal-mortality rate three times that of women aged 20-to-24.

Maternal-mortality rates have declined significantly in almost all developed countries in recent years. Table 3 shows such trends for selection of countries.

Sri Lanka is an interesting success story. From a level of 522 in 1950-1955, the maternal-mortality rate, excluding abortions, fell to 260 ten years later, and to 87 in 1980.[4] No doubt the fact that 85 percent of the births in Sri Lanka are attended by trained attendants, and 76 percent take place in institutions, provides at least part of the explanation. Over the same period, the total fertility rate fell from 5.3 in 1953 to 3.8 in 1977; and contraceptive prevalence rose from 32 percent in 1975 to 48 percent in 1981-1982.[5]

As overall maternal mortality has fallen, it has usually been deaths from sepsis that have declined first. In Sri Lanka, in 1950-1955 one-quarter of the maternal deaths were due to sepsis. By 1977, the proportion had fallen to ten percent.[4] In China, where overall rates have fallen to 49 in 1984, deaths from sepsis now account for only some six percent of all maternal deaths. Such declines reflect both improvements in the standard of delivery care, such as, for example, the emphasis on the three *cleans* (*clean* hands, *clean* delivery surface, and *clean* cord care) and the lower case fatality resulting from the availability of antibiotics.[6] Deaths from hemorrhage are usually slower to decline. The short-time between the onset of serious bleeding and death means that access to lifesaving interventions is crucial.

Hypertensive disorders of pregnancy (HDP) remain one of the more common morbid conditions of pregnancy. The death rate due to HDP seems to fall more slowly than that from sepsis. The prevalence of HDP and eclampsia varies widely, as seen in the results from the WHO collaborative study (Table 4). It is noteworthy that the fall of mortality from HDP in such countries as Sweden was not a function of a decline in the incidence of eclampsia but was the result of the decline in the case-fatality rate.[7]

Severe anemia in pregnancy contributes greatly to maternal morbidity and mortality. In rural India, in 1981, anemia was given as the second most-important cause of maternal mortality, after hemorrhage, where it is usually a contributing factor.[8] Together, these two causes accounted for 41 percent of maternal deaths. In one study from India, the risk of a maternal death was increased 14-fold when the woman had a hemoglobin level of less than 8 gm percent.[9]

On the basis of a review of all information available in 1979, it was estimated that, in 1975, there were some 230 million anemic women in the world; about half the nonpregnant women live in developing countries, and two-thirds of those pregnant. The highest proportion of women with hemoglobin concentrations below the WHO norm is in Asia, followed by Oceania and Africa.[10]

MALARIA AND PREGNANCY

In addition to the nutritional anemia of pregnant women, in many areas of the developing world malaria will lower the hemoglobin level by 1.5 g percent[11] and result in a 150 to 250 gram lowering of birthweight.[12] Malaria during pregnancy, among primagravida women, greatly increases the risk of cerebral malaria and death. The risks of chloroquine to the fetus are exceedingly low, and more than offset by the dangers that untreated malaria has for both mother and infant. However, with increasing prevalence and higher levels of resistance of the malaria parasites to chloroquine, the management of malaria during pregnancy becomes increasingly complex. The safety of the newer anti-malarial drugs has not been established with respect to effects on the fetus.[11]

UNWANTED PREGNANCY AND ABORTION

A considerable proportion of the very-high fertility observed, particularly in developing countries, is unwanted. If all women who said they wanted no more children were actually able to stop childbearing, the number of births would be reduced by an average of 35 percent in Latin America, 33 percent in Asia, and 17 percent in Africa.[13]

The incidence of abortion and its consequences and complications represents a public health problem of major dimensions in a large number of countries, regardless of whether the procedure is legally available and accessible. In all settings, its occurrence and persistence reflect the failure to satisfy the fertility regulating desires and needs of women. That failure may represent a combination of societal actions or inaction (policies, access to information, and services, etc.), personal health behavior and choice, and contraceptive failure.

Even an estimate of the incidence of legally induced abortion is difficult to obtain, while estimates of illegally induced abortion are generally unreliable. However, estimates based on either official reporting or secondary data sources suggest that there are some 33 million legally induced abortions performed annually (with a low of 30 million and a high of 40 million). The Soviet Union and China account for fully 25 million of these cases.[14] The estimates of illegally induced abortion are highly speculative. The total number of abortions is estimated to be between 40 and 60 million. On a global basis, that level of abortion would suggest there are from 24 to 32 induced abortions for every 100 known pregnancies.[13]

The effect on maternal mortality of a change in the legal status of abortion has been well-documented in several countries. In Romania, where abortion had been widely available and practiced after it was made illegal, both the birth rate and the maternal-mortality rate rose sharply. The maternal-mortality rate has stayed high, with 80 percent of maternal deaths being abortion-related, while the birth rate has gradually returned to the low levels of the early 1960s (Table 3). In Cuba, between 1968 (when abortions were first permitted in hospitals) and 1976, about half of the decline in maternal mortality, from 85 to 46, was attributed to the decline in abortion-associated deaths.[15]

BREAST-FEEDING AND FERTILITY

Breast-feeding has been recognized as a unique and critical factor in the health and well-being of both the mother and the infant. Although much maligned as a means of fertility regulation, the weight of demographic and epidemiologic data supports the conclusion that any changes in breast-feeding practices that reduce the present high incidence and long duration of breast-feeding, and the high frequency of suckling, will have a profound effect on fertility. Thus, if in Bangladesh, for example, the breast-feeding patterns were to change to those typical of industrialized countries, the already high-fertility rates could be expected to rise by over 50 percent. To maintain fertility at current levels, contraceptive use would have to increase from nine percent to about 52 percent.[16] When feeding is provided on demand, particularly without any supplementation before four-to-six months, breast-feeding prolongs the period of postpartum amenorrhoea.[17]

LONG-TERM REPRODUCTIVE MORBIDITY

Long-term morbidity and disability are many women's legacy from inadequate or unskilled maternity care, unregulated fertility, and sexually transmitted diseases. If, singly or in combination, these conditions do not lead to a maternal death, they frequently result in serious physical suffering and social consequences for the woman. In physical terms, the consequences are measured in terms of pelvic inflammatory disease (PID), ectopic pregnancy, infertility, vesico-vaginal and recto-vaginal fistula, and uterine prolapse. The social and personal consequences are very much a reflection of the responsiveness, sensitivity, and supportiveness provided by the husband, the family, and the community. The long-term morbidity contributes to family disruption, divorce, and the ostracism and stigmatization of the women concerned.

Although information on long-term reproductive morbidity is difficult to obtain, in many circumstances information on ectopic pregnancy serves as a useful indicator of the combination of conditions, i.e., sexually transmitted disease, post-abortal, and puerperal sepsis.[18] Both in developed and developing countries the incidence of ectopic pregnancy is increasing dramatically. Over a 17-year period, the rate has tripled in Finland.[19] Whereas in 1967, one in 142 pregnancies was ectopic; in 1983, one in 50 was ectopic. Ectopic pregnancies place a burden on hospital services, in terms of the capacity for emergency operative facilities, skilled staff, and blood transfusion services, the latter being greatly complicated by the problem of AIDS in many parts of the world.

The health and health-service implications of infertility are emerging more clearly. In several countries, and in many subgroups, primary and secondary infertility may be as high as 15 percent to 20 percent, with consequently heavy demands placed on health services and unjustifiably heavy burdens placed on women, who account for only a portion of the infertility.[20] Care for the infertile couple in many countries is ad hoc, both expensive and frustrating for all concerned. Sexually transmitted diseases, and inadequate access to diagnostic and therapeutic services for the control of infections, are major factors in excessive levels of infertility in many countries.

LOW BIRTHWEIGHT AND PRETERM DELIVERY

The birthweight of an infant is the single most-important determinant of its chances of survival, healthy growth, and development. Because birthweight is conditioned by the health and nutritional status of the mother, the proportion of low birthweight (LBW) infants closely reflects the health status of the communities into which they are born.

Low birthweight can be caused by short gestation and/or by retarded intra-uterine growth. Although etiologically distinct, both have an important effect on fetal and neonatal mortality. A review carried out in 1984 led to an estimate of 20 million LBW infants, or 16 percent of those born in 1982. This constitutes a fall, in both relative and absolute terms, when compared to estimates for 1979 of 21 million LBW infants, making up 16.8 percent of the 122 million born that year.[21]

The incidence of LBW, by region, ranges from 31.1 percent in South Asia and 19.7 percent in Asia as a whole, to 14.0 percent in Africa, 10.1 percent in Latin America, 6.8 percent in North America, and 6.5 percent in Europe. There is no evidence of any improvement in South Asia, the region where the problem is most acute. Rates in that region remain between 20 percent and 50 percent.[19]

The major factors associated with low birthweight in developing countries include the pre-pregnancy weight and height of the mother; weight gain during pregnancy; infections, particularly malaria, anemia, parity, and sex of the infant, and racial factors (Table 5). In the industrialized countries, infection plays a less-important role and cigarette-smoking a much more important role, accounting for one-third of the low birthweight.[22]

PERINATAL MORBIDITY AND MORTALITY

Information on perinatal mortality is often unreliable and difficult to obtain because of incompleteness of reporting and variations in the definitions used. Under-reporting of perinatal, or even neonatal mortality, is far more common than the under-reporting of infant mortality, and may have contributed to the failure of health authorities to recognize both the importance of the problem and the possible options for action.

High perinatal mortality rates of 80 to 100 per 1,000 live births are found among the least developed and most disadvantaged countries; and, moderately high rates i.e., 40 to 60/1,000 live births are found in most developing countries. In most developed countries, and a number of developing countries with strong programs of maternal health care, the perinatal mortality rate is in the low 20s; and, in a few instances, such as Japan, the Nordic countries, and the Federal Republic of Germany, the rate is below ten. Because birthweight itself is such a major determinant of perinatal mortality, comparisons of perinatal mortality must make an adjustment for differences in birthweight distributions.[23] Even in many of the least developed countries as much as 40 percent to 50 percent of the infant mortality occurs during the first month of life, largely in the first week.

Decline in perinatal mortality is in large part a function of the health of the mother and the quality of pregnancy, delivery, and newborn care. Perinatal mortality rates within a country, therefore, are a very sensitive indicator of program interventions and are useful as an indicator of the quality of care in different populations and areas of a country. The timing of a perinatal death, i.e., antepartum, intrapartum, and postpartum, also provides a good measure of the quality of the maternal health-care services. In European countries with perinatal mortality rates around 10/1000 live births, the ratio of fresh stillbirths to macerated stillbirths is 0.2. In two developing countries where special studies were carried out, the ratios were 1.5 and 1.7, suggesting inadequate referral and management of pregnancies at risk of complications.[21]

In a number of developed countries, and a few small developing countries, perinatal mortality has decreased by half over the period from 1965 through 1980 (Table 6). Investment in high technology is not the only way such declines have come about. Regionalization of perinatal care, the application of a risk approach, and a greater understanding of the pathophysiological basis of perinatal morbidity and mortality, with better management of pregnancy and delivery, have, in many instances, contributed to this decline without major investments in facilities and equipment. Even within a four year period of time, with no increase in medical or maternity expenditures, over a 50 percent reduction of perinatal mortality and stillbirth rates was accomplished through a primary health care programme among plantation workers and their families in South India (Table 7).[24] In contrast to postneonatal infant mortality, social, economic, and environmental improvements have far less of an impact during this period, except insofar as they affect maternal health and low birthweight.

INFANT AND CHILD MORTALITY

While not as great as the differentials in maternal mortality, the differences between the infant and child mortality in the poorest countries and the most privileged are up to 30-fold. On average, one in 12 infants in the developing countries dies before reaching the age of one, compared to one in 71 in the industrialized countries. For children under five, the ratios are one in eight compared to one in 56.

Differentials are not confined to comparisons between countries, for even within developed countries there are two-to-threefold differences in infant, neonatal and, postneonatal mortality rates between the most- and least-socially advantaged groups.

In 1986, WHO reported over 14 million children died before reaching their fifth birthday, two-thirds of them aged less than one year. Ninety-nine percent of all infant and child deaths in the world are in the developing countries, although these countries account for only 85 percent of all children under the age of five.

Nevertheless, considerable progress has been made over the last 30 years. Despite the fact that the annual number of births has increased from 86 million in 1950 to 130 million in 1986, the annual number of infant deaths has fallen from 16 million in 1950 to some 14 million in 1986. The infant mortality rate for developing countries, as a whole, fell from 188 in 1950 to 92 in 1980, and 81 in 1986; the under-five mortality rate fell from 295 in 1950 to 142 in 1980, and 124 in 1986. The UN Population Division projects a further reduction of some 30 percent in the infant mortality rate of developing countries between 1985 and 2000, to a level of 61. A similar fall is projected for the developed countries, to a level of 11 in 2000.

The main killers of young children in high-mortality countries are the infectious diseases (Table 8).

INFANT AND CHILD DISEASE MORBIDITY

In many developing country societies, the common pattern is that of repeated infectious diseases during childhood, with as much as 30 percent to 40 percent of a child's life spent suffering gastrointestinal, respiratory, or other infections.

In 1974, when the Expanded Programme on Immunization (EPI) was established by the WHO, less than five percent of infants in the developing world were fully immunized. In 1987, 45 percent of the infants in the developing world now receive the third dose of DPT or polio, and more than 60 percent receive at least the first dose. However, vaccine coverage in the developing world is the lowest for the two EPI diseases which cause the highest number of deaths—measles and neonatal tetanus. These two diseases account for over 80 percent of the 3.4 million deaths annually attributable to the EPI target diseases. Measles immunization is at the level of 35 percent, while immunization of pregnant women against tetanus is at the level of 16 percent.[25]

Measles affects 70 million children yearly in the developing countries. About two million of these cases end fatally. Protein energy malnutrition commonly increases the risk of death and is often an important factor in growth retardation. Although the case-mortality rate in developed countries is not high, complications are not infrequent. About one percent of cases are hospitalized, and encephalitis affects one case in 2000, with frequent sequelae of permanent brain damage and mental retardation. Case-fatality rates are often over one percent in the developing world.

Mortality from neonatal tetanus in some areas of the world has been as high as from 100 to 260/1,000 live births. In Haiti, the introduction and improvements in the training of traditional birth attendants had reduced those rates by as much as half that in 1962. The subsequent introduction of immunization of pregnant women, and later of all women, in an outreach program eliminated the disease as a public health problem.[26] Similar marked reduction in neonatal tetanus was found in China with the simple adherence to the principles of the "three cleans" in the training of the traditional birth attendants: clean hands, clean delivery surface, and clean cutting and care of the umbilical cord. (WHO 1985)

Of an expected 850,000 deaths from pertussis, approximately 30 percent have been prevented through immunization. Of an expected 365,000 cases of poliomyelitis, nearly 40 percent have been prevented. In a follow-up of the EPI program in Indonesia, the decline in the morbidity rate of diphtheria corresponded to the level of coverage achieved with two doses of DPT.[27]

DIARRHEAL DISEASE MORTALITY AND MORBIDITY

The incidence and case-mortality rates for diarrheal disease have been difficult to obtain, and difficult to compare over time and between different countries. Nevertheless, the Diarrheal Control Programme of WHO has summarized the results of 193 surveys in 49 countries, in which the standardized WHO/CDD methodology was used (Table 9). The median number of diarrheal episodes per year for children, globally, is estimated to be 3.6, with the Americas-region surveys showing a median of 6.2 and the Western Pacific surveys having a median of 2.2. Globally, it is estimated that one-third of the child deaths are associated with diarrhea.[28]

NUTRITIONAL PATTERNS OF CHILDREN

It is estimated that 40 million preschool children in developing countries are living in conditions of acute malnutrition, and more than three times that number in a chronic state of insufficient nutrition and associated illness that is hampering their growth.[29] Growth patterns of children and their trends over time have frequently been used as indicators of health and nutrition status. The most-widely used indicator, weight-for-age, has been used as a measure of protein-energy malnutrition. Interpretations of trends in nutritional status, based on weight-for-age, are complicated by the fact that weight-for-age is a composite of both stunting and wasting.

Anthropometric indicators for stunting (height-for-age) and for wasting (weight-for-height) provide a much clearer picture of the health status of children. *Wasting*, a highly sensitive indicator, varies widely by season and quickly reflects the impact of acute illnesses such as measles and diarrheal diseases. *Stunting* reflects more the accumulated health and nutritional legacy of a child.

Trends in stunting have been analyzed from nine countries in different parts of the world.[30] In seven, there was an improvement and in two a deterioration (Table

10). For all regions except Asia, the prevalence of protein-energy malnutrition among children under five appears to be decreasing over the last few decades (Table 11).

BREAST-FEEDING TRENDS AND CHILD HEALTH

The nutritional and infection protecting properties of breast milk have been amply demonstrated. The decline of breast-feeding has been associated with an increase in infant morbidity and mortality, especially among the more disadvantaged communities of both the developed and developing world. Among the direct results are an increase in diarrhoeal diseases in infants fed breast-milk substitutes.[31]

In developed countries, changing lifestyles, particularly involvement of women in the work force, changes in family structure, and developments in food technology, appear to have been important contributors to the decline in breast-feeding, which took place between the 1940s and the early 1970s. In developed countries, many of the potentially adverse effects on child health of the decline have been countered by improved sanitation, clean water, communicable disease control, family planning services, and general socio-economic improvements. However, a similar erosion of breast-feeding in the developing world could have a disastrous impact on health and family planning.

Early initiation of breast-feeding consistently appears as a key factor in the establishment and duration of breast-feeding.[32] While there is strong evidence that early mother-to-child, skin-to-skin contact, and demand feeding are important factors in enhancing breast-feeding,[33] many of the maternity and health care routines limit, rather than facilitate, these practices.

In reviewing the worldwide patterns of breast-feeding, WHO described a typology that appeared to conform to the dynamic changes in patterns according to stage of development and population subgroups within a country. Time-trend analysis from a few countries has confirmed the sequential nature of that pattern, with a sharp decline in breast-feeding in the urban higher-income groups first, followed by other groups, and then a resurgence of breast-feeding again initiated among the higher-income urban groups.

COVERAGE OF MCH, INCLUDING FAMILY PLANNING

Almost everywhere, there is a dearth of systematic, comprehensive, and critical reviews and evaluations of program coverage, performance, and effectiveness. Wide variations in the proportion of women receiving prenatal care exist both between and within geographic areas. In Africa, the proportions range from 33 percent to 90 percent; in Latin America, from 20 percent to 81 percent; and, in Asia, from five percent to 98 percent.[34]

Maternal Care

In a significant number of cases, and especially in rural areas, the percentage of women receiving prenatal care (by a trained attendant) exceeds the percentage receiving skilled intrapartum care. This discrepancy between high levels of prenatal care coverage and somewhat lower levels of supervised delivery care coverage, in some instances, may be related to the geographic inaccessibility due to lack of transport, and the distances and time necessary to travel once a woman goes into labor. But, in many settings, cultural preference and distances may play an equal, if not greater, role. Hassouna has described how even the majority of non-professional health workers are delivered by a traditional birth attendant in Cairo, despite the availability and their knowledge of the delivery care facilities.[35] A similar preference for traditional birth attendants, who are more like family birth attendants, has been noted in Zimbabwe.

On the basis of available information, it is possible to build up estimates for the coverage of maternity care in the various regions of the world. These estimates show that only some 55 percent of the births in the world are attended by trained personnel. Even fewer take place in an institution. This means that some 58 million of the 128 million infants born in 1983 were delivered with the help of untrained traditional birth attendants, family members, or by the mother alone.

In the developed world, nearly all births are attended by trained personnel, but in the developing world, where 85 percent of the world's births take place, fewer than half were so attended. The coverage of child health care is extremely difficult to quantify. If one uses immunization protection as a measure, many countries have shown spectacular progress. However, the use of immunization coverage, as a surrogate for overall infant and child health care coverage, is only possible in situations where immunizations are provided almost exclusively by the organized health services. Social mobilization and mass campaigns, while admirably raising the level of protection in a relatively short period of time, and intended to lead to sustainability through the health system, do not really reflect overall care for children. Thus, for example, a recent evaluation of MCH services in Tanzania suggested that, apart from immunization coverage, which ranged from 70 percent for BCG to 30 percent for measles, the programs were having limited, if any, impact on the main problems of mothers and children.[37]

FAMILY PLANNING

From only a few countries with family planning programs in the beginning of the 1960s, currently 120 governments now support such programs either directly or indirectly. About 95 percent of people in the developing world live in countries which provide some form of public support for family planning programs, generally as part of MCH programs. Contraceptive prevalence, as a measure of family-planning program effectiveness, has increased. In over 75 countries, with 60 percent of the world's women, contraceptive prevalence rates of 30 percent or above prevail. However, in over 50 countries, with 20 percent of the world's women, prevalence rates are below ten percent.[38]

Despite the apparently high contraceptive-prevalence rates in some countries, there does not appear to be a commensurate change in fertility. This somewhat paradoxical observation has been attributed to high discontinuation and failure rates of certain contraceptive methods and, at times, to over-reporting of acceptor rates in some programs. Another contributing factor to an apparent lack of effect on birth rates, despite an increased rate of contraceptive prevalence, is the use of such methods by older couples who are already at a low risk of pregnancy.[39] The World Fertility Survey has shown a marked discrepancy in many countries between current fertility, numbers of unwanted births per woman, and contraceptive prevalence. In Africa, only 23 percent of women not wanting any more births are practicing contraception; in Asia it is 43 percent; and in Latin America, 57 percent. Evidently, in many circumstances and in many countries, either the methods and/or the services are not accessible and/or acceptable in physical, cultural, or personal terms. As a consequence, deaths from illegally induced abortion continue to constitute from 25 percent to 50 percent of maternal mortality in many countries.

The pattern of use of different methods of contraception, often a consequence of availability, varies widely. (Table 12) For example, in Thailand, of the 65 percent of women practicing family planning, fully 90 percent are protected from unwanted pregnancies by such methods as sterilization, oral or injectable hormonal contraceptives, or IUDs. On the other hand, in Bulgaria, although 76 percent practice family planning, these effective methods are being used by less than ten percent of contracepting women. Globally, about 325 million couples, out of 800 million of reproductive age, are using an effective method of contraception, namely:

135 million – sterilization
70 million – IUD
55 million – oral hormonal contraceptives
37 million – condoms
30 million – injectable hormonal contraceptives, barrier methods, and other modern methods

Another 20 million to 40 million use traditional methods, such as periodic abstinence or withdrawal.[40]

PRIMARY HEALTH CARE AND MCH,
INCLUDING FAMILY PLANNING (FP)

Primary health care (PHC) has inherent to it the concept of placing the appropriate technologies at the most appropriate level of the system. Over the last several years, both research and experience have shown that many of the appropriate technologies in MCH/FP can be transferred successfully to families and communities. Such successful transfers have included: community-based distribution of contraceptives and of oral rehydration salts; home preparation of ORT; growth monitoring and follow-up action by women's organizations, teachers, and others; home-based monitoring of pregnancy, and of child health and growth through the use of home-based records; and the identification and referral by traditional birth attendants of pregnancies at potential risk of complications.

Since some of the essential technologies for MCH/FP cannot be made available at the PHC level, they must be available and accessible at the level of first referral. Thus, for example, without the availability of the skills, supplies, and equipment for an assisted delivery, cesarean section, the provision of blood, etc, little progress will be made in significantly lowering the very-high maternal-mortality rates found in many countries.

If the different levels of care are not integrated and mutually supportive—although all the technologies may be appropriately placed—there will be only a limited impact, particularly in such areas as maternal health.

The field of MCH/FP experienced the debate, for many years, as to whether and how to integrate the MCH and FP components. In most countries, that debate has been resolved, although functional integration continues to elude many countries, in large part due to the legacy of discrepancies in policies, resource allocation (including external resources), management support, training, etc. More recently, major advances in the development and adaptation of other appropriate MCH/FP technologies have come about, such as those related to immunization and oral rehydration therapy. However, many countries have failed to learn the lessons of the MCH and FP debate, once again developing vertical structures for the delivery of these services.

Does the emphasis on one technology or program area have a beneficial spillover effect, a detrimental, or no effect on other aspects of MCH/FP? A recent evaluation of MCH services in Tanzania suggested that, apart from immunization coverage, which ranged from 70 percent for BCG to 30 percent for measles, the programs were having limited, if any, impact on the main problems of mothers and children.[37] There was no "spillover" effect.

The needs for the future in maternal and child health, including family planning, have been aptly summarized in the WHO Expert Committee report on MCH/FP.[41] "If the focus of health care is to shift from the hospital to the community, and from selected coverage to total coverage, community and family health, particularly MCH care, must be made the central objective of basic and continuing education for all members of the health team. Moreover, to ensure the integration of MCH care into the general community health services, the MCH content should be incorporated into the curricula for the basic and postgraduate preparation of health personnel in universities and professional or vocational schools. This calls for a vast expansion and reorientation of the educational system for health personnel, and for basic changes in the philosophies of medicine, nursing, and allied health professions, coupled with the reformulation and reshaping of curricula and methods of teaching."

TABLE 1

INFANT, TODDLER AND CHILD MORTALITY RATES, RATIOS (M/F) AND PREFERENCE FOR SEX OF CHILDREN

Country	Infant	Toddler	Child	Index of Son Preference
Senegal	1.16	0.99	1.00	1.5
Nepal	1.03	0.89	0.95	4.0
Bangladesh	1.03	0.73	0.84	3.3
Pakistan	1.05	0.63	0.68	4.9
Cameroon	1.07	1.04	0.99	1.2
Egypt	1.01	0.71	0.94	1.5
Turkey	1.10	0.62	0.94	1.4
Ivory Coast	1.24	1.19	1.11	1.2
Indonesia	1.30	1.15	1.31	1.1
Morocco	1.06	0.88	1.11	1.2
Kenya	1.10	1.17	1.02	1.1
Ghana	1.22	1.15	0.95	1.0
Colombia	1.19	0.75	0.83	1.0
Tunisia	1.02	1.05	1.25	1.3
Mexico	1.25	0.86	0.88	1.2
Thailand	1.08	1.42	0.65	1.4
Syria	0.92	1.05	0.64	2.3
Sri Lanka	1.24	0.68	0.87	1.5
Jordan	0.85	0.81	0.99	1.9
Venezuela	1.27	1.14	0.90	0.8
Fiji	1.19	0.92	1.04	1.3
Jamaica	1.36	1.07	1.17	0.7
Malaysia	1.31	1.41	1.19	1.2
Portugal	1.49	1.52	0.59	1.0

SOURCE: World Health Organization. Evaluation of the Strategy for Health for All. Seventh Report of the World Health Situation. Geneva, WHO, 1987, and World Fertility Survey.

NOTES: a) Countries are ordered by level of under five mortality

b) Index of son preference (from the World Fertility Survey) - Ratio of the number of mothers who prefer the next child to be male to the number of mothers who prefer the next child to be female

TABLE 2
ESTIMATES OF MATERNAL MORTALITY

Region	Live births (millions)	Maternal Mortality Rate (per 100,000 live births)	Maternal deaths (thousands)
Africa	23.4	640	150
Asia	73.9	420	308
Latin America	12.6	270	34
Oceania	0.2		2
Developing Countries	110.1	450	494
Developed Countries	18.2	30	6
World	128.3	390	500

SOURCE: World Health Organization. Evaluation of the Strategy for Health for All. Seventh Report of the World Health Situation. Geneva, WHO, 1987, and World Fertility Survey.

TABLE 3
CHANGES IN MATERNAL MORTALITY IN SELECTED COUNTRIES

Country	1965	1975	Change	Latest
USA	32	13	-59%	9 (1980)
France	23	20	-13%	13 (1980)
Fed. Rep. Germany	69	40	-42%	11 (1983)
Czechoslovakia	35	18	-49%	8 (1982)
Greece	46	19	-59%	12 (1982)
Portugal	85	43	-48%	5 (1984)
Japan	88	29	-67%	15 (1983)
Romania	86	121	+41%	149 (1984)
Romania excl. abortion	65	31	-52%	21 (1984)

SOURCE: World Health Organization Maternal Mortality data bank.

TABLE 4

PROPORTION OF MOTHERS WITH PRE-ECLAMPSIA AND ECLAMPSIA

	Pre-eclampsia (per cent)	Eclampsia (per cent)
Viet Nam	1.5	0.34
Burma	4.4	0.40
Thailand	7.5	0.93
China	8.3	0.17

SOURCE: World Health Organization, Hypertensive Disorders of Pregnancy, Technical Report Series No. 758, WHO, Geneva, 1987.

TABLE 5

FACTORS ASSOCIATED WITH INTRA-UTERINE GROWTH RETARDATION AND PRE-TERM DELIVERY

	Relative Risk of Intra-uterine Growth Retardation	Relative Risk of Pre-term Deilvery
Maternal height		
< 157.5 - 158 cm	1.27	1.0
Pregnancy weight		
< 49.5 kg	1.84	
< 54.0 kg		1.25
Primiparity	1.23	?
Previous LBW infant	2.75	
Previous pre-term infant		3.08
Pregnancy weight gain		
< 7 kg (well nourished)	1.98	?
100 kcal/day supplement		
undernourished women	0.47	
well-nourished women	0.82	
Smoking	2.42	1.41
Alcohol -> 2 drinks/day	1.78	?

SOURCE: Belsey MA: The epidemiology of infertility. Bulletin of the World Health Organization, 54:319-341, 1976.

TABLE 6

PERINATAL MORTALITY RATES (PER 1,000 LIVE BIRTHS)
FOR SELECTED COUNTIRES, 1965 - 1984

Year	Sweden	Singapore	England & Wales	France	Japan	Mauritius
1965	19.9	25.8	27.3	28.2	30.1	82.0
1970	16.5	21.7	23.8	23.7	21.7	60.9
1975	11.3	16.7	19.9	18.3	16.0	61.6
1980	8.7	13.5	13.4	13.0	-	39.5
1984	6.8	10.4	10.1	11.3	8.0	32.1

SOURCE: Edouard L: The epidemiology of perinatal mortality, World Health Statistics
Quarterly, 383:289-301, 1985.

TABLE 7

COMPREHENSIVE LABOR - WELFARE SCHEME ESTATES: DATA ON STILLBIRTH
AND PERINANTAL MORTALITY RATES* (PER 1,000 LIVE BIRTHS)

Year	Still birth rate	Perinatal mortality rate
1979	69.8	109.7
1980	44.3	82.5
1981	36.6	73.2
1982	27.9	47.7

SOURCE: Kramer MS: Determinants of Low Birth Weight: A methodologic and meta-analysis,
Bulletin of the World Health Organization, 1987.

* Total population covered by the CLWS was over 250,000

TABLE 8

CAUSES OF DEATH OF CHILDREN UNDER FIVE

Cause	Million p.a.
Acute diarrhea and related causes	5.0
Malaria	3.0
Measles	2.1
Neonatal tetanus	0.8
Pertussis	0.6
Acute respiratory infections	4.0
Typhoid fever	0.5

SOURCE: World Health Organization.

TABLE 9

SUMMARY OF RESULTS OF 193 DIARRHEA MORTALITY, MORBIDITY, AND TREATMENT SURVEYS OF CHILDREN AGED 0 - 4 YEARS, 1981 - 1986

WHO Region	Number of Surveys (countries)		Mortality rates/1,000 children (Median) All Causes	Diarhhea- Associated	Percentage of deaths Diarrhea Associated	Annual Incidence (episodes/ child/year)
AFR	40	(17)	32.0	11.5	41.1	4.7
AMR	6	(06)	11.0	3.9	34.9	6.2
EMR	32	(09)	15.7	6.7	43.2	3.8
SEA	67	(09)	13.7	3.6	28.3	3.2
WPR	48	(08)	8.4	2.2	22.4	2.2
Total	193	(49)	18.0	5.6	36.0	3.6

SOURCE: World Health Organization. Programme for Control of Diarrheal Diseases. Interim progamme report 1986. WHO document No. WHO/CDD/87.26.

TABLE 10

AVERAGE ANNUAL CHANGE IN PREVALENCE OF STUNTING

Country	Year 1	Year 2	Per cent change
Egypt	1978	1980	-2.95
Nicaragua	1965 - 7	1980 - 2	-1.69
Thailand	1975	1984	-1.41
El Salvador	1965	1975	-1.05
Lesotho	1976	1981	-1.04
Colombia	1965 - 6	1977 - 80	-0.47
Sri Lanka	1975 - 6	1978	-0.50
Sierra Leone	1974 - 5	1977 - 8	+0.92
Kenya	1978 - 9	1982	+1.03

For all regions except Asia, the prevalence of protein-energy malnutrition among children under five appears to be decreasing over the last few decades.

SOURCE: Filmore, C, 1986.

TABLE 11

ESTIMATED PROTEIN-ENERGY MALNUTRITION PREVALENCE BY REGION, DETERMINED AS A PERCENTAGE OF CHILDREN WITH LOW WEIGHT FOR AGE

Country	1963 - 1973	1973 - 1983
Africa	31.1%	25.5%
Americas	25.9%	17.7%
Asia	50.6%	54.0%
Oceania	22.0%	11.5%

SOURCE: Filmore, C, 1986.

TABLE 12

CONTRACEPTION: ESTIMATED PERCENTAGE OF MARRIED WOMEN OF REPRODUCTIVE AGE PRACTICING CONTRACEPTION, 1980 - 1981

	Percent
World total	45
Total excluding China	38
Developing regions:	
Total	38
Total excluding China	24
Africa	11
Asia	42
East Asia	69
South Asia	24
Latin America	43
Developed regions:	
Total	68

SOURCE: United Nations. Recent levels and trends of contraceptive use as asessed in 1983. New York, UN, 1984.

REFERENCES

1. World Health Statistics Annual, 1985. Based on the findings of the World Fertility Survey.

2. Maternal Mortality. A tabulation of available information. Second edition. WHO document No. FHE/86.3, 1986.

3. World Fertility Survey, Bangladesh. Geveva, WHO, 1987.

4. Chen LC et al. Maternal Mortality in Rural Bangladesh. Studies in Family Planning, 5(11):334-341, 1974.

5. Sri Lanka, Ministry of Health, Family Health Bureau. Medium Term Plan. Family Health Program, 1985-1989. Colombo, The Ministry, 1984.

6. Zhang L, Ding H. China: Analysis of cause and rate of regional maternal death in 21 provinces, municipalities and autonomous regions. Chinese Journal of Obstetrics and Gynaecology, 21(4):195-197, 1986.

7. Hobert U. Maternal mortality in Sweden. Umea, Sweden, Umea University, 1985.

8. Registrat General, India, 1981 quoted in: Bhasker Rao, A: Maternal mortality in India. A Review. Paper presented to the Interregional Meeting on the Prevention of Maternal Mortality, Geneva, 11-15 Nov 1985. WHO document no. FHE/PMM/85.9.4, 1985.

9. Shotri A. Risk Approach Studies in Maternal and Child Health in Pune, India (in press).

10. Royston E. The prevalence of nutritional anaemia in women in developing countries: A critical review of available information. World Health Statistics Quarterly, 35:52-91, 1982.

11. Buck AA, quoted in Royston, E. The prevalence of nutritional anaemia in women in developing countries: A critical review of available information. World Health Statistics Quarterly, 35:52-91, 1982.

12. WHO Expert Committee on Malaria, Eighteenth report. Technical Report Series No. 735, Geneva, WHO, 1986.

13. Maine D et al. Prevention of maternal deaths in developing countries: programme options and practical considerations. Paper prepared for the International Safe Motherhood Conference, Nairobi, Feb. 10-13, 1987 (1986).

14. Tietze C, Henshaw SW. Induced abortion. A world review 1986. 6th ed. New York, Alan Guttmacher Institute, 1986.

15. Rodriguez Castro R. Complicaciones del aborto a Corto Plazo, in: Reproduction Humana y Regulacion de la fertilidad, Simposio Cuba-OMS, Havana, 1978.

16. World Health Organization and U.S. National Research Council, Breast-feeding and fertility regulation: current knowledge and programme policy implications. Bulletin of the World Health Organization, 61(3):371-382, 1983.

17. De Chateau P et al. A study of factors promoting and inhibiting lactation. Developmental Medicine and Child Neurology, 19:575, 1977.

18. Muir DG, Belsey MA. Pelvic inflammatory disease and its consequences in the developing world. Am J Obstet Gynecol 138(7)part 2, 913-928, 1980.

19. Makinen JI. Ectopic Pregnancy in Finland 1976-83: a massive increase, Brit Med J, 294, 240-241, 1987.

20. Belsey MA. The epidemiology of infertility. Bulletin of the World Health Organization, 54:319-341, 1976.

21. The incidence of low birth weight: an update.Weekly Epidemiological Record,59(27)205-211, 1984.

22. Kramer MS. Determinants of Low Birth Weight: A methodologic and meta-analysis, Bulletin of the World Health Organization, 1987.

23. Edouard L. The epidemiology of perinatal mortality, World Health Statistics Quarterly, 383:289-301, 1985.

24. Laing R. Health and Health Services for Plantation Workers: Four case studies, Evaluation and Planning Centre for Health Care, London School of Hygiene and Tropical Medicine (London) p 39, 1986.

25. World Health Organization. Expanded Programme of Immunization, 1987.

26. Berggren W. A tetanus control program in Haiti, Am Journal Trop Med, 1974.

27. Kim-Farley R et al. Assessing the impact of the expanded programme on immunization: the example of Indonesia. Bulletin of the World Health Organization, 65(2):203-206, 1987.

28. World Health Organization. Programme for Control of Diarrheal Diseases. Interim programme report 1986. WHO document No. WHO/CDD/87.26.

29. World Health Organization, Global nutritional status. Anthropometric indicators. WHO document no. NUT/AUTREF/87.3,1987.

30. Filmore C. Protein-energy malnutrition trends in nine countries (unpublished document),1986.

31. Victoria CG et al. Evidence for the protection by breast-feeding against infant deaths from infectious diseases in Brazil. Lancet ii(Aug 8):319-322, 1987.

32. Slopar KS et al. Increasing breastfeeding in a community. Archives of Diseases in Childhood. 52:700, 1977.

33. The dynamics of breastfeeding. WHO Chronicle. 37(1):6-10, 1983.

34. Royston E and Ferguson J. The coverage of maternity care: a critical review of available information. World Health Statistics Quarterly, 38:267-288, 1985.

35. Hassouna WA. Health sector assessment study. Health Services Researcher, S1:4, 1982.

36. Mutambirwa J. The role of traditional medicine in Zimbabwe. Presentation at Zimbabwe National MCH Workshop, June, 1983.

37. Shears P, Mkerenga R. Evaluating the impact of mother and child health services at village level: a survey in Tanzania, and lessons for elsewhere. Annals of Tropical Pediatrics 5:55-59, 1985.

38. United Nations. Recent levels and trends of contraceptive use as assessed in 1983. New York, UN, 1984.

39. Amin, R et al. Fertility, contraceptive use and socioeconomic context in Bangladesh. Paper prepared for the annual meeting of the Population Association of America, Boston, Mar 28-30, 1985.

40. Mauldin WP, Segal SJ. Prevalence of contraceptive use in developing countries. A chart book. New York: Rockefeller Foundation, 1986.

41. New trends and approaches in the delivery of maternal and child care in health services. Sixth report of the WHO Expert Committee on Maternal and Child Health. Technical Report Series No 600, Geneva, WHO, 1976.

APPENDIX

Ⅱ DEFINITIONS

Helen M. Wallace

Uniformity in nomenclature and in definition of terms is essential for the purposes of program planning and program evaluation for the professional health worker, in the field of MCH and handicapped children. The data used in the evaluation of patient care and services cannot be collected and analyzed uniformly, unless the meaning of the terms used is uniform and commonly understood. Neither can comparisons be made between countries, states, local communities, or hospitals without uniformity in the definition, collection, and analysis of data. The definitions which follow are some of those commonly used in the field of MCH.

1. Live Birth:
The complete expulsion or extraction from the mother of a product of conception, irrespective of the duration of pregnancy, which, after such separation, breathes or shows any other evidence of life, such as beating of the heart, pulsation of the umbilical cord, or definite movement of voluntary muscles, whether or not the cord has been cut or the placenta is attached.

2. Crude Birth Rate:
Annual total number of live births per 1,000 population.

3. Age-Specific Birth Rate:
Number of live births to mothers of a given age, to the female population of that age. Expressed as the total number of live births to mothers in a five-year age group per 1,000 women in that age group.

4. **Women of Reproductive Age:**
   The total number of women aged 15 through 49, resident in a given country, on July 1 of a given year, irrespective of marital status or fertility.

5. **General Fertility Rate:**
   Number of live births per 1,000 women aged, 15-44 years.

6. **Crude Death Rate:**
   Annual number of deaths per 1,000 population.

7. **Infant:**
   A baby born alive, from the time of birth until the first birthday.

8. **Infant Death:**
   Death in a child under one-year of age.

9. **Infant Mortality Rate:**
   Number of deaths in infants under one year of age (from birth to first birthday), per 1,000 live births.

10. **Neonatal:**
    Period from birth to "under-28 days" of life.

11. **Neonatal Death:**
    Death in a child less than 28 completed days of age.

12. **Neonatal Mortality Rate:**
    Number of deaths of babies less than 28 completed days of age, per 1,000 live births.

13. **Postneonatal:**
    Period from 28th day of life to the first birthday.

14. **Postneonatal Death:**
    Death in a child more than 28 completed days of life, and under one year of age.

15. **Postneonatal Mortality Rate:**
    Number of deaths of babies from 28th day of life to the first birthday, per 1,000 live births.

16. **Fetal Death:**
    Death prior to the complete expulsion or extraction from the mother of a product of conception, irrespective of the duration of pregnancy; the death is indicated by the fact that after such separation, the fetus does not breathe or show any other evidence of life, such as beating of the heart, pulsation of the umbilical cord, or definite movement of voluntary muscles.

17. Perinatal: [1]

Perinatal deaths refer to the sum of spontaneous fetal deaths occurring after 20-weeks gestation, plus infant deaths occurring during the first 27 days following birth (neonatal deaths).

The recommendations of both the World Health Organization and the U.S. Public Health Conference on Records and Statistics are the basis for the three Perinatal mortality measures generally used in the U.S.

Perinatal Definition I refers only to fetal deaths of 28 weeks or more gestation, and infant deaths of less than seven days.

Perinatal Definition II refers to fetal deaths of 20 weeks or more gestation, and infant deaths under 28 days of age.

Perinatal Definition III includes fetal deaths of 20 weeks gestation or more, and infant deaths of less than seven days.

Definition I is generally used for international comparisons.

Measures of perinatal mortality can be experienced as either a *rate* or a *ratio*. The *perinatal mortality rate* is defined as the number of perinatal deaths per 1,000 live births and fetal deaths. The *perinatal mortality ratio* is the number of perinatal deaths per 1,000 live births.

18. Low Birthweight:

Weight of 2,500 grams (5.5 pounds) or less at birth.

19. Maternal Death [2]

The death of a woman while pregnant, or within 42 days of termination of pregnancy, irrespective of the duration and site of pregnancy, from any cause related to, or aggravated, by the pregnancy or its management, but not from accidental or incidental causes. Maternal deaths can be direct or indirect. *Direct deaths* are those resulting from obstetric complications of pregnancy, labor, and puerperium; from interventions, omissions, incorrect treatment; or from a chain of events resulting from any of the above. *Indirect deaths* are those resulting from previous existing disease, or disease that developed during pregnancy and which was not due to direct obstetric causes but which was aggravated by physiologic effects of pregnancy.

20. Newer Mortality Rates Proposed by UNICEF: [3]

Child Mortality Rate (CMR) The probability of dying between exact age one and exact age five, commonly calculated as the number of deaths of children between exact ages one and five during a given period, divided by the annual average number of children reaching age one during the same period, and expressed per 1,000 children.

Child Death Rate (CDR) Death rate between exact ages one to five; number of deaths of children between exact ages one and five during a given period, divided by the average population between exact ages one and five during the same period, and expressed per thousand population.

Infant and Child Mortality Rage (ICMR) The probability of dying between birth and exact age five, commonly calculated as the number of deaths of children under five years of age during a given period, divided by the average annual number of births during the same period, and expressed per thousand live births.

REFERENCES

1. National Center for Health Statistics. Perinatal Mortality in the United States: 1950-81. Monthly Vital Statistics Report Vol. 34, No. 12, Supplement. 16 pages. March 31, 1986.

2. World Health Organization. International Classification of Diseases. Manual of International Statistical Classification of Diseases, Injuries, and Causes of Death. 9th revision. Geneva, 1977.

3. Goldstone, L.

    A. A New Index of Infant & Child Mortality. October 22, 1985. Typewritten. 10 pages.

    B. Infant & Child Mortality. A disparity Analysis (second thoughts). February, 1987. Typewritten. 6 pages. UNICEF, New York, New York.